Dermatologic Principles and Practice in Oncology
Conditions of the Skin, Hair, and Nails in Cancer Patients

Dermatologic Principles and Practice in Oncology

Conditions of the Skin, Hair, and Nails in Cancer Patients

Edited by

MARIO E. LACOUTURE, MD

Associate Member
Dermatology Service
Memorial Sloan-Kettering Cancer Center
Associate Professor
Department of Dermatology
Cornell University
New York, NY
USA

WILEY Blackwell

Library of Congress Cataloging-in-Publication Data
Dermatologic principles and practice in oncology : conditions of the skin, hair, and nails in cancer patients / [edited by] Mario E. Lacouture.
        p. ; cm.
    Includes bibliographical references and index.
    ISBN 978-0-470-62188-2 (hardback : alk. paper) – ISBN 978-1-118-59060-7 – ISBN 978-1-118-59061-4 – ISBN 978-1-118-59062-1 – ISBN 978-1-118-59063-8
    I. Lacouture, Mario E.
    [DNLM: 1. Skin Diseases–etiology.   2. Skin Diseases–psychology.   3. Antineoplastic Agents–adverse events.
4. Neoplasms–complications.   5. Skin Care–nursing.   6. Skin Manifestations. WR 140]
    RC280.S5
    616.99'477–dc23
                                    2013013054

Cover image: © authors and editor, middle image: istockphoto.com
Cover design by Matt Kuhns

Printed in Singapore

10 9 8 7 6 5 4 3 2 1

Contents

Contents

Section 5 Late Cutaneous Events from Cancer Treatment

Section 6 Dermatologic Practice in Oncology

List of Contributors

Asha Acharya PhD
Technical Resources International, Inc.
Bethesda, MD, USA

Najla Al-Dawsari MD, FAAD
Consultant Dermatologist
Dhahran Health Center
Saudi Aramco Medical Service Organization
Saudi Arabia

Raed O. Alhusayen MBBS, MSCE, FRCPC
Clinical Associate
Division of Dermatology
Sunnybrook Health Sciences Centre
Toronto, Canada

Iris Amitay-Laish MD
Dermatologist
Department of Dermatology
Rabin Medical Center, Beilinson Hospital
Petah Tikva, Israel

Milan J. Anadkat MD
Associate Professor
Division of Dermatology
Center for Advanced Medicine
Washington University School of Medicine
St. Louis, MO, USA

Yevgeniy Balagula MD
Clinical Research Fellow
Dermatology Service
Memorial Sloan-Kettering Cancer Center
New York, NY, USA

Robert Baran MD
Honorary Professor of the University of
Franche-Comté
Nail Disease Center
Cannes, France;
Consultant Dermatologist
Cancer Institute Gustave Roussy
Villejuif, France

Christine B. Boers-Doets MSc
Department of Clinical Oncology
Leiden University Medical Center
Leiden, The Netherlands

Judy H. Borovicka MD
Clinical Research Fellow
Northwestern University Feinberg School of
Medicine
Chicago, IL, USA

Jeffrey P. Callen MD
Professor of Medicine (Dermatology)
Chief, Division of Dermatology
University of Louisville School of Medicine
Louisville, KY, USA

David Cella PhD
Professor and Chair, Department of Medical
Social Sciences
Northwestern University Feinberg School of
Medicine
Robert H. Lurie Comprehensive Cancer Center of
Northwestern University
Chicago, IL, USA

Alice Chen MD, FACP
Senior Investigator
Cancer Therapy Evaluation Program
National Cancer Institute
Rockville, MD, USA

Jennifer Nam Choi MD
Assistant Professor, Department of Dermatology,
Yale University School of Medicine
New Haven, CT, USA

Emily Y. Chu MD, PhD
Staff Clinician
Dermatology Branch, Center for Cancer Research
National Cancer Institute, National Institutes of
Health
Bethesda, MD, USA

Kathryn T. Ciccolini RN, BSN, OCN
Office Practice Nurse
Dermatology Service
Memorial Sloan-Kettering Cancer Center
New York, NY, USA

Jonathan Cotliar MD
Associate Professor
Departments of Dermatology and Medicine
Robert H. Lurie Comprehensive Cancer Center
Northwestern University Feinberg School of
Medicine
Chicago, IL, USA

Amy J. Derick MD
Clinical Instructor of Dermatology
Northwestern University Feinberg School of
Medicine
Chicago, IL, USA;
Derick Dermatology LLC
Barrington, IL, USA

Maura Dickler MD
Associate Member
Breast Cancer Medicine Service
Department of Medicine
Memorial Sloan-Kettering Cancer Center
New York, NY, USA

Reinhard Dummer MD
Vice-Chairman
Department of Dermatology
University Hospital Zurich
Zurich, Switzerland

Robert Eilers Jr. MD
Resident Physician
Department of Dermatology
University of Michigan
Ann Arbor, MI, USA

Bernard Fouilloux MD
Consultant Dermatologist (Oncology Section)
Hôpital Nord
Saint-Etienne, France

Francine Foss MD
Professor of Medicine and Dermatology
Yale University School of Medicine
New Haven, CT, USA
Consultant Dermatologist
Dhahran Health Center
Saudi Aramco Medical Service Organization
Saudi Arabia

Claus Garbe MD
Professor of Dermatology
Head, Division of Dermatooncology
Department of Dermatology
University Medical Center
Tuebingen, Germany

Amit Garg MD
Hofstra School of Medicine and North Shore-LIJ
Health System
Manhasset, New York, USA

Jennifer R.S. Gordon MD
Clinical Research Fellow
Northwestern University Feinberg School of
Medicine
Chicago, IL, USA

Emmy Graber MD
Assistant Professor of Dermatology;
Director, Cosmetic and Laser Center
Boston University School of Medicine
Boston, MA, USA

Ann Cameron Haley MMS, PA-C
Clinical Research Assistant
Northwestern University Feinberg School of
Medicine
Chicago, ILUSA

Axel Hauschild MD
Department of Dermatology
University Hospital Schleswig-Holstein Campus
Kiel, Germany

Molly A. Hinshaw MD
Dermatopathologist
Troy and Associates, Brookfield, WI, USA;
Associate Clinical Professor of Dermatology
University of Wisconsin School of Medicine and
Public Health
Wisconsin, WI, USA

Stephanie W. Hu MD
Dermatology Resident
Ronald O. Perelman Department of Dermatology
New York University School of Medicine
New York, NY, USA

James I. Ito MD
Professor and Chief
Division of Infectious Diseases
City of Hope Comprehensive Cancer Center
Duarte, CA, USA

Katharina C. Kaehler MD
Senior Consultant Dermatooncology
Department of Dermatology
University Hospital Schleswig-Holstein Campus
Kiel, Germany

Zahra Kassam MBBS, FRCR (UK),
FRCP(C), MSc
Staff Radiation Oncologist
Stronach Regional Cancer Centre
Southlake Regional Health Centre;
Princess Margaret Cancer Center
Toronto, ON, Canada

Caroline C. Kim MD
Assistant Professor, Harvard Medical School;
Director, Pigmented Lesion Clinic;
Associate Director, Cutaneous Oncology Program,
Department of Dermatology
Beth Israel Deaconess Medical Center
Boston, MA, USA

Sandra R. Knowles BScPhm
Assistant Professor
University of Toronto, Toronto, Canada;
Sunnybrook Health Sciences Centre
Toronto, Canada

Heidi H. Kong MD, MHSc
Investigator and Head, Clinical Research Section
Dermatology Branch, Center for Cancer Research
National Cancer Institute, National Institutes of
Health
Bethesda, MD, USA

Mario E. Lacouture MD
Associate Member
Dermatology Service
Memorial Sloan-Kettering Cancer Center;
Associate Professor
Department of Dermatology
Cornell University
New York, NY, USA

Nicole E. Larsen
Northwestern University Feinberg School of
Medicine
Robert H. Lurie Comprehensive Cancer Center of
Northwestern University
Chicago, IL, USA

Seppo W. Langer MD, PhD
Head, Thoracic and Neuroendocrine Section
Department of Oncology
Copenhagen University Hospital – Rigshospitalet
Copenhagen, Denmark

Erica H. Lee MD
Assistant Attending
Dermatology Service
Memorial Sloan-Kettering Cancer Center
New York, NY, USA

Mee-young Lee MSN
Nurse Practitioner
Cutaneous Oncology Program
Department of Hematology Oncology
Beth Israel Deaconess Medical Center
Boston, MA, USA

Larissa Leister MD
Attending Physician
Department of Dermatology
University Hospital Essen
Essen, Germany

Elisabeth Livingstone MD
Attending Physician
Department of Dermatology
University Hospital Essen
Essen, Germany

Charles L. Loprinzi MD
Regis Professor of Breast Cancer Research
Mayo Clinic
Rochester, MN, USA

Katherine Szyfelbein Masterpol
MD
Department of Dermatology
Assistant Professor in Dermatology
Boston University School of Medicine
Boston, MA, USA

Christine Mateus MD
Cancer Institute Gustave Roussy
Villejuif, France

Beth N. McLellan MD
Assistant Professor of Dermatology
The Ronald O. Perelman Department of
Dermatology
New York University School of Medicine
New York, NY, USA

Roger von Moos MD
Associate Professor of Oncology
University of Zurich
Zurich, Switzerland

Amanda R. Moraska MD
Anesthesiology Institute
Cleveland Clinic
Cleveland, OH, USA

Patricia L. Myskowski MD
Attending Physician, Dermatology Service
Memorial Sloan-Kettering Cancer Center;
Professor of Dermatology
Weill Cornell Medical College
New York, NY, USA

Kishwer S. Nehal MD
Director of Mohs Surgery
Dermatology Service
Memorial Sloan-Kettering Cancer Center
New York, NY, USA

Elise A. Olsen MD
Professor of Dermatology and Medicine
Duke University Medical Center
Durham, NC, USA

Cindy England Owen MD
Assistant Professor of Medicine (Dermatology)
University of Louisville School of Medicine
Louisville, KY, USA

Devika Patel MD
Resident in Dermatology
Department of Dermatology
Henry Ford Hospital
Detroit, MI, USA

Tejesh Patel MD
Assistant Professor
Department of Dermatology
University of Tennessee Health Science Center
Memphis, TN, USA

Caroline Robert MD, PhD
Chief of Dermatology Department
Cancer Institute Gustave Roussy
Villejuif, France

Alyx Rosen MD
Clinical Research Fellow
Dermatology Service
Memorial Sloan-Kettering Cancer Center
New York, NY, USA

Steven T. Rosen MD
Division of Hematology/Oncology
Northwestern University Feinberg School of
Medicine;
Robert H. Lurie Comprehensive Cancer Center of
Northwestern University
Chicago, IL, USA

Dirk Schadendorf MD
Full Professor of Dermatology, Director and
Chair of Department of Dermatology
University Hospital Essen
Essen, Germany

Ann Setser
Setser Health Consulting LLC
Chesterfield, MO, USA

Neil H. Shear MD, FRCPC
Professor of Medicine (Dermatology, Clinical
Pharmacology) and Pharmacology
University of Toronto
Toronto, Canada

Vincent Sibaud MD
Department of Oncodermatology and Clinical
Research Unit
Claudius Regaud Institute
Cancer Comprehensive Center
Toulouse, France

Tomas Skacel MD, PhD
Lecturer in Oncology
1st Dept Medicine, 1st Medical Faculty
Charles University Prague
Czech Republic

Stephen T. Sonis DMD, DMSc
Senior Surgeon Brigham and Women's Hospital
and the Dana-Farber Cancer Institute;
Clinical Professor of Oral Medicine
Harvard School of Dental Medicine
Boston, MA, USA

Shannon C. Trotter
Assistant Clinical Professor
Director, Pigmented Lesion Clinic
Division of Dermatology
Ohio State University
Columbus, OH, USA

James L. Troy MD
Clinical Professor of Dermatology and Director
of Dermatopathology
Dermatology Medical College of Wisconsin
Milwaukee, WI, USA

Lynne I. Wagner PhD
Associate Professor
Department of Medical Social Sciences
Northwestern University Feinberg School of
Medicine;
Robert H. Lurie Comprehensive Cancer Center of
Northwestern University
Chicago, IL, USA

Dennis P. West PhD, FCCP, CIP
Professor in Dermatology and Pediatrics
Northwestern University Feinberg School of
Medicine
Robert H. Lurie Comprehensive Cancer Center of
Northwestern University
Chicago, IL, USA

Rebecca K.S. Wong MB, ChB, MSc,
FRCP
Professor
Department of Radiation Oncology
University of Toronto, Princess Margaret Hospital
University Health Network
Toronto, Canada

Caroline Yeager AB
Department of Dermatology
Duke University Medical Center
Durham, NC, USA

Gil Yosipovitch MD
Professor of Dermatology Neurobiology and
Anatomy
Wake Forest University Health Sciences
Winston-Salem, NC, USA

Lisa Zimmer MD
Senior Attending Physician
Department of Dermatology
University Hospital Essen
Essen, Germany

Preface

This book is intended for oncology, nursing, and dermatology students, educators, and practitioners. Any of the modalities used against cancer: surgery, radiation, medical therapies, or therapeutic transplants, may have an effect on skin and its appendages, which can not only affect quality of life, health, but may also impact cost and dose intensity of therapy, all of which may affect clinical outcome. Although the focus is mainly on dermatologic adverse events of medical therapy, the effects of radiation, transplants, and surgeries will also be explored, with an emphasis on accurate diagnosis and effective management. In addition, basic dermatologic nomenclature, pathology, and adverse event grading will be included for readers who have not had these as part of their curriculum or training. As dermatologic conditions may appear before or after the diagnosis of cancer, paraneoplastic conditions that may herald an underlying malignancy, as well as late effects of therapy, respectively, are also described herein by leaders in the field.

The skin is the human body's largest organ, a self-renewing tissue whose functions include thermoregulation, sensation, immunity, fluid and organ preservation, and vitamin D synthesis. These various functions, along with its multiple layers and the formation of appendages, such as hair and nails, allows for a complexity that is nowhere more manifest than in the oncology setting. Contributing authors have a unique expertise in the diagnosis and treatment of dermatologic conditions in people living with cancer. This vast expertise will undoubtedly assist in mitigating the various untoward events that can affect cancer patients and survivors, both physically and psychosocially.

In order to make this book rapidly accessible whenever a patient presents with a dermatologic condition, chapters have principally been divided into the mechanism of action of medical therapies, when appropriate. In addition, cutaneous structures have also been taken into consideration, with a separate chapter for hair, nails, and mucosae. Basic dermatologic procedures and appearance-related interventions have also been included, to expand the therapeutic options that may improve the quality of life and cutaneous health of our patients. The ultimate goal of this book is to help optimize the treatment of cancer, by minimizing the effects of dermatologic conditions on quality of life and maximizing therapeutic consistency.

Acknowledgment

We are very grateful to cancer patients, survivors, and their families, who have generously donated their time, thoughts, and have allowed us to photograph and discuss their symptoms them at a difficult time in their lives. We are privileged to have participated in their care. We are grateful to the support staff who enable us to deliver care to people touched by cancer. And we thank the readers for allowing us to participate in the care and understanding of their patients' dermatologic conditions.

Mario E. Lacouture MD
Associate Member
Department of Medicine
Memorial Sloan-Kettering Cancer Center
New York, NY, USA

1 Dermatology and Oncology

1 Epidemiology and Burden of Disease

Beth N. McLellan[1], Devika Patel[2] and Mario E. Lacouture[3,4]

[1]The Ronald O. Perelman Department of Dermatology, New York University School of Medicine, New York, NY, USA
[2]Department of Dermatology, Henry Ford Hospital, Detroit, MI, USA
[3]Dermatology Service, Memorial Sloan-Kettering Cancer Center, New York, NY, USA
[4]Department of Dermatology, Cornell University, New York, NY, USA

Introduction

Due to recent advances in cancer therapies, patients are now living longer than ever before. For all diagnosed cancers, the 5-year relative survival has increased from 50% in 1975–1977 to 66% in 1996–2004 [1]. From 1990 to 2003, all-site cancer deaths in the United States decreased by 1% per year and these declines were especially pronounced for some of the most common malignancies including breast, prostate, colorectal, and lung cancers [2]. In the United States in 2009, there were 1 479 350 new cancers expected to be diagnosed [1], of which 52–87% were treated with surgery, 24–35% with chemotherapy, and 47–51% with radiation therapy (based on 2002 data for breast, lung, and colorectal cancers) [3]. Fifty to sixty thousand hematopoietic stem cell transplants are performed worldwide per year [4].

The large number of people being diagnosed with cancer in combination with increased survival rates have led to an increased number of patients living with a history of cancer, estimated to be 11.1 million in 2005 in the United States [1], of which 270 000 are survivors of pediatric cancers [5]. The increased number of patients living with and after cancer has revealed a number of dermatologic issues specific to this population: affecting cutaneous health, causing a financial burden, decreasing health-related quality of life, and impairing consistent drug dosing.

Dermatologic health in cancer patients and survivors

The relationship between the skin, hair, and nails and internal malignancies is manifested in various ways and in all phases of a patient's experience with cancer (Figure 1.1) . Even before a diagnosis of cancer is made, the skin may be affected by genetic syndromes with an increased cancer risk, environmental carcinogens leading to both skin conditions and internal malignancies, or paraneoplastic syndromes. Before treatment begins, patients can be affected by a number of dermatologic problems, most commonly tinea pedis/onychomycosis, pruritus, and xerosis [6]. After the diagnosis of cancer is made, cancer treatments (systemic agents, radiation, therapeutic transplants, and surgeries) can result in a number of skin, hair, and nail adverse events (AEs) that develop either as a result of idiosyncratic reactions or as an effect on rapidly proliferating cells (of which the skin, hair, and nails are prototypical structures).

The number of dermatologic AEs of chemotherapeutic agents is large and continues to expand as new agents come into use (see Appendix 1.1). In 2008, of approximately 384 000 routine AEs for phase I and II studies were reported to the Cancer Therapy Evaluation Program (CTEP) via the Clinical Data Update System (CDUS), 30 834 (8.04%) were dermatologic in nature (personal communication, Clinical Data Update System). Actual numbers of dermatologic AE to therapy may be higher than these estimates because of underreporting and inaccurate grading of AEs [14]. These inaccuracies have at least partly been brought about by difficulty applying existing grading systems to distinct dermatologic AEs, as has been demonstrated with other toxicities [15]. Another difficulty is grading AEs that are of low grade but prolonged duration [16]. Improved reporting of dermatologic AE is expected as focused grading scales are created [17].

In addition to the primary dermatologic toxicity of therapy, secondary skin infections are a frequent complication. In one study of patients receiving epidermal growth factor receptor inhibitors (EGFRIs), 38% of patients showed evidence of infection at sites of dermatologic toxicities [18]. Treatment modalities other than chemotherapy including radiation therapy, cancer-related surgery, and hematologic transplants are associated with distinct dermatologic toxicities and secondary infections (Figure 1.2).

Financial burden

In addition to the psychosocial effects (discussed in Chapter 6), dermatologic AEs also result in a financial cost to patients. Overall costs of treating cancer have increased by 75% from 1995 to

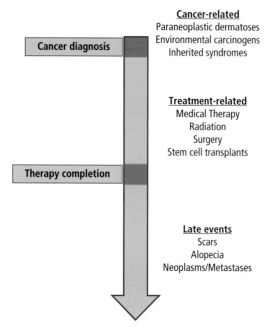

Figure 1.1 Dermatologic events in the life of the cancer patient and/or survivor [7]. GVHD, graft versus host disease. Adapted from Agha, 2007 [7].

2004 [3]. A portion of this cost can be attributed to supportive dermatologic care. Median medical costs per patient treated for head and neck or nonsmall cell lung cancer with radiochemotherapy are $39 313 per patient with mucositis/pharyngitis and $20 798 per patient without mucositis/pharyngitis [19]. Much of the increased cost was attributed to increased length of hospital stay [19]. For dermatologic AEs in patients treated with EGFRIs or platelet-derived growth factor receptor (PDGFR) and vascular endothelial growth factor receptor (VEGFR) inhibitors, mean cost of treatment for dermatologic toxicities was $2496 per patient [20]. Costs associated with stem cell transplantation can be increased by as much as $28,100 by development of acute graft versus host disease (GVHD) [21]. It is plausible that a prophylactic approach to managing treatment-induced AEs could decrease these associated costs.

Health-related quality of life

All of the described dermatologic toxicities due to cancer treatment can have a significant impact on a patient's health-related quality of life (HRQL). Patients most frequently report dermatologic AE as carrying a negative impact and of being unanticipated prior to therapy, with 67% of patients reporting that dermatologic AEs are worse than their initial belief [22]. Fifty-eight percent of patients rate chemotherapy-induced alopecia as the most traumatic side effect from their therapy and 8% of patients would decline chemotherapy because of fear of hair loss [23]. In a study of breast cancer patients receiving radiation therapy, the skin

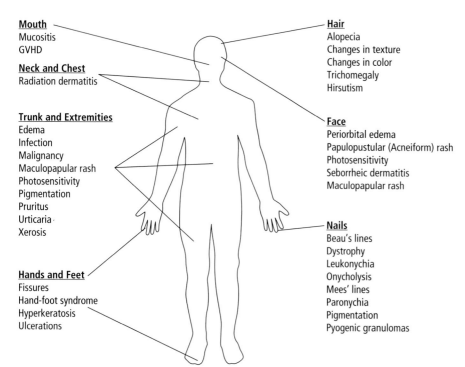

Figure 1.2 Locations of therapy-induced dermatologic toxicities.

changes induced by radiotherapy were found to negatively impact physical well-being, body image, emotional well-being, functional well-being, and treatment satisfaction [24]. Scars resulting from oncologic surgical procedures can lead to psychologic problems in 15% of survivors of childhood cancers [25]. In a prospective study measuring the frequency and impact on quality of life of dermatologic toxicities in women receiving chemotherapy, 34% of women reported dermatologic AEs as most important during treatment and they were the most common significant contributor to overall HRQL [26]. Of those who develop dermatologic AEs, 69% feel significantly limited in their daily activities [26].

Dosing of chemotherapy

Perhaps the most imposing challenge offered by dermatologic AE is their ability to result in dose modifications of anticancer therapies. Although the effects of anticancer therapy dose modification on progression-free survival or overall survival have not been evaluated, one can surmise that by reducing dose intensity, clinical outcome will be negatively affected. Studies linking the frequency and severity of dermatologic AEs to a longer median survival underscore the importance of managing dermatologic events, as patients who develop these untoward events are those most likely to benefit from their antineoplastic therapy [27]. Most notably, the papulopustular (acneiform) eruption to the EGFRIs (e.g., erlotinib, cetuximab, and panitumumab) has been shown to correlate with increased progression-free and overall survival in a variety of solid tumors [28,29].

In patients receiving cetuximab for example, up to 11.3% will develop a grade 3 or higher skin rash, necessitating dose reductions [30]. The development of mucositis is shown to lead to a twofold increased risk of chemotherapy dose reduction and limits the ability to give methotrexate for prevention of GVHD following autologous stem cell transplants [31]. Effectively recognizing and treating dermatologic toxicities to chemotherapy can minimize dose reductions and treatment interruptions as shown in the STEPP trial in which 12 doses were delayed in the prophylactic skin treatment arm, compared to 21 doses in the reactive arm [32].

Conclusions

The increasing number of cancer patients and survivors has led to an increased awareness of the HRQL components and treatment-related dermatologic manifestations seen in this patient population. These dermatologic toxicities are diverse and can have an enormous impact on the cutaneous health of patients, overall costs of treatment, healthcare-related quality of life, and consistent anticancer therapy. The recognition of all of these factors has led to a new field within dermatology: supportive oncodermatology, which is focused on the addressing the aforementioned dermatologic issues facing cancer patients and survivors.

References

1 American Cancer Society. (2009) Cancer Facts and Figures 2009. Available from: http://www.cancer.org/downloads/STT/500809web.pdf (accessed 15 April 2010).
2 Byers, T. (2008) Changes in cancer mortality. In: V.T. DeVita, T.S. Lawrence & S.A. Rosenberg (eds), *Cancer Principles and Practice of Oncology*, 8th ed., pp. 275–282. Lippincott Williams & Wilkins, Philadelphia.
3 Warren, J.L., Yabroff, K.R., Meekins, A. *et al.* (2008) Evaluation of trends in the cost of initial cancer treatment. *Journal of the National Cancer Institute*, **100**, 888–897.
4 Center for International Blood and Marrow Transplant Research. (2008) 2008 Biennial Report Appendix G – Part 1. Available from: http://bloodcell.transplant.hrsa.gov/RESEARCH/Biennial_Report/PDFs/2008_Biennial_Report_CWBYCTP_Sec3G1.pdf (accessed 16 April 2010).
5 Oeffinger, K.C., Mertens, A.C., Sklar, C.A. *et al.* (2006) Chronic health conditions in adult survivors of childhood cancer. *New England Journal of Medicine*, **355**, 1572–1582.
6 Kiliç, A., Gül, Ü. & Soylu, S. (2007) Skin findings in nternal malignant diseases. *International Journal of Dermatology*, **46**, 1055–1060.
7 Agha, R., Kinahan, K., Bennett, C.L. & Lacouture, M.E. (2007) Dermatologic challenges in cancer patients and survivors. *Oncology*, **21**, 1462–1472.
8 Litt, J.Z. (2009) *Litt's Drug Eruption Reference Manual*, 15th ed., Informa Healthcare, New York.
9 Kantarjian, H., Giles, F., Wunderle, L. *et al.* (2006) Nilotinib in imatinib-resistant CML and Philadelphia chromosome-positive ALL. *New England Journal of Medicine*, **354**, 2542–2551.
10 Iwamoto, F.M., Lamborn, K.R., Robins, H.I. *et al.* (2010) Phase II trial of pazopanib (GW786034), an oral multi-targeted angiogenesis inhibitor, for adults with recurrent glioblastoma (North American Brain Tumor Consortium Study 06-02). *Neuro-Oncology*, **12**, 855–861.
11 Teneriello, M.G., Tseng, P.C., Crozier, M. *et al.* (2009) Phase II evaluation of nanoparticle albumin-bound paclitaxel in platinum-sensitive patients with recurrent ovarian, peritoneal, or fallopian tube cancer. *Journal of Clinical Oncology*, **27**, 1426–1431.
12 Molife, L.R., Attard, G., Fong, P.C. *et al.* (2010) Phase II, two-stage, single-arm trial of the histone deacetylase inhibitor (HDACi) romidepsin in metastatic castration-resistant prostate cancer (CRPC). *Annals of Oncology*, **21**, 109–113.
13 Montero, A.J., Estrov, Z., Freireich, E.J. *et al.* (2006) Phase II study of low-dose interleukin-11 in patients with myelodysplastic syndrome. *Leukemia and Lymphoma*, **47**, 2049–2054.
14 Bauer, K.A., Hammerman, S., Rapoport, B. & Lacouture, M.E. (2008) Completeness in the reporting of dermatologic adverse drug reactions associated with monoclonal antibody epidermal growth factor report inhibitors in phase II and III colorectal cancer clinical trials. *Clinical Colorectal Cancer*, **7**, 209–214.
15 Basch, E. (2010) The missing voice of patients in drug-safety reporting. *New England Journal of Medicine*, **362**, 865–869.
16 Edgerly, M. & Fojo, T. (2008) Is there room for improvement in the era of targeted therapies? *Journal of the National Cancer Institute*, **100**, 240–242.
17 Lacouture, M.E., Maitland, M.L., Segaert, S. *et al.* (2010) A proposed EGFR inhibitor dermatologic adverse event-specific grading scale

from the MASCC skin toxicity study group. *Supportive Care in Cancer*, **18**, 509–522.

18 Eilers, R.E. Jr, Gandhi, M., Patel, J.D. *et al.* (2010) Dermatologic infections in cancer patients treated with epidermal growth factor receptor inhibitor therapy. *Journal of the National Cancer Institute*, **102**, 47–53.

19 Nonzee, N.J., Dandade, N.A., Patel, U. *et al.* (2008) Evaluating the supportive care costs of severe radiochemotherapy-induced mucositis and pharyngitis: results from a Northwestern University Costs of Cancer Program pilot study with head and neck and nonsmall cell lung cancer patients who received care at a county hospital, a Veterans Administration hospital, or a comprehensive cancer care center. *Cancer*, **113**, 1446–1452.

20 Borovicka, J.H., Hensley, J.R., Calahan, C. *et al.* (2010) Economic burden associated with the management of dermatologic toxicities induced by targeted anticancer therapies. Presented at American Academy of Dermatology 68th Annual Meeting, March 2010.

21 Redaelli, A., Botteman, M.F., Stephens, J.M. *et al.* (2004) Economic burden of acute myeloid leukemia: a literature review. *Cancer Treatment Reviews*, **30**, 237–247.

22 Gandhi, M., Oishi, K., Zubal, B. & Lacouture, M.E. (2010) Unanticipated toxicities from anticancer therapies: survivors' perspectives. *Supportive Care in Cancer*, **18**, 1461–1468.

23 McGarvey, E.L., Baum, L.D., Pinkerton, R.C. & Rogers, L.M. (2001) Psychological sequelae and alopecia among women with cancer. *Cancer Practice*, **9**, 283–289.

24 Schnur, J.B., Oullette, S.C., DiLorenzo, T.A. Green, S. & Montgomery, G.H. (2011) A qualitative analysis of acute skin toxicity among breast cancer radiotherapy patients. *Psycho-Oncology*, **20**, 260–268.

25 Pinter, A.B., Hock, A., Kajtar, P. & Dóber, I. (2003) Long-term follow-up of cancer in neonates and infants: a national survey of 142 patients. *Pediatric Surgery International*, **19**, 233–239.

26 Hackbarth, M., Haas, N., Fotopoulou, C., Lichtenegger, W. & Sehouli, J. (2008) Chemotherapy-induced dermatological toxicity: frequencies and impact on quality of life in women's cancers. Results of a prospective study. *Supportive Care in Cancer*, **16**, 267–273.

27 Li, T. & Perez-Soler, R. (2009) Skin toxicities associated with epidermal growth factor receptor inhibitors. *Targeted Oncology*, **4**, 107–119.

28 Wacker, B., Nagrani, T., Weinberg, J., Witt, K., Clark, G. & Cagnoni, P.J. (2007) Correlation between development of rash and efficacy in patients treated with the epidermal growth factor receptor tyrosine kinase inhibitor erlotinib in two large phase III studies. *Clinical Cancer Research*, **13**, 3913–3921.

29 Peréz-Soler, R. & Saltz, L. (2005) Cutaneous adverse effects with HER1/EGFR-targeted agents: is there a silver lining? *Journal of Clinical Oncology*, **23**, 5235–5246.

30 Su, X., Lacouture, M.E., Jia, Y. & Wu, S. (2009) Risk of high-grade skin rash in cancer patients treated with cetuximab: an antibody against epidermal growth factor receptor: systemic review and meta-analysis. *Oncology*, **77**, 124–133.

31 Murphy, B.A. (2007) Clinical and economic consequences of mucositis induced by chemotherapy and/or radiation therapy. *Journal of Supportive Oncology*, **5**, 13–21.

32 Lacouture, M.E., Mitchell, E.P., Piperdi, B. *et al.* (2010) Skin toxicity evaluation protocol with panitumumab (STEPP), a phase II, open-label, randomized trial evaluating the impact of a pre-emptive skin treatment regimen on skin toxicities and quality of life in patients with metastatic colorectal cancer. *Journal of Clinical Oncology*, **28**, 1351–1357.

33 Kwak, E.L., Bang, Y.J., Gamidge, D.R., *et al.* (2010) Anaplastic lymphoma kinase inhibition in non-small-cell lung cancer. *New England Journal of Medicine*, **363**, 1693–1703.

34 Mitchell, E.P. (2013) Targeted therapy for metastatic colorectal cancer: role of afibercept. *Clinical Colorectal Cancer*, **12**, 73–85.

35 Robinson, B.G., Paz-Ares, L., Krebs, A., Vasselli, J. & Haddad, R. (2010) Vandetanib (100 mg) in patients with locally advanced or metastatic hereditary medullary thyroid cancer. *Journal of Clinical Endocrinology and Metabolism*, **95**, 2664–2671.

36 Cortes, J.E., Kantarijan, H., Shah, N.P., *et al.* (2012) Ponatinib in refractory Philadelphia chromosome-positive leukemias. *New England Journal of Medicine*, **367**, 2075–2088.

37 Rini, B.I., Escudier, B., Tomczak, P. *et al.* (2011) Comparative effectiveness of axitinib versus sorafenib in advanced renal cell carcinoma (AXIS): a randomized phase 3 trial. *Lancet*, **378**, 1931–1939.

38 Smith, D.C., Smith, M.R., Sweeny, C. *et al.* (2013) Cabozantinib in patients with advanced prostate cancer: results of a phase II randomized discontinuation trial. *Journal of Clinical Oncology*, **31**, 412–419.

39 Cortes, J.E., Kim, D.W., Kantarjian, H.M. *et al.* (2012) Bosutinib versus imatinib in newly diagnosed chronic-phase chronic myeloid leukemia: results from the BELA trial. *Journal of Clinical Oncology*, **30**, 3486–3492.

40 Demetri, G.D., Reichardt, P., Kang, Y.K. *et al.* (2013) Efficacy and safety of regorafenib for advanced gastrointestinal stromal tumours after failure of imatinib and sunitinib (GRID): an international, multicentre, randomised, placebo-controlled, phase 3 trial. *Lancet*, **381**, 295–302.

41 Chapman, P.B., Hauschild, A., Robert, C. *et al.* (2011) Improved survival with vemurafenib in melanoma with BRAF V600E mutation. *New England Journal of Medicine*, **364**, 2507–2516.

42 Anderson, L., Schmieder, G.J., Werschler, W.P. *et al.* (2009) Randomized, double-blind, double-dummy, vehicle-controlled study of ingenol mebutate gel 0.025% and 0.05% for actinic keratosis. *Journal of the American Academy of Dermatology*, **60**, 934–943.

43 Von Hoff, D.D, LoRusso, P.M., Rudin C.M. *et al.* (2009) Inhibition of hedgehog pathway in advanced basal-cell carcinoma. *New England Journal of Medicine*, **361**, 1164–1172.

44 Axelson, M., Liu, K., Jiang, X. *et al.* (2013) U.S. Food and Drug Administration approval: vismodegib for recurrent, locally advanced, or metastatic basal cell carcinoma. *Clinical Cancer Research*, **19**, 2289–2293.

45 Bissler, J.J., Kingswood, J.C., Radzikowska, E. *et al.* (2013) Everolimus for angiomyolipoma associated with tuberous sclerosis complex or sporadic lymphangioleiomyomatosis (EXIST-2): a multicentre, randomized, double blind, placebo-controlled trial. *Lancet*. Epub ahead of print.

46 Hodi, F.S., O'Day, S.J., McDermott, D.F. *et al.* (2010) Improved survival with ipilimumab in patients with metastatic melanoma. *New England Journal of Medicine*, **363**, 711–723.

47 Swain, S.M., Kim, S.B., Cortés, J. *et al.* (2013) Pertuzumab, trastuzumab, and docetaxel for HER2-positive metastatic breast cancer (CLEOPATRA study): overall survival results from a randomised, double-blind, placebo-controlled, phase 3 study. *Lancet Oncology*, **14**, 461–471.

Appendix 1.1 Anticancer agents and associated adverse events affecting the skin, mucosa, hair, and nails. Based on data from Litt JZ, 2009 [8].

Drug	Skin	Mucosal/ENT	Hair	Nails
Alkylating agents				
Busulfan	Churg–Strauss syndrome, bullous dermatitis, eccrine squamous syringometaplasia, macular erythema (>10%), erythema multiforme (<1%), exanthems, Kaposi sarcoma, pigmentation (1–10%), purpura, urticaria (>10%), vasculitis, xerosis	Cheilitis, dysgeusia, mucositis, pigmentation	Alopecia (>10%)	Pigmentation
Thiotepa	Allergic reactions (1–10%), angioedema, eccrine squamous syringometaplasia, leukoderma, pigmentation (1–10%), pruritus (1–10%), rash (1–10%), urticaria (3%)	Stomatitis (<1%)	Alopecia (1–10%)	
Mechlorethamine	Acanthosis nigricans, angioedema, bullous dermatitis, cellulitis, cyst, dermatitis, erythema multiforme (<1%), exanthems (<1%), fungal dermatitis, herpes zoster (>10%), pigmentation, pruritus, purpura, squamous cell carcinoma, SJS, urticaria, xerosis	Dysgeusia (1–10%), tinnitus	Alopecia (1–10%)	
Melphalan	Angioedema, eccrine squamous syringometaplasia, edema, exanthem (4%), petechiae, pruritus (1–10%), purpura, rash (1–10%), scleroderma, urticaria, vasculitis (1–10%), vesiculation (1–10%)	Mucositis	Alopecia (1–10%)	Beau lines
Chlorambucil	Angioedema, edema, exanthem, facial erythema, herpes simplex, herpes zoster, Kaposi sarcoma, lupus erythematosus, necrosis, perianal irritation, photosensitivity, pruritus, psoriasis, purpura, rash (1–10%), Sézary syndrome, SJS, TEN, urticaria	Oral lesions	Alopecia	
Cyclophosphamide	Allergic reaction, angioedema, carcinoma, dermatitis, dermatitis herpetiformis, dermatofibromas, eccrine squamous syringometaplasia, edema, eosinophilic pustular folliculitis, erythema multiforme (<1%), exanthem, facial burning, graft versus host reaction, hand-foot syndrome, herpes zoster, lupus erythematosus, lymphoma, myxedema, neutrophilic eccrine hidradenitis, pemphigus, photo-recall, pigmentation (<1%), pruritus, purpura, scleroderma, SJS, TEN (<1%), urticaria, vasculitis	Gingival pigmentation, mucositis (10%)	Alopecia (universal and severe in one-third)	Beau lines, dystrophy, leukonychia, onychodermal band, pigmentation (<1%)
Ifosfamide	Allergic reaction (1–10%), dermatitis (1–10%), pigmentation (1–10%)	Oral lesions, sialorrhea (<1%), stomatitis (<1%)	Alopecia (50–100%)	Ridging (1–10%)
Carmustine	Dermatitis (<1%), eccrine squamous syringometaplasia, erythema, exanthems, telangiectasia, tenderness	Stomatitis (1–10%)	Alopecia (1–10%)	
Streptozocin	Edema, exanthems, pruritus, purpura, TEN			
Dacarbazine	Actinic keratoses, angioedema, erythema, exanthems, fixed eruption, photo-recall, photosensitivity (<1%), rash (1–10%), urticaria, vasculitis	Dysgeusia (1–10%), stomatitis (48%)	Alopecia (1–10%)	Pigmentation
Temozolomide	Allergic reactions, edema, hand-foot syndrome, Kaposi sarcoma, peripheral edema (11%), pruritus (8%), rash (8%)		Alopecia	
Etoposide	Allergic reactions (1–2%), diaphoresis, eccrine squamous syringometaplasia, erythema, erythema multiforme, exanthems, facial edema, hand-foot syndrome, neutrophilic eccrine hidradenitis, photo-recall, pigmentation, pruritus, purpura, rash, SJS, urticaria	Dysgeusia, mucositis (>10%), tinnitus, tongue edema	Alopecia (8–66%)	Beau lines, onychopathy
BCNU	Dermatitis (<1%), eccrine squamous syringometaplasia, erythema, exanthems, pigmentation, telangiectasia, tenderness	Stomatitis (1–10%)	Alopecia (1–10%)	

(Continued)

Drug	Skin	Mucosal/ENT	Hair	Nails
Antimetabolites				
Methotrexate	Acne, acral erythema, allergic reactions, angiomas, bullous dermatitis, capillaritis, carcinoma, dermatitis, dermatofibromas, eccrine squamous syringometaplasia, edema, eosinophilic pustular folliculitis, erosion of psoriatic plaques, erythema (>10%), erythema multiforme, exanthems (15%), furunculosis, herpes simplex, herpes zoster, lymphadenopathy, lymphoma, melanoma, molluscum contagiosum, necrosis, nodular eruption, non-Hodgkin lymphoma, photo-recall, photosensitivity (5%), pigmentation (1–10%), pruritus (1–5%), purpura, Raynaud phenomenon, SJS, telangiectasia, TEN (<1%), urticaria, vasculitis (>10%)	Aphthous stomatitis, dysgeusia, gingivitis (>10%), glossitis (>10%), mucositis	Alopecia (1–6%), pigmented bands	Discoloration, paronychia, pigmentation
Pemetrexed	Allergic reactions, desquamation (22%), edema, photo-recall, pressure necrosis, pruritus, purpura, rash (42%), vasculitis	Aphthous stomatitis, gingivitis, mucositis (5–17%)		
Capecitabine	Dermatitis (37%), diaphoresis (0.2%), edema (9%), erythema, exfoliative dermatitis (31–37%), hand-foot syndrome (7–58%), lupus erythematosus, photo-recall (<1%), photosensitivity, pigmentation, pruritus, purpura (0.2%), pyogenic granuloma, ulcerations, vesiculation, vitiligo, xerosis	Mucositis, oral candidiasis (0.2%), stomatitis (24%)	Alopecia (<1%)	Hyponychial dermatitis, nail loss, onychomadesis, paronychia, subungual hyperkeratosis
Cytarabine	Allergic reactions (<1%), angioedema (<1%), dermatitis, diaphoresis, edema (<1%), erythema, exanthems, lichenoid eruption, lupus erythematosus, peripheral edema, photosensitivity, purpura, urticaria, vasculitis	Dysgeusia, tinnitus, xerostomia (1–10%)		
Gemicitabine	Acral necrosis, allergic reactions (4%), cellulitis, dermatitis, diaphoresis, edema (13%), erysipelas, exanthems, hand-foot syndrome, linear IgA dermatosis, lipodermatosclerosis, livedo reticularis, necrotizing vasculitis, petechiae (16%), photo-recall (<74%), pruritus (13%), pseudolymphoma, rash (30%), Raynaud phenomenon, scleroderma, SJS, TEN	Dysgeusia, mucositis, stomatitis (11%)	Alopecia (15%)	
6-Mercaptopurine	Dermatitis (2%), edema, exanthems (<1%), herpes zoster, lichenoid eruption, lupus erythematosus, melanoma, neoplasms, palmar-plantar erythema, petechiae, photo-recall, photosensitivity, pigmentation (1–10%), pruritus, purpura, TEN, urticaria, vasculitis	Glossitis (<1%), mucositis (1–10%), oral lesions (1–5%), stomatitis (1–10%)	Alopecia	Nail loss
6-TG	Exanthems, malignancies, palmar erythema, petechiae, photosensitivity (<1%), pruritus, psoriasis, purpura, rash (1–10%)	Stomatitis (1–10%), xerostomia	Alopecia	
Fludarabine	Edema (>10%), exanthems, herpes simplex, paraneoplastic pemphigus, petechiae, rash (>10%), squamous cell carcinoma	Dysgeusia (<1%), stomatitis (>10%)	Alopecia (1–10%)	
Cladribine	Allergic reactions, diaphoresis (1–10%), edema (6%), eosinophilic cellulitis, erythema (6%), erythroderma, exanthems (27–50%), halogenoderma, herpes, petechiae (8%), pruritus (6%), purpura (10%), rash (27%), SJS, TEN, transient acantholytic dermatosis, urticaria, vasculitis			

Drug	Skin	Mucosal/ENT	Hair	Nails
Topoisomerase-interacting agents				
Irinotecan	Allergic reactions (9%), diaphoresis (16%), edema (10.2%), exanthems, hand-foot syndrome, photosensitivity, pigmentation, pruritus, pyogenic granuloma, rash (<21%)	Dysgeusia, mucositis (2%), sialorrhea	Alopecia (13–60.5%)	
Topotecan	Allergic reactions, erythema (<1%), fixed eruption, neutrophilic eccrine hidradenitis, purpura (<1%), scleroderma	Mucositis, stomatitis (24%)	Alopecia (59%)	Pigmentation
Doxorubicin	Actinic keratoses, allergic reactions (<1%), angioedema, cellulitis, dermatitis, dermatitis herpetiformis, diaphoresis, exanthems, exfoliative dermatitis, fixed eruption, hand-foot syndrome, inflammation, intertrigo, keratoderma, necrosis, photo-recall, pigmentation, pruritus, psoriasis, purpura, rash, Raynaud phenomenon, scleroderma, toxic erythema, urticaria (<1%)	Ageusia, mucositis, oral lesions, pigmentation, stomatitis (>10%), tongue pigmentation	Alopecia (>10%)	Beau lines, melanonychia, Muehrcke lines
Daunorubicin	Angioedema, dermatitis, erythema, exanthems, exfoliative dermatitis, folliculitis, hand-foot syndrome, hypomelanosis, neutrophilic eccrine hidradenitis, pigmentation, pruritus, rash (<1%), urticaria (<1%)	Mucositis	Alopecia (>10%)	Pigmentation (<1%)
Idarubicin	Acral erythema, bullous dermatitis, exanthems (<1%), neutrophilic dermatosis, photo-recall, rash (>10%), urticaria (>10%)	Mucositis (50%)	Alopecia (77%)	Pigmentation
Mitoxantrone	Allergic reactions (<1%), diaphoresis (1–10%), edema (>10%), erythema, fungal dermatitis (>15%), necrosis, petechiae (>10%, bluish pigmentation, purpura (>10%), rash (<1%), ulcerations, urticaria, vitiligo		Alopecia (20–60%)	
Dactinomycin	Acne (>10%), actinic keratoses, bullous pemphigoid, cellulitis, dermatitis, erythema, erythema multiforme, exanthems, folliculitis, reactivation of keratoses, lichenoid eruption, photo-recall (>10%), pigmentation, pruritus, pustules, TEN, urticaria	Cheilitis, oral lesions, ulcerative stomatitis (>5%)	Alopecia (>10%)	
Teniposide	Facial edema, rash, urticaria	Mucositis, stomatitis (3%)	Alopecia (31%)	
Epidermal growth factor receptor/Anaplastic lymphoma kinase/Vasuclar endothelial growth factor inhibitors				
Erlotinib	Acne, acute generalized exanthematous pustulosis, erythema (18%), fissures, folliculitis, papulopustular eruption, photosensitivity, pruritus (13%), rash (75%), telangiectasia, xerosis (12%)	Aphthous stomatitis (17%)	Alopecia, eyelash hypertrichosis, trichomegaly	Paronychia, pyogenic granulomas
Gefitinib	Acne (39–52%), acute generalized exanthematous pustulosis, desquamation (39%), erosive pustular dermatosis, exanthems, folliculitis, glucagonoma syndrome, hand-foot syndrome, pigmentation, pruritus, pyoderma gangrenosum, rash (52%), rosacea, scaling, seborrhea, ulcerations, urticaria, xerosis	Epistaxis, oral ulceration, stomatitis	Abnormal texture, alopecia, hypertrichosis	Paronychia (6%), pyogenic granulomas, nail changes (17%)
Cetuximab	Acne (88%), allergic reactions, burning, erythema, exanthems, fissures, folliculitis, papulopustular eruption, peripheral edema (10%), pruritus (10%), rash, transient acantholytic dermatosis, xerosis	Stomatitis (11%)	Alopecia (5%)	Nail changes (16%), paronychia
Panitumumab	Acne (57%), eczema, erythema (65%), exfoliative dermatitis (25%), fissures (20%), peripheral edema (12%), photosensitivity, pigmentation, pruritus (57%), rash (22%), telangiectasia, xerosis (10%)	Oral mucositis (6%)	Hair changes	Nail changes, paronychia (25%), pyogenic granulomas
Crizotinib [33]	Edema (16%)			
Ziv-aflibercept [34]		Stomatitis (20%)		

(Continued)

Drug	Skin	Mucosal/ENT	Hair	Nails
Multikinase small molecule tyrosine kinase inhibitors				
Imatinib	Acne, acute febrile neutrophilic dermatosis, acute generalized exanthematous pustulosis, carcinoma, dermatomyositis, eccrine squamous syringometaplasia, edema (1–5%), erythema, exanthems, exfoliative dermatitis, hypomelanosis, lichen planus, mycosis fungoides, necrolysis, neutrophilic eccrine hidradenitis, palmar-plantar hyperkeratosis, petechiae (1–10%), photosensitivity, pigmentation, pityriasis rosea, pruritus (6–10%), psoriasis, rash (32–39%), SJS, TEN, urticaria, vasculitis	Oral lichenoid eruption	Follicular mucinosis	Dystrophy, pigmentation
Dasatinib	Acne, dermatitis, hyperhidrosis, photosensitivity, pigmentation, pruritus (11%), rash (39%), urticaria, xerosis	Dysgeusia, mucositis (16%)	Alopecia	
Nilotinib [9]	Pruritus (17%), rash (22%), xerosis (12%)		Alopecia (6%)	
Sunitinib	Bullous dermatitis, edema, hand-foot syndrome, peripheral edema (17%), pigmentation, pyoderma gangrenosum, rash (14–38%, xerosis (17%)	Dysgeusia (21–43%), glossodynia (15%), mucositis (29–53%), stomatitis	Alopecia (5–12%), pigmentation	
Sorafenib	Acne (1–10%), inflammation of actinic keratoses, desquamation (40%), eczema (<1%), eruptive facial cysts, erythema (>10%), erythema multiforme (<1%), folliculitis (<1%), hand-foot syndrome (30%), hyperkeratosis, pruritus (19%), rash (40%), seborrheic dermatitis, squamous cell carcinoma, urticaria (<1%), vasculitis, xerosis (11%)	Angular stomatitis, cheilitis, dysphagia (1–10%), glossodynia (1–10%), mucositis (1–10%), rhinorrhea (<1%), xerostomia (1–10%)	Alopecia (27%)	Splinter hemorrhages
Pazopanib [10]	Decubitus ulcer (3%), edema (3%), flushing (3%), hand-foot syndrome (3%), hyperhidrosis (3%), hypopigmentation (3%), pruritus (3%), xerosis (3%)	Epistaxis (11%)		
Vandetanib [35]	Rash (26%), photosensitivity (16%)			
Ponatinib [36]	Rash (32%), acneiform dermatitis (14%), dry skin (14%), erythema nodosum (2%), melanoma (1%)			
Axitinib [37]	Palmar-plantar erythrodysaesthesia (27%), rash (13%)	Mucosal inflammation (15%), stomatitis (15%)	Alopecia (4%)	
Cabozantinib [38]	Rash (13%), palmar-plantar erythrodysethesia (30%)	stomatitis (11%), mucosal inflammation (21%)		
Bosutinib [39]	Rash (20%)			
Regorafenib [40]	Hand-foot skin reaction (56%), rash (18%)	Oral mucositis (38%)	Alopecia (24%)	

Drug	Skin	Mucosal/ENT	Hair	Nails
Antimicrotubule agents				
Paclitaxel	Allergic reactions (15%), angioedema, desquamation (7%), edema (21%), erythema, exanthems (<1%), fixed eruption, folliculitis, hand-foot syndrome, lupus erythematosus, photo-recall (<1%), photosensitivity, pigmentation, pruritus (<1%), purpura, pustules, rash (12%), scleroderma, SJS, urticaria	Mucositis (>10%), oral lesions (3–8%), stomatitis (2–39%)	Alopecia (87–100%), alopecia areata	Nail changes, leukonychia, Mees lines, paronychia, pigmentation (2%), subungual hyperkeratosis, thickening
Docetaxel	Allergic reactions, angioedema, edema (1–20%), erythema (0.9%), exanthems, fixed eruption, hand-foot syndrome, lupus erythematosus, photo-recall, photosensitivity, pigmentation, pruritus, radiodermatitis, rash (0.9%), scleroderma, seborrheic keratoses, squamous syringometaplasia, SJS, TEN, urticaria, xerosis	Dysgeusia, dysphagia, mucositis, nasal septal perforation, stomatitis (5–42%)	Alopecia (80%)	Beau lines, discoloration, dystrophy, hyponychial dermatitis, nail loss, paronychia, pigmentation, subungual abscess, subungual hemorrhage, subungual hyperkeratosis, transverse superficial loss of nail plate
Albumin-bound paclitaxel [11]			Alopecia (86.9%)	
Vincristine	Actinic keratoses, allergic reactions angioedema, dermatitis herpetiformis, edema, erythroderma, exanthems, hand-foot syndrome, pigmentation, pruritus, rash (1–10%), Raynaud phenomenon, urticaria	Dysgeusia (1–10%), oral lesions (1–10%), oral ulceration (1–10%), stomatitis (<1%)	Alopecia (20–70%)	Beau lines, leukonychia, Mees lines, Muehrcke lines, onychodermal band, pigmentation
Vinblastine	Acne, acral necrosis, angioedema, bullous dermatitis (<1%), cellulitis, dermatitis (1–10%), erythema, erythema multiforme, exanthems, photo-recall, photosensitivity (1–10%), pigmentation, purpura, Raynaud phenomenon (1–10%), ulcerations, urticaria	Dysgeusia (>10%), oral lesions (1–5%), oral vesiculation, ototoxicity, stomatitis (>10%)	Alopecia (>10%), hair changes	
Vinorelbine	Angioedema, erythema, hand-foot syndrome, pigmentation, pruritus, rash (<5%), TEN, vasculitis	Dysgeusia (>10%), mucositis, stomatitis (>10%)	Alopecia (12%)	
Estramustine	Acne, allergic reactions, angioedema, edema (>10%), exanthems, facial flushing, pigmentation (<1%), pruritus (2%), purpura (3%), rash (1%), urticaria, xerosis (2%)		Alopecia (<1%)	

(Continued)

Drug	Skin	Mucosal/ENT	Hair	Nails
Histone deacetylase, proteasome inhibitors, retinoids, and demethylating agents				
Vorinostat	Angioedema (9%), exfoliative dermatitis (9%), peripheral edema (13%), pruritus (12%)	Dysgeusia (28%), xerostomia (16%)	Alopecia (19%)	
Romidepsin [12]	Skin and subcutaneous disorder (4%)	Dry mouth (4%)		
Arsenic trioxide	Acral desquamation, carcinoma, bullous dermatitis, dermatitis, dermatofibrosarcoma protuberans, edema, ephelides, erythema, erythema multiforme, erythema nodosum, exanthems, exfoliative dermatitis, fixed eruption, follicular keratosis, herpes simplex, herpes zoster, hyperhidrosis, hyperkeratosis of the palms and soles (40%), hypomelanosis, keratoses, leukomelanosis, lichen planus, livedo reticularis, melanoma, melanosis, merkel cell carcinoma, morphea, palmar-plantar erythema, palmar-plantar hyperhidrosis, parapsoriasis, photo-recall, photosensitivity, pityriasis rosea, pruritus, psoriasis, purpura, rash, Raynaud phenomenon, SJS, ulcerations, urticaria, vitiligo, xerosis	Dysgeusia, oral mucosal eruption (8%), oral pigmentation, stomatitis	Alopecia	Leukonychia, Mees lines, pigmentation
All-trans retinoic acid	Acne (1%), acute febrile neutrophilic dermatosis, bullous dermatitis, burning (10–40%), carcinoma, cellulitis (1–10%), crusting, dermatitis, desquamation (14%), diaphoresis (20%), edema (29%), erythema (1–49%, erythema nodosum, facial edema (1–10%), flaking (23%), hyperkeratosis (78%), hypomelanosis (5%), irritation (5%), pallor (1–10%), palmar-plantar desquamation (1–10%), photosensitivity (10%), pigmentation (5%), pruritus (10–40%), pyogenic granuloma, rash (54%), retinoic acid–APL syndrome (25%), scaling (10–40%), shivering (63%), stinging (1–26%), ulcerations (penile), vasculitis, vesiculobullous eruption, xerosis (49–100%)	Cheilitis (10%), gingivitis (<1%), xerostomia (10%)	Alopecia areata (14%)	
Bexarotene	Acne (<10%), allergic granulomatous angiitis, bacterial infections (1.2–13.2%), burning, cold extremities, dermatitis, erythema, exanthems (<10%), exfoliative dermatitis (10–28%), facial edema, irritation, necrosis, nodular eruption (<10%), peripheral edema (13.1%), photosensitivity, pruritus (20–30%), pustules, rash (16.7%), stinging, ulcerations (<10%), vasculitis, vesiculobullous eruption (<10%), xerosis	Cheilitis (<10%), gingivitis (<10%), xerostomia (<10%)	Alopecia (4–11%)	
Miscellaneous agents				
L-Asparaginase	Allergic reactions, angioedema, diaphoresis, edema, exanthems, pruritus (<1%), TEN, urticaria (1–15%)	Aphthous stomatitis (1–10%), oral lesions (26%)	Alopecia	
Bleomycin	Acral necrosis, acral sclerosis, allergic reactions, angioedema, bullous dermatitis (1–5%), calcification, dermatitis, digital gangrene, eccrine squamous syringometaplasia, erythema, erythema gyratum, exanthems, fixed eruption, flagellate erythema/pigmentation, hand-foot syndrome, hyperkeratosis of the palms and soles, intertrigo, neutrophilic eccrine hidradenitis, nodular eruption, palmar nodules, photo-recall, pigmentation (50%), pruritus (>5%), rash, Raynaud phenomenon (>10%), scleroderma, SJS, striae, urticaria, vesiculation, xerosis.	Glossitis, oral papillomatosis, oral ulceration, stomatitis (>10%), tongue erosions	Alopecia (50%), graying of the hair	Beau lines, dystrophy, reduced growth, nail loss, onychodystrophy
Procarbazine	Allergic reactions (<1%), angioedema, dermatitis (<1%), diaphoresis, edema, exanthems (4–9%), exfoliative dermatitis, fixed eruption, herpes zoster, petechiae, photosensitivity, pigmentation (1–10%), pruritus (<1%), purpura, rash, TEN, urticaria (9%)	Oral lesions (1–5%), stomatitis (>10%), xerostomia	Alopecia (1–10%)	

Drug	Skin	Mucosal/ENT	Hair	Nails
Miscellaneous agents				
Thalidomide	Bullous dermatitis (5%), burning, dermatitis, desquamation, diaphoresis, edema, erythema, erythema multiforme, erythema nodosum, erythroderma, exanthems, exfoliative dermatitis, facial erythema, nodular eruption, palmar erythema, pruritus, psoriasis, purpura, pustuloderma, rash (11–50%), SJS, TEN, ulcerations, urticaria (3%), vasculitis, xerosis	Xerostomia	Alopecia	Brittle nails
Lenalidomide	Acute febrile neutrophilic dermatosis, diaphoresis (8%), erythema (5.4%), peripheral edema (20%), pruritus (42%), rash (36%), xerosis (14%)	Dysgeusia (6%), rhinitis (7%), stomatitis, xerostomia (7%)		
Vemurafenib [41]	Keratoacanthomas (6%), cutaneous squamous cell carcinoma (12%), rash (10%), pruritus (6%)		Alopecia (8%)	
Ingenol mebutate [42]	Erythema (34%), flaking/scaling (29%), crusting (9.2%), erosion/ulceration (1.9%), hypopigmentation/hyperpigmentation (19.8%), scarring (0.6%)			
Vismodegib [43,44]	Xerosis	Keratitis (3%), corneal abrasion (3%)	Alopecia (63.8%)	
Everolimus [45]	Acne-like skin lesions (22%), eczema (10%)	Stomatitis (48%), mouth ulceration (19%), apthous stomatitis (19%)		
Biotherapy				
Interferon-a2a Interferon-a2b	Acne (1%), acral sclerosis, allergic reactions, angioedema, atrophie blanche, Behçet disease, bullous dermatitis, dermatitis, dermatitis herpetiformis, dermatomyositis, diaphoresis (22%), eczema, edema (11%), erythema, erythema nodosum, exanthems, fungal dermatitis (<1%), halo dermatitis, herpes simplex (1%), Kaposi sarcoma, keratoses, lichen myxedematosus, lichen planus, lichenoid eruption, linear IgA dermatosis, livedo reticularis, lupus erythematosus, melanoma, necrosis, nodular eruption, pemphigus, photo-recall, photosensitivity (<1%), pigmentation (<1%), capillaritis, pityriasis versicolor, pruritus (13%), psoriasis, purpura, rash (44%), Raynaud phenomenon, sarcoidosis, scleroderma, seborrheic dermatitis, telangiectasia, ulcerations, urticaria (<3%), vasculitis, vitiligo, xerosis (17%)	Ageusia, anosmia, aphthous stomatitis, dysgeusia (25%), oral lichen planus, oral pemphigus, sialopenia, stomatitis (1–10%), xerostomia (>10%)	Alopecia (1–10%), alopecia areata, curly hair, hypertrichosis, pigmentation, straight hair	
Interleukin 2	Allergic granulomatous angiitis, allergic reactions (<1%), angioedema, bullous dermatitis, bullous pemphigoid, dermatitis, desquamation, edema (47%), erythema (41%), erythema multiforme, erythema nodosum, erythroderma, exanthems, exfoliative dermatitis (14%), intertrigo, Kaposi sarcoma, linear IgA dermatosis, necrosis, pemphigus, petechiae (4%), photosensitivity, pruritus (48%), psoriasis, purpura (4%), rash (26%), sarcoidosis, scleroderma, SJS, TEN, urticaria (2%), vasculitis, vitiligo, xerosis (15%)	Aphthous stomatitis, dysgeusia (7%), glossitis, oral mucosal eruption, oral ulceration, stomatitis 932%), xerostomia	Alopecia (<1%)	

(Continued)

Drug	Skin	Mucosal/ENT	Hair	Nails
Monoclonal antibodies				
Trastuzumab	Acne (2%), allergic reactions (3%), angioedema (<1%), cellulitis (<1%), diaphoresis, edema (8%), hand-foot syndrome, herpes simplex (2%), herpes zoster (1%), peripheral edema (10%), photosensitivity, rash (18%), ulcerations (1%)	Stomatitis (<1%)	Alopecia	Dystrophy
Bevacizumab	Exfoliative dermatitis, pigmentation, ulcerations, xerosis, hand-foot syndrome	Dysgeusia, oral ulceration, stomatitis, xerostomia	Alopecia	Changes
Rituximab	Angioedema (>10%), dermatitis, diaphoresis, exanthems, herpes zoster, Kaposi sarcoma, necrosis, paraneoplastic pemphigus, peripheral edema, pruritus (10%), rash (10%), SJS, TEN, urticaria (10%)	Orogenital ulceration, otitis, perianal ulcerations, rhinitis		
Alemtuzumab	Abscess, allergic reactions (<1%), angioedema (<1%), angioedema (<1%), bullous dermatitis (<1%), cellulitis (<1%), facial edema (<1%), hematomas (<1%), herpes simplex, herpes zoster, peripheral edema (13%), pruritus, purpura (8%), rash, squamous cell carcinoma (<1%), urticaria	Dysgeusia(<1%), gingivitis (<1%), sinusitis, stomatitis (14%), stomatodynia		
Gemtuzumab	Herpes simplex (22%), peripheral edema (21%), petechiae (21%), rash (23%)	Mucositis (<4–25%), stomatitis (32%)		
Ibritumomab	Allergic reactions (2%), angioedema (5%), bullous dermatitis, diaphoresis (4%), erythema multiforme, exfoliative dermatitis, peripheral edema (8%), petechiae (3%), pruritus (9%), purpura (7%), rash (8%), SJS, TEN, urticaria (4%)	Mucositis	Alopecia	
Tositumomab	Allergic reactions, angioedema, carcinoma, diaphoresis (8%), peripheral edema (9%), pruritus, rash (17%)	Rhinitis (10%)		
Ipilimumab [46]	Vitiligo (2.3%), rash (19.1%), pruritus (24%)		Alopecia	
Pertuzumab [47]	Pruritus (6%), dry skin (6%), acneiform rash (13%)	Mucosal inflammation (7%)		
Endocrine agents				
Tamoxifen	Dermatomyositis, diaphoresis, edema (2–6%), exanthems (3%), lupus erythematosus, photo-recall, pruritus, purpura, radiodermatitis, rash (1–10%), sarcoma, urticaria, vasculitis, xerosis (7%)	Dysgeusia, vaginal pruritus, xerostomia (7%)	Alopecia, hirsutism, hypertrichosis, pigmentation	
Toremifene	Dermatitis, diaphoresis (20%), edema (5%), pigmentation, pruritus			
Raloxifene	Capillaritis, diaphoresis (3.1%), edema, peripheral edema (3–5%), rash (5.5%), vitiligo	Vaginitis (4.3%)		
Anastrozole	Angioedema, diaphoresis, erythema multiforme, lupus erythematosus, peripheral edema (10.1%), pruritus (2–5%), rash (7.5%), shivering, SJS, urticaria	Vaginal dryness (1.7%), xerostomia	Alopecia (2–5%)	
Letrozole	Diaphoresis (<5%), exanthems (5%), pruritus (2%), psoriasis (5%), rash (1–10%), TEN, vesiculation (5%)		Alopecia (<5%)	
Exemestane	Diaphoresis (6–12%), edema (7%), hyperhidrosis, peripheral edema (9%), pruritus (2–5%), rash (2–5%)		Alopecia (2–5%)	
Fulvestrant	Diaphoresis (5%), edema (9%), rash (7%)	Vaginitis		

Drug	Skin	Mucosal/ENT	Hair	Nails
Endocrine agents				
Leuprolide	Acne, allergic granulomatous angiitis, dermatitis (5%), dermatitis herpetiformis, diaphoresis, edema (1–10%), exanthems, lupus erythematosus, nodular eruption, photosensitivity, pigmentation (<5%), pruritus (<5%), purpura (<1%), rash (1–10%), stickiness, urticaria, xerosis (<5%)	Dysgeusia(<5%), vaginitis,	Alopecia (<5%), hypertrichosis (<1%)	
Flutamide	Bullous dermatitis, diaphoresis, edema (4%), erythema, exanthems, lupus erythematosus, photosensitivity, rash (3%), TEN, urticaria			
Bicalutamide	Angioedema, carcinoma, diaphoresis (6%), edema (2–5%), exanthems (<1%), herpes zoster, pruritus (2–5%), rash (6%), urticaria, xerosis (2–5%)	Xerostomia	Alopecia	
Nilutamide	Diaphoresis (6%), edema (2%), pruritus (2%), rash (5%), urticaria, xerosis (5%)	Xerostomia (2%0	Alopecia	
Fluoxymesterone	Acne (>10%), dermatitis, edema (>10%), exanthems, furunculosis, lichenoid eruption, lupus erythematosus, pruritus, psoriasis, purpura, seborrhea, striae, urticaria	Stomatitis	Alopecia, hirsutism (1–10%)	
Estradiol	Acanthosis nigricans, acne (5%), allergic granulomatous angiitis, angioedema, bullous dermatitis, chloasma (<1%), dermatitis, eczema, edema (<1%), erythema multiforme, erythema nodosum, exanthems, exfoliative dermatitis, fixed eruption (<1%), hyperkeratosis, livedo reticularis, lupus erythematosus, Mucha–Habermann disease, osteoma cutis, papulovesicular eruption, photosensitivity, pigmentation, porphyria cutanea tarda, pruritus, pseudolymphoma, purpura, rash (<1%), Raynaud phenomenon, scleroderma, spider nevi, striae, telangiectasia, urticaria, vasculitis, vesiculation	Gingival hyperplasia/hypertrophy, mucosal eruption, pigmentation, vulvovaginal candidiasis	Alopecia (9%), hirsutism (<5%), straight hair	
Octreotide	Allergic granulomatous angiitis, allergic reactions, cellulitis (1–4%), diaphoresis, edema (1–10%), exanthems, petechiae (1–4%), pruritus (1–4%), purpura (1–4%), rash (<1%), Raynaud phenomenon (1–4%), urticaria (1–4%)	Vaginitis (1–4%), xerostomia	Alopecia (<1%)	
Megestrol	Acne, acute generalized exanthematous pustulosis, angioedema, dermatitis, diaphoresis (31%), edema, erythema multiforme, erythema nodosum, exanthems, hemorrhage, melasma, pruritus, rash, telangiectasia, urticaria		Alopecia, hirsutism	
Medroxyprogesterone acetate	Acne (1–5%), allergic reactions (<1%), angioedema, chloasma (1–10%), diaphoresis (<31%), edema (>10%), erythema nodosum, exanthems, hemorrhage, Mucha–Habermann disease, photosensitivity, pigmented purpuric eruption, pruritus (1–10%), rash (1–5%), scleroderma (<1%), striae, urticaria, xerosis (<1%)	Bromhidrosis (<1%), vaginitis (1–5%)	Alopecia (1–5%), hirsutism (<1%)	

(Continued)

Drug	Skin	Mucosal/ENT	Hair	Nails
Agents for management of hematologic reactions				
Epoetin Alfa	Acne, angioedema (1–5%), dermatitis, edema (17%), erythroderma, exanthems, lichenoid eruption, photosensitivity, pruritus, rash (1–10%), urticaria		Alopecia, alopecia totalis, hypertrichosis	
Darbepoetin	Edema (21%), pruritus (8%), rash (7%), urticaria			
Filgastrim Sargramostin	Abscess, acne, acral erythema, acute febrile neutrophilic dermatosis, allergic granulomatous angiitis, allergic reactions (19%), diaphoresis, edema, erythema, erythema nodosum, exanthems (5–63%), exfoliative dermatitis (10%), folliculitis, graft versus host reaction, lichenoid eruption, linear IgA dermatosis, lupus erythematosus, neutrophilic eccrine hidradenitis, palmar-plantar pustulosis, pruritus (1–5%), psoriasis, pyoderma gangrenosum, rash (<40%), urticaria, vasculitis	Dysgeusia, mucositis (40%), stomatitis (>10%)	Alopecia (>10%)	
Pegfilgastrim	Acute febrile neutrophilic dermatosis, allergic reactions (<1%), peripheral edema, pyoderma gangrenosum, rash (<1%), urticaria (<1%)	Dysgeusia, mucositis, stomatitis	Alopecia	
Oprelvekin [13]	Peripheral edema (4%), rash (1%)	Tearing (1%)		
Low molecular weight heparin	Allergic reactions (1–10%), angioedema (<1%), baboon syndrome, burning, dermatitis, erythema, erythema nodosum exanthems, fixed eruption, hemorrhage, livedo reticularis, necrosis, peripheral edema, petechiae, pruritus (<1%), purpura (>10%), rash, scleroderma, toxic dermatitis, TEN, ulcerations, urticaria (<1%), vasculitis	Gingivitis (>10%)	Alopecia	Discoloration
Warfarin	Abscess, acral purpura, angioedema (<1%), bullous dermatitis, dermatitis, exanthems, exfoliative dermatitis, hematomas, hemorrhage, livedo reticularis, necrosis (>10%), pruritus (<1%), purple toe syndrome, purplish erythema of the feet and toes (<1%), purpura, rash (<1%), ulcerations, urticaria, vasculitis, vesiculation	Oral ulceration (<1%), tongue hemorrhage	Alopecia (>10%)	

APL, acute promyelocytic leukemia; Ig, immunoglobulin; SJS, Stevens–Johnson syndrome; TEN, toxic epidermal necrolysis.

2 The History of Supportive Oncodermatology

Yevgeniy Balagula[1], Steven T. Rosen[2,3] and Mario E. Lacouture[1]

[1]Dermatology Service, Memorial Sloan-Kettering Cancer Center, New York, NY, USA
[2]Division of Hematology/Oncology, Northwestern University Feinberg School of Medicine, Chicago, IL, USA
[3]Robert H. Lurie Comprehensive Cancer Center of Northwestern University, Chicago, IL, USA

The vast array of anticancer treatment modalities including surgical interventions, radiotherapy, stem cell transplantation, conventional cytotoxic chemotherapy, and novel targeted agents has drastically changed the lives of oncology patients throughout the last century. Nevertheless, this remarkable progress in therapeutics has not been devoid of significant systemic adverse events (AEs) affecting hematopoietic, gastrointestinal, and dermatologic organ systems. While the advent of systemic antibiotics and blood transfusions has reduced the high morbidity associated with bone marrow suppression and an altered immune system, AE affecting the skin and its adnexae have not attracted the same attention, and there has been a relative paucity of effective management strategies.

The major shift in chemotherapeutics in the last decade has been driven by the development of "targeted" agents. Although this has resulted in improved patient survival and a lower incidence of acute nonspecific AE, a wide spectrum of dermatologic toxicities affecting the majority of patients has been recognized. Their significant burden on patients' quality of life (QoL), with impact on consistent administration of anticancer therapy, has heightened the importance of dermatologic health in cancer patients. Subsequent multidisciplinary research efforts have made considerable strides toward elucidating underlying mechanisms, better understanding of impact on QoL, and the development of evidence-based management strategies, leading to the emergence of "supportive oncodermatology" – a discipline dedicated to dermatologic health in cancer patients undergoing therapy, as well as cancer survivors (Figure 2.1).

Evolution of anticancer therapeutics

Evidence of cancer identified in Peruvian and Egyptian mummies dates back to approximately 2500 BC. The early treatment approach consisted of tumor eradication with a hot iron [1]. The Ebers papyrus, 1500 BC, contains descriptions of arsenic paste used against ulcerated tumors [2], and surgical removal of breast carcinomas was performed by Celsus in 30 BC to 38 AD [3]. Besides physical destruction, oral remedies were also used, with Pliny the Elder (AD 23–79) utilizing several compounds (e.g., amygdaline or vitamin B17) [4]. An array of chemicals including mercury, lead, iron, potassium, and iodine were utilized by Paracelsus (1493–1541) to treat a spectrum of internal diseases including cancer [5].

Only 2 months after the discovery of X-rays in November 1895 by William Conrad Röntgen, Emil Grubbe, at the time a Chicago medical student, was allegedly the first to utilize radiation to treat breast cancer [6]. The first successful application of radiotherapy for a dermatologic indication (a giant hairy nevus) was performed by Leopold Freund in 1896 [7]. The term "chemotherapy" was coined by the Nobel laureate Paul Ehrlich (1854–1915), with the era of modern chemotherapy emerging in the 1940s when nitrogen mustard, a nonspecific DNA alkylating agent, was shown to induce regression in lymphoma patients [8,9].

As the list of chemotherapy agents continued to expand, it was realized that combining different agents yielded better results. In 1965, a combination of methotrexate, vinca alkaloid (vincristine), 6-mercaptopurine, and prednisone (POMP) was demonstrated to achieve long-term remissions in children with acute lymphocytic leukemia [10]. The addition of 5-fluorouracil to the arsenal of chemotherapeutics in 1957 was a significant step forward in the treatment of solid malignancies [11]. Driven by discoveries of intricate mechanisms responsible for tumorigenesis, an abundance of chemotherapy agents were synthesized and approved in the latter part of the twentieth century, including alkylating agents (busulfan), plant alkaloids (paclitaxel), antitumor antibiotics (doxorubicin), antimetabolites (capecitabine), and topoisomerase inhibitors (irinotecan).

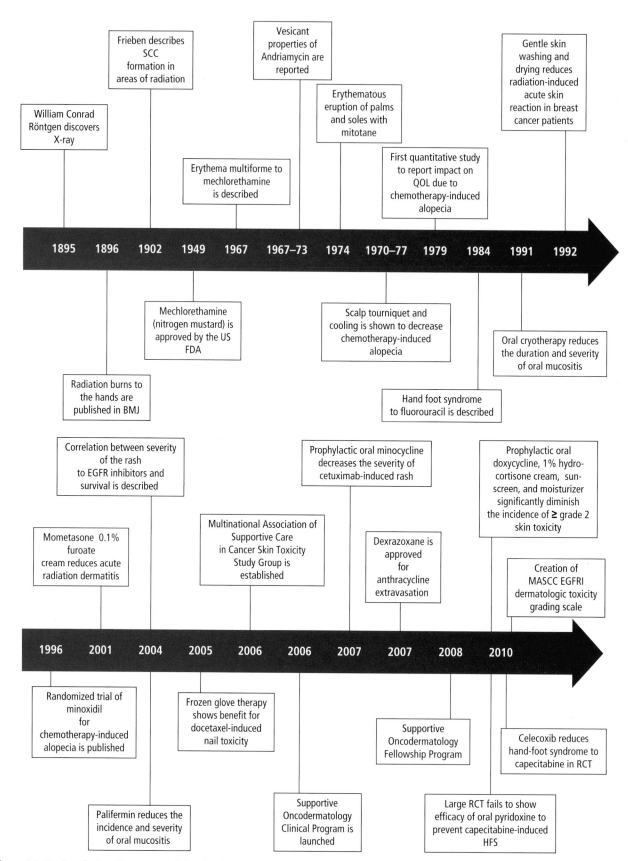

Figure 2.1 Timeline of selected key events and clinical trials in supportive oncodermatology. BMJ, *British Medical Journal*; EGFR, epidermal growth factor receptor; EGFRI, epidermal growth factor receptor inhibitor; FDA, Food and Drug Administration; HFS, hand-foot syndrome; MASCC, Multinational Association of Supportive Care in Cancer; QOL, quality of life; RCT, randomized controlled trial; SCC, squamous cell carcinoma.

The last two decades of the twentieth century were highlighted by the identification and improved understanding of carcinogenic mutations involving cell membrane tyrosine kinase receptors and intracellular signaling pathway enzymes. The ability to inhibit specific molecular targets launched oncology into an era of "targeted therapy." Agents such as rituximab, a chimeric monoclonal IgG1 antibody targeting the B-cell CD20 surface receptor, were at the forefront of therapy for patients with non-Hodgkin lymphoma [12,13]. Subsequently, a wide spectrum of agents inhibiting cell membrane epidermal growth factor receptors (EGFRs), tyrosine kinases of the Raf-Mek-Erk cascade, and other mitogen activated protein kinase (MAPK) signaling pathways have been synthesized [14].

Spectrum of dermatologic adverse events stemming from conventional cytotoxic chemotherapy agents

An early insightful observation was made in the sixteenth century by Paracelsus, who noted: "All things are poison and nothing is without poison, only the dose permits something not to be poisonous" [15]. The rapid evolution of anticancer therapeutics has been paralleled by the concomitant emergence of an expanding spectrum of dermatologic AEs, with at least 50 distinct AEs affecting the skin and its adnexae which have been described in association with more than 30 therapies or agents [16–19].

The hematologic and gastrointestinal AEs associated with nitrogen mustard were evident since its introduction in the 1940s. In contrast, a maculopapular rash has only rarely been reported with this agent [20], and in 1967 the first case report of erythema multiforme was published in the *Archives of Internal Medicine* [21]. In 1974, Zuehlke presented a clinical syndrome as a reaction to mitotane, characterized by an erythematous eruption on the palms and soles [22]. Almost a decade later, a similar presentation was documented in a patient with acute myelogenous leukemia undergoing treatment with a combination of doxorubicin, vincristine, and cytarabine [23]. In 1984, this distinct clinical presentation was also attributed to a protracted infusion of 5-fluorouracil and doxorubicin, now termed palmar-plantar erythrodysesthesia [24]. Liposomal doxorubicin and capecitabine (a prodrug that is enzymatically converted to 5-fluorouracil) have also been identified as triggers of what is currently referred to as hand-foot syndrome (HFS) [25]. The first large randomized double-blind placebo-controlled trial for the prevention of HFS was published in 2010 [26]. However, it failed to demonstrate efficacy of oral pyridoxine in prevention of capecitabine-associated HFS.

Oral mucositis, usually manifesting within the first week of therapy and characterized by erythema, edema, and ulceration of the oropharyngeal mucosa, has been reported to affect 40–70% of patients receiving standard chemotherapy regimens [27], of which 10% are severe (grade 3–4) [28,29]. The incidence of severe mucositis is 30–50% in the setting of high-dose conditioning

chemotherapy in preparation for hematopoietic stem cell transplantation [30]. It is associated with clinically significant sequelae including pain, nutritional deficiencies, weight loss, feeding tube placement, infection, and increases the risk of hospitalization [27,31,32]. In 1991, oral cryotherapy, utilizing ice chips placed in the mouth for 30 minutes during 5-fluorouracil infusion, was shown to be a simple but effective intervention diminishing the severity and duration of oral mucositis [33]. In 2004, a randomized double-blind placebo-controlled phase III trial demonstrated that palifermin, a recombinant human keratinocyte growth factor, significantly reduced the incidence and duration of severe mucositis compared with placebo in recipients of autologous stem cell transplantation undergoing intensive conditioning therapy (63% vs. 98%, p < 0.001) [34]. These results have led to the approval of this intravenous agent for the prevention of mucositis in this patient population. Oral glutamine in a novel proprietary formulation has also been shown to diminish severe oral mucositis significantly in a 2007 randomized trial of patients receiving anthracycline-based chemotherapy (1.2% vs. 6.7%, p = 0.005) [35].

In addition to cutaneous and mucosal surfaces, adnexal structures (e.g., hair, nails) can also be significantly affected by conventional cytotoxic chemotherapy agents. Since the initial description of chemotherapy-induced alopecia (CIA) in the 1950s [36,37], this particular adverse event has remained one of the most significant and prevalent toxicities [38]. Fifty-eight percent of women undergoing alopecia-inducing therapy consider it the most distressing AE and 8% would potentially avoid chemotherapy in anticipation of this toxicity [39]. Multiple agents are known to cause alopecia, including paclitaxel (>80%), doxorubicin (60–100%), cyclophosphamide (>60%), and 5-fluorouracil (10–50%) [40]. The use of cold caps has been attempted in numerous trials, but has not been widely adopted [41,42]. In 1996, a randomized trial of topical 2% minoxidil demonstrated some benefit in reducing the duration of CIA in breast cancer patients [43].

Any component of a nail unit (nail plate, nail bed, and periungual tissues) can be affected by multiple cytotoxic agents with resultant manifestations such as leukonychia, onycholysis, Beaus lines, and paronychia [44,45]. For example, docetaxel commonly results in nail toxicities affecting up to 88% of patients [46]. Additionally, taxanes (paclitaxel and docetaxel) can induce painful subungual hemorrhages that contribute to separation of the nail plate from the nail bed (onycholysis), and subsequent development of a painful subungual abscess, which can cause cessation of therapy [47]. Frozen gloves, worn by patients during docetaxel infusion, have been demonstrated to represent an effective strategy diminishing the incidence (51% vs. 11%, p = 0.0001) and severity of nail toxicity [48].

Necrotizing and irritating properties of certain intravenous chemotherapy agents can cause significant tissue destruction upon their extravasation. Localized pain, edema, necrosis, and ulceration have been reported in association with early agents such as nitrogen mustard (1940s) and doxorubicin (1970s)

[8,49,50]. Significant morbidity from anthracycline-associated soft tissue necrosis prompted investigations that attempted to describe the clinical course, histopathology, and management as early as 1976 [51]. At present, partly because of improved intravascular access, extravasation injuries are observed in up to 6% of patients undergoing intravenous treatments, but nevertheless may have significant clinical sequelae [52]. The first antidote for anthracycline extravasation has been approved by the Food and Drug Adminstration (FDA) in 2007, more than 30 years after the recognition of its necrotizing properties [53]. Dexrazoxane, a topoisomerase II inhibitor and iron chelator, was shown to significantly reduce the incidence of necrosis requiring surgery.

Radiation and surgery-induced mucocutaneous toxicities

Less than a year after the discovery of ionizing radiation, in 1896 radiation-induced burns affecting the hands were reported in the *British Medical Journal* [54]. In 1902, Frieben described a squamous cell carcinoma arising on the dorsal hand of a radiation technician [55], and, after the discovery of radium, experiments in 1900 showed that when in contact with skin, inflammation was induced [56,57]. At present, radiotherapy is a fundamental component of numerous treatment protocols and both acute and chronic mucocutaneous AEs are frequently observed. Acute toxicities range from radiation dermatitis, characterized by erythema, edema, moist desquamations, and ulceration in severe cases, to oropharyngeal mucositis. Severe mucositis can affect up to 56% of patients treated with altered fractionation radiation [32], and acute radiation dermatitis is seen in up to 90% of breast and head and neck cancer patients [58,59]. Although improved patient responses may be obtained through utilization of combination therapies, concomitant administration of epidermal growth factor receptor inhibitors (EGFRIs), or conventional cytotoxic chemotherapy agents with radiation enhances the severity of mucocutaneous toxicities, which has been referred to as "radiation enhancement" [60,61]. Telangiectasias, fat necrosis, skin fibrosis, pigmentary changes, and atrophy represent the changes of chronic radiation dermatitis, which may manifest several years after the initial insult [62,63]. While numerous topical and systemic interventions for prevention and management of acute radiation dermatitis have been investigated, there is currently insufficient clinical evidence to support the use of any specific agent [64]. However, the use of high potency corticosteroids has been demonstrated to be effective in ameliorating the severity of acute skin reactions [64,65].

Radiation and surgical interventions can sever delicate lymphatic channels with subsequent accumulation of interstitial fluids and the development of lymphedema. The cumulative 5-year incidence of lymphedema in breast cancer survivors can reach 42% [66]. The vast majority of breast cancer survivors (80%) develop lymphedema within 2 years of diagnosis, with signs and symptoms that can persist for more than a decade following surgery [67].

Mucocutaneous toxicities induced by novel targeted agents

Following the approval of the tyrosine kinase inhibitor imatinib in 2001, numerous agents have been approved by regulatory agencies, and their AE profiles have emerged. EGFRIs represent one such class of agents. The most characteristic cutaneous toxicity of these agents, which has become known as a class effect, is a papulopustular (acneiform) rash, which affects up 90% of treated patients [68]. Other commonly observed dermatologic toxicities include xerosis, pruritus, nail and hair alterations, paronychia, and mucosal changes [69]. With the introduction of sorafenib and sunitinib, small molecule multikinase inhibitors (MKIs) for treatment of renal cell carcinomas and gastrointestinal stromal tumors, a new entity that clinically mimics HFS has been described. In an attempt to distinguish this from HFS associated with conventional cytotoxic agents, it has been referred to as hand-foot skin reaction (HFSR) [70]. Similar to EGFRIs, MKIs are associated with a wide spectrum of mucocutaneous toxicities including xerosis, pruritus, seborrheic dermatitis-like rash, scalp dysesthesias, alopecia, subungual hemorrhages, and mucosal inflammation [71].

Emergence of supportive oncodermatology and future directions

The remarkable deveopments in cancer therapies have been possible, at least in part, because of improved management of toxicities from cancer treatment. In the late 1950s, the utilization of transfusions has led to a reduction in hemorrhagic complications in leukemic patients [72]. In addition, prompt empiric antibiotic therapy in immunosuppressed patients has resulted in a significant decrease in early mortality from infectious complications [73]. In contrast, mucocutaneous toxicities have not attracted the same level of interest. There has been a relative paucity of research efforts to quantify the impact of dermatologic toxicities on patients' QoL and their management strategies [42].

The spectrum of dermatologic toxicities resulting from an array of novel targeted therapies, which affect the majority of treated patients in cosmetically sensitive areas, and the continued emergence of new mucocutaneous AE, has highlighted the importance of dermatologic health in cancer patients throughout the last decade. As a result, significant progress has been made in our understanding of the underlying mechanisms of certain toxicities and the ability to diminish their severity and quantify their impact on patients' QoL. Since 2007, multiple randomized controlled trials have been conducted investigating the management strategies of EGFRI-induced papulopustular rash and provide evidence-based data supporting the prophylactic use of antibiotics to mitigate the significant impact of this specific toxicity [74–77]. In 2006, a referral center at the Robert H. Lurie Comprehensive Cancer Center and the Department of Dermatology of Northwestern University in Chicago was created through the multidisciplinary effort of dermatologists, oncologists, and ophthalmologists [78]. Specializing in dermatologic health of cancer patients, this SERIES (Skin and Eye Reactions to Inhibitors of EGFR and kinaseS) clinic has set the stage for specialized dermatologic care for cancer patients. Similarly, in the same year, the Multinational Association for Supportive Care in cancer (MASCC) established the Skin Toxicity Study group which serves to motivate continued research efforts and to develop effective management approaches. Only two years following its inception, a comprehensive classification system was created, the MASCC EGFR Inhibitor Skin Toxicity tool, which it is hoped will improve the ability to quantify the impact of EGFRI-associated toxicities in the setting of clinical trials and routine care [79]. Multidisciplinary efforts have also yielded several management guidelines for dermatologic toxicities associated with EGFRIs and MKIs [69,80,81].

This global effort has contributed to the emergence of supportive oncodermatology as a new discipline within dermatology, which specifically addresses dermatologic health in cancer patients and survivors. One of the fundamental principles of oncodermatology is to ensure timely and early intervention to maintain QoL and anticancer therapy dose intensity. Driven by a multidisciplinary approach and improved global awareness of dermatologic health in cancer patients, significant progress has been made in our understanding of mucocutaneous AEs, their impact on patient care, and treatment strategies. However, much remains to be accomplished and future efforts should emphasize the development of accurate classification schemes, further understanding of underlying pathophysiology, management strategies, and identifying potential risk factors, which will assist in selecting the most appropriate patient population for pre-emptive therapy. The field of supportive oncodermatology can facilitate improved awareness of dermatologic toxicities and research efforts, with the mutual goal of maximizing patient QoL and optimizing utilization of potentially life-prolonging anticancer interventions.

References

1 Wright, J.C. (1984) Cancer chemotherapy: past, present, and future: Part I. *Journal of the National Medical Association*, **76**, 773–784.

2 Slaughter, D. (1959) An introduction to cancer and cancer diagnosis. In: J.B. Field (ed), *Cancer-Diagnosis and Treatment*, pp. 1–11. Little, Brown, Boston.

3 Pack, G. & Ariel, I. (1968) *The History of Cancer Therapy. Cancer Management: A Special Graduate Course on Cancer Sponsored by the American Cancer Society. Inc.*, p. 2. J.B. Lippincott, Philadelphia.

4 Moss, R.W. (1999) *The Cancer Industry*, Equinox Press, State College, PA.

5 Robinson, V. (1929) *Pathfinders in Medicine*, Medical Life Press, New York.

6 Grubbe, E.H. (1933) Priority in the therapeutic use of X-rays. *Radiology*, **21**, 156–162.

7 Freund, L. (1897) Ein mit Rontgen-strahlen behandelter Fall von Naevus pigmentosis piliferus. *Wiener Medizinische Wochenschrift*, **10**, 428–433.

8 Goodman, L., Wintrobe, M., Dameshek, W., Goodman, M., Gilman, A. & McLennan, M. (1946) Nitrogen mustard therapy: use of methyl-bis(beta-chloroethyl)amine hydrochloride and tris(beta-chloroethyl) amine hydrochloride for Hodgkin's disease, lymphosarcoma, leukemia and certain allied and miscellaneous disorders. *Journal of the American Medical Association*, **132**, 126–132.

9 Gilman, A. & Philips, F.S. (1946) The biological actions and therapeutic applications of the B-chloroethyl amines and sulfides. *Science*, **103**, 409–436.

10 Frei, E.I. (1965) The effectiveness of combinations of antileukemic agents in inducing and maintaining remission in children with acute leukemia. *Blood*, **26**, 642–656.

11 Heidelberger, C., Chaudhuri, N.K., Danneberg, P. et al. (1957) Fluorinated pyrimidines: a new class of tumour-inhibitory compounds. *Nature*, **179**, 663–666.

12 Todd, P.A. & Brogden, R.N. (1989) Muromonab CD3: a review of its pharmacology and therapeutic potential. *Drugs*, **37**, 871–899.

13 Zhang, Q., Chen, G., Liu, X. & Qian, Q. (2007) Monoclonal antibodies as therapeutic agents in oncology and antibody gene therapy. *Cell Research*, **17**, 89–99.

14 Roberts, P.J. & Der, C.J. (2007) Targeting the Raf-MEK-ERK mitogen-activated protein kinase cascade for the treatment of cancer. *Oncogene*, **26**, 3291–3310.

15 Wolff, J. (1907) *Die Lehre von der Krebskrankheit von den altesten Zeiten bis zur Gegenwart*, G. Fischer, Jena.

16 Heidary, N., Naik, H. & Burgin, S. (2008) Chemotherapeutic agents and the skin: an update. *Journal of the American Academy of Dermatology*, **58**, 545–570.

17 Lacouture, M.E., Laabs, S.M., Koehler, M. et al. (2009) Analysis of dermatologic events in patients with cancer treated with lapatinib. *Breast Cancer Research and Treatment*, **114**, 485–493.

18 Chin, S.N., Trinkaus, M., Simmons, C. et al. (2009) Prevalence and severity of urogenital symptoms in postmenopausal women receiving endocrine therapy for breast cancer. *Clinical Breast Cancer*, **9**, 108–117.

19 Roche. (2004) Vesanoid (tretinoin) package insert. Available at: http://www.accessdata.fda.gov/drugsatfda_docs/label/2004/20438s004lbl.pdf (accessed on 22 March 2013).

20 Goodman, L.S. & Gilman, A. (1960) *The Pharmacological Basis of Therapeutics*, 2nd ed., p. 1423. Macmillan Co, New York.

21 Brauer, M.J., McEvoy, B.F. & Mitus, W.J. (1967) Hypersensitivity to nitrogen mustards in the form of erythema multiforme: a unique adverse reaction. *Archives of Internal Medicine*, **120**, 499–503.

22 Zuehlke, R.L. (1974) Erythematous eruption of the palms and soles associated with mitotane therapy. *Dermatologica*, **148**, 90–92.

23 Burgdorf, W.H., Gilmore, W.A. & Ganick, R.G. (1982) Peculiar acral erythema secondary to high-dose chemotherapy for acute myelogenous leukemia. *Annals of Internal Medicine*, **97**, 61–62.

24 Lokich, J.J. & Moore, C. (1984) Chemotherapy-associated palmar-plantar erythrodysesthesia syndrome. *Annals of Internal Medicine*, **101**, 798–799.

25 Janusch, M., Fischer, M., Marsch, W., Holzhausen, H.J., Kegel, T. & Helmbold, P. (2006) The hand-foot syndrome: a frequent secondary manifestation in antineoplastic chemotherapy. *European Journal of Dermatology*, **16**, 494–499.

26 Kang, Y.K., Lee, S.S., Yoon, D.H. et al. (2010) Pyridoxine is not effective to prevent hand-foot syndrome associated with capecitabine therapy: results of a randomized, double-blind, placebo-controlled study. *Journal of Clinical Oncology*, **28**, 3824–3829.

27 Scully, C., Epstein, J. & Sonis, S. (2003) Oral mucositis: a challenging complication of radiotherapy, chemotherapy, and radiochemotherapy: part 1, pathogenesis and prophylaxis of mucositis. *Head and Neck*, **25**, 1057–1070.

28 Keefe, D.M., Schubert, M.M., Elting, L.S. et al. (2007) Updated clinical practice guidelines for the prevention and treatment of mucositis. *Cancer*, **109**, 820–831.

29 Raber-Durlacher, J.E., Elad, S. & Barasch, A. (2010) Oral mucositis. *Oral Oncology*, **46**, 452–456.

30 Sonis, S.T., Elting, L.S., Keefe, D. et al. (2004) Perspectives on cancer therapy-induced mucosal injury: pathogenesis, measurement, epidemiology, and consequences for patients. *Cancer*, **100**, 1995–2025.

31 Cheng, K.K., Leung, S.F., Liang, R.H., Tai, J.W., Yeung, R.M. & Thompson, D.R. (2009) Severe oral mucositis associated with cancer therapy: impact on oral functional status and quality of life. *Supportive Care in Cancer*, **18**, 1477–1485.

32 Trotti, A., Bellm, L.A., Epstein, J.B. et al. (2003) Mucositis incidence, severity and associated outcomes in patients with head and neck cancer receiving radiotherapy with or without chemotherapy: a systematic literature review. *Radiotherapy and Oncology: Journal of the European Society for Therapeutic Radiology and Oncology*, **66**, 253–262.

33 Mahood, D.J., Dose, A.M., Loprinzi, C.L. et al. (1991) Inhibition of fluorouracil-induced stomatitis by oral cryotherapy. *Journal of Clinical Oncology*, **9**, 449–452.

34 Spielberger, R., Stiff, P., Bensinger, W. et al. (2004) Palifermin for oral mucositis after intensive therapy for hematologic cancers. *New England Journal of Medicine*, **351**, 2590–2598.

35 Peterson, D.E., Jones, J.B. & Petit, R.G. 2nd (2007) Randomized, placebo-controlled trial of Saforis for prevention and treatment of oral mucositis in breast cancer patients receiving anthracycline-based chemotherapy. *Cancer*, **109**, 322–331.

36 Rees, R.B., Bennett, J.H. & Bostick, W.L. (1955) Aminopterin for psoriasis. *A. M. A. Archives of Dermatology*, **72**, 133–143.

37 Bierman, H.R., Kelly, K.H., Knudson, A.G. Jr, Maekawa, T. & Timmis, G.M. (1958) The influence of 1,4-dimethyl sulfonoxy-1,4-dimethylbutane (CB 2348, Dimethyl Myleran) in neoplastic disease. *Annals of the New York Academy of Sciences*, **68**, 1211–1222.

38 Wang, J., Lu, Z. & Au, J.L. (2006) Protection against chemotherapy-induced alopecia. *Pharmaceutical Research*, **23**, 2505–2514.

39 McGarvey, E.L., Baum, L.D., Pinkerton, R.C. & Rogers, L.M. (2001) Psychological sequelae and alopecia among women with cancer. *Cancer Practice*, **9**, 283–289.

40 Trueb, R.M. (2009) Chemotherapy-induced alopecia. *Seminars in Cutaneous Medicine and Surgery*, **28**, 11–14.

41 Mols, F., van den Hurk, C.J., Vingerhoets, A.J. & Breed, W.P. (2009) Scalp cooling to prevent chemotherapy-induced hair loss: practical and clinical considerations. *Supportive Care in Cancer*, **17**, 181–189.

42 Grevelman, E.G. & Breed, W.P. (2005) Prevention of chemotherapy-induced hair loss by scalp cooling. *Annals of Oncology*, **16**, 352–358.

43 Duvic, M., Lemak, N.A., Valero, V. et al. (1996) A randomized trial of minoxidil in chemotherapy-induced alopecia. *Journal of the American Academy of Dermatology*, **35**, 74–78.

44 Payne, A.S., James, W.D. & Weiss, R.B. (2006) Dermatologic toxicity of chemotherapeutic agents. *Seminars in Oncology*, **33**, 86–97.

45 Gilbar, P., Hain, A. & Peereboom, V.M. (2009) Nail toxicity induced by cancer chemotherapy. *Journal of Oncology Pharmacy Practice*, **15**, 143–155.

46 Winther, D., Saunte, D.M., Knap, M., Haahr, V. & Jensen, A.B. (2007) Nail changes due to docetaxel: a neglected side effect and nuisance for the patient. *Supportive Care in Cancer*, **15**, 1191–1197.

47 Minisini, A.M., Tosti, A., Sobrero, A.F. et al. (2003) Taxane-induced nail changes: incidence, clinical presentation and outcome. *Annals of Oncology*, **14**, 333–337.

48 Scotté, F., Tourani, J.M., Banu, E. et al. (2005) Multicenter study of a frozen glove to prevent docetaxel-induced onycholysis and cutaneous toxicity of the hand. *Journal of Clinical Oncology*, **23**, 4424–4429.

49 Wang, J.J., Cortes, E., Sinks, L.F. & Holland, J.F. (1971) Therapeutic effect and toxicity of adriamycin in patients with neoplastic disease. *Cancer*, **28**, 837–843.

50 Tan, C., Etcubanas, E., Wollner, N. et al. (1973) Adriamycin: an antitumor antibiotic in the treatment of neoplastic diseases. *Cancer*, **32**, 9–17.

51 Rudolph, R., Stein, R.S. & Pattillo, R.A. (1976) Skin ulcers due to adriamycin. *Cancer*, **38**, 1087–1094.

52 Apisarnthanarax, N. & Duvic, M. (2000) Dermatologic complications of cancer chemotherapy. In: R.C. Bast, D.W. Kufe, R.E. Pollock, R.R. Weichselbaum, J.F. Holland & E. Frei (eds), *Cancer Medicine*, 5th ed., Chapter 144. Decker, Hamilton, ON.

53 Mouridsen, H.T., Langer, S.W., Buter, J. et al. (2007) Treatment of anthracycline extravasation with Savene (dexrazoxane): results from two prospective clinical multicentre studies. *Annals of Oncology*, **18**, 546–550.

54 Stevens, L. (1896) Injurious effects on the skin. *British Medical Journal*, **1**, 998.

55 Frieben, H. (1902) Demonstration eines Cancroid des rechten Handruckens, das sich nach langdauernder Einwirkung von Rontgenstrahlen entwickelt hatte. *Fortschritte auf dem Gebiete der Röntgenstrahlen und der Nuklearmedizin*, **6**, 106–111.

56 Walkoff, F. (1900) Unsichtbare, photographisch wirksame Strahlen. *Photographische Rundschau*, **14**, 189–191.

57 Giesel, F. (1900) Ueber radioactive Stoffe. *Berichte der Deutschen Chemischen Gesellschaft*, **33**, 3569–3571.

58 Harper, J.L., Franklin, L.E., Jenrette, J.M. & Aguero, E.G. (2004) Skin toxicity during breast irradiation: pathophysiology and management. *Southern Medical Journal*, **97**, 989–993.

59 Bernier, J., Bonner, J., Vermorken, J.B. et al. (2008) Consensus guidelines for the management of radiation dermatitis and coexisting acne-like rash in patients receiving radiotherapy plus EGFR inhibitors for the treatment of squamous cell carcinoma of the head and neck. *Annals of Oncology*, **19**, 142–149.

60 Guillot, B., Bessis, D. & Dereure, O. (2004) Mucocutaneous side effects of antineoplastic chemotherapy. *Expert Opinion on Drug Safety*, **3**, 579–587.

61 Tejwani, A., Wu, S., Jia, Y., Agulnik, M., Millender, L. & Lacouture, M.E. (2009) Increased risk of high-grade dermatologic toxicities with radiation plus epidermal growth factor receptor inhibitor therapy. *Cancer*, **115**, 1286–1299.

62 Meric, F., Buchholz, T.A., Mirza, N.Q. et al. (2002) Long-term complications associated with breast-conservation surgery and radiotherapy. *Annals of Surgical Oncology*, **9**, 543–549.

63 Hymes, S.R., Strom, E.A. & Fife, C. (2006) Radiation dermatitis: clinical presentation, pathophysiology, and treatment 2006. *Journal of the American Academy of Dermatology*, **54**, 28–46.

64 Salvo, N., Barnes, E., van Draanen, J. et al. (2010) Prophylaxis and management of acute radiation-induced skin reactions: a systematic review of the literature. *Current Oncology*, **17**, 94–112.

65 Miller, R.C., Schwartz, D.J., Sloan, J.A. et al. (2011) Mometasone furoate effect on acute skin toxicity in breast cancer patients receiving radiotherapy: a phase III double-blind, randomized trial from the North Central Cancer Treatment Group N06C4. *International Journal of Radiation Oncology, Biology, Physics*, **79**, 1460–1466.

66 Norman, S.A., Localio, A.R., Potashnik, S.L. et al. (2009) Lymphedema in breast cancer survivors: incidence, degree, time course, treatment, and symptoms. *Journal of Clinical Oncology*, **27**, 390–397.

67 Oliveri, J.M., Day, J.M., Alfano, C.M. et al. (2008) Arm/hand swelling and perceived functioning among breast cancer survivors 12 years post-diagnosis: CALGB 79804. *Journal of Cancer Survivorship*, **2**, 233–242.

68 Perez-Soler, R., Delord, J.P., Halpern, A. et al. (2005) HER1/EGFR inhibitor-associated rash: future directions for management and investigation outcomes from the HER1/EGFR inhibitor rash management forum. *The Oncologist*, **10**, 345–356.

69 Burtness, B., Anadkat, M., Basti, S. et al. (2009) NCCN task force report: management of dermatologic and other toxicities associated with EGFR inhibition in patients with cancer. *Journal of the National Comprehensive Cancer Network*, **7** (Suppl. 1), S5–S21; quiz S2–4.

70 Yang, C.H., Lin, W.C., Chuang, C.K. et al. (2008) Hand-foot skin reaction in patients treated with sorafenib: a clinicopathological study of cutaneous manifestations due to multitargeted kinase inhibitor therapy. *British Journal of Dermatology*, **158**, 592–596.

71 Lacouture, M.E., Reilly, L.M., Gerami, P. & Guitart, J. (2008) Hand foot skin reaction in cancer patients treated with the multikinase inhibitors sorafenib and sunitinib. *Annals of Oncology*, **19**, 1955–1961.

72 Freireich, E.J., Schmidt, P.J., Schneiderman, M.A. & Frei, E. 3rd. (1959) A comparative study of the effect of transfusion of fresh and preserved whole blood on bleeding in patients with acute leukemia. *New England Journal of Medicine*, **260**, 6–11.

73 Pizzo, P.A. (1984) Granulocytopenia and cancer therapy:past problems, current solutions, future challenges. *Cancer*, **54**, 2649–2661.

74 Scope, A., Agero, A.L., Dusza, S.W. et al. (2007) Randomized double-blind trial of prophylactic oral minocycline and topical tazarotene for cetuximab-associated acne-like eruption. *Journal of Clinical Oncology*, **25**, 5390–5396.

75 Jatoi, A., Rowland, K., Sloan, J.A. et al. (2008) Tetracycline to prevent epidermal growth factor receptor inhibitor-induced skin rashes: results of a placebo-controlled trial from the North Central Cancer Treatment Group (N03CB). *Cancer*, **113**, 847–853.

76 Jatoi, A., Green, E.M., Rowland, K.M. Jr, Sargent, D.J. & Alberts, S.R. (2009) Clinical predictors of severe cetuximab-induced rash: observations from 933 patients enrolled in north central cancer treatment group study N0147. *Oncology*, **77**, 120–123.

77 Lacouture, M.E., Mitchell, E.P., Piperdi, B. et al. (2010) Skin toxicity evaluation protocol with panitumumab (STEPP): a phase II, open-label, randomized trial evaluating the impact of a pre-emptive skin treatment regimen on skin toxicities and quality of life in patients with metastatic colorectal cancer. *Journal of Clinical Oncology*, **28**, 1351–1357.

78 Lacouture, M.E., Basti, S., Patel, J. & Benson, A. 3rd (2006) The SERIES clinic: an interdisciplinary approach to the management of toxicities of EGFR inhibitors. *Journal of Supportive Oncology*, **4**, 236–238.

79 Lacouture, M.E., Maitland, M.L., Segaert, S. et al. (2010) A proposed EGFR inhibitor dermatologic adverse event-specific grading scale from the MASCC skin toxicity study group. *Supportive Care in Cancer*, **18**, 509–522.

80 Lacouture, M.E., Wu, S., Robert, C. et al. (2008) Evolving strategies for the management of hand-foot skin reaction associated with the multitargeted kinase inhibitors sorafenib and sunitinib. *The Oncologist*, **13**, 1001–1011.

81 Melosky, B., Burkes, R., Rayson, D., Alcindor, T., Shear, N. & Lacouture, M. (2009) Management of skin rash during EGFR-targeted monoclonal antibody treatment for gastrointestinal malignancies: Canadian recommendations. *Current Oncology*, **16**, 16–26.

3 Structure and Function of the Integumentary System and the Dermatology Lexicon

Emmy Graber[1] and Amit Garg[2]

[1]Boston University School of Medicine, Boston, MA, USA
[2]Hofstra School of Medicine North Shore-LIJ Health System, New York, USA

Introduction

The integument, comprised of three layers of skin and its appendages, represents the largest organ of the body (Figure 3.1). In its most basic of functions, the integument serves to protect the body from the external environment and to maintain an internal homeostasis of temperature, fluid, and nutrients. The ability to diagnose and treat skin disease in oncology patients may be enhanced by the clinician's understanding of the structure and function of the integumentary system and by an appreciation of the primary and sequential lesions that arise as a result of aberrances of its components. Certain conditions have a predilection for the palms and soles rather than other locations on the body. The skin on the palms and soles is thicker than on other areas, lacks sebaceous glands, but is copious in eccrine (sweat) glands. There are no hair follicles on the palms and soles. However, cutaneous nerves abound in these areas. In this chapter, we introduce the essential components of the integument and describe the dermatology lexicon of morphologic terms.

Skin

Epidermis

The epidermis is a continually renewing structure made up primarily of ectodermally derived keratinocytes and organized into four layers: the stratum germinativum, stratum spinosum, stratum granulosum, and the stratum corneum. Its thickness varies depending on location, being thinnest on the eyelids (0.05 mm) and thickest on the palms and soles (1.5 mm). Mitotically active basal layer keratinocytes attached to the basement membrane differentiate upward until reaching a terminally differentiated stage in which they are called corneocytes. These anucleate corneocytes comprise the keratinized stratum corneum, the lipid (ceramide) and protein (loricrin) rich surface barrier of the skin. The epidermal barrier regulates desquamation, permeation of water and environmental solubles, activity of antimicrobial peptides, and initiation of cytokine-mediated inflammation, among other critical functions. Keratinocytes throughout the epidermis are tightly intercalated through calcium-dependent cell surface adhesion molecules known as desmosomes.

Immigrant cells of the epidermis include melanocytes, Langerhans cells and Merkel cells. Melanocytes are neural crest-derived dendritic cells largely residing in the basal layer of the epidermis. These cells synthesize pigment and are primarily responsible for imparting color to the skin. Langerhans cells are the marrow derived dendritic antigen presenting cells of the epidermis whose cytoplasm contains characteristic racket-shaped structures known as Birbeck granules. Tumor antigens presented by Langerhans cells mount a tumor-specific immune response and, as such, these cells have been evaluated as vehicles of antitumor and vaccine therapies. Merkel cells are slow-adapting type I mechanoreceptors located in sites of high tactile sensitivity, including the lips, oral cavity, digits, and around hair follicles. Merkel cell carcinoma has been a focus of attention in dermatology and oncology given its aggressive and recalcitrant nature.

Dermal–epidermal junction

The dermal–epidermal junction, also known as the basement membrane zone, is the interface between the epidermis and the uppermost portion of the dermis. This junction contains interconnecting layers of proteins (hemidesmosomes, basal lamina, lamina densa, anchoring fibrils) that secure the epidermis to the dermis and form a semipermeable barrier. Blistering

Dermatologic Principles and Practice in Oncology: Conditions of the Skin, Hair, and Nails in Cancer Patients, First Edition. Edited by Mario E. Lacouture.
© 2014 John Wiley & Sons, Inc. Published 2014 by John Wiley & Sons, Inc.

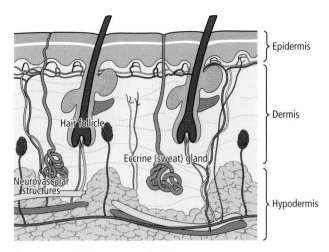

Figure 3.1 Basic skin anatomy and cellular structures.

diseases, some of which are induced by medications, are caused by antibody mediated disruptions to basement membrane zone proteins resulting in clefts separating the epidermis and dermis.

Dermis

The dermis provides pliability, elasticity, and tensile strength to the skin, with a thickness ranging from 0.3 mm on the eyelid and 3.0 mm on the back. It is organized into two portions:
1. The upper papillary dermis, which hugs the epidermis and is made up of loosely arranged collagen fibers; and
2. The reticular dermis, which makes up almost the entire thickness of the dermis.
The connective tissue matrix of the reticular dermis is composed of interwoven bundles of densely packed helical collagen fibrils surrounded by elastic fibers. Type I collagen makes up 80–90% of dermal collagen. The matrix also contains glycoproteins, proteoglycans, and glycosaminoglycans that form the water binding ground substance of the dermis. Vascular and nerve networks as well as appendages are also housed in the dermis.

The predominant cell types within the dermis include fibroblasts, macrophages, mast cells, and circulating cells of the immune system. Mesenchymally derived fibroblasts synthesize and degrade connective tissue matrix proteins which provide the structural framework for the dermis. Bone marrow derived macrophages differentiate into circulating monocytes and migrate to the dermis before differentiating further in tissue. Macrophages in the skin serve a number of important functions including antigen processing and presentation, phagocytosis, and wound healing. Mast cells are integral to the initiation of immediate-type hypersensitivity reactions in the skin (e.g., urticaria). Preformed histamine, which is initially confined to secretory granules within mast cells, is the major mediator of these reactions, although tryptase, chymase, carboxypeptidase, and other mast cell mediators are frequently involved.

Vasculature

Oxygen and nutrition delivery, temperature and blood pressure regulation, wound repair, and immunologic progression represent just some of the roles of the cutaneous vasculature. There are two main horizontal plexuses of vessels that run through the upper and lower portions of the dermis. The vasculature tree in the skin advances from arterioles to precapillary sphincters to arterial and venous capillaries which become postcapillary venules, and ultimately venules. Cutaneous vessels of various sizes can be affected by inflammatory diseases (e.g., leukocytoclastic vasculitis, urticaria) or by bland occlusive vasculopathies (e.g., antiphospholipid antibody syndrome).

Lymph channels of the skin regulate interstitial pressure through resorption of released fluids and debris from vessels and tissue. Lymphatics begin as blind endings in the papillary dermis and drain into a horizontal plexus of lymph vessels that run below the papillary dermal venous plexus. Lymph flows vertically downward through the dermis to a deeper collecting plexus located at the base of the dermis. Cancer patients are susceptible to pathologic conditions involving the lymphatic vessels, including lymphedema and lymphangitis. Additionally, the importance of lymphatics in the progression and spread of cancer is now well documented.

Nerves

The skin contains a network of sensory and sympathetic autonomic fibers which regulate a number of critical functions in the skin. Cutaneous nerves arise segmentally from spinal nerves and follow a pattern in the skin similar to the vasculature. Pencillate sensory fibers and specialized corpuscular structures function as the receptors of touch, pain, temperature, and itch. The type and density of these receptors vary, and this accounts for the differences in sensation and acuity across body sites.

After primary infection with the varicella zoster virus, the virus migrates along sensory nerve fibers to the satellite cells of dorsal root ganglia and becomes dormant. The virus may become reactivated by conditions of decreased cellular immunity and result in herpes zoster, a dermatomal eruption of grouped vesicles on an erythematous base.

Subcutaneous tissue

Beneath the dermis lies a layer of subcutaneous adipose tissue, also known as the panniculus, which is subject to a number of inflammatory and neoplastic disorders. The subcutaneous tissue insulates and cushions the body and serves as one of its energy reserves. It is federated with the dermis through networks of vessels, nerves, and appendages. Synthesis and storage of fat result from accumulation of lipid within adipocytes and from proliferation of existing adipocytes. Regulatory feedback signaling in this process is mediated by leptin, a hormone secreted by adipocytes. Adipocytes are organized into lobules separated by septa of fibrous connective tissue containing vessels, lymphatics, and inflammatory cells.

Appendages

Eccrine sweat glands

Eccrine sweating represents a physiologic response to increased body temperature. There are 2–4 million eccrine glands, capable of producing up to 10 L of sweat per day distributed over almost the entire body surface. They are most numerous on the forehead, axillae, palms, and soles. The eccrine sweat gland is made up of a secretory coil and a duct. Clear (secretory), dark (mucoid), and myoepithelial cells comprise the secretory coil to generate an ultrafiltrate of an isotonic precursor fluid in response to cholinergic stimulation. The duct reabsorbs sodium and chloride to produce hypotonic sweat which is secreted on the surface of the skin.

Apocrine sweat glands

The physiologic role of apocrine sweat glands in humans is unclear. These glands are found in the axillae, perineum, and areolae, and begin to secrete a milky odorless fluid around the time of puberty. Though sweat secreted by apocrine glands is odorless, it emits odor when acted upon by bacteria upon reaching the surface of the skin. Apocrine glands have a coiled structure located at the border of the deep dermis and the subcutaneous fat. This coiled structure extends upward into a straight tubular structure that drains into the mid-portion of the hair follicle and shares a common secretory opening to the surface with sebaceous glands.

Sebaceous glands

Sebaceous glands are composed of lobules of lipid-producing sebocytes lining sebaceous ducts associated with hair follicles throughout the body. A sebaceous gland and the associated hair follicle are termed a pilosebaceous unit. Nonhair-bearing sites including the mouth (Fordyce spots), the eyelids (meibomian glands), the nipples (Montgomery glands), and the genitals (Tyson glands) also have sebaceous glands. The greatest density of these glands is noted on the face and scalp. Only the palms and soles, which also have no hair follicles, are completely devoid of sebaceous glands.

Sebaceous glands release lipids through holocrine secretion, a process in which the entire cell disintegrates to extrude its contents. Human sebum reaching the surface of the skin consists of a mixture of lipids including cholesterol, squalene, triglycerides, and free fatty acids. Sebum is speculated to maintain hydration of the skin's surface, to keep the skin soft, and to protect it from infection by bacteria and fungi, perhaps because of its immunoglobulin A content.

Hair

Hair in humans has cosmetic and social significance, and this accounts for the considerable psychologic impact among patients suffering from hair loss (alopecia).

The hair follicle is divided into the infundibulum and the isthmus which comprise the upper portion of the follicle, as well as the suprabulbar area and the bulb which make up the lower follicle. While the upper follicle is permanent, the lower follicle regenerates with each follicular cycle. Rapidly dividing keratinocytes in the bulb's matrix form the hair shaft. Also residing within the matrix are melanocytes which produce pigment that forms the basis of hair color. The cuticle of the hair shaft covers and protects the hair once it exits the shaft.

Hair follicles perpetually cycle through three phases: anagen (growth), catagen (involution), and telogen (rest). On the scalp, about 90% of the approximately 100,000 follicles are in anagen and the rest primarily in telogen. Hairs are in the anagen phase for about 3 years, the catagen phase for a few days, and the telogen phase for about 3 months. Approximately 1% of telogen hairs (100–150 hairs) are normally shed from the scalp daily. Scalp hairs in anagen grow at a rate of 0.37–0.44 mm/day or approximately 1 cm/month. Chemotherapeutics represent the most common causes of anagen effluvium. As most hair follicles are in the anagen stage at any given time, anagen effluvium affects the majority of scalp hair.

Hair is further classified according to size. Terminal hairs are at least 60 μm in diameter and are found on the scalp, eyebrows, and eyelashes at birth. The length of the terminal hair is determined by the duration of the anagen growth phase. Vellus hairs are less than 30 μm in diameter and typically do not achieve a length greater than 2 cm. These hairs are found throughout the body and become terminal hairs in the beard area, trunk, axillae, and genitalia under the influence of male sex hormones at puberty.

The bottom of the hair root is known as the hair matrix. The hair matrix cells divide and move up the follicle, differentiating into either hair cells or inner epithelial sheath cells (hair lining). Interspersed amongst matrix stem cells are melanocytes, which produce hair pigment. The pigment is synthesized from the amino acid tyrosine (catalyzed by the enzyme phenol-oxidase) and transformed to dopa and then to dopaquinone. Further transformation of dopaquinone proceeds in two directions: either directly to indolquinone or through the addition of the amino acid cysteine. Further polymerization of indolquinone alone produces the dark pigment, eumelanin. Polymerization of indolquinone and dopaquinone with an added cysteine produces the yellow pigment, pheomelanin. Hair matrix cells phagocytose eumelanin or pheomelanin from dendritic elongations of melanocytes. This is how hair assumes its color: black if eumelanin is dominant, and yellow or red if pheomelanin is the major pigment.

Nails

In addition to serving an aesthetic purpose, nails enhance tactile senses and the biomechanics of fingers and toes. Nails can be affected in a number of disease states or responses to therapy, and a basic appreciation for the structure and function of nails may aid the clinician in detecting abnormal physiologic states.

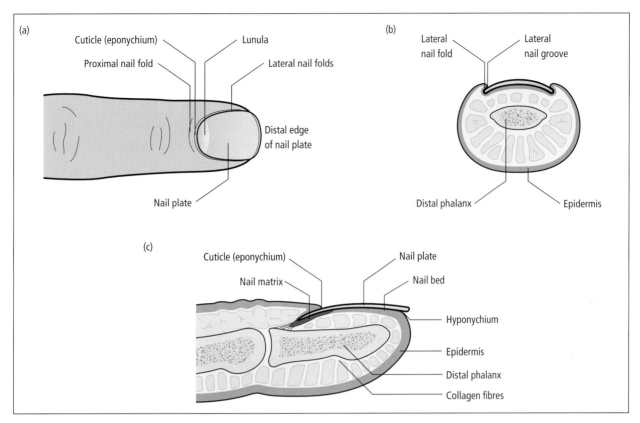

Figure 3.2 Basic nail anatomy; (a) dorsal view (b) cross-section (c) sagittal view.

The nail apparatus consists of the nail plate, proximal nail fold, nail matrix, nail bed, and the hyponychium (Figure 3.2). The nail plate is a keratinized structure attached to the nail bed and surrounded by the nail folds. The proximal nail fold forms the cuticle which firmly attaches to the proximal portion of the nail plate. The lunula, the whitish colored half-moon-shaped area on the proximal part of fingernails, represents the visible portion of the nail matrix, the structure in which keratins comprising the dorsal portion of the nail plate are synthesized. The nail bed, which contributes to formation of the ventral nail plate, extends distally from the lunula. The distal nail plate separates from the underlying skin at the hyponychium.

The nail plate grows throughout life. The total regeneration time for fingernails and toenails is approximately 6 and 12 months, respectively. Given the slow nail growth rate, diseases of the nail matrix may only become evident months after onset. For the same reason, the nail plate requires a similar amount of time to appear normal after disease remission or with treatment. Systemic illness, malnutrition, and treatment with antimitotic drugs are common medical reasons associated with slowed nail plate growth rate.

Morphology

The first step in formulating a relevant differential diagnosis involves understanding and using a standard terminology in describing lesions and eruptions. For example, once an eruption has been described as red to plum-colored edematous plaques on the forearms in a patient with acute myelogenous leukemia, the experienced physician puts Sweet syndrome at the top of the differential diagnosis.

The process of examining and describing skin lesions may be likened to that of viewing a painting. First, one takes in the whole "canvas," viewing the patient from a few feet away and appreciating the distribution and arrangement of an eruption. Then, one looks more closely at the "mountains" making up the landscape, specifying precise primary morphology and color. Finally, one examines the details of the "canvas," taking in the texture and brush strokes, assessing for the presence and quality of scale, for example.

Raised lesions

Papule

A papule is a solid elevated lesion less than 0.5 cm in size in which a significant portion projects above the plane of the surrounding skin. Papules can be further described as: sessile, pedunculated, dome-shaped, flat-topped, rough, smooth, filiform, mammillated, or umbilicated (Figure 3.3, Figure 3.4, and Figure 3.5).

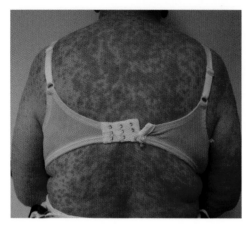

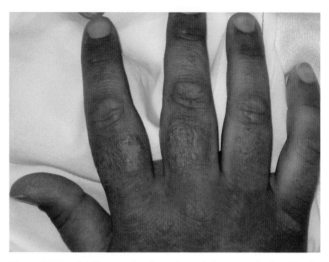

Figure 3.3 Blanchable pink erythematous macules, papules, and plaques coalescing most prominently over the trunk. A morbilliform drug reaction to a penicillin antibiotic.

Figure 3.5 Purplish flat-topped scaly papules and plaques on the dorsal hands. Chronic graft versus host disease.

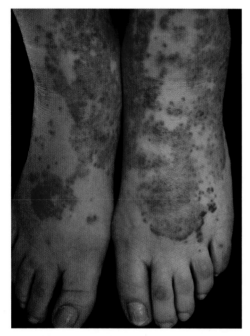

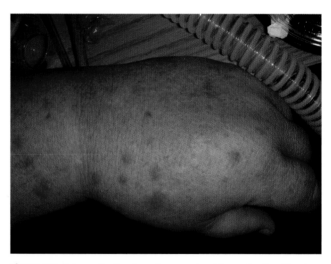

Figure 3.4 Palpable purpuric papules and plaques on the dorsal feet, ankles, and lower extremities. Leukocytoclastic vasculitis secondary to co-trimoxazole in a cancer patient.

Figure 3.6 Red–purple edematous plaques and nodules on the dorsal hands. Acute febrile neutrophilic dermatosis (Sweet syndrome) in a cancer patient. Photograph © Amit Garg.

Plaque

A plaque is a plateau-like elevation that has a greater width than height. By definition, plaques have a diameter larger than 0.5 cm. Plaques may be characterized further by their size, shape, color, and surface change (Figure 3.3, Figure 3.4, Figure 3.5, Figure 3.6, Figure 3.7, and Figure 3.8).

Nodule

A nodule is a solid palpable lesion that has a diameter larger than 0.5 cm (Figure 3.8 and Figure 3.9). Depth, rather than diameter,

differentiates a nodule from a large papule or plaque. Depending on their anatomic level in the skin, nodules are of five types:
1. Epidermal
2. Epidermal–dermal
3. Dermal,
4. Dermal–subdermal, and
5. Subcutaneous.

Features of a nodule that may help reveal a diagnosis include whether it is warm, hard, soft, fluctuant, movable, fixed, or painful. Similarly, different surfaces of nodules, such as smooth, keratotic,

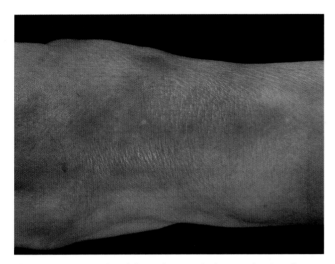

Figure 3.7 A sclerotic bound down plaque on the forearm. Chronic graft versus host disease. Photograph © Amit Garg.

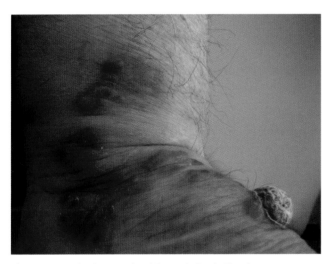

Figure 3.8 Purple plaques and nodules on the hands. Kaposi sarcoma. Photograph © Amit Garg.

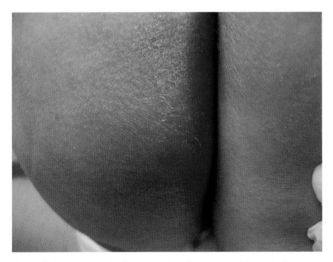

Figure 3.9 A warm tender fluctuant red erythematous nodule on the buttock. An abscess in a patient receiving chemotherapy.

ulcerated, or fungating, also help direct diagnostic considerations. The term "tumor" is sometimes also included under the heading of a nodule and is a general term for any mass, benign or malignant.

Cyst

A cyst is an encapsulated cavity or sac lined with a true epithelium that contains fluid or semisolid material. Depending on the nature of the contents, cysts may be hard, doughy, or fluctuant.

Wheal

A wheal is a swelling of the skin that is evanescent, disappearing within 24 hours. These lesions, also commonly known as hives, are the result of edema produced by the escape of plasma through vessel walls in the dermis. Wheals may be tiny papules or giant plaques, and they may take various shapes (round, oval, serpiginous, or annular), often in the same patient. Borders of a wheal are well demarcated.

Angioedema is another type of edematous reaction but is deeper and firmer than wheals. It is most prominent in areas with very loose dermis and subcutaneous tissue such as the lip, eyelid, or scrotum.

Depressed lesions

Erosion

An erosion results from loss of the epidermal or mucosal epithelium. It appears as a raw, moist, circumscribed, slightly depressed lesion. Erosions may result from trauma, detachment of epidermal layers, rupture of vesicles or bullae, or epidermal necrosis. Unless they become secondarily infected, erosions do not scar.

Ulcer

An ulcer is a defect in which the epidermis and at least the upper portion of the dermis has been destroyed (Figure 3.10 and Figure

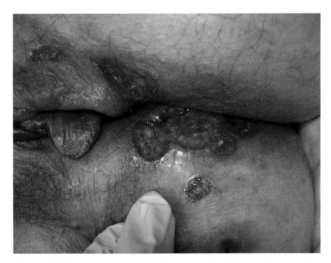

Figure 3.10 Red erythematous ulcers forming scalloped borders (demonstrating grouping) in the perineum. Herpes simplex virus infection in an immunocompromised cancer patient.

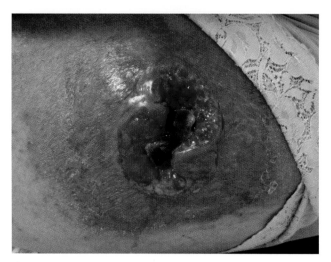

Figure 3.11 Red erythematous ulcerated nodule or tumor with greenish exudates. Cutaneous T-cell lymphoma, with superimposed *Pseudomonas* infection. Photograph © Amit Garg.

3.11). Breach of the dermis and destruction of adnexal structures impede healing and result in formation of a scar. Borders of an ulcer may be rolled, undermined, punched out, jagged, or angular. The base of an ulcer may be clean, ragged, or necrotic. Discharge may be purulent, granular, or malodorous. Surrounding skin may be red, purple, pigmented, reticulated, indurated, sclerotic, or infarcted.

Atrophy

Atrophy refers to the dwindling of the skin. An atrophic epidermis is glossy, translucent, and wrinkled. Atrophy of the dermis or subcutis results in depression of the skin.

Poikiloderma

As a morphologic term, poikiloderma refers to the combination of atrophy, telangiectasia, and varied pigmentary changes (hyper- and hypo-) over an area of skin. This combination of features imparts a dappled appearance to the skin.

Flat lesions

Macule

A macule is flat and perceptible only as an area of color different from the surrounding skin (Figure 3.3). It is 0.5 cm or less.

Patch

A patch is similar to a macule; it is a flat area of skin or mucous membranes with a different color from its surrounding skin. A patch is larger than 0.5 cm, and also differs from a macule by having surface change such as fine scale.

Sclerosis

Sclerosis refers to a circumscribed or diffuse hardening of the skin that results from dermal fibrosis. It is detected more easily by palpation, on which the skin may feel board-like and bound down.

Erythema

Erythema represents the blanchable pink–red color of skin or mucous membrane due to dilatation of arteries and veins in the dermis. It exists in different colors, which should be specified precisely. Describing erythema with the color it most closely resembles provides a meaningful clue to diagnosis. Plum-colored erythema, for example, may direct the clinical towards a diagnosis of Sweet syndrome in the cancer patient. "Beefy" red erythema and pustules suggests a diagnosis of cutaneous candidiasis in the immunosuppressed individual. Purplish erythema of flat-topped papules and plaques may suggest chronic graft versus host reaction in the appropriate context.

Erythroderma

Erythroderma is a generalized deep redness of the skin involving more than 90% of the body surface. The type of scaling or desquamation, which follows establishment of the generalized erythema, provides a clue to the primary process. Generalized exfoliation after erythema subsides is often noted after a medication reaction.

Fluid-filled lesions

Vesicle and bulla

Vesicles and bullae arise from cleavage at various levels of the epidermis (intraepidermal) or of the dermal–epidermal interface (subepidermal). A vesicle is a fluid-filled cavity smaller than or equal to 0.5 cm, whereas a bulla (blister) is larger than 0.5 cm. Bullae are further characterized as tense or flaccid. Clear, serous, hemorrhagic, or pus-filled contents may be visualized when the cavity wall is thin and translucent enough.

Pustule

A pustule is a circumscribed raised cavity in the epidermis or infundibulum containing pus. The purulent exudate, composed of leukocytes with or without cellular debris, may contain bacteria or be sterile. The exudate may be white, yellow, or greenish-yellow in color, the latter two more suggestive of an infectious etiology (Figure 3.12).

Furuncle

A furuncle is a deep necrotizing folliculitis with suppuration. It presents as an inflamed follicle-centered nodule with a central pustule or necrotic plug. Several furuncles may coalesce to form a carbuncle.

Abscess

An abscess is a localized accumulation of purulent material so deep in the dermis or subcutaneous tissue that the pus is usually

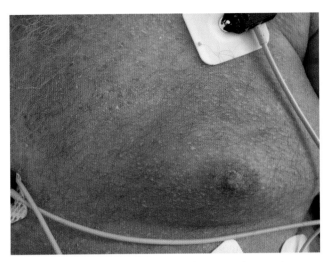

Figure 3.12 Numerous scattered pustules overlying an erythematous base distributed diffusely over the trunk. Acute generalized exanthematous pustulosis secondary to a cephalosporin antibiotic is the diagnosis.

not visible on the surface of the skin. An abscess is a pink erythematous warm tender fluctuant nodule.

Surface changes

Scale

A scale is a flat plate or flake arising from the outermost layer of the epidermis (Figure 3.5). When epidermal differentiation is disordered, casting of stratum corneum becomes apparent as scale. Not all scales are similar, and a clinician with a well-trained eye can obtain diagnostically useful information from the type of scale present. For example, scales split off from the epidermis in finer scales or in sheets may suggest a drug reaction in the appropriate clinical context. Lacy white scale overlying flat-topped violaceous papules and plaques may suggest a lichenoid reaction such as occurs in chronic graft versus host disease.

Crust

Crusts are hardened deposits that result when serum, blood, or purulent exudate dries on the surface of the skin. The color of crust is a yellow–brown when formed from dried serous secretion; turbid yellowish-green when formed from purulent secretion, usually suggestive of infection; and reddish-black when formed from hemorrhagic secretion.

Eschar

The presence of an eschar implies tissue necrosis, gangrene, or other ulcerating process. It is an adherent hard black crust on the surface of the skin.

Purpura and vascular lesions

Purpura

Extravasation of red blood from cutaneous vessels into skin or mucous membranes results in reddish-purple lesions included under the term purpura. Purpura is nonblanching under the pressure of two glass slides, unlike erythema caused by vascular dilatation (Figure 3.4).

Petechiae are small pinpoint purpuric macules. Ecchymoses are larger, bruise-like purpuric patches. These lesions correspond to a noninflammatory extravasation of blood. A lesion that is purpuric and palpable ("palpable purpura") suggests the presence of an inflammatory insult to the vessel walls (e.g., leukocytoclastic vasculitis) as a cause of extravasation of blood.

Infarct

An infarct is an area of cutaneous necrosis resulting from occlusion of blood vessels in the skin. A cutaneous infarct presents as a dusky red plaque which becomes grey to black in color.

Shape, configuration, arrangement, and distribution of lesions

The shape, arrangement, and pattern of distribution of lesions are important morphologic characteristics that aid in diagnosis. For example, a few tense blisters on the trunk may elicit a broad differential diagnosis, but the same blisters on the palms and soles of the feet might suggest a reaction to chemotherapy in the appropriate clinical context.

Target A target lesion has at least three distinct zones of color.

Annular A lesion that is annular has an edge that differs from the center, for example by being raised, scaly, or of a different color.

Polycyclic A polycyclic eruption forms from coalescence of annular or arcuate (incompletely annular) lesions.

Reticular A reticular pattern appears net-like or lacy, comprised of regularly spaced rings or partial rings that spare intervening skin.

Linear A linear arrangement resembles a straight line.

Scattered Scattered lesions are irregularly distributed.

Herpetiform Herpetiform lesions are clustered together.

Dermatomal Lesions in a dermatomal distribution are unilateral and lie in the distribution of a single spinal afferent nerve root.

Lymphangitic A lymphangitic distribution spreads along the distribution of a lymph vessel.

Photo exposed A photo (sun) exposed distribution predominantly involves areas not covered by clothing, including the face, dorsal hands, and a triangular area corresponding to the opening of a V-neck shirt on the upper chest.

Acral Acral locations include the hands, feet, wrists, and ankles.

Intertriginous Skin folds in which two skin surfaces are in contact represent intertriginous areas of the body: the axillae, inguinal folds, inner thighs, inframammary skin, and under an abdominal pannus.

Generalized Widespread involvement on the skin is referred to as generalized.

Conclusions

The ability to diagnose a rash accurately is not specific to dermatologists. Any clinician who makes the effort to study the skin and learn the dermatologic lexicon can develop a functional appreciation of the fundamentals of diagnosis. For the cancer patient and survivor, recognition of dermatologic disease may represent an opportunity to intervene early on for associated disease states, including infections, inflammatory reactions, immunologic responses, progression of disease, and adverse reactions to therapy.

4 Types of Dermatologic Reactions

Raed O. Alhusayen[1,3], Sandra R. Knowles[2,4] and Neil H. Shear[1,2,3,4]

[1]Division of Dermatology, Sunnybrook Health Sciences Centre, Toronto, Canada
[2]Division of Clinical Pharmacology and Toxicology, Sunnybrook Health Sciences Centre, Toronto, Canada
[3]Department of Medicine, University of Toronto, Toronto, Canada
[4]Department of Pharmacology and Toxicology, University of Toronto, Canada

Adverse drug reactions are responsible for 6% of all hospital admissions [1]. Furthermore, the incidence of severe or fatal drug reactions during hospital stays are 7% and 0.62%, respectively [2]. Drug reactions can present in a variety of ways, although cutaneous drug eruptions are one of the most common manifestations.

The diagnostic approach for a patient with a possible drug-induced eruption should include a focused history and physical examination. A skin biopsy and laboratory tests might be warranted. Apart from the history of the skin involvement, enquiry about accompanying systemic symptoms, especially fever, is extremely helpful in assessing the cause and the severity of the clinical presentation. Peripheral eosinophilia, although not necessarily present, supports the diagnosis of a drug reaction [3]. In this article, we review the common types of generalized cutaneous drug reactions and provide an approach to diagnosing patients with suspected drug reactions.

Exanthematous eruptions

The most common presentation of drug reactions is the simple exanthematous reaction, also known as "drug eruption," maculopapular or morbilliform eruption [4]. The peak incidence occurs 7–10 days after starting the offending drug, but it is much shorter on re-exposure [5]. The erythematous nonscaly papules and plaques usually start on the upper trunk, and then spread to the rest of the body [3]. Mucosae are usually spared [4,6]. Pruritus is a very common feature but there are no systemic symptoms. Resolution, usually within 7–14 days, occurs with a change in color from bright red to a brownish red, which may be followed by desquamation. The underlying mechanism is a T-cell mediated type IV hypersensitivity reaction [7]. The common culprits are sulphonamide and beta-lactam antibiotics, anticonvulsants, and allopurinol [3,8]. Among chemotherapeutic agents, this reaction has been reported following exposure to fluorouracil, cytarabine, etoposide, chlorambucil, hydroxyurea, melphalan, and procarbazine [9].

Another more serious presentation is drug hypersensitivity syndrome (HSS), also known as drug reaction with eosinophilia and systemic symptoms (DRESS). In addition to the cutaneous involvement, patients are systemically unwell, with fever and internal involvement [10]. Although most patients have an exanthematous eruption, more serious cutaneous manifestations such as an erythrodermic eruption or Stevens–Johnson syndrome (SJS) and/or toxic epidermal necrolysis (TEN) – like lesions may be evident. The liver is usually involved, as indicated by elevated liver enzymes [11,12]. Abdominal pain may be present, although most patients do not have symptoms of internal organ involvement. Facial edema is a typical characteristic of drug HSS [13]. Patients describe the skin lesions as asymptomatic or painful, rather than itchy. Eosinophilia and atypical lymphocytosis are predominant features [4]. Some patients may become hypothyroid due to an autoimmune thyroiditis approximately 2 months after the first symptoms appear [11,14]. In patients with a history of HSS, re-exposure to the offending agent may cause development of symptoms within 1 day. Although symptoms resolve in most patients after discontinuation of the drug, there are some patients who develop autoimmune disease and/or production of autoantibodies after resolution of HSS [15]. The most commonly offending drugs in HSS are aromatic anticonvulsants (phenytoin, phenobarbital, carbamazepine), allopurinol, sulphonamide antibiotics, lamotrigine, dapsone, minocycline, nevirapine, and abacavir [16,17]. There have been reports of HSS caused by chlorambucil and imatinib [18,19].

Dermatologic Principles and Practice in Oncology: Conditions of the Skin, Hair, and Nails in Cancer Patients, First Edition. Edited by Mario E. Lacouture.
© 2014 John Wiley & Sons, Inc. Published 2014 by John Wiley & Sons, Inc.

Urticarial eruptions

Drug-induced urticaria can develop within minutes to hours of ingesting the offending medication. The erythematous plaques are extremely itchy and although the eruption can last as long as the offending drug is continued, the individual lesions do not last more than 24 hours [20]. The underlying mechanism is a type I immunoglobulin E (IgE) mediated hypersensitivity reaction [7]. During the acute presentation, it is critical to rule out anaphylaxis, also an IgE-mediated reaction. Compared with urticaria alone, patients with anaphylaxis have airway and circulatory compromise secondary to extravascular leakage and edema, manifesting as dyspnea and hypotension [21,22]. If not immediately treated, patients may progress into anaphylactic shock. Sulphonamides, beta-lactam antibiotics, muscle relaxants, and IV contrast media are common causes of drug-induced urticaria and anaphylaxis [4,21]. Type I reactions are rarely observed, but have been documented with mitomycin, taxanes, procarbazine, L-asparaginase and daunorubicin [23].

Angioedema presents within minutes to days as deep-seated edematous plaques on the skin, associated with massive swelling of the lips and/or other mucous membranes. Compared with urticaria, lesions are skin-colored and sometimes painful, rather than red and itchy [21]. Aspirin and other nonsteroidal anti-inflammatory drugs (NSAIDs) induce angioedema through the inhibition of cyclo-oxygenase (COX-1) enzyme, resulting in edema through the release of leukotrienes [24]. Angiotensin-converting enzyme (ACE) inhibitors cause a delayed, sometimes after years, form of angioedema through the accumulation of bradykinin, a potent vasodilator [25,26]. Angioedema may also be representative of an IgE-mediated reaction; it is often found concurrently with urticaria.

Serum sickness-like reaction is another serious drug eruption occurring 1–3 weeks after drug initiation. In addition to the urticarial lesions, patients have systemic symptoms, including fever and arthralgia [27]. Unlike serum sickness, there is neither immune complex deposition nor hypocomplementemia [16]. Cefaclor is the most commonly cited cause, although this reaction has also been reported with rituximab, minocycline, and bupropion [16,28–30].

Lichenoid eruptions

Patients with lichenoid drug reactions present with purplish flat-topped papules but the white lacy fine scales, known as Wickham striae, are usually absent [31]. Lichenoid eruptions tend to be generalized rather than localized, as with lichen planus. The sparing of mucous membranes and nails and the presence of eosinophils in the infiltrate support a diagnosis of lichenoid drug eruption over lichen planus [31,32]. The reaction can develop after several years of starting the offending drug, and might take months to resolve after the medication is discontinued, which

makes it difficult to diagnose. Several groups of antihypertensive medications have been implicated in lichenoid drug eruptions, including ACE inhibitors, beta-blockers, calcium channel blockers, furosemide, and thiazide diuretics [32–49]. Lichen planus-like eruptions have also been reported with tumor necrosis factor-alfa (TNF) antagonists, such as infliximab, etanercept, and adalimumab [50,51]. Furthermore, lichen planus-like lesions have been widely reported with the use of imatinib mesylate [35].

Acneiform eruptions

In these eruptions, which resemble acne vulgaris, patients develop follicular papules, pustules, and nodules. These eruptions have the same distribution as acne vulgaris, with a predilection for the face, upper chest, and back, although other areas like scalp, buttocks, and extremities can be involved. Comedones, which are the hallmark of acne vulgaris, are notably absent in acneiform eruptions [3]. Several medications can cause an acneiform eruption, including lithium, phenytoin, isoniazid, and steroids [52,53].

Among the anticancer agents, epidermal growth factor inhibitors are a common cause of the acneiform eruption. Depending on the specific agent, the incidence ranges from 25% with gefitinib to 90% with cetuximab and panitumumab [54]. The lag time of the eruption is about 1 week after starting the medication and reaches maximum intensity in about 4 weeks. Two features seem to be more common in acneiform eruptions caused by this group of drugs: the higher prevalence of pruritus and the predominance of pustules [54–56]. The acneiform eruption is associated with a better prognosis compared with patients who do not develop the reaction [54,57,58]. Apart from epidermal growth factor inhibitors, several medications used in the oncology setting can cause an acneiform eruption including granulocyte colony stimulating factor (G-CSF), cyclosporine, dactinomycin, corticosteroids, cyclophosphamide, and mTOR inhibitors [53,59–61].

Pustular eruptions (acute generalized exanthematous pustulosis)

Patients develop large patches and plaques of erythema studded with tiny pustules 1–5 days after starting the offending drug [3,4,62]. The eruption is accentuated in flexural areas. It is associated with fever, leukocytosis with neutrophilia, and eosinophilia, but there is no organ involvement [63]. An important feature is the nonfollicular distribution of the pustules. Differentiating acute generalized exanthematous pustulosis (AGEP) from pustular psoriasis based on clinical findings may be difficult. A biopsy showing eosinophils, necrotic keratinocytes, a mixed interstitial and mid-dermal perivascular infiltrate, and absence of tortuous or dilated blood vessels favors AGEP over pustular psoriasis [64]. Beta-lactam antibiotics, macrolides, quinolones, sulphonamides, antimalarials, diltiazem, and terbinafine are common causes of AGEP [65]. Also, there have been case reports of AGEP caused by imatinib [66,67].

Bullous eruptions

Bullous eruptions are the most serious of the delayed drug eruptions. It is best to think of SJS and TEN as two points within a spectrum. The area of skin detachment differentiates SJS from TEN. SJS, TEN, and SJS–TEN overlap are defined by detachment of less than 10%, more than 30%, and 10–30% of the skin surface area, respectively [68]. The syndrome begins within 4–8 weeks from starting the offending drug. A prodrome of fever, malaise, and arthralgia often precedes the skin eruption [16,69]. The skin lesions start with tender patches that rapidly progress into flaccid bullae and skin detachment. Involvement of mucous membranes, with widespread erosions and hemorrhagic crusting, is very common, and internal organs may be involved [70,71]. The skin pathology shows full thickness necrosis of the epidermis [72]. The mortality rate can be very high (>90%) and it is best predicted using the SCORTEN tool, which is based on a set of clinical and laboratory criteria measured at presentation [73]. Allopurinol is the most common drug cause, accounting for 17% of all cases [74]. Other common medications include aromatic anticonvulsants, sulphonamide antibiotics, NSAIDs, nevirapine, and lamotrigine [75]. Although erythema multiforme, characterized by well-developed target lesions, is sometimes included within the SJS–TEN spectrum, it is best discussed as a separate entity to avoid confusion. With the exception of some cases of SJS in children, which are caused by mycoplasma infection, SJS and TEN are caused by drugs, whereas erythema multiforme is caused by infections [76,77].

Drug-induced linear IgA disease is a less serious autoimmune subepidermal blistering disease, with erythematous plaques and large tense blisters at the periphery [78]. In the majority of patients, the mucous membranes of the mouth and eyes are involved [79]. A skin histopathology and immunofluorescence shows subepidermal bullae with neutrophilic infiltrate and linear deposition of IgA at the dermo-epidermal junction [80]. Differentiating between drug-induced and idiopathic linear IgA based on clinical findings is not possible, so history is critical. In drug-induced linear IgA disease, the eruption usually develops 1–5 days after starting the offending drug and it resolves within 2 weeks of discontinuation [81]. Vancomycin is the most commonly cited cause [82,83].

Pemphigus is an autoimmune blistering disease in which autoantibodies attack adhesion molecules in the epidermis, leading to acantholysis and bulla formation. The target antigens, desmogleins, are components of desmosomes [80]. The target antigen in pemphigus foliaceus, desmoglein 1, is located in a more superficial layer of the epidermis and its expression is restricted to the skin, leading to superficial erosions on the skin with sparing

of the mucous membranes [80]. In pemphigus vulgaris, in addition to desmoglein 1, autoantibodies target desmoglein 3, which is located in the suprabasilar epidermal region and expressed in the mucous membranes and skin, leading to deeper erosions involving the skin and mucous membranes [84]. The clinical presentation of drug-induced pemphigus depends on the offending drug. Medications containing a thiol group (e.g., penicillamine and captopril) usually result in a foliaceus picture and lack the production of autoantibodies; the onset of the reaction is usually about 1 year after starting the offending medication [80,85]. Conversely, non-thiol drugs (e.g., beta-lactams and dipyrone) result in a picture indistinguishable from idiopathic pemphigus vulgaris [80,85]. It is more appropriate to call this type drug-triggered pemphigus, as the symptoms do not resolve after discontinuing the offending drug. On the other hand, bullous pemphigoid is characterized by pruritic tense blisters on an urticarial base. The involvement of mucous membranes is less common in bullous pemphigoid than in pemphigus [86]. The target antigens are bullous pemphigoid 1 and 2, which are components of the adhesion molecules that attach the basal layer of keratinocytes in the epidermis to the basement membrane [80]. Histopathology and immunofluorescence studies show subepidermal blistering with eosinophilic infiltrate and linear deposition of IgG and C3 along the basement membrane zone [80]. Although most cases of bullous pemphigoid are not drug-induced, the medications most commonly implicated in drug-induced bullous pemphigoid are furosemide, beta-lactams, penicillamine, and ACE inhibitors, NSAIDs, and influenza vaccine [87–89].

Drug-induced vasculitis

Leukocytoclastic vasculitis is a form of small vessel vasculitis that is limited to the skin [90]. Patients develop nonblanching purpuric papules on the lower extremities, which can ulcerate. Usually it has a rapid onset and resolves in few weeks, but sometimes it progresses into a chronic course with recurrent episodes. The eruption might be associated with generalized malaise and arthralgia, but, by definition, other organs are not affected. Obtaining a skin biopsy is essential to differentiate leukocytoclastic vasculitis from other vasculitides and other nonvasculitic dermatoses. The pathology shows extravasation of red blood cells, neutrophilic infiltrate, nuclear dust, and fibrin deposition around dermal blood vessels [90,91]. If Henoch–Schönlein purpura is suspected, it is important to perform a perilesional skin biopsy for immunofluorescence histologic assay to rule out IgA deposition [91]. Drugs are responsible for about 20% of cases of leukocytoclastic vasculitis [90]. Other causes include infections, connective tissue disease, inflammatory bowel disease, and lymphoproliferative disorders [92]. The presence of eosinophils in the infiltrate supports a drug etiology [93]. The average interval from initiation of drug therapy to onset of drug-induced vasculitis is 7–21 days [4]. In oncology, colony-stimulating factors, epidermal growth factor inhibitors, interferons, methotrexate, and rituximab have been reported as causing leukocytoclastic vasculitis [94–96]. Other commonly offending drugs include NSAIDs, beta-lactams, and isotretinoin [97,98].

Another less commonly described entity is protoplasmic-staining antineutrophil cytoplasmic antibodies (p-ANCA) positive drug-induced vasculitis [99]. In addition to the ANCA positivity, internal organ involvement distinguishes it from leukocytoclastic vasculitis. The eruption can develop several months to years after starting the offending drug. Hydralazine, allopurinol, propylthiouracil, minocycline, and phenytoin are commonly cited offending drugs [94,98].

Erythroderma

The term erythroderma refers to the involvement of at least 90% of the skin with erythema and exfoliation [100]. Due to the involvement of a large surface area, patients can struggle with temperature control, electrolyte imbalance, and hypoproteinemia. The enlargement of lymph nodes is common. Drugs are only responsible for small percentage of erythroderma cases [101,102]. The most common cause is an underlying dermatosis, such as psoriasis, pityriasis rubra pilaris, or atopic dermatitis [102,103]; rarely, it can be the first presentation of cutaneous lymphoma [101,104]. Obtaining a skin biopsy is required for all patients with no previous history of underlying dermatosis. The pathology of drug-induced erythroderma might show similar features to cutaneous T-cell lymphoma with lichenoid infiltrate and atypical lymphocytes, but it demonstrates necrotic keratinocytes and lacks Pautrier microabscesses [100,105]. In 30% of cases, an underlying cause cannot be identified [106]. More than 60 drugs have been reported in association with erythroderma [103]. In oncology, erythroderma has been reported in association with systemic retinoids, cisplatin, carboplatin, erythropoietin, and fluorouracil [103].

Approach to patients with suspected drug eruption

In an attempt to reach the right diagnosis, we utilize information obtained from the history, physical examination, and laboratory tests. Usually, we are required to make a diagnosis and make management decisions before some important information becomes available. Despite the availability of various tests, often a definite diagnosis cannot be confirmed. Unless it is a straightforward case, it is important to resist the temptation to give a definitive diagnosis. Instead, we suggest presenting differential diagnoses and using a ranking or attribution system to express the possibility of each diagnosis. This is especially important when discussing the cause of an eruption in which drugs are only one among several possible causes or in determining the culprit drug among a list of medications.

To facilitate the thinking process in diagnosing patients with suspected drug eruptions, we present a simple multistep approach. The steps have a logical flow, building on pieces of information as they become available, which resembles real-life situations. We also provide diagnostic algorithms to assist in navigating through the differential diagnoses (Figure 4.1, Figure 4.2, Figure 4.3, Figure 4.4, Figure 4.5, Figure 4.6 and Figure 4.7).

Step 1: Recognizing the morphology

We advise against obtaining a detailed history prior to examining the patient. Determining the morphology will allow for a focused pertinent history and will assist in ordering relevant investigations. The major morphologic groups are exanthematous, urticarial, lichenoid, pustular, purpuric, bullous, and erythrodermic. The presence of severe facial edema in the setting of exanthematous eruption supports a diagnosis of HSS [13]. Relative sparing of palms and soles favors a simple exanthematous drug eruption over acute graft versus host disease (GVHD) [107].

In urticarial eruptions, additional symptoms such as hypotension or nausea/vomiting suggest a more serious diagnosis, namely anaphylaxis. The presence of mucous membrane involvement is also observed with angioedema [21]. The depth and color of skin lesions are also important. Lesions of urticaria and serum sickness-like reaction are erythematous and superficial, whereas those of angioedema are skin-colored and deep-seated. Urticarial lesions that heal with post-inflammatory hyperpigmentation or purpura should raise the possibility of urticarial vasculitis [108]. Sweet syndrome and neutrophilic eccrine hidradenitis (NEH) can present with urticarial lesions or well-defined, juicy, dusky red papules and plaques scattered on the skin [109,110].

In lichenoid eruptions, involvement of mucous membranes is seen in lichen planus and lichenoid variant of GVHD, but is less likely in lichenoid drug eruptions [31]. Severe ulcerative lichen planus can be seen in association with thymoma [111].

The first step in assessing pustular eruptions is determining whether the pustules are follicular or nonfollicular. Acne, acneiform eruptions, and folliculitis have follicular pustules and papules. Both acne and acneiform eruptions can have nodules and scarring, but comedones are only present in acne [3]. Nonfollicular pustules on an erythematous base are seen in pustular psoriasis and AGEP. AGEP pustules tend to be small, whereas lesions of pustular psoriasis vary in size [4,112].

Purpuric eruptions can be classified into punctate and livedoid, meaning "net-like" [91]. Punctate palpable purpura is a sign of small-vessel vasculitis, and nonpalpable punctate lesions are seen in low platelet situations, like idiopathic thrombocytopenic purpura or disorders of platelet dysfunction [113,114]. Meningococcemia and disseminated intravascular coagulation (DIC) skin lesions include nonpalpable purpura, pustules, hemorrhagic bullae, and necrotic lesions. Livedoid purpura and necrotic lesions over fatty regions like buttocks and female breasts are seen in warfarin-induced skin necrosis [115]. Livedoid purpura and ulcerated nodules over muscles are associated with polyarteritis nodosa and other medium vessel vasculitides [90,91].

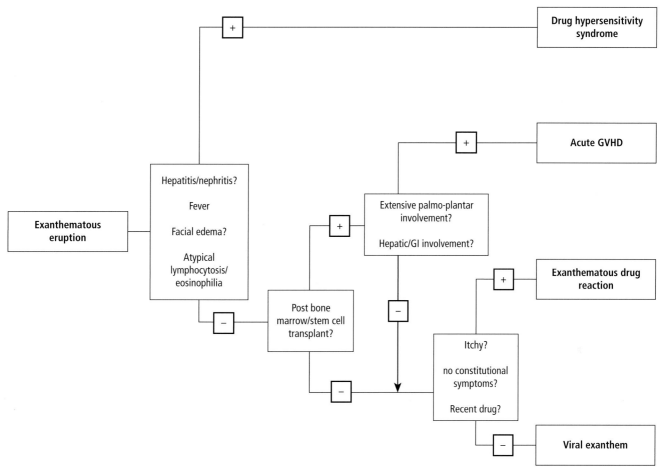

Figure 4.1 Algorithm for the diagnosis of exanthematous (maculopapular or morbilliform) eruptions. +, present; –, absent.

It is best to divide bullous eruptions into tense or flaccid bullae. Tense bullae on an erythematous base favor a diagnosis of bullous pemphigoid or linear IgA. In linear IgA, the bullae might have an annular configuration surrounding the central erythematous plaque. Tense bullae on a normal base with scarring and milia support a diagnosis of epidermolysis bullosa acquisita [80]. Photodistributed tense bullae on normal skin are seen in porphyria cutanea tarda and pseudoporphyria [116]. Other common lesions of porphyria cutanea tarda are facial hypertrichosis and scarring, which are absent in pseudoporphyria [116]. Flaccid bullae and erosions with mucous membrane involvement favor diagnoses of SJS–TEN or pemphigus vulgaris. In SJS–TEN, the mucous membrane involvement manifests as diffuse hemorrhagic crusting of the lips, whereas ulcerations of the buccal mucosa and gingivitis are more commonly seen in pemphigus vulgaris. The oral lesions observed in a rare type of pemphigus, paraneoplastic pemphigus, can mimic those of SJS–TEN. Similarly, severe cases of acute GVHD can present with a picture similar to TEN [107]. Flaccid bullae and erosions with sparing of mucous membranes are seen in staphylococcal scalded skin syndrome (SSSS) and pemphigus foliaceus. While the erosions in SSSS are widespread and moist on an ery-

thematous base, those of pemphigus foliaceus are brownish and keratotic.

Patients with erythroderma secondary to an underlying dermatosis might show classic signs of that dermatosis [100]. If the erythroderma is secondary to psoriasis, nail pitting and psoriasiform plaques might be seen. Excoriations and accentuation in flexural areas suggests an underlying atopic dermatitis, whereas the presence of keratotic papules on the dorsa of the hands, and the severe involvement of the head and neck area, are more commonly seen pityriasis rubra pilaris. In cases of erythroderma secondary to cutaneous lymphoma, one might find tumors, enlarged lymph nodes, and hepatosplenomegaly.

Step 2: Associated symptoms and systemic involvement

Regardless of the morphology of the skin eruption, the presence of systemic involvement points to a severe drug eruption or a nondrug-related condition. It is important to ask about pruritus, fever, weight loss, night sweats, malaise, and organ-specific systemic involvement. The history should also include drug intake (prescription and nonprescription medications, as well as herbal preparations), past medical and surgical history, and known allergies.

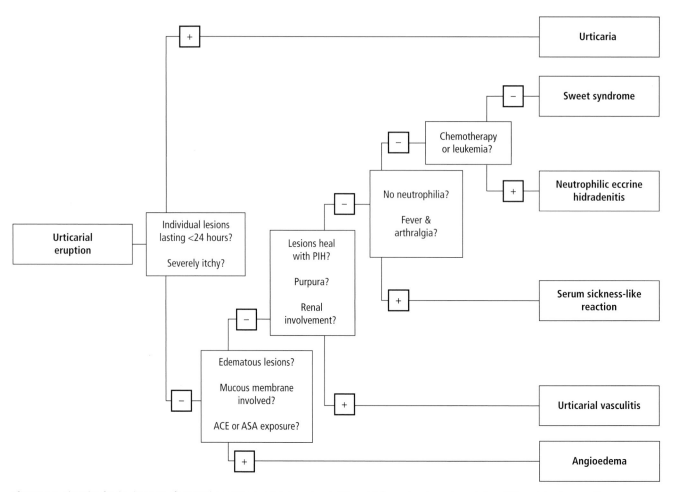

Figure 4.2 Algorithm for the diagnosis of urticarial eruptions. +, present; −, absent. PIH, post-inflammatory hyperpigmentation: ACE, angiotensin-converting enzyme inhibitor; ASA, acetylsalicylic acid.

In exanthematous eruptions, the presence of pruritus and the absence of systemic involvement are in keeping with diagnosis of simple exanthematous drug eruption [4]. Viral exanthems (e.g., respiratory syncytial virus, adenovirus, measles) have identical morphology to exanthematous drug eruptions [9]. The presence of prodromal symptoms supported by exposure history and the absence of pruritus favors a diagnosis of viral exanthem. The presence of painful rather than pruritic lesions, systemic symptoms (e.g., fever) and internal organ involvement (e.g., elevated liver enzymes) in a patient starting new medications 2–8 weeks prior to presentation, should raise the question of HSS [10]. In addition, eosinophilia or atypical lymphocytosis can be seen in the peripheral blood of HSS patients [12]. Following bone marrow, hematopoietic stem cell, or solid organ transplant, GVHD should be considered. When present, the triad of dermatitis, hepatitis, and enteritis strongly supports a diagnosis of GVHD [107]. Compared with drug eruptions, skin lesions tend to be tender or asymptomatic rather than pruritic [107].

In urticarial eruptions, individual skin lesions lasting less than 24 hours, in association with severe pruritus, differentiates urticaria from other diagnoses [108]. Association with certain physical triggers (e.g., cold or water) need to be explored. Nonpruritic urticaria-like lesions are seen in angioedema, serum sickness-like reactions, urticarial vasculitis, Sweet syndrome, and NEH. In addition to the skin lesions, patients with serum sickness-like reactions have fever and arthralgia [16]. Medication history especially of NSAIDs or ACE inhibitors use should be sought in patients with angioedema [21,25]. In urticarial vasculitis, presence of systemic involvement, especially renal disease, in addition to history of connective tissue disease is sometimes seen, but not necessarily present [108]. In addition to the well-demarcated skin lesions, patients with Sweet syndrome usually have fever and neutrophilia [109]. Conversely, patients with NEH do not have visceral involvement, but a history of underlying hematologic malignancy or the use of some medications known to cause NEH (e.g., G-CSF) is usually found [110].

In patients with lichenoid eruptions sparing the mucous membranes, history of medication intake should be sought carefully. In pustular eruptions, patients with nonfollicular pustules present acutely and they are usually systematically ill and febrile. The history of psoriasis supports the diagnosis of pustular

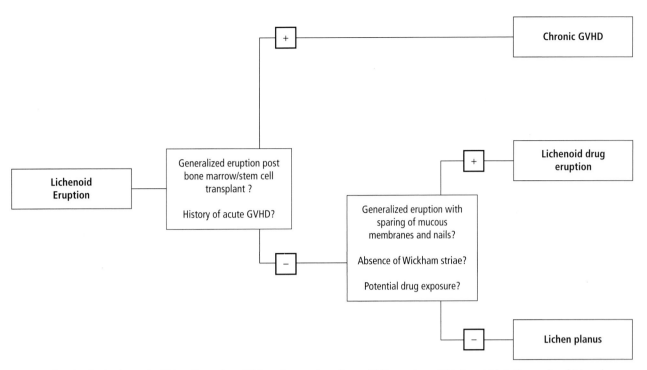

Figure 4.3 Algorithm for the diagnosis of lichenoid eruptions. GVHD, graft versus host disease. Wickham striae, whitish lines visible in the papules of lichen planus. +, present; −, absent.

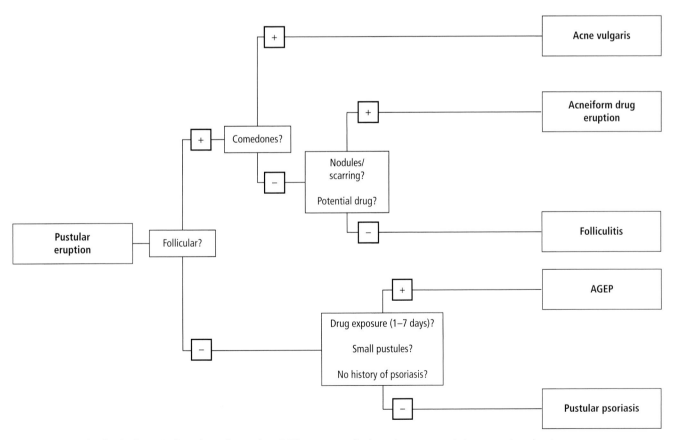

Figure 4.4 Algorithm for the diagnosis of papulopustular eruptions. AGEP, acute generalized exanthematous pustulosis. +, present; −, absent.

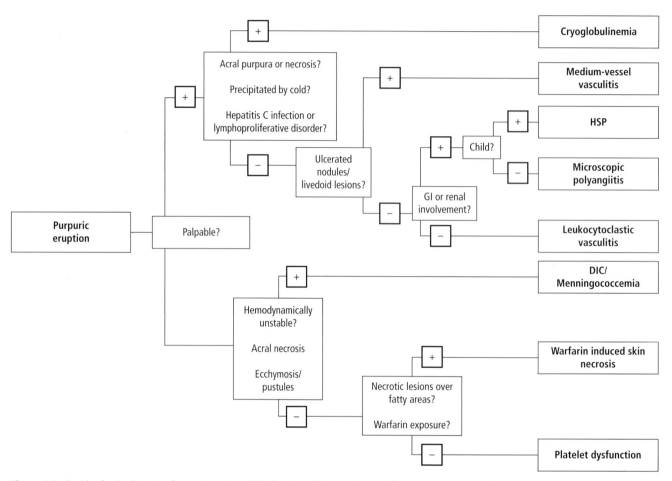

Figure 4.5 Algorithm for the diagnosis of purpuric eruptions. DIC, disseminated intravascular coagulation; HSP, Henoch–Schönlein purpura. +, present; −, absent.

psoriasis, while a recent (i.e., 1–5 days) history of ingesting a new medication raises the possibility of AGEP. Medications known to exacerbate psoriasis include anti-TNF-alfa therapy (e.g., inflix-imab, etanercept, adalimumab), lithium, G-CSF, radiotherapy, beta-blockers, and antimalarial agents [3,4,117,118]. Neutrophilic leukocytosis is seen in both AGEP and pustular psoriasis, but eosinophilia would suggest AGEP [63,112]. In patients with follicular pustules that lack comedones, the history should focus on drugs that can cause acneiform eruptions. History of previous folliculitis is also helpful if recurrent folliculitis is suspected.

Among bullous eruptions, SJS–TEN and SSSS present acutely, while others have a more protracted course. SJS–TEN is a clinical diagnosis. It is based on the acute development of prodromal symptoms, skin detachment, and hemorrhagic crusting of mucous membranes in a patient who started a high-risk medication 2–8 weeks prior to presentation. SSSS develops in very young children or adults who cannot clear the offending staphylococcal exotoxins due to renal impairment or immuno-suppression [119]. Pruritus distinguishes bullous pemphigoid from other primary bullous disorders. Drug history should be obtained in patients with a first-time presentation suggestive of pemphigus, bullous pemphigoid, or porphyria. Porphyria

work-up should be ordered, as appropriate, as it differentiates porphyria from pseudoporphyria [115]. If epidermolysis bullosa acquisita is suspected, ruling out a potential underlying malig-nancy is advised [120].

In patients with palpable purpura, it is important to determine whether the involvement is limited to the skin or involves other organs. Leukocytoclastic vasculitis, apart from an occasionally elevated erythrocyte sedimentation rate, lacks systemic involvement. Its main differential diagnosis, Henoch–Schönlein purpura, is usually associated with gastrointestinal, and less commonly renal, involvement [91,92]. Similar to urticaria, history in leukocytoclastic vasculitis should attempt to identify potential underlying causes. Isolated thrombocytopenia is seen in idiopathic thrombocytopenic purpura [114]. Lung and sinus involvement and C-ANCA positivity are the hallmarks of Wegener granulomatosis [91]. P-ANCA positivity and multior-gan, especially renal, involvement is observed in microscopic polyangiitis and in a rare subset of drug-induced vasculitis, so it is essential to take a careful drug history [113]. Patients with polyarteritis nodosa usually have muscle aches and abdominal complaints [92,113]. In the setting of cold-precipitated livedoid eruptions on ankles and lower legs, a cryoglobulins level should

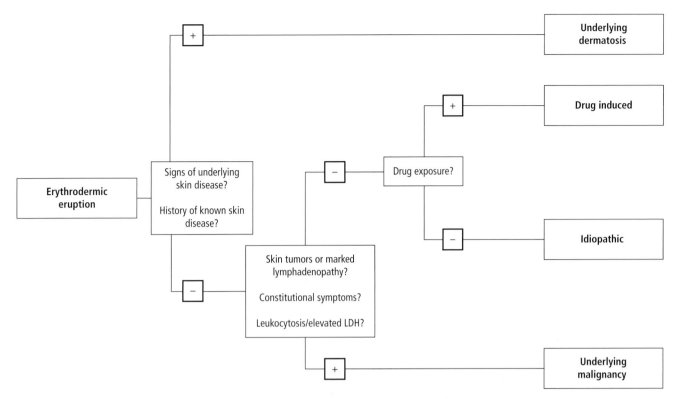

Figure 4.6 Algorithm for the diagnosis of erythrodermic eruptions. LDH, lactate dehydrogenase. +, present; –, absent.

be obtained. Monoclonal (type I) cryoglobulinemia is associated with lymphoproliferative disorders [91]. Patients with meningococcemia and DIC, in addition to having polymorphic skin lesions, have an acute presentation and they are extremely ill and hemodynamically unstable.

In erythrodermic patients, the history should focus on underlying dermatoses and medication intake. The absence of a known underlying cause, and the presence of fever, night sweats, weight loss, marked lymphadenopathy, hepatosplenomegaly, or elevated lactate dehydrogenase levels, should raise the concern of a paraneoplastic association [101,104,105].

Step 3: Histopathologic assessment

Skin biopsies might guide the management by adding or excluding certain diseases from the differential diagnosis list. In most cases, clinicopathologic correlation is required.

Among the exanthematous eruptions, biopsy may be useful in diagnosing acute GVHD, showing vacuolar interface changes with various degrees of scattered necrotic keratinocytes depending on the severity of the condition [107]. In the most severe cases, full thickness necrosis of the epidermis, similar to TEN, is seen [9]. Exanthematous drug eruption can show superficial lymphocytic infiltrate with or without spongiosis. The presence of eosinophils supports a drug-induced cause [4].

Skin biopsies of lesions of urticaria show sparse numbers of neutrophils and eosinophils in the dermis [108]. The presence of vasculitis is the hallmark of urticarial vasculitis [92,108]. Both

Sweet syndrome and NEH show dense neutrophilic infiltrate in the dermis, but in NEH there is accentuation around eccrine glands with a varying degree of eccrine gland necrosis [109,110].

Several histopathologic features, when present, are helpful in distinguishing lichenoid drug eruption from lichen planus. The presence of eosinophils, higher degree of necrotic keratinocytes, and focal parakeratosis are suggestive of a lichenoid drug eruption [31,32]. Lichen planus and lichenoid GVHD have identical features, but suprabasilar vacuolization can be seen in the latter [9,107].

In pustular lesions, a skin biopsy would confirm the follicular basis of the eruption if it was not clear clinically. Both AGEP and pustular psoriasis show subcorneal collections of neutrophils. The presence of eosinophils and necrotic keratinocytes is more commonly seen in AGEP, whereas the presence of torturous blood vessels in the superficial dermis favors pustular psoriasis [64].

Histopathology and immunofluorescence are extremely helpful in bullous eruptions. Although SJS–TEN is a clinical diagnosis, a skin biopsy is sometimes performed to confirm the diagnosis. The pathology shows full thickness necrosis of the epidermis with no discernable inflammatory infiltrate [72]. Immunobullous disorders are divided into intraepidermal and subepidermal, based on the location of the bullae. The pemphigus group demonstrates intraepidemal blistering, while the blistering seen with other disorders is subepidermal. Immunofluorescence shows intercellular epidermal deposition in pemphigus, but it might be

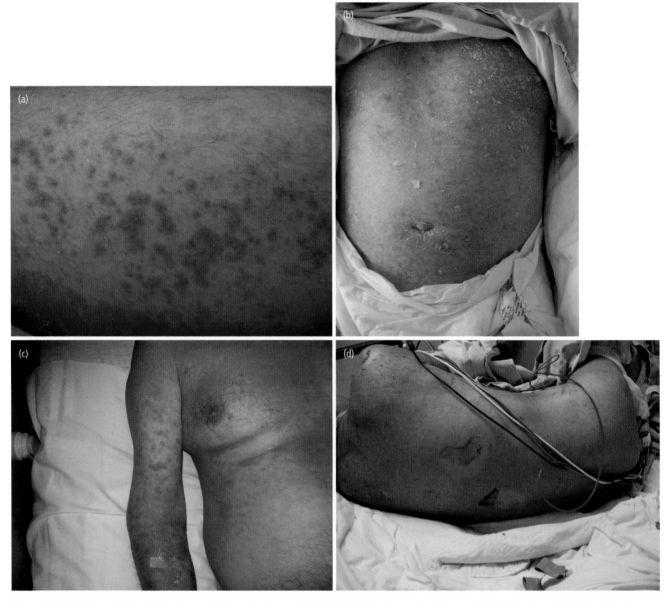

Figure 4.7 Clinical presentation of (a) acute generalized exanthemtous pustulosis (AGEP); (b) graft versus host disease; (c) leukemia cutis; and (d) toxic epidermal necrolysis (TEN).

negative in some drug-induced cases [80,121]. Bullous pemphigoid shows subepidermal blistering with eosinophilic infiltrate and immunofluorescence microscopy demonstrates linear deposition of IgG and C3 along the dermo-epidermal junction [80,84]. Epidermolysis bullosa acquisita can have similar features to bullous pemphigoid, but special tests, like salt split skin test, can differentiate the two if needed [80]. Subepidermal blistering, neutrophilic infiltrate, and linear deposition of IgA characterize linear IgA disease [84]. Both porphyria and pseudoporphyria show cell-poor subepidermal blistering and a nonspecific immunofluorescence pattern, but the increased thickness of blood vessel walls in the dermis is more commonly seen in porphyria [122].

Extravasation of RBCs, neutrophilic infiltrate with nuclear dusting, and fibrin deposition in blood vessel walls characterize vasculitis [91,113]. If Henoch–Schönlein purpura is suspected, a perilesional biopsy should be obtained for immunofluorescence. It should show deposition of IgA [91]. Granuloma formation or involvement of blood vessels in the subcutis is usually seen in medium vessel vasculitis [91,92].

The skin biopsy in erythroderma does not always give a definite answer about the cause of erythroderma [102,106]. Performing multiple biopsies from different sites should be considered. The presence of a lichenoid reaction with necrotic keratinocytes and the lack of features suggestive of an underlying dermatosis are in keeping with a drug etiology [100,105].

Step 4: Determining the offending drug

In patients receiving multiple drugs, rank the medications, based on the relative probability of each one of them possibly causing the drug eruption. The Naranjo scale is sometimes used to determine the probability that an observed adverse reaction is caused by a drug [123]. Based on the score obtained from a short questionnaire, the reaction is classified as definite, probable, possible, or doubtful. Regardless of the method used, several factors should be employed in determining the probability of each medication being responsible for the adverse reaction. The first factor is determining the most likely timeframe, given the type of skin eruption. In cases of drug challenge, many reactions often occur much more rapidly than on initial exposure. The second factor is determining the timing of each medication that was started within the accepted timeframe for the specified drug eruption. Trends in laboratory parameters should also be tracked during the critical period. The third factor is assessing the association of a given medication to cause the observed reaction. This is based largely on previous knowledge and searching the literature. By analyzing the information obtained from these three factors, it should be possible to develop a reasonable ranking of the potential offending drugs.

Several diagnostic tests are available to assess drug causality [124]. The concept behind the *in vivo* tests is rechallenging the patient with the potential medication. This rechallenge could be performed by systemic intake (usually oral), skin prick intradermal, and/or skin patch testing [124–126]. The *ex vivo* tests assess the behavior of the patient's immune cells when incubated with the suspected drug. Examples of these tests include macrophage migration inhibition factor and lymphocyte toxicity assay [124,127]. *Ex vivo* tests are only available in larger centers, and the use of some of them is limited to research purposes.

Conclusions

In conclusion, drug eruptions can present in a variety of ways. The first step in evaluating patients with a suspected drug eruption is to identify the morphology of the skin eruption. The presence of systemic symptoms point to a severe drug reaction or a nondrug-related cause. A thorough history and review of the literature are important in prioritizing the possible offending drugs.

References

1 Goettler, M., Schneeweiss, S. & Hasford, J. (1997) Adverse drug reaction monitoring: cost and benefit considerations. Part II: cost and preventability of adverse drug reactions leading to hospital admission. *Pharmacoepidemiology and Drug Safety*, **6** (Suppl. 3), S79–S90.

2 Lazarou, J., Pomeranz, B.H. & Corey, P.N. (1998) Incidence of adverse drug reactions in hospitalized patients: a meta-analysis of prospective studies. *Journal of the American Medical Association*, **279**, 1200–1205.

3 Nigen, S., Knowles, S.R. & Shear, N.H. (2003) Drug eruptions: approaching the diagnosis of drug-induced skin diseases. *Journal of Drugs in Dermatology*, **2**, 278–299.

4 Valeyrie-Allanore, L., Sassolas, B. & Roujeau, J.C. (2007) Drug-induced skin, nail and hair disorders. *Drug Safety: An International Journal of Medical Toxicology and Drug Experience*, **30**, 1011–1030.

5 Bircher, A.J. & Scherer, K. (2010) Delayed cutaneous manifestations of drug hypersensitivity. *Medical Clinics of North America*, **94**, 711–725, x.

6 Cotliar, J. (2007) Approach to the patient with a suspected drug eruption. *Seminars in Cutaneous Medicine and Surgery*, **26**, 147–154.

7 Pichler, W.J., Adam, J., Daubner, B., Gentinetta, T., Keller, M. & Yerly, D. (2010) Drug hypersensitivity reactions: pathomechanism and clinical symptoms. *Medical Clinics of North America*, **94**, 645–664, xv.

8 Romano, A., Blanca, M., Torres, M.J. *et al.* (2004) Diagnosis of nonimmediate reactions to beta-lactam antibiotics. *Allergy*, **59**, 1153–1160.

9 Mays, S.R., Kunishige, J.H., Truong, E., Kontoyiannis, D.P. & Hymes, S.R. (2007) Approach to the morbilliform eruption in the hematopoietic transplant patient. *Seminars in Cutaneous Medicine and Surgery*, **26**, 155–162.

10 Bocquet, H., Bagot, M. & Roujeau, J.C. (1996) Drug-induced pseudolymphoma and drug hypersensitivity syndrome (Drug Rash with Eosinophilia and Systemic Symptoms: DRESS). *Seminars in Cutaneous Medicine and Surgery*, **15**, 250–257.

11 Kano, Y. & Shiohara, T. (2009) The variable clinical picture of drug-induced hypersensitivity syndrome/drug rash with eosinophilia and systemic symptoms in relation to the eliciting drug. *Immunology and Allergy Clinics of North America*, **29**, 481–501.

12 Jeung, Y.J., Lee, J.Y., Oh, M.J., Choi, D.C. & Lee, B.J. (2010) Comparison of the causes and clinical features of drug rash with eosinophilia and systemic symptoms and Stevens-Johnson syndrome. *Allergy, Asthma and Immunology Research*, **2**, 123–126.

13 Shiohara, T., Inaoka, M. & Kano, Y. (2006) Drug-induced hypersensitivity syndrome (DIHS): a reaction induced by a complex interplay among herpesviruses and antiviral and antidrug immune responses. *Allergology International*, **55**, 1–8.

14 Gupta, A., Eggo, M.C., Uetrecht, J.P. *et al.* (1992) Drug-induced hypothyroidism: the thyroid as a target organ in hypersensitivity reactions to anticonvulsants and sulfonamides. *Clinical Pharmacology and Therapeutics*, **51**, 56–67.

15 Kano, Y., Ishida, T., Hirahara, K. & Shiohara, T. (2010) Visceral involvements and long-term sequelae in drug-induced hypersensitivity syndrome. *Medical Clinics of North America*, **94**, 743–759, xi.

16 Knowles, S.R. & Shear, N.H. (2007) Recognition and management of severe cutaneous drug reactions. *Dermatologic Clinics*, **25**, 245–253, viii.

17 Cornejo-Garcia, J.A., Blanca-Lopez, N., Dona, I. *et al.* (2009) Hypersensitivity reactions to non-steroidal anti-inflammatory drugs. *Current Drug Metabolism*, **10**, 971–980.

18 Vaida, I., Roszkiewicz, F., Gruson, B., Makdassi, R. & Damaj, G. (2009) Drug rash with eosinophilia and systemic symptoms after

chlorambucil treatment in chronic lymphocytic leukaemia. *Pharmacology*, **83**, 148–149.

19 Le, N.P., Viseux, V., Chaby, G., Billet, A., Denoeux, J.P. & Lok, C. (2006) [Drug reaction with eosinophilia and systemic symptoms (DRESS) following imatinib therapy]. *Annales de Dermatologie et de Venereologie*, **133**, 686–688.

20 Kozel, M.M., Mekkes, J.R., Bossuyt, P.M. & Bos, J.D. (1998) The effectiveness of a history-based diagnostic approach in chronic urticaria and angioedema. *Archives of Dermatology*, **134**, 1575–1580.

21 Limsuwan, T. & Demoly, P. (2010) Acute symptoms of drug hypersensitivity (urticaria, angioedema, anaphylaxis, anaphylactic shock). *Medical Clinics of North America*, **94**, 691–710, x.

22 Kanji, S. & Chant, C. (2010) Allergic and hypersensitivity reactions in the intensive care unit. *Critical Care Medicine*, **38**, S162–S168.

23 Guillot, B., Bessis, D. & Dereure, O. (2004) Mucocutaneous side effects of antineoplastic chemotherapy. *Expert Opinion on Drug Safety*, **3**, 579–587.

24 Sanchez-Borges, M., Capriles-Hulett, A. & Caballero-Fonseca, F. (2003) Cutaneous reactions to aspirin and nonsteroidal antiinflammatory drugs. *Clinical Reviews in Allergy and Immunology*, **24**, 125–136.

25 Hoover, T., Lippmann, M., Grouzmann, E., Marceau, F. & Herscu, P. (2010) Angiotensin converting enzyme inhibitor induced angio-oedema: a review of the pathophysiology and risk factors. *Clinical and Experimental Allergy: Journal of the British Society for Allergy and Clinical Immunology*, **40**, 50–61.

26 Nussberger, J., Cugno, M. & Cicardi, M. (2002) Bradykinin-mediated angioedema. *New England Journal of Medicine*, **347**, 621–622.

27 King, B.A. & Geelhoed, G.C. (2003) Adverse skin and joint reactions associated with oral antibiotics in children: the role of cefaclor in serum sickness-like reactions. *Journal of Paediatrics and Child Health*, **39**, 677–681.

28 Knowles, S.R., Shapiro, L. & Shear, N.H. (1996) Serious adverse reactions induced by minocycline: report of 13 patients and review of the literature. *Archives of Dermatology*, **132**, 934–939.

29 McCollom, R.A., Elbe, D.H. & Ritchie, A.H. (2000) Bupropion-induced serum sickness-like reaction. *Annals of Pharmacotherapy*, **34**, 471–473.

30 Schutgens, R.E. (2006) Rituximab-induced serum sickness. *British Journal of Haematology*, **135**, 147.

31 Halevy, S. & Shai, A. (1993) Lichenoid drug eruptions. *Journal of the American Academy of Dermatology*, **29**, 249–255.

32 Tilly, J.J., Drolet, B.A. & Esterly, N.B. (2004) Lichenoid eruptions in children. *Journal of the American Academy of Dermatology*, **51**, 606–624.

33 Bodmer, M., Egger, S.S., Hohenstein, E., Beltraminelli, H. & Krahenbuhl, S. (2006) Lichenoid eruption associated with the use of nebivolol. *Annals of Pharmacotherapy*, **40**, 1688–1690.

34 Massa, M.C., Jason, S.M., Gradini, R. & Welykyj, S. (1991) Lichenoid drug eruption secondary to propranolol. *Cutis: Cutaneous Medicine for the Practitioner*, **48**, 41–43.

35 Kuraishi, N., Nagai, Y., Hasegawa, M. & Ishikawa, O. (2010) Lichenoid drug eruption with palmoplantar hyperkeratosis due to imatinib mesylate: a case report and a review of the literature. *Acta Dermato-Venereologica*, **90** (1), 73–76. Review.

36 Gómez Fernández, C., Sendagorta Cudós, E., Casado Verrier, B., Feito Rodríguez, M., Suárez Aguado, J. & Vidaurrázaga Díaz de

Arcaya, C. (2010) Oral lichenoid eruption associated with imatinib treatment. *European Journal of Dermatology*, **20** (1), 127–128.

37 Kawakami, T., Kawanabe, T. & Soma, Y. (2009) Cutaneous lichenoid eruption caused by imatinib mesylate in a Japanese patient with chronic myeloid leukaemia. *Acta Dermato-Venereologica*, **89** (3), 325–326.

38 Sendagorta, E., Herranz, P., Feito, M. *et al.* (2009) Lichenoid drug eruption related to imatinib: report of a new case and review of the literature. *Clinical and Experimental Dermatology*, **34** (7), e315–e316. Review.

39 Wahiduzzaman, M. & Pubalan, M. (2008) Oral and cutaneous lichenoid reaction with nail changes secondary to imatinib: report of a case and literature review. *Dermatology Online Journal*, **14** (12), 14. Review.

40 Chan, C.Y., Browning, J., Smith-Zagone, M.J., Martinelli, P.T. & Hsu, S. (2007) Cutaneous lichenoid dermatitis associated with imatinib mesylate. *Dermatology Online Journal*, **13** (2), 29.

41 Pascual, J.C., Matarredona, J., Miralles, J., Conesa, V. & Borras-Blasco, J. (2006) Oral and cutaneous lichenoid reaction secondary to imatinib: report of two cases. *International Journal of Dermatology*, **45** (12), 1471–1473.

42 Dalmau, J., Peramiquel, L., Puig, L., Fernández-Figueras, M.T., Roé, E. & Alomar, A. (2006) Imatinib-associated lichenoid eruption: acitretin treatment allows maintained antineoplastic effect. *British Journal of Dermatology*, **154** (6), 1213–1216.

43 Scheinfeld, N. (2006) Imatinib mesylate and dermatology. Part 2: a review of the cutaneous side effects of imatinib mesylate. *Journal of Drugs in Dermatology*, **5** (3), 228–231. Review.

44 Prabhash, K. & Doval, D.C. (2005) Lichenoid eruption due to imatinib. *Indian Journal of Dermatology, Venereology and Leprology*, **71** (4), 287–288.

45 Ena, P., Chiarolini, F., Siddi, G.M. & Cossu, A. (2004) Oral lichenoid eruption secondary to imatinib (Glivec). *Journal of Dermatological Treatment*, **15** (4), 253–255.

46 Roux, C., Boisseau-Garsaud, A.M., Saint-Cyr, I., Hélénon, R., Quist, D. & Delaunay, C. (2004) [Lichenoid cutaneous reaction to imatinib]. *Annales de Dermatologie et de Venereologie*, **131** (6–7 Pt 1), 571–573. [in French].

47 Lim, D.S. & Muir, J. (2002) Oral lichenoid reaction to imatinib (STI 571, Gleevec). *Dermatology (Basel, Switzerland)*, **205** (2), 169–171.

48 Lim, D. & Muir, J. (2002) Lichenoid eruption to STI 571. *American Journal of Hematology*, **70** (2), 179.

49 Lim, D. & Muir, J. (2001) Imatinib for chronic myeloid leukaemia: a NICE mess. *Lancet*, **358** (9296), 1903.

50 Asarch, A., Gottlieb, A.B., Lee, J. *et al.* (2009) Lichen planus-like eruptions: an emerging side effect of tumor necrosis factor-alpha antagonists. *Journal of the American Academy of Dermatology*, **61**, 104–111.

51 Kerbleski, J.F. & Gottlieb, A.B. (2009) Dermatological complications and safety of anti-TNF treatments. *Gut*, **58**, 1033–1039.

52 Fung, M.A. & Berger, T.G. (2000) A prospective study of acute-onset steroid acne associated with administration of intravenous corticosteroids. *Dermatology (Basel, Switzerland)*, **200**, 43–44.

53 Momin, S.B., Peterson, A. & Del Rosso, J.Q. (2010) A status report on drug-associated acne and acneiform eruptions. *Journal of Drugs in Dermatology*, **9**, 627–636.

54 Agero, A.L., Dusza, S.W., Benvenuto-Andrade, C., Busam, K.J., Myskowski, P. & Halpern, A.C. (2006) Dermatologic side effects

associated with the epidermal growth factor receptor inhibitors. *Journal of the American Academy of Dermatology*, **55**, 657–670.

55 Segaert, S. & Van Cutsem, E. (2005) Clinical signs, pathophysiology and management of skin toxicity during therapy with epidermal growth factor receptor inhibitors. *Annals of Oncology*, **16**, 1425–1433.

56 Shah, N.T., Kris, M.G., Pao, W. *et al.* (2005) Practical management of patients with non-small-cell lung cancer treated with gefitinib. *Journal of Clinical Oncology*, **23**, 165–174.

57 Hammond-Thelin, L.A. (2008) Cutaneous reactions related to systemic immunomodulators and targeted therapeutics. *Dermatologic Clinics*, **26**, 121–159, ix.

58 Hu, J.C., Sadeghi, P., Pinter-Brown, L.C., Yashar, S. & Chiu, M.W. (2007) Cutaneous side effects of epidermal growth factor receptor inhibitors: clinical presentation, pathogenesis, and management. *Journal of the American Academy of Dermatology*, **56**, 317–326.

59 Lee, P.K. & Dover, J.S. (1996) Recurrent exacerbation of acne by granulocyte colony-stimulating factor administration. *Journal of the American Academy of Dermatology*, **34**, 855–856.

60 el Shahawy, M.A., Gadallah, M.F. & Massry, S.G. (1996) Acne: a potential side effect of cyclosporine A therapy. *Nephron*, **72**, 679–682.

61 Laing, M.E., Laing, T.A., Mulligan, N.J. & Keane, F.M. (2006) Eosinophilic pustular folliculitis induced by chemotherapy. *Journal of the American Academy of Dermatology*, **54** (4), 729–730.

62 Mockenhaupt, M. (2009) Severe drug-induced skin reactions: clinical pattern, diagnostics and therapy. *Journal der Deutschen Dermatologischen Gesellschaft*, **7**, 142–160.

63 Choi, M.J., Kim, H.S., Park, H.J. *et al.* (2010) Clinicopathologic manifestations of 36 Korean patients with acute generalized exanthematous pustulosis: a case series and review of the literature. *Annals of Dermatology*, **22**, 163–169.

64 Kardaun, S.H., Kuiper, H., Fidler, V. & Jonkman, M.F. (2010) The histopathological spectrum of acute generalized exanthematous pustulosis (AGEP) and its differentiation from generalized pustular psoriasis. *Journal of Cutaneous Pathology*, **37**, 1220–1229.

65 Sidoroff, A., Dunant, A., Viboud, C. *et al.* (2007) Risk factors for acute generalized exanthematous pustulosis (AGEP): results of a multinational case–control study (EuroSCAR). *British Journal of Dermatology*, **157**, 989–996.

66 Schwarz, M., Kreuzer, K.A., Baskaynak, G., Dorken, B. & le Coutre, P. (2002) Imatinib-induced acute generalized exanthematous pustulosis (AGEP) in two patients with chronic myeloid leukemia. *European Journal of Haematology*, **69**, 254–256.

67 Brouard, M.C., Prins, C., Mach-Pascual, S. & Saurat, J.H. (2001) Acute generalized exanthematous pustulosis associated with STI571 in a patient with chronic myeloid leukemia. *Dermatology (Basel, Switzerland)*, **203**, 57–59.

68 Bastuji-Garin, S., Rzany, B., Stern, R.S., Shear, N.H., Naldi, L. & Roujeau, J.C. (1993) Clinical classification of cases of toxic epidermal necrolysis, Stevens-Johnson syndrome, and erythema multiforme. *Archives of Dermatology*, **129**, 92–96.

69 Lissia, M., Mulas, P., Bulla, A. & Rubino, C. (2010) Toxic epidermal necrolysis (Lyell's disease). *Burns: Journal of the International Society for Burn Injuries*, **36**, 152–163.

70 Wetter, D.A. & Camilleri, M.J. (2010) Clinical, etiologic, and histopathologic features of Stevens-Johnson syndrome during an 8-year period at Mayo Clinic. *Mayo Clinic Proceedings*, **85**, 131–138.

71 Yamane, Y., Aihara, M. & Ikezawa, Z. (2007) Analysis of Stevens-Johnson syndrome and toxic epidermal necrolysis in Japan from 2000 to 2006. *Allergology International*, **56**, 419–425.

72 Nagy, N. & McGrath, J.A. (2010) Blistering skin diseases: a bridge between dermatopathology and molecular biology. *Histopathology*, **56**, 91–99.

73 Bastuji-Garin, S., Fouchard, N., Bertocchi, M., Roujeau, J.C., Revuz, J. & Wolkenstein, P. (2000) SCORTEN: a severity-of-illness score for toxic epidermal necrolysis. *Journal of Investigative Dermatology*, **115**, 149–153.

74 Halevy, S., Ghislain, P.D., Mockenhaupt, M. *et al.* (2008) Allopurinol is the most common cause of Stevens-Johnson syndrome and toxic epidermal necrolysis in Europe and Israel. *Journal of the American Academy of Dermatology*, **58**, 25–32.

75 Mockenhaupt, M., Viboud, C., Dunant, A. *et al.* (2008) Stevens-Johnson syndrome and toxic epidermal necrolysis: assessment of medication risks with emphasis on recently marketed drugs: The EuroSCAR-study. *Journal of Investigative Dermatology*, **128**, 35–44.

76 Birch, J., Chamlin, S., Duerst, R. & Jacobsohn, D. (2008) *Mycoplasma pneumoniae* and atypical Stevens-Johnson syndrome in a hematopoietic stem cell transplant recipient. *Pediatric Blood and Cancer*, **50**, 1278–1279.

77 Lam, N.S., Yang, Y.H., Wang, L.C., Lin, Y.T. & Chiang, B.L. (2004) Clinical characteristics of childhood erythema multiforme, Stevens-Johnson syndrome and toxic epidermal necrolysis in Taiwanese children. *Journal of Microbiology, Immunology, and Infection*, **37**, 366–370.

78 Guide, S.V. & Marinkovich, M.P. (2001) Linear IgA bullous dermatosis. *Clinics in Dermatology*, **19**, 719–727.

79 Kelly, S.E., Frith, P.A., Millard, P.R., Wojnarowska, F. & Black, M.M. (1988) A clinicopathological study of mucosal involvement in linear IgA disease. *British Journal of Dermatology*, **119**, 161–170.

80 Mihai, S. & Sitaru, C. (2007) Immunopathology and molecular diagnosis of autoimmune bullous diseases. *Journal of Cellular and Molecular Medicine*, **11**, 462–481.

81 Navi, D., Michael, D.J. & Fazel, N. (2006) Drug-induced linear IgA bullous dermatosis. *Dermatology Online Journal*, **12**, 12.

82 Billet, S.E., Kortuem, K.R., Gibson, L.E. & El Azhary, R. (2008) A morbilliform variant of vancomycin-induced linear IgA bullous dermatosis. *Archives of Dermatology*, **144**, 774–778.

83 Waldman, M.A., Black, D.R. & Callen, J.P. (2004) Vancomycin-induced linear IgA bullous disease presenting as toxic epidermal necrolysis. *Clinical and Experimental Dermatology*, **29**, 633–636.

84 Patricio, P., Ferreira, C., Gomes, M.M. & Filipe, P. (2009) Autoimmune bullous dermatoses: a review. *Annals of the New York Academy of Sciences*, **1173**, 203–210.

85 Goldberg, I., Kashman, Y. & Brenner, S. (1999) The induction of pemphigus by phenol drugs. *International Journal of Dermatology*, **38**, 888–892.

86 Hodge, L., Marsden, R.A., Black, M.M., Bhogal, B. & Corbett, M.F. (1981) Bullous pemphigoid: the frequency of mucosal involvement and concurrent malignancy related to indirect immunofluorescence findings. *British Journal of Dermatology*, **105**, 65–69.

87 Lee, J.J. & Downham, T.F. (2006) Furosemide-induced bullous pemphigoid: case report and review of literature. *Journal of Drugs in Dermatology*, **5**, 562–564.

88 Bialy-Golan, A. & Brenner, S. (1996) Penicillamine-induced bullous dermatoses. *Journal of the American Academy of Dermatology*, **35**, 732–742.

89 Walsh, S.R., Hogg, D. & Mydlarski, P.R. (2005) Bullous pemphigoid: from bench to bedside. *Drugs*, **65**, 905–926.

90 Chen, K.R. & Carlson, J.A. (2008) Clinical approach to cutaneous vasculitis. *American Journal of Clinical Dermatology*, **9**, 71–92.

91 Kawakami, T. (2010) New algorithm (KAWAKAMI algorithm) to diagnose primary cutaneous vasculitis. *Journal of Dermatology*, **37**, 113–124.

92 Carlson, J.A., Cavaliere, L.F. & Grant-Kels, J.M. (2006) Cutaneous vasculitis: diagnosis and management. *Clinics in Dermatology*, **24**, 414–429.

93 Bahrami, S., Malone, J.C., Webb, K.G. & Callen, J.P. (2006) Tissue eosinophilia as an indicator of drug-induced cutaneous small-vessel vasculitis. *Archives of Dermatology*, **142**, 155–161.

94 Doyle, M.K. & Cuellar, M.L. (2003) Drug-induced vasculitis. *Expert Opinion on Drug Safety*, **2**, 401–409.

95 Kim, M.J., Kim, H.O., Kim, H.Y. & Park, Y.M. (2009) Rituximab-induced vasculitis: a case report and review of the medical published work. *Journal of Dermatology*, **36**, 284–287.

96 Torner, O., Ruber, C., Olive, A. & Tena, X. (1997) Methotrexate related cutaneous vasculitis. *Clinical Rheumatology*, **16**, 108–109.

97 Dwyer, J.M., Kenicer, K., Thompson, B.T. *et al.* (1989) Vasculitis and retinoids. *Lancet*, **2**, 494–496.

98 Cuellar, M.L. (2002) Drug-induced vasculitis. *Current Rheumatology Reports*, **4**, 55–59.

99 Gao, Y. & Zhao, M.H. (2009) Review article: drug-induced anti-neutrophil cytoplasmic antibody-associated vasculitis. *Nephrology (Carlton, Victoria)*, **14**, 33–41.

100 Sehgal, V.N., Srivastava, G. & Sardana, K. (2004) Erythroderma/exfoliative dermatitis: a synopsis. *International Journal of Dermatology*, **43**, 39–47.

101 Sigurdsson, V., Toonstra, J., Hezemans-Boer, M. & van Vloten, W.A. (1996) Erythroderma: a clinical and follow-up study of 102 patients, with special emphasis on survival. *Journal of the American Academy of Dermatology*, **35**, 53–57.

102 Botella-Estrada, R., Sanmartin, O., Oliver, V., Febrer, I. & Aliaga, A. (1994) Erythroderma: a clinicopathological study of 56 cases. *Archives of Dermatology*, **130**, 1503–1507.

103 Rothe, M.J., Bernstein, M.L. & Grant-Kels, J.M. (2005) Life-threatening erythroderma: diagnosing and treating the "red man". *Clinics in Dermatology*, **23**, 206–217.

104 Wieselthier, J.S. & Koh, H.K. (1990) Sézary syndrome: diagnosis, prognosis, and critical review of treatment options. *Journal of the American Academy of Dermatology*, **22**, 381–401.

105 Sentis, H.J., Willemze, R. & Scheffer, E. (1986) Histopathologic studies in Sézary syndrome and erythrodermic mycosis fungoides: a comparison with benign forms of erythroderma. *Journal of the American Academy of Dermatology*, **15**, 1217–1226.

106 Hasan, T. & Jansen, C.T. (1983) Erythroderma: a follow-up of fifty cases. *Journal of the American Academy of Dermatology*, **8**, 836–840.

107 Hausermann, P., Walter, R.B., Halter, J. *et al.* (2008) Cutaneous graft-versus-host disease: a guide for the dermatologist. *Dermatology (Basel, Switzerland)*, **216**, 287–304.

108 Poonawalla, T. & Kelly, B. (2009) Urticaria: a review. *American Journal of Clinical Dermatology*, **10**, 9–21.

109 Cohen, P.R. (2009) Neutrophilic dermatoses: a review of current treatment options. *American Journal of Clinical Dermatology*, **10**, 301–312.

110 Bachmeyer, C. & Aractingi, S. (2000) Neutrophilic eccrine hidradenitis. *Clinics in Dermatology*, **18**, 319–330.

111 Calista, D. (2001) Oral erosive lichen planus associated with thymoma. *International Journal of Dermatology*, **40**, 762–764.

112 Lyons, J.H., III (1987) Generalized pustular psoriasis. *International Journal of Dermatology*, **26**, 409–418.

113 Carlson, J.A. (2010) The histological assessment of cutaneous vasculitis. *Histopathology*, **56**, 3–23.

114 Lotti, T. (1994) The purpuras. *International Journal of Dermatology*, **33**, 1–10.

115 Nazarian, R.M., Van Cott, E.M., Zembowicz, A. & Duncan, L.M. (2009) Warfarin-induced skin necrosis. *Journal of the American Academy of Dermatology*, **61**, 325–332.

116 Green, J.J. & Manders, S.M. (2001) Pseudoporphyria. *Journal of the American Academy of Dermatology*, **44**, 100–108.

117 Borras-Blasco, J., Navarro-Ruiz, A., Borras, C. & Castera, E. (2009) Adverse cutaneous reactions induced by TNF-alpha antagonist therapy. *Southern Medical Journal*, **102**, 1133–1140.

118 Fry, L. & Baker, B.S. (2007) Triggering psoriasis: the role of infections and medications. *Clinics in Dermatology*, **25**, 606–615.

119 Stanley, J.R. & Amagai, M. (2006) Pemphigus, bullous impetigo, and the staphylococcal scalded-skin syndrome. *New England Journal of Medicine*, **355**, 1800–1810.

120 Chamberlain, A.J., Cooper, S.M., Allen, J. *et al.* (2004) Paraneoplastic immunobullous disease with an epidermolysis bullosa acquisita phenotype: two cases demonstrating remission with treatment of gynaecological malignancy. *Australasian Journal of Dermatology*, **45**, 136–139.

121 Brenner, S., Bialy-Golan, A. & Anhalt, G.J. (1997) Recognition of pemphigus antigens in drug-induced pemphigus vulgaris and pemphigus foliaceus. *Journal of the American Academy of Dermatology*, **36**, 919–923.

122 Maynard, B. & Peters, M.S. (1992) Histologic and immunofluorescence study of cutaneous porphyrias. *Journal of Cutaneous Pathology*, **19**, 40–47.

123 Naranjo, C.A., Busto, U., Sellers, E.M. *et al.* (1981) A method for estimating the probability of adverse drug reactions. *Clinical Pharmacology and Therapeutics*, **30**, 239–245.

124 Shear, N.H. (1990) Diagnosing cutaneous adverse reactions to drugs. *Archives of Dermatology*, **126**, 94–97.

125 Friedmann, P.S. & Ardern-Jones, M. (2010) Patch testing in drug allergy. *Current Opinion in Allergy and Clinical Immunology*, **10**, 291–296.

126 Kranke, B. & Aberer, W. (2009) Skin testing for IgE-mediated drug allergy. *Immunology and Allergy Clinics of North America*, **29**, 503–516.

127 Mayorga, C., Sanz, M.L., Gamboa, P.M. *et al.* (2010) *In vitro* diagnosis of immediate allergic reactions to drugs: an update. *Journal of Investigational Allergology and Clinical Immunology*, **20**, 103–109.

5 Grading Dermatologic Adverse Events in Clinical Trials Using CTCAE v4.0

Alice Chen[1], Asha Acharya[2] and Ann Setser[3]

[1]Cancer Therapy Evaluation Program, National Cancer Institute, Rockville, MD, USA
[2]Technical Resources International, Inc., Bethesda, MD, USA
[3]Setser Health Consulting LLC, Chesterfield, MO, USA

With the advent of newer chemotherapeutic and targeted agents over the last 10 years in oncology therapy, dermatologic toxicities has become more prevalent and a growing concern in the management of cancer patients. Assessment and management of dermatologic toxicities has become an important part of oncology care requiring collaboration between oncologists, dermatologists, and internists. This partnership requires an accurate catalog and grading of dermatologic adverse events (AEs) for effective communication, better delivery of agents, interagent comparisons, and appropriate supportive measures.

The International Conference on Harmonization of Technical Requirements for Registration of Pharmaceutical for Human Use's E2C Guideline defines adverse drug reaction (ADR) based on preapproval and postmarketing setting as follows:

In the *pre-approval clinical experience* with a new medicinal product or its new usages, particularly as the therapeutic dose(s) may not be established: all noxious and unintended responses to a medicinal product related to any dose should be considered adverse drug reactions. The phrase "responses to a medicinal products" means that a causal relationship between a medicinal product and an adverse event is at least a reasonable possibility, i.e., the relationship cannot be ruled out.

Regarding *marketed medicinal products*, a well-accepted definition of an adverse drug reaction in the post-marketing setting is found in WHO Technical Report 498 [1972] and reads as follows: A response to a drug which is noxious and unintended and which occurs at doses normally used in man for prophylaxis, diagnosis, or therapy of disease or for modification of physiological function.

The old term "side effect" has been used in various ways in the past, usually to describe negative (unfavorable) effects, but also positive (favorable) effects. It is recommended that this term no longer be used and particularly should not be regarded as synonymous with adverse event or adverse reaction [1].

The most widely used severity grading scale, the National Cancer Institute's (NCI) Common Terminology Criteria for Adverse Events (CTCAE) is a descriptive terminology that can be utilized for AE reporting. An AE is a term that is a unique representation of a specific event used for medical documentation and scientific analyses. A grading (severity) scale is provided for each AE term. Each CTCAE v4.0 AE term is a Medical Dictionary for Regulatory Activities (MedDRA) Lowest Level Term (LLT).

The NCI CTCAE v3.0 predated the wide use of epidermal growth factor receptor (EGFR) inhibitors and other targeted agents, and was inadequate for reporting type and grade of dermatologic AEs seen in recent years. This potentiated underreporting, inconsistent and inaccurate grading of distinctive dermatologic AEs. The Multinational Association of Supportive Care in Cancer (MASCC) Skin Toxicity Study Group [2] proposed a new tool, the MASCC EGFRI Skin Toxicity Tool (MESTT), for grading the dermatologic toxicities seen with EGFR inhibitors. The Skin and Subcutaneous Tissue Disorders Working Group used this as a guide during the CTCAE v4.0 revision in 2009 [3].

Common Terminology Criteria for Adverse Events

The purpose of the CTCAE is to provide standards for the description and exchange of safety information in oncology research. It comprised a list of AE terms commonly encountered in oncology therapeutic trials, accompanied by a severity grading scale for each AE. It is used to define protocol parameters (such as maximum tolerated dose and dose-limiting toxicity), to provide eligibility assessments, and to guide dose modification during the conduct of a clinical trial. The CTCAE facilitates the evaluation

Dermatologic Principles and Practice in Oncology: Conditions of the Skin, Hair, and Nails in Cancer Patients, First Edition. Edited by Mario E. Lacouture.
© 2014 John Wiley & Sons, Inc. Published 2014 by John Wiley & Sons, Inc.

of new cancer therapies and treatment modalities, and the comparison of safety profiles between interventions. Since its inception, the objective of the CTCAE is to standardize AE reporting within the NCI oncology research community, across trials, groups, and modalities. The CTCAE lists AE terms for signs, symptoms, and abnormal diagnostic tests seen in oncology interventions. Each AE term is associated with a five-point grading scale to measure severity of clinical findings. The grading scale provides consistency and guidance for documentation of AEs, and provides a framework to compare AEs across interventions and studies.

In 2007, CTCAE v3.0 was evaluated as a standard terminology within the NCI Cancer Biomedical Informatics Grid® (caBIG®) initiative. CaBIG® is an open-source open-access information network enabling cancer researchers to share tools, data, applications, and technologies according to agreed-upon standards and identified needs. Recommendations for changes to the CTCAE v3.0 were made to maximize compliance with vocabulary standards. Cancer Therapy Evaluation Program (CTEP) and Center for Biomedical Informatics and Information Technology (CBIIT) organized a CTCAE revision project involving participants from the oncology community with multidisciplinary domain expertise. The NCI Enterprise Vocabulary Services helped provided a definition for each term. One of the goals of the revision is to convert CTCAE to allow for greater compliance with vocabulary standards.

In May 2009, CTCAE v4.0 was published [3]. The major change in this version is that each CTCAE term is a MedDRA term. MedDRA is a clinically validated dictionary used internationally by regulatory authorities and the regulated biopharmaceutical industry throughout the entire medical terminology regulatory process, from premarketing to postmarketing activities, for data entry, retrieval, evaluation, and presentation. The MedDRA dictionary is organized by System Organ Class (SOC) divided into High Level Group Terms (HLGT), High Level Terms (HLT), Preferred Terms (PT), and finally into Lower Level Terms (LLT). MedDRA does not provide severity grading of the terms. It is the AE classification dictionary endorsed by the International Conference on Harmonisation of Technical Requirements for Registration of Pharmaceuticals for Human Use (ICH). MedDRA is used in the United States, the European Union, and Japan. Europe and Japan currently mandates its use for safety reporting.

CTCAE grade scale

The importance of CTCAE is its severity grading scale and focus on adverse drug reactions seen with oncology drugs. MedDRA is a list of terms that does not differentiate between normal physiologic events (puberty) and adverse drug reactions (diarrhea). MedDRA provides no scale of severity. A serious AE is any untoward medical occurrence that at any dose results in death or is life threatening. The term "life threatening" in the definition of "serious" refers to an event in which the patient was

at risk of death at the time of the event; it does not refer to an event that hypothetically might have caused death if it were more severe. For example, a serious AE is that which requires inpatient hospitalization or prolongation of existing hospitalization, or results in persistent or significant disability/incapacity. The terms "severe" and "serious" are not synonymous. "Severe" is often used to describe the intensity (severity) of a specific event (as in mild, moderate, or severe rash); the event itself, however, may be of relatively minor medical significance (such as alopecia). This is not the same as "serious," which is based on patient/event outcome or action criteria usually associated with events that pose a threat to a patient's life or functioning. Seriousness (not severity) serves as a guide for defining regulatory reporting obligations. CTCAE uses a template of general characteristics for each grade providing the foundation for unique severity criterion for each CTCAE AE term (Table 5.1).

Attribution

An attribution is an assessment of whether an AE is likely caused by the agent(s) being tested. When assessing whether an AE is related to a medical treatment or procedure, the following attribution categories are utilized by CTEP NCI for assessment of AEs (Table 5.2).

Changes in CTCAE V4.0

Some changes result from the conversion of all CTCAE v3.0 terms to single MedDRA terms. Significant changes to CTCAE v4.0 dermatologic AEs grading scales are the inclusion of the percentage of body surface area (BSA) (Figure 5.1) involvement as a major discriminating factor between grades and the inclusion of psychosocial impact on the patient. New terms were also added to provide more accurate description of the toxicities that used to be reported as "CTCAE other, specify." "CTCAE other, specify" had remained, although is not a MedDRA term, to allow unknown AEs to be reported (e.g., hypertrichosis as seen with the EGFR inhibitors). In CTCAE v3.0, AEs are grouped by categories. In CTCAE v4.0, AEs are grouped by MedDRA Primary SOC. The SOCs are the highest level of the MedDRA hierarchy and are identified by anatomic or physiologic system, etiology, or purpose (e.g., SOC Investigations for laboratory test results). CTCAE terms are grouped by MedDRA Primary SOCs. Within each SOC, AEs are listed and accompanied by descriptions of severity (grade).

Refined grading to correlate with clinical management

Some CTCAE v3.0 AE grading descriptors are very brief. As dermatologic toxicities are seen more frequently and are becoming more of a clinical management issue requiring change in therapy dose, grading criteria were expanded on many of the CTCAE v4.0

Table 5.1 General characteristics of Common Terminology Criteria for Adverse Events (CTCAE) grading scale.

Grade	General characteristics
1. Mild	Minor; no specific medical intervention indicated; asymptomatic laboratory finding only; radiographic finding only; marginal clinical relevance; mild symptoms and intervention not indicated; non-prescription intervention indicated
2. Moderate	Intervention indicated; minimal, local, noninvasive intervention indicated; limiting instrumental ADL. Though many of the dermatologic manifestations have little clinical significance, they cause significant psychosocial impact to the patients. AEs that could cause significant psychosocial impact to the patient are graded as 2
3. Severe	Medically significant but not life-threatening; impatient or prolongation of hospitalization indicated; important medical events that do not result in hospitalization but may jeopardize the participant or may require intervention either to prevent hospitalization or to prevent the event from becoming life-threatening or potentially resulting in death; limiting basic self care ADL; disabling resulting in persistent or significant disability or incapacity*
4. Life-threatening	Life-threatening consequences; urgent intervention indicated; urgent operative intervention indicated; participant is at risk of death at time of event if immediate intervention is not undertaken
5	Death related to AE

ADL, activities of daily living; AE, adverse event.
*Disabling was a descriptor for Grade 4 in CTCAE v3.0. A semicolon indicates "or" within the description of the grade. Instrumental ADL refers to a higher functioning level such as preparing meals, shopping for groceries or clothes, using the telephone, or managing money. Self-care ADL refers to basic dialy function like bathing, dressing and undressing, feeding self, using the toilet, or taking medications. Not all grades are appropriate for all AEs. Therefore, some AEs are listed with fewer than five options for grade selection.

Table 5.2 Attribution categories to agent.

Definite	The adverse event is *clearly related* to the agent(s)
Probable	The adverse event is *likely related* to the agent(s)
Possible	The adverse event *may be related* to the agent(s)
Unlikely	The adverse event is *doubtfully related* to the agent(s)
Unrelated	The adverse event is *clearly NOT related* to the agent(s). Requires documentation of other causes

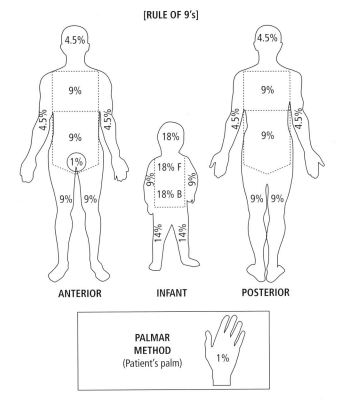

dermatologic AEs (see Appendix 5.1). Some examples are alopecia, rash acneiform, and skin hyperpigmentation.

Alopecia

Alopecia was the most common dermatologic toxicity seen with chemotherapy before the wide use of targeted therapies. The degree of hair loss varies according to the agent(s), route of administration, dosage, and schedule of administration per regimen. In a review by Koo *et al.* [4], regimens with the highest incidence of complete alopecia included the following: epirubicin + paclitaxel (100%), doxorubicin + cyclophosphamide (50–96%), epirubicin + verapamil (75%), docetaxel (74%), doxorubicin + cyclophosphamide + vincristine (72%), and doxorubicin (61–70%). Despite active research, only AS101 and minoxidil were able to reduce the severity or shorten the duration of chemotherapy-induced alopecia (CIA) but could not prevent CIA [5]. The CTCAE v4.0 defined alopecia as a "disorder characterized by a decrease in density of hair compared to normal

Figure 5.1 Body surface area calculation using the rule of 9's (commonly used to assess percentage of involvement and to help guide treatment decisions in burn patients). Head 9%; chest (front) 9%; abdomen (front) 9%; upper/mid/low back and buttocks 18%; each arm 9%; each palm 1%; groin 1%; each leg 18% total (front 9%, back 9%).

for a given individual at a given age and body location" [3]. In CTCAE v3.0, differentiation between Grade 1 and 2 was very subjective (see Appendix 5.1). In CTCAE v4.0, objective measurement of the lost of normal hair was used to determine severity. Taking into account that alopecia, although not clinically significant, has psychosocial impact for many patients, if this exists it will be graded as Grade 2 in terms of severity.

Rash acneiform

Acneiform-like rash is a common AE induced by the agents that target the human EGFR such as erlotinib [6,7], afatinib, cetuximab, panitumumab [8,9], and sorafenib [10]. Accurate assessment of the severity (grade) of the rash allows for management of the rash and oncologic therapy. This is a "disorder characterized by an eruption of papules and pustules, typically appearing in face, scalp, upper chest and back." The CTCAE v3.0 term was Rash: acne/acneiform; the grading for this AE changed significantly. In CTCAE v3.0, Grades 1 and 2 were determined by the need for intervention. If there were serious symptoms regardless of degree or amount of skin involved, it would be graded as Grade 3, which could result in alteration of dosing in a clinical trial. In CTCAE v4.0, the percentage of BSA involved determines the grade, providing a degree of clinical significance. Also, if the acneiform rash affects the higher level function (instrumental activities of daily living (ADL)), the rash is considered moderately severe and is graded as Grade 2. To be more clinically relevant, Grade 3 is >30% BSA involvement or the presence of infection. This requires holding the investigational agent and dose reduction at the resumption of treatment. Grade 4 was added in CTCAE v4.0, using the generic definition if the toxicity leads to "life-threatening consequences" [3]. Grade 4 also includes "superinfection with IV antibiotics indicated."

Skin hyperpigmentation

This is defined as a "disorder characterized by darkening of the skin due to excessive melanin deposition" [3]. In CTCAE v3.0, the degree of darkening was used for grading. As hyperpigmentation is largely cosmetic and its effects psychologic, in CTCAE v4.0, the "% of BSA involved" and the psychosocial impact was taken into consideration for grading. This toxicity should not lead to withholding agent or dose reduction; this toxicity could only be graded as 1 or 2.

Split of embedded terms

To better distinguish severity indicators from clinical findings, some terms previously embedded within descriptions of grade for a single CTCAE v3.0 term were listed as unique CTCAE v4.0 terms and associated with severity scales specific to the finding (Table 5.3). Examples include Rash/Desquamation in CTCAE v3.0 split into three CTCAE v4.0 terms: Rash maculo-papular; Erythroderma; and Bullous dermatitis; and CTCAE v3.0's Nail changes are split into three CTCAE v4.0 terms: Nail discoloration, Nail ridging, and Nail loss.

Rash maculopapular

Among rashes, maculo-papular rash was found to be the most common AE caused by vemurafenib, everolimus, temsirolimus [11], and sorafenib [12]. The term "Rash maculo-papular" is an exact wording of a MedDRA term. This is a "disorder characterized by the presence of macules (flat) and papules (elevated). Also, known as morbilliform rash, it is one of the most common cutaneous AEs, frequently affecting the upper trunk, spreading centripetally and associated with pruritus" [3]. In CTCAE v3.0, symptoms were used to distinguish Grade 1 and 2. Desquamation involving percentage of BSA (< or ≥50% BSA) was used to distinguish Grades 2 and 3. In version CTCAE 4.0, the percentage of BSA involvement is used to distinguish Grades 1–3. In addition, Grades 2 and 3 again incorporate ADLs to distinguish between the two grades. Lastly, it was felt this rash does not lead to life-threatening condition or death so Grades 4 and 5 are removed.

Erythroderma

A variety of drugs and malignancies, including solid tumors and lymphoproliferative diseases, can cause erythroderma. Among the malignancies, cutaneous T-cell lymphoma is the most common cause of erythroderma. In cases of paraneoplastic erythroderma, the cutaneous finding of erythroderma may occur as the only symptom of a malignancy. Erythema and exfoliative dermatitis are some of the most common dermatologic AEs of sorafenib, used in treatment of metastatic renal cell carcinoma and hepatocellular carcinoma [13]. Polyzos et al. [14] have reported patients manifesting diffuse erythroderma within minutes of infusion with oxaliplatin. This is a new term in CTCAE v4.0.defined as "a disorder characterized by generalized inflammatory erythema and exfoliation. The inflammatory process involves >90% of the body surface area" [3]. Since, by definition, >90% of BSA had to be involved, percentage of involvement is not used to assist with the grading. Instead, symptoms and ability to perform ADL is used to distinguish between Grades 2 and 3. Grade 4 requires intensive care unit or burn unit admission due to life-threatening nature of the toxicity.

Bullous dermatitis

Bullous dermatitis is another new AE term added to CTCAE v4.0. It is "a disorder characterized by inflammation of the skin characterized by the presence of bullae which are filled with fluid" [3]. It allows for Grade 1 blistering that may not be of clinical significance by the amount of involvement. If the location causes any change in the ability of the patient to function, the grade would increase depending on the limitation of function to Grade 2 or 3. In addition, percentage of BSA involvement is used to help describe severity and possibly change management. Oteri et. al. [15] have reported a case of bullous dermatitis induced by the EGFR inhibitor erlotinib.

Table 5.3 Split and embedded terms.

CTCAE Version	AE Term	Grade 1	Grade 2	Grade 3	Grade 4	Grade 5
3.0	Rash/desquamation	Macular or papular eruption or erythema without associated symptoms	Macular or papular eruption or erythema with pruritus or other associated symptoms; localized desquamation or other lesions covering <50% of BSA	Severe, generalized erythroderma or macular, papular or vesicular eruption; desquamation covering ≥50% BSA	Generalized exfoliative, ulcerative, or bullous dermatitis	Death
4.0	Rash maculo-papular	Macules/papules covering <10% BSA with or without symptoms (e.g., pruritus, burning, tightness)	Macules/papules covering 10–30% BSA with or without symptoms (e.g., pruritus, burning, tightness); limiting instrumental ADL	Macules/papules covering >30% BSA with or without associated symptoms; limiting self-care ADL	–	–
4.0	Erythroderma	–	Erythema covering >90% BSA without associated symptoms; limiting instrumental ADL	Erythema covering >90% BSA with associated symptoms (e.g., pruritus or tenderness); limiting self-care ADL	Erythema covering >90% BSA with associated fluid or electrolyte abnormalities; ICU care or burn unit indicated	Death
4.0	Bullous dermatitis	Asymptomatic; blisters covering <10% BSA	Blisters covering 10–30% BSA; painful blisters; limiting instrumental ADL	Blisters covering >30% BSA; limiting self-care ADL	Blisters covering >30% BSA; associated with fluid or electrolyte abnormalities; ICU care or burn unit indicated	Death
3.0	Nail changes	Discoloration; ridging (koilonychias); pitting	Partial or complete loss of nail(s); pain in nailbed(s)	Interfering with ADL	–	–
4.0	Nail discoloration	Asymptomatic; clinical or diagnostic observations only; intervention not indicated	–	–	–	–
4.0	Nail ridging	Asymptomatic; clinical or diagnostic observations only; intervention not indicated	–	–	–	–
4.0	Nail loss	Asymptomatic separation of the nail bed from the nail plate or nail loss	Symptomatic separation of the nail bed from the nail plate or nail loss; limiting instrumental ADL	–	–	–

ADL, activities of daily living; BSA, body surface area.

Nail discoloration, nail ridging, and nail loss

These three terms are split from Nail changes in CTCAE v3.0. It was felt that these are unique changes with different clinical significance. Nail discoloration and ridging are mild AEs and do not require any changes in drug treatment. However, patients notice these changes so it is important to document in clinical trials to alleviate patients' concerns. Nail loss could impair higher level of function (instrumental ADL); therefore, Grade 2 descriptor is provided. This is especially relevant in the Accelerated Titration Design Phase I trials [16] in which an attributed Grade 2 AE changes the accelerated titration escalation (100%) to a standard Fibonacci escalation.

New adverse events

Skin and subcutaneous tissue clinical findings recently identified with targeted therapy resulted in the addition of terms to CTCAE never before listed. With the wider use of CTCAE outside of the oncology field, some AEs were added to provide for this wider use (see Appendix 5.2).

Hypertrichosis

Hypertrichosis is a "disorder characterized by hair density or length beyond the accepted limits of normal in a particular body region, for a particular age or race" [3]. Hypertrichosis of the face and eyelash trichomegaly has been encountered after treatment with cetuximab [17], erlotinib [18–20], panitumumab, and gefitinib [21]. Treatment involves waxing, laser treatments, or trimming of the eyelashes. Due to relationship to these targeted agents, this AE was added to CTCAE v4.0. Because this disorder does not lead to severe or life-threatening conditions or death, hypertrichosis cannot be graded as Grades 3–5. The difference between Grades 1 and 2 largely depend on the rate of hair growth and the ability for the patient to manage the hair growth. In addition, any significant psychosocial impact would be graded as Grade 2.

Hypohidrosis

Hypohidrosis is defined as a "disorder characterized by reduced sweating" [3]. This toxicity has been seen with antimuscarinic anticholinergic agents, EGFR inhibitors, carbonic anhydrase inhibitors, and tricyclic antidepressants. As it is a significant AE reported with therapeutic agents, it was added to CTCAE v4.0. Because this condition can lead to life-threatening conditions and possibly death, Grades 2–5 descriptions are provided. Hypohidrosis from drug therapy leading to heat stroke would be Grade 4.

Lipohypertrophy

Lipohypertrophy is a "disorder characterized by hypertrophy of the subcutaneous adipose tissue usually at the site of multiple subcutaneous injections like insulin" [3]. The percentage of BSA

is used to differentiate between grades. The other difference is if it limits the daily function and the need for medications to manage pain. This condition could not lead to life-threatening condition or death so Grades 4 or 5 are not possible.

Periorbital edema

Periorbital edema is defined as a "disorder characterized by swelling due to an excessive accumulation of fluid around the orbits of the face" [3]. It is commonly seen with multikinase inhibitors including imatinib, dasatinib, and nilotinib. Grade 1 does not require any intervention; Grade 2 requires only topical intervention. If the condition is severe enough to require operative intervention, it is graded as Grade 3.

Moved to different SOC

In CTCAE v3.0, AEs are grouped by CTCAE v3.0 categories. In CTCAE v4.0, MedDRA SOC organizes the terms and their placement is dictated by the placement of that term in MedDRA's Primary SOC. CTCAE v4 has 26 SOCs. Some skin conditions that are associated with infection are listed in the Infection SOC (Table 5.4 and Table 5.5) in CTCAE v4.0.

Papulopustular rash

Papulopustular rash occurs in the majority (45–100%) of patients receiving EGFR inhibitors [22]. In most cases, it is mild, transient, and well tolerated, but in 8–12% of patients it may be sufficiently severe and persistent to necessitate intervention. Given the increasing use of these agents and the occurrence of this toxicity, papulopustular rash was added to CTCAE v4.0 under the Infection SOC. It is defined as a "disorder characterized by an eruption consisting of papules (a small, raised pimple) and pustules (a small pus filled blister), typically appearing in face, scalp, and upper chest and back unlike acne, this rash does not present with whiteheads or blackheads, and can be symptomatic, with itchy or tender lesions" [3]. The percentage of involvement regardless of symptoms of pruritus or tenderness provided differentiation of Grades 1–3. Other differentiating criteria include presence of psychosocial impact or limitation of daily function. If superinfection were present, the AE would be graded as 3 or 4 depending on the need for IV antibiotics.

Rash pustular

A pustular rash is "characterized by a circumscribed and elevated skin lesion filled with pus" [3]. These lesions vary greatly in size and shape and can be generalized or localized to the hair follicles or sweat glands. Severe pustular eruption have been associated with imatinib and voriconazole during treatment of chronic myeloid leukemia [23]. There are two grades for this AE because this could not lead to life-threatening condition or death without another cause (i.e., systemic infection) being present. The major difference between the grades is the use of oral or IV antibiotics.

Table 5.4 Skin adverse events listed under Infection System Organ Class.

CTCAE v4.0 AE Term	Grade 1	Grade 2	Grade 3	Grade 4	Grade 5
Papulopustular rash	Papules and/or pustules covering <10% BSA, which may or may not be associated with symptoms of pruritus or tenderness	Papules and/or pustules covering 10–30% BSA, which may or may not be associated with symptoms of pruritus or tenderness; associated with psychosocial impact; limiting instrumental ADL	Papules and/or pustules covering >30% BSA, which may or may not be associated with symptoms of pruritus or tenderness; limiting self-care ADL; associated with local superinfection with oral antibiotics indicated	Papules and/or pustules covering any % BSA, which may or may not be associated with symptoms of pruritus or tenderness and are associated with extensive superinfection with IV antibiotics indicated; life-threatening consequences	Death
Rash pustular	–	Localized; local intervention indicated (e.g., topical antibiotic, antifungal, or antiviral)	IV antibiotic, antifungal, or antiviral intervention indicated; radiologic or operative intervention indicated	–	–
Paronychia	Nail fold edema or erythema; disruption of the cuticle	Localized intervention indicated; oral intervention indicated (e.g., antibiotic, antifungal, antiviral); nail fold edema or erythema with pain; associated with discharge or nail plate separation; limiting instrumental ADL	Surgical intervention or IV antibiotics indicated; limiting self care ADL	–	–

Table 5.5 Skin adverse events listed under Injury, Poisoning, and Procedural Complications.

CTCAE v4.0 AE Term	Grade 1	Grade 2	Grade 3	Grade 4	Grade 5
Dermatitis radiation	Faint erythema or dry desquamation	Moderate to brisk erythema; patchy moist desquamation, mostly confined to skin folds and creases; moderate edema	Moist desquamation in areas other than skin folds and creases; bleeding induced by minor trauma or abrasion	Life-threatening consequences; skin necrosis or ulceration of full thickness dermis; spontaneous bleeding from involved site; skin graft indicated	Death
Injection site reaction	Tenderness with or without associated symptoms (e.g., warmth, erythema, itching)	Pain; lipodystrophy; edema; phlebitis	Ulceration or necrosis; severe tissue damage; operative intervention indicated	Life-threatening consequences; urgent intervention indicated	Death

Paronychia

This is "characterized by an infectious process involving the soft tissues around the nail" [3]. The intervention indicated defines the three grades (none, surgical, or IV antibiotics). Again, the ability to perform instrumental or self-care ADLs also provides the differentiation between Grades 2 and 3. This is a local condition and the condition itself could not lead to life-threatening condition or death so could not be graded as 4 or 5.

CTCAE vs. MESTT

A study was designed to assess the correlation between the severity grading of the dermatologic toxicities associated with tyrosine kinase inhibitors (TKIs) using the NCI CTCAE v4.0 and the MESTT [24]. One hundred patients were interviewed at the National Cancer Centre Singapore with the criteria of being treated with erlotinib, gefitinib, lapatinib, sorafenib, or sunitinib for 2 weeks and had experienced some degree of dermatologic toxicity. Dermatologic toxicities are graded using CTCAE and MESTT, respectively, by a single observer. Eighty-five percent experienced xerosis, 72% had pruritus, 65% had papulopustular rash, 33% experienced nail changes, and 24% had alopecia. Good correlation was observed between the scales, but there is a tendency for the MESTT to report higher toxicity grades for rash, xerosis, and paronychia.

Conclusions

Many novel therapies focus on new targets. New targeted therapies results in new toxicities not previously seen with the older chemotherapeutic agents. One of the more common toxicities seen with the targeted agents involved the skin, hair, and nails. Recently, the MASCC Skin Toxicity Study Group published proposed EGFR inhibitor dermatologic AE-specific grading scale [2]. This grading system is used to assist with the revision of dermatologic AEs listed in the CTCAE v4.0. Addition of new AEs accommodate for new toxicities seen with the targeted agents. Some toxicity in CTCAE v3.0 was split to better define a number of distinct rashes. In addition, the grading system was updated to reflect the newer management of these toxicities. An attempt was made to grade for more clinical and management relevance. These grading criteria, developed by the working groups, are taken into consideration as this grading leads to management, changes in dose, or withdrawal of agents. Significant attention was focused on the delineation of Grades 2 and 3 because the management of these two grades in phase I trials usually means holding the agent and dose reduction in future dosing. As new agents come into development, new toxicities will appear. CTCAE now has a governance group that will determine if there is a need for next revision. In addition, with wider use of CTCAE v4.0, additional revisions will become obvious. Recommendations are always welcome and may be submitted to ncictcaehelp@mail.nih.gov. This is important because the changes for CTCAE v5 will be partially driven by the recommendations received. Complete lists of the CTCAE v4.0 AEs can be found at http://evs.nci.nih.gov/ftp1/CTCAE/About.html.

References

1 ICH (2003) Internation Conference of Harmonisation of Technical Requirements for Requirements for registration of pharmaceuticals for Human Use: ICH harmonised tripartite guideline post-approval safety data management: definitions and standards for expedited reporting E2D, Current Step 4 version, dated 12 November 2003.

2 Lacouture, M.E., Maitland, M.L., Segaert, S. *et al.* (2010) A proposed EGFR inhibitor dermatologic adverse event-specific grading scale from the MASCC skin toxicity study group. *Supportive Care in Cancer*, **18**, 509–522.

3 Common Terminology Criteria for Adverse Events (CTCAE) Version 4.0 (2009) Available from: http://www.acrin.org/Portals/0/Administration/Regulatory/CTCAE_4.02_2009-09-15_Quick Reference_5x7.pdf (accessed 25 April 2013).

4 Koo, L.C., Davis, S.T., Suttle, A.B. *et al.* (2002) Incidence of chemotherapy-induced alopecia by chemotherapy regimen: a review of published randomized trials. *Proceedings of the American Society for Clinical Oncology*, **21**, 2876.

5 Wang, J., Lu, Z. & Au, J.L. (2006) Protection against chemotherapy-induced alopecia. *Pharmaceutical Research*, **23**, 2505–2514.

6 Saif, M.W., Merikas, I., Tsimboukis, S. & Syrigos, K. (2008) Erlotinib-induced skin rash. Pathogenesis, clinical significance and management in pancreatic cancer patients. *Journal of the Pancreas*, **9**, 267–274.

7 Tsimboukis, S., Merikas, I., Karapanagiotou, E.M. *et al.* (2009) Erlotinib-induced skin rash in patients with non-small-cell lung cancer: pathogenesis, clinical significance, and management. *Clinical Lung Cancer*, **10**, 106–111.

8 Mydin, A.R. & Armstrong, J.G. (2007) Acneiform rash secondary to cetuximab plus head and neck radiotherapy. *Radiotherapy and Oncology*, **85**, 171.

9 Tomkova, H., Kohoutek, M., Zabojnikova, M. *et al.* (2010) Cetuximab-induced cutaneous toxicity. *Journal of the European Academy of Dermatology and Venereology*, **24**, 692–696.

10 Fleta-Asin, B., Vano-Galvan, S., Ledo-Rodriguez, A. *et al.* (2009) Facial acneiform rash associated with sorafenib. *Dermatology Online Journal*, **15**, 7.

11 Buckner, J.C., Forouzesh, B., Erlichman, C. *et al.* (2010) Phase I, pharmacokinetic study of temsirolimus administered orally to patients with advanced cancer. *Investigational New Drugs*, **28**, 334–342.

12 Escudier, B., Eisen, T., Stadler, W.M. *et al.* (2007) Sorafenib in advanced clear-cell renal-cell carcinoma. *New England Journal of Medicine*, **356**, 125–134.

13 Bilac, C., Muezzinoglu, T., Ermertcan, A.T. *et al.* (2009) Sorafenib-induced erythema multiforme in metastatic renal cell carcinoma. *Cutaneous and Ocular Toxicology*, **28**, 90–92.

14 Polyzos, A., Tsavaris, N., Gogas, H. *et al.* (2009) Clinical features of hypersensitivity reactions to oxaliplatin: a 10-year experience. *Oncology*, **76**, 36–41.

15 Oteri, A., Cattaneo, M.T., Filipazzi, V. *et al.* (2009) A case of bullous dermatitis induced by erlotinib. *The Oncologist*, **14**, 1201–1204.

16 Simon, R., Freidlin, B., Ruinstein, L. *et al.* (1997) Accelerated titration designs for phase I clinical trials in oncology. *Journal of the National Cancer Institute*, **89**, 1138–1147.

17 Bouche, O., Brixi-Benmansour, H., Bertin, A. *et al.* (2005) Trichomegaly of the eyelashes following treatment with cetuximab. *Annals of Oncology*, **16**, 1711–1712.

18 Carser, J.E. & Summers, Y.J. (2006) Trichomegaly of the eyelashes after treatment with erlotinib in non-small cell lung cancer. *Journal of Thoracic Oncology*, **1**, 1040–1041.

19 Lane, K. & Goldstein, S.M. (2007) Erlotinib-associated trichomegaly. *Ophthalmic Plastic and Reconstructive Surgery*, **23**, 65–66.

20 Vergou, T., Stratigos, A.J., Karapanagiotou, E.M. *et al.* (2010) Facial hypertrichosis and trichomegaly developing in patients treated with the epidermal growth factor receptor inhibitor erlotinib. *Journal of the American Academy of Dermatology*, **63**, e56–e58.

21 Pascual, J.C., Banuls, J., Belinchon, I. *et al.* (2004) Trichomegaly following treatment with gefitinib (ZD1839). *British Journal of Dermatology*, **151**, 1111–1112.

22 Li, T. & Perez-Soler, R. (2009) Skin toxicities associated with epidermal growth factor receptor inhibitors. *Targeted Oncology*, **4**, 107–119.

23 Gambillara, E., Laffitte, E., Widmer, N. *et al.* (2005) Severe pustular eruption associated with imatinib and voriconazole in a patient with chronic myeloid leukemia. *Dermatology (Basel, Switzerland)*, **211**, 363–365.

24 Chan, A. & Tan, E.H. (2011) How well does the MESTT correlate with CTCAE scale for the grading of dermatological toxicities associated with oral tyrosine kinase inhibitors? *Supportive Care in Cancer*, **19**, 1667–1674.

Appendix 5.1 Refined grading to correlate with clinical presentation and management.

CTCAE Version	AE Term	Grade 1	Grade 2	Grade 3	Grade 4	Grade 5
3.0	Hair loss/alopecia (scalp or body)	Thinning or patchy	Complete	–	–	–
4.0	Alopecia	Hair loss of <50% of normal for that individual that is not obvious from a distance but only on close inspection; a different hair style may be required to cover the hair loss but it does not require a wig or hair piece to camouflage	Hair loss of ≥50% normal for that individual that is readily apparent to others; a wig or hair piece is necessary if the patient desires to completely camouflage the hair loss; associated with psychosocial impact	–	–	–
3.0	Rash: acne/acneiform	Intervention not indicated	Intervention indicated	Associated with pain, disfigurement, ulceration, or desquamation	–	Death
4.0	Rash acneiform	Papules and/or pustules covering <10% BSA, which may or may not be associated with symptoms of pruritus or tenderness	Papules and/or pustules covering 10–30% BSA, which may or may not be associated with symptoms of pruritus or tenderness; associated with psychosocial impact; limiting instrumental ADL	Papules and/or pustules covering >30% BSA, which may or may not be associated with symptoms of pruritus or tenderness; limiting self-care ADL; associated with local superinfection with oral antibiotics indicated	Papules and/or pustules covering any % BSA, which may or may not be associated with symptoms of pruritus or tenderness and are associated with extensive superinfection with IV antibiotics indicated; life-threatening consequences	Death
3.0	Hyperpigmentation	Slight or localized	Marked or generalized	–	–	–
3.0	Telangiectasias	Few	Moderate number	Many and confluent	–	–
4.0	Telangiectasias	Telangiectasias covering <10% BSA	Telangiectasias covering >10% BSA; associated with psychosocial impact	–	–	–
3.0	Induration/fibrosis	Increased density on palpation	Moderate impairment of function not interfering with ADL; marked increase in density and firmness on palpation with or without minimal retraction	Dysfunction interfering with ADL; very marked density, retraction or fixation	–	–

(Continued)

CTCAE Version	AE Term	Grade 1	Grade 2	Grade 3	Grade 4	Grade 5
4.0	Fat atrophy *and* skin atrophy	Covering <10% BSA and asymptomatic	Covering 10–30% BSA and associated with erythema or tenderness; limiting instrumental ADL	Covering >30% BSA; associated with erythema or tenderness; limiting self-care ADL	–	–
3.0	Rash: Hand-foot syndrome	Minimal skin changes or dermatitis (e.g., erythema) without pain	Skin changes (e.g., peeling, blisters, bleeding, edema) or pain, not interfering with function	Ulcerative dermatitis or skin changes with pain interfering with function	–	–
4.0	Palmar-plantar erythrodysesthesia syndrome	Minimal skin changes or dermatitis (e.g., erythema, edema, or hyperkeratosi) without pain	Skin changes (e.g., peeling, blisters, bleeding, edema, or hyperkeratosis) with pain; limiting instrumental ADL	Severe skin changes (e.g., peeling, blisters, bleeding, edema, or hyperkeratosis) with pain; limiting self-care ADL	–	–
3.0	Skin breakdown/ decubitus ulcer *and* Ulceration	–	Local wound care; medical intervention indicated	Operative debridement or other invasive intervention indicated (e.g., hyperbaric oxygen)	Life-threatening consequences; major invasive intervention indicated (e.g., tissue reconstruction, flap, or grafting)	–
4.0	Skin Ulceration	Combined area of ulcers <1 cm; nonblanchable erythema of intact skin with associated warmth or edema	Combined area of ulcers 1–2 cm; partial thickness skin loss involving skin or subcutaneous fat	Combined area of ulcers >2 cm; full-thickness skin loss involving damage to or necrosis of subcutaneous tissue that may extend down to fascia	Any size ulcer with extensive destruction, tissue necrosis, or damage to muscle, bone, or supporting structures with or without full thickness skin loss	Death
4.0	Skin hyperpigmentation	Hyperpigmentation covering <10% BSA; no psychosocial impact	Hyperpigmentation covering >10% BSA; associated psychosocial impact	–	–	–
3.0	Hypopigmentation	Slight or localized	Marked or generalized	–	–	–
4.0	Skin Hypopigmentation	Hypopigmentation or depigmentation covering <10% BSA; no psychosocial impact	Hypopigmentation or depigmentation covering >10% BSA; associated psychosocial impact	–	–	–
3.0	Urticaria	Intervention not indicated	Intervention indicated for <24 h	Intervention indicated for ≥24 h	–	–
4.0	Skin urticaria	Combined area of ulcers <1 cm; nonblanchable erythema of intact skin with associated warmth or edema	Combined area of ulcers 1–2 cm; partial thickness skin loss involving skin or subcutaneous fat	Combined area of ulcers >2 cm; full-thickness skin loss involving damage to or necrosis of subcutaneous tissue that may extend down to fascia	Any size ulcer with extensive destruction, tissue necrosis, or damage to muscle, bone, or supporting structures with or without full thickness skin loss	Death
3.0	Bruising	Localized or in a dependent area	Generalized	–	–	–

CTCAE Version	AE Term	Grade 1	Grade 2	Grade 3	Grade 4	Grade 5
4.0	Purpura	Combined area of lesions covering <10% BSA	Combined area of lesions covering 10–30% BSA; bleeding with trauma	Combined area of lesions covering >30% BSA; spontaneous bleeding	–	–
3.0	Rash: erythema multiforme (e.g., Stevens–Johnson syndrome, toxic epidermal necrolysis)	–	Scattered, but not generalized eruption	Severe (e.g., generalized rash or painful stomatitis); IV fluids, tube feedings, or TPN indicated	Life-threatening; disabling	Death
4.0	Stevens–Johnson syndrome	–	–	Skin sloughing covering <10% BSA with associated signs (e.g., erythema, purpura, epidermal detachment and mucous membrane detachment)	Skin sloughing covering 10 - 30% BSA with associated signs (e.g., erythema, purpura, epidermal detachment and mucous membrane detachment)	Death
4.0	Toxic epidermal necrolysis	–	–	–	Skin sloughing covering ≥30% BSA with associated symptoms (e.g., erythema, purpura, or epidermal detachment)	Death
3.0	Photosensitivity	Painless erythema	Painful erythema	Erythema with desquamation	Life-threatening	Death
4.0	Photosensitivity	Painless erythema and erythema covering <10% BSA	Tender erythema covering 10–30% BSA	Erythema covering >30% BSA and erythema with blistering; photosensitivity; oral corticosteroid therapy indicated; pain control indicated (e.g., narcotics or NSAIDs)	Life-threatening consequences; urgent intervention indicated	Death
3.0	Pruritus/itching	Mild or localized	Intense or widespread	Intense or widespread and interfering with ADL	–	–
4.0	Pruritus	Mild or localized; topical intervention indicated	Intense or widespread; intermittent; skin changes from scratching (e.g., edema, papulation, excoriations, ichenification, oozing/crusts); oral intervention indicated; limiting instrumental ADL	Intense or widespread;constant; limiting self carevADL or sleep; oral corticosteroid or immunosuppressive therapy indicated	–	–
3.0	Dry skin	Asymptomatic	Symptomatic, not interfering with ADL	Symptomatic, interfering with ADL	–	–
4.0	Dry skin	Covering <10% BSA and no associated erythema or pruritus	Covering 10–30% BSA and associated with erythema or pruritus; limiting instrumental ADL	Covering >30% BSA and associated with pruritus; limiting self-care ADL	–	–

ADL, activities of daily living; BSA, body surface area; NSAID, nonsteroidal anti-inflammatory drug; TPN, total parenteral nutrition.
A semicolon indicates "or" within the description of the grade. A single dash (–) indicates a grade is not available. Instrumental ADL refer to preparing meals, shopping for groceries or clothes, using the telephone, managing money, etc. Self-care ADL refer to bathing, dressing and undressing, feeding self, using the toilet, taking medications, and not bedridden. Not all grades are appropriate for all AEs. Therefore, some AEs are listed with fewer than five options for grade selection.

Appendix 5.2 New adverse events in CTCAE v4.0 for the Skin and subcutaneous tissue disorders section.

CTCAE v4.0 AE Term	Grade 1	Grade 2	Grade 3	Grade 4	Grade 5
Hypertrichosis	Increase in length, thickness or density of hair that the patient is either able to camouflage by periodic shaving or removal of hairs or is not concerned enough about the overgrowth to use any form of hair removal	Increase in length, thickness or density of hair at least on the usual exposed areas of the body [face (not limited to beard/moustache area) plus/minus arms] that requires frequent shaving or use of destructive means of hair removal to camouflage; associated with psychosocial impact	–	–	–
Hypohidrosis	–	Symptomatic; limiting instrumental ADL	Increase in body temperature; limiting self-care ADL	Heat stroke	Death
Lipohypertrophy	Asymptomatic and covering <10% BSA	Covering 10–30% BSA and associated tenderness; limiting instrumental ADL	Covering >30% BSA and associated tenderness and narcotics or NSAIDs indicated; lipohypertrophy; limiting self-care ADL	–	–
Periorbital edema	Soft or nonpitting	Indurated or pitting edema; topical intervention indicated	Edema associated with visual disturbance; increased intraocular pressure, glaucoma or retinal hemorrhage; optic neuritis; diuretics indicated; operative intervention indicated	–	–
Scalp pain	Mild pain	Moderate pain; limiting instrumental ADL	Severe pain; limiting self-care ADL	–	–
Hyperhidrosis	Limited to one site (palms, soles, or axillae); self-care interventions	Involving >1 site; patient seeks medical intervention; associated with psychosocial impact	Generalized involving sites other than palms, soles, or axillae; associated with electrolyte/hemodynamic imbalance	–	–
Hirsutism	In women, increase in length, thickness, or density of hair in a male distribution that the patient is able to camouflage periodic shaving, bleaching, or removal of hair	In women, increase in length, thickness or density of hair in a male distribution that requires daily shaving or consistent destructive means of hair removal to camouflage; associated with psychosocial impact	–	–	–
Bullous dermatitis	Asymptomatic; blisters covering <10% BSA	Blisters covering 10–30% BSA; painful blisters; limiting instrumental ADL	Blisters covering >30% BSA; limiting self-care ADL	Blisters covering >30% BSA; associated with fluid or electrolyte abnormalities; ICU care or burn unit indicated	Death

CTCAE v4.0 AE Term	Grade 1	Grade 2	Grade 3	Grade 4	Grade 5
Erythroderma	–	Erythema covering >90% BSA without associated symptoms; limiting instrumental ADL	Erythema covering >90% BSA with associated symptoms (e.g., pruritus or tenderness); limiting self-care ADL	Erythema covering >90% BSA with associated fluid or electrolyte abnormalities; ICU care or burn unit indicated	Death
Erythema multiforme	Target lesions covering <10% BSA and not associated with skin tenderness	Target lesions covering 10 - 30% BSA and associated with skin tenderness	Target lesions covering >30% BSA and associated with oral or genital erosions	Target lesions covering >30% BSA; associated with fluid or electrolyte abnormalities; ICU care or burn unit indicated	Death
Body odor	Mild odor; physician intervention not indicated; self-care interventions	Pronounced odor; psychosocial impact; patient seeks medical intervention	–	–	–
Pain of skin	Mild pain	Moderate pain; limiting instrumental ADL	Severe pain; limiting self-care ADL		

6 Psychosocial Issues in Oncology: Clinical Management of Psychosocial Distress, Health-Related Quality of Life, and Special Considerations in Dermatologic Oncology

Lynne I. Wagner and David Cella

Northwestern University Feinberg School of Medicine, Robert H. Lurie Comprehensive Cancer Center of Northwestern University, Chicago, IL, USA

The challenges that cancer imposes on psychological, emotional, and social well-being have been increasingly recognized as an important area for clinical and research attention since the 1970s, when the field of psycho-oncology was established. The expanding evidence base documenting the psychosocial effects of cancer warranted a 2008 report from the Institute of Medicine (IOM): Cancer care for the whole patient: Meeting psychosocial health needs [1]. According to the IOM, "cancer care today often provides state-of-the-science biomedical treatment, but fails to address the psychological and social (psychosocial) problems associated with the illness." This chapter reviews principles of psychosocial care of adults with cancer with a focus on the unique concerns for dermatologic populations.

Psychosocial distress

Distress is common among the general population. According to Kessler and Wang [2], over 25% of adults met diagnostic criteria for a mental disorder in the past year and 46.4% of the population met criteria for an episode in their lifetime. Hoffman *et al.* [3] examined National Health Interview survey data from 4636 adult cancer survivors and found survivors had a significantly elevated risk of experiencing distress (OR = 1.4) in comparison to 122 220 healthy controls.

It has been estimated that 13–25% of cancer survivors have significant symptoms of depression with elevated risk years after cancer diagnosis, depression is a common reason for mental health referral, and survivors have an increased likelihood of hospitalization for depression [4–6]. Clinical features of depression are described in Table 6.1. Fatigue, sleep difficulties,

and appetite loss are key symptoms of depression and also common among adults with cancer. Emotional and cognitive symptoms can be more informative than physical symptoms in assessing for depression among adults with cancer. Cancer survivors also have an increased risk for anxiety, including health-related anxiety, fear of cancer recurrence or progression, and post-traumatic stress. Approximately 9–29% of cancer survivors have been estimated to have significant symptoms of anxiety [6,7]. While few adults with cancer meet criteria for post-traumatic stress disorder, 20–30% demonstrated evidence of subclinical post-traumatic stress symptoms [8]. Clinical features of anxiety disorders are described in Table 6.2. Cancer survivors have also demonstrated a significantly higher risk for suicide. Based on surveillance epidemiology and end results (SEER) data, adults with cancer have a suicide rate of 31.4 per 100 000 compared to the general US population at 16.7 per 100 000 [9,10].

Distress among dermatologic samples

Patients with malignant dermatologic conditions contend with psychosocial concerns as outlined above in addition to cosmetic consequences of disease and associated impairments in physical, emotional, and social function. Health-related quality of life (HRQL) has been defined as the extent to which one's usual or expected physical, emotional, and social well-being are affected by a medical condition or its treatment [11]. HRQL and psychosocial concerns among adults with melanoma, squamous cell carcinoma (SCC), and cutaneous lymphoma are reviewed. This is followed by a discussion of psychosocial considerations

Dermatologic Principles and Practice in Oncology: Conditions of the Skin, Hair, and Nails in Cancer Patients, First Edition. Edited by Mario E. Lacouture.
© 2014 John Wiley & Sons, Inc. Published 2014 by John Wiley & Sons, Inc.

Table 6.1 Psychosocial needs (Adapted from Institute of Medicine 2008).

General need	Dermatology-specific need
Information about illness, treatments, treatment adverse events	Education on dermatologic toxicities associated with cancer treatments (e.g., hand-foot syndrome)
Support coping with emotions associated with illness and treatment	Cognitive behavioral strategies to manage uncertainty, chronicity of condition
Support in managing illness	Relaxation strategies to manage pruritus
Behavior modification to minimize impact of disease	Behavioral interventions to promote adherence to home-based regimens
Practical resources	Resources for costs associated with transportation (e.g., phototherapy)
Help in managing disruptions in work, school, and family life	Communicating with others about cosmetic manifestations of disease and/or treatment adverse events
Financial assistance	Resources for costs associated with over-the-counter emollients, medications

Table 6.2 Clinical presentation of mood and anxiety disorders.

	Depression	Anxiety disorders
Emotional	Sadness	Tense, "on edge," uneasy
	Loss of interest or pleasure	Feeling of impending doom
	Excessive irritability	
Cognitive	Hopelessness	Worry
	Helplessness	Rumination
	Excessive feelings of guilt	Hypervigilance
	Difficulty concentrating	Avoidance
		Re-experiencing of distressing event (e.g., cancer diagnosis or treatment)
Physical	Fatigue	Autonomic hyperarousal
	Sleep difficulties	Muscle tension
	Increase or decrease in appetite and/or weight	Headaches
	Psychomotor slowing or restlessness	Gastrointestinal distress
Behavioral	Decreased social activities	Frequent contact with healthcare providers
	Decreased pleasurable activities	Frequent requests for repetition of health information (e.g., medication instructions)
		Excessive healthcare utilization

for cancer patients experiencing dermatologic adverse events (AEs) from anticancer treatment.

Treatment for metastatic melanoma is largely focused on the goal of palliation, therefore treatment-related AEs and HRQL are important considerations in treatment decision making and evaluating new treatment regimens [12–14]. Cormier *et al.* [15] reviewed the literature and conducted expert clinician and patient interviews to identify the most salient HRQL concerns. The most common concerns included lymphedema, limits to physical activity, financial difficulties, distress, feeling overwhelmed, and interference in functional well-being. These findings were used to create a melanoma-specific HRQL instrument, the Functional Assessment of Cancer Therapy (FACT) – Melanoma. Early stage melanoma patients (stages I and II) were primarily concerned with cosmetic effects associated with surgical treatment whereas patients with advanced melanoma (stage III) were concerned about postoperative AEs, such as lymphedema. These findings underscore the importance of tailoring assessment of psychosocial concerns to the patient's stage of disease.

Cutaneous basal cell carcinoma (BCC) and SCC, nonmelanoma skin cancers, while nonfatal are also associated with psychosocial and HRQL concerns. Chren *et al.* [16] examined skin-related quality of life among patients with BCC and SCC and found post-treatment HRQL was predicted by pre-treatment skin-related quality of life, lower comorbidity index score, and better emotional function. Pretreatment skin-related quality of life was

associated with patient, tumor, and treatment characteristics. Participants who were married, more educated, reported higher annual income, and with fewer comorbid illnesses had better pretreatment HRQL. In addition, participants with smaller tumors that were not located on the head and neck had better HRQL prior to treatment. Research on HRQL following treatment for BCC and SCC is mixed, with some studies demonstrating benefits to HRQL following treatment [16], while others have not documented significant change in HRQL from pre- to post-treatment [17]. Rhee *et al.* [18,19] found no change in overall HRQL from pre- to post-treatment among patients with cervicofacial skin cancer; however, improvements were observed in emotional well-being, particularly for employed patients younger than 65 years of age. These findings emphasize the importance of psychosocial factors in this population. Rhee *et al.* [20] identified the need for an HRQL measure for patients with nonmelanoma skin cancers and have developed and validated the

Skin Cancer Index to assess emotional well-being, social function, and appearance-related concerns.

The current World Health Organization–European Organisation for Research and Treatment of Cancer (WHO EORTC) classification of cutaneous lymphomas with primary cutaneous manifestations includes 13 entities [21,22]. Cutaneous lymphomas are associated with a multitude of dermatologic symptoms and can have a profound effect on HRQL. Sampogna et al. [23] reported the most common symptoms include pruritus, sensitive skin, worry about progression, concerns about social interactions, frustration, and impairment in sexual function. Sampogna et al. also found fatigue, pain, and insomnia were commonly reported. Based on qualitative interviews, patients reported the most common concerns that interfere with HRQL include pruritus, fatigue, uncertainty about disease progression, depression, and the effect of disease on family members [24,25]. Participants frequently discussed frustration because of the chronicity of their disease and burdensome treatment requirements, such as daily application of topical medications or frequent visits to the medical center for phototherapy. Quantitative ratings of the most important HRQL issues confirmed these findings and indicated sleep difficulties, sensitive skin, worry about the seriousness of their illness, and feeling bothered by one's skin condition were also important to HRQL. Expert clinicians generally identified similar concerns as important to HRQL. These findings were used to develop the FACT-CTCL, a patient-reported outcomes measure to assess HRQL [24,25]. Demierre et al. [26] documented greater impairments in HRQL among patients with advanced disease. Treatment response is often evaluated based on relief of key dermatologic symptoms, such as pruritus and visible skin plaques or tumors, among patients with all stages of disease [27].

Several studies have documented a high prevalence of distress among dermatologic populations with nonmalignant disease [28–31], with increased risk of distress among patients who do not experience benefit from dermatologic intervention [32], suggesting dermatologic symptomatology may contribute to elevated distress. The presence of psychiatric disorders were associated with higher impairments in functioning and higher levels of symptom burden on the Skindex-29 [33], a patient-reported outcomes measure to assess the effects of skin disease on quality of life [31]. Documentation of distress among nonmalignant dermatologic populations underscores the need to address psychosocial issues in patients with malignant dermatologic conditions, given the added complexity of managing a potentially terminal disease.

Dermatologic AEs from cancer treatment

Research on the psychosocial and HRQL aspects of dermatologic toxicities has documented AEs on well-being. Wagner and Lacouture [34] interviewed 20 patients and 12 expert clinicians on the HRQL effects of epidermal growth factor receptor inhibitors (EGFRIs). Physical well-being was compromised by skin burning, irritation and sensitivity, pruritus, and interference with sleep quality resulting from skin discomfort. Patients also identified sensitivity to the sun, changes to facial appearance, avoidance of social activities, disruption in function caused by paronychia, concern about changes in hair texture or hair loss, and the effects on family members as significant concerns. Quantitative ratings of items that are important to HRQL were consistent with themes that emerged from qualitative interviews [24,25]. Expert clinicians did not identify skin sensitivity, irritation and concerns about hair loss, disrupted social function, and depression as important to patient HRQL. While these concerns were not the most salient according to participants' quantitative ratings, excerpts from qualitative interviews provided insight into the effects on social well-being. For example, a few participants discussed how their changed physical appearance because of facial rash required that they either disclose their cancer diagnosis or attribute their rash to another cause. Participants also discussed the social discomfort associated with skin rash because of fears of contagion. With regard to emotional well-being, many participants described the dermatologic toxicities as a physical reminder of their cancer diagnosis and this reminder induced distress and anxiety about the future. Wagner et al. [24,25] have developed a FACT-EGFRI instrument to quantify the most salient concerns from the patient's perspective and the measure includes 18 items to assess skin, nail, and hair AEs.

Patients receiving sunitinib, a tyrosine kinase inhibitor, for renal cell carcinoma have reported significantly better overall quality of life in comparison to those receiving interferon alfa [35]. However, patients receiving sunitinib had a significantly higher rate of Grade 3 or 4 hand-foot skin reaction (HFSR). In a local study, we have analyzed qualitative interview data from seven patients receiving a tyrosine kinase inhibitor for renal cell carcinoma. When asked to identify AEs that interfere with HRQL, many participants have identified symptoms of HFSR as interfering with HRQL. Patients describe these symptoms as "blisters" or "callouses" on their hands, feet, or other areas of their body, which are painful and interfere with functions such as wearing shoes, walking, and handling objects (D. Cella and L.I. Wagner, unpublished data). A survey of 11 patients treated with sorafenib or sunitinib showed that HFSR has a substantial effect on overall HRQL and physical symptoms are the most critical in this population [36]. HFSR has been associated with other anticancer treatments. HFSR associated with capecitabine is a dose-limiting toxicity and there are limited supportive interventions available to prevent or treat this symptom [37,38].

Prospective assessment of chemotherapy-induced dermatologic AEs demonstrated that dermatologic symptoms are common following treatment of advanced women's cancers. Hackbarth et al. [39] examined 91 women with advanced stage gynecologic malignancies (breast 43%, ovarian 35%, cervical 13%, endometrial 6%, other 3%) receiving chemotherapy. The overall incidence of dermatologic AEs was 86.8% and 34.1% of participants identified skin changes as the most unpleasant AEs of treatment, higher than gastrointestinal side effects and weakness. Alopecia was reported by 75.8% of the sample, 23.1% reported nail changes, and 18.7% developed palmo-plantar erythrodyesesthesia, or HFSR. Among this group, 53% had Grade 3 HFSR using the Common Terminology Criteria for Adverse Events (CTCAE) grading system. Of participants with Grade 3 HFSR, 88.9% reported severe limitations in work or other daily activities. Based on these findings, Hackbarth et al. recommend pretreatment education and counseling on the risk of dermatologic AEs and advised providers to evaluate the potential for dermatologic AEs when selecting treatment regimens.

Alopecia is a well-known AE of chemotherapy and the effect of alopecia on HRQL and psychosocial function has been documented. Lemieux et al. [40] conducted a review of 38 articles on alopecia and HRQL among studies examining patients with breast cancer. Chemotherapy-induced alopecia frequently ranked among the most distressing side effects of chemotherapy. Alopecia ranked in the top three most troubling symptoms, even among participants receiving high-dose chemotherapy. According to Lemieux et al. [40], two studies have documented chemotherapy refusal among a subgroup of participants (8%) because of the risk of alopecia. Hair loss was described as traumatizing and distressing, and two studies reviewed reported alopecia was more difficult than losing a breast. Consistent with other dermatologic AEs, alopecia negatively affects social function. Alopecia is a visible reminder of disease and may result in a loss of privacy regarding medical status as others may easily observe this AE. Lemieux et al. [40] reported evidence that alopecia negatively affects self-esteem and body image. Hesketh et al. [41] summarized literature on the AEs of alopecia on HRQL, including anxiety, depression, negative body image, lowered self-esteem, and reduced sense of well-being. Recommendations for healthcare providers are provided, including education and patient self-care strategies throughout treatment in accordance with each phase of hair loss and regrowth.

A survey of 379 cancer survivors who participated in a survivors' workshop demonstrated that dermatologic conditions continued to compromise HRQL after treatment completion [42]. The majority of the sample included breast cancer survivors (66%) and was predominantly female (89%). A significant proportion of the sample reported concern about hair loss prior to treatment (47% reported being "very concerned") and concerns about skin irritation and dry skin were more salient post-treatment (23–24%). Survivors identified dry skin (63%), nail problems (51%), and itching (36%) as particularly problematic and compromised HRQL. Of note, survivors were either unaware of potential dermatologic AEs or underestimated the effects of dermatologic AEs on HRQL prior to treatment. Concerns about dermatologic toxicities increased following treatment indicating that dermatologic well-being is an important consideration in enhancing quality of cancer survivorship. Long-term dermatologic concerns have also been documented among childhood cancer

survivors. Kinahan et al. [43] examined a sample of 78 childhood cancer survivors and found that 59% reported current concerns regarding a dermatologic condition associated with cancer treatment. Childhood cancer survivors surveyed were on average 29.7 years of age and 19.2 years (range 6–46 years) post-diagnosis. The most prevalent concerns attributable to cancer treatment included scarring (33.3%), alopecia (12.8%), and new diagnosis of skin cancer (11.5%). Fifty percent of participants reported seeking care from a dermatologist for these concerns. While these findings are based on a nonrepresentative sample, results support the need for a large-scale longitudinal assessment of childhood cancer survivors' dermatology-specific HRQL. Oeffinger et al. [44] examined a sample of 10 397 childhood cancer survivors and 3034 siblings and documented an increased risk of second cancers among survivors, including melanoma and nonmelanoma skin cancers. Research to date examining childhood cancer survivors supports the need for clinicians to attend to dermatologic concerns among long-term survivors.

Risk factors for distress

Risk factors for distress include younger age at cancer diagnosis, female, nonmarried, lower socioeconomic status, and having pre-existing depression, anxiety, or substance abuse [1]. The intensity of anticancer treatment and site of cancer can be risk factors for elevated distress, particularly if treatment is disfiguring [1]. Distress has been associated with lower quality of life, decreased employment functioning, decreased adherence to medical regimens, increased medical costs, increased health risk behaviors, and decreased health protective behaviors [1]. Spelten et al. [45] found that 7–70% of cancer survivors either stop working or report a change in work status at the time of diagnosis.

Cancer treatments commonly used for dermatologic malignancies or resulting in dermatologic AEs have been associated with impairments in emotional well-being. Based on the severity of depression associated with interferon [46], Musselman et al. [47] evaluated paroxetine and found prophylactic treatment with paroxetine reduced depression associated with treatment. A case-report study identified a potential risk of depression associated with tyrosine kinase inhibitors (TKI) [48]; however, Pirl et al. [49] were unable to identify an association based on a prospective assessment of 29 nonsmall cell lung cancer patients receiving a TKI. Isotretinoin is an effective treatment for acne and is occasionally used in oncology settings for the management of dermatologic toxicities or as one agent in a multiagent anticancer regimen. Marqueling and Zane [50] conducted a systematic review of the literature on depression and isotretinoin among acne patients. Marqueling and Zane reviewed nine studies and did not identify a statistically significant increase in depression diagnosis or symptoms of depression. Given the consequences of unrecognized and untreated depression and suicidal behavior, patients who receive treatments associated with an increased risk for mood disturbances should receive routine monitoring of emotional function.

Clinical management of distress

Physicians substantially underestimate distress among adults with cancer [51–53]. Detmar et al. [54] surveyed members of the American Society of Clinical Oncology and found one-third of respondents do not routinely screen patients for distress and physicians defer to patients to raise concerns about distress. The National Comprehensive Cancer Network (NCCN) has assembled an expert panel on distress and has published guidelines on the clinical management of distress (www.nccn.org; [55]).

Many tools are available and have been used to identify distressed cancer patients, including the NCCN Distress Thermometer [55], the Personal Health Questionnaire-9 , the Hospital Anxiety and Depression Scale, and the Brief Symptom Inventory-18 [56,57]. Chochinov et al. [58] have published recommendations on conducting clinical interviews to identify depressed cancer patients. In the first published randomized clinical trial evaluating outcomes associated with web-based screening for distress, Carlson et al. [59] randomized 585 breast cancer patients and 549 lung cancer patients to minimal screening, full screening, or full screening followed by triage for psychosocial care. Participants who received screening followed by triage for psychosocial care had improved psychosocial well-being 3 months later in comparison to participants who received minimal screening.

Measuring distress and health-related quality of life in dermatologic oncology

The assessment of psychosocial concerns and HRQL among patients with dermatologic AE and malignancies should include standardized measures of distress, described above, measurement of overall HRQL, and the assessment of dermatologic-specific concerns. Table 6.3 presents a list of standardized measures for the assessment of general HRQL, dermatology-specific quality of life, disease-specific concerns, and distress. Both et al. [60] reviewed generic and dermatology-specific HRQL instruments and provided a detailed description of commonly used measures. As described above, dermatology-specific and disease-specific scales should assess symptom burden, interference in functional abilities, and psychosocial effects of illness including illness-specific distress and worry about illness and the future. For example, the Dermatology Quality of Life Scales (DQOLS) includes subscales within the Psychosocial domain to assess psychosocial aspects of HRQL including embarrassment, despair, irritableness, and distress. The Activities domain assesses everyday activities, summer activities, social activities, and sexual function.

Psychosocial interventions in oncodermatology

Psychosocial intervention with oncodermatology patients should address common psychosocial issues among oncology patients, including anxiety and depression, as well as strategies to address psychosocial aspects unique to dermatologic malignancies or dermatologic AEs, such as embarrassment and concerns about appearance. By providing education on known dermatologic AEs during treatment and training in a skin care management program [61], patients may experience a greater sense of control and experience less symptom-related distress. When appropriate, psychosocial intervention should also include nonpharmacologic strategies for symptom management. Given the impairments in social function observed among patients with dermatologic malignancies or treatment-related AEs, psychosocial intervention should incorporate behavioral activation and increased social activities for patients who are socially isolated. Skills training could include a review of communication skills to address the unique challenges patients face with regard to discussing cosmetic effects of illness or treatment AEs to facilitate increased social activities. Patients who experience social anxiety could learn cognitive restructuring techniques to cope with concerns about others' opinions about their appearance and the significance of others' opinions. Cognitive strategies for coping with rumination and worry could be reviewed for patients who struggle with fear of progression and uncertainty about the future. Symptom reframing, which involves educating and coaching patients on how to interpret troubling symptoms, may help to reduce symptom-related distress. For example, if patients are educated on dermatologic toxicities associated with cancer treatment and encouraged to view dermatologic symptoms as benign and common, patients will experience less distress in response to symptom burden and will be better able to cope. Frith et al. [62] interviewed 19 women regarding chemotherapy-induced alopecia and found key interview themes that supported the role of "anticipatory coping." Anticipatory coping involves affective and behavioral rehearsal prior to hair loss and results in increased feelings of control over this challenging experience. Strategies for coping with reminders of illness are especially important for dermatologic populations, who may experience frequent reminders due to cosmetic effects of disease or treatment-related symptoms. Patients with low grade conditions, such as stage I–II cutaneous lymphoma, may benefit from learning strategies for coping with the chronicity of their condition. Intervention for dermatologic populations should also include behavioral strategies to promote adherence and persistence when appropriate for patients for whom treatment includes daily application of topical medications or adherence to use of sunscreen and protective clothing.

Verhoeven et al. [63] apply a cognitive behavioral model for understanding chronic pain to chronic pruritus. Verhoeven et al. examined a sample of 235 patients with dermatitis or psoriasis and found that a cognitive style of catastrophizing, higher levels

Table 6.3 Patient-reported outcomes measures for use in supportive oncodermatology.

Domain	Instrument	Scales
Generic health-related quality of life measure	Functional Assessment of Cancer Therapy – General (FACT-G)	Physical well-being
		Functional well-being
		Emotional well-being
		Social well-being
	Medical Outcomes Study Short-Form-36, SF-36	Role limitations due to physical problem
		Bodily pain
		General health
		Vitality
		Social functioning
		Role limitations due to emotions
		Mental health
		Health transition
Dermatology-specific measure	Skindex-29, Skindex-16, Skindex-17	Emotions
		Functioning
		Symptoms
	Dermatology Life Questionnaire Index (DLQI)	Symptoms
		Daily activities
		Leisure
		Work/school
		Personal relationships
		Treatment
	Dermatology-Specific Quality of Life (DSQL)	Physical symptoms
		Daily activities
		Social activities
		Work/school experiences
		Self-perception
		SF-36 vitality subscale
		SF-36 mental subscale
	Dermatology Quality of Life Scale (DQOLS)	Psychosocial
		Activities
		Symptoms
Melanoma	FACT-Melanoma	Melanoma-specific concerns
Cutaneous basal cell carcinoma	Skin Cancer Index	Emotion
		Social
		Appearance
Squamous cell carcinoma	Skin Cancer Index	Emotion
		Social
		Appearance
Cutaneous lymphoma	FACT-Cutaneous T-cell Lymphoma (FACT-CTCL)	Cutaneous lymphoma-specific concerns
Side effects of epidermal growth factor receptor inhibitors	FACT-EGFRI	Skin adverse events
		Hair adverse events
		Nail adverse events
Hand-foot syndrome	Hand-foot syndrome-18	Hand-specific items
		Foot-specific items
Psychosocial distress	NCCN Distress Thermometer	Distress rating
		Problem checklist
	Hospital Anxiety and Depression Scale	Depression
		Anxiety
	Personal Health Questionnaire-9	Depression
	Brief Symptom Inventory	Somatization
		Depression
		Anxiety

of activity avoidance, and heightened physiologic reactivity (per self-report) predicted more itching and lower disease-related quality of life. These findings suggest that teaching cognitive behavioral strategies to manage symptoms can address catastrophizing, activity avoidance, and can teach strategies to promote physiologic relaxation thus reducing the level of physiologic reactivity which may exacerbate symptom burden.

Conclusions

Psychosocial distress is common among adults with cancer and those with dermatologic malignancies or dermatologic AEs from treatment face unique issues because of associated challenges to maintaining normal social function. Psychosocial and HRQL concerns have been studied among populations with dermatologic malignancies and standardized measures exist to quantify the effects of disease and treatment-related AEs on physical, function, emotional, and social well-being. Psychosocial interventions have been demonstrated to reduce distress and improve well-being among adults with cancer. Cognitive behavioral strategies have potential utility to reduce disease burden and improve quality of life among dermatologic oncology populations. According to the IOM [1], "it is not possible to deliver good-quality cancer care without using existing approaches, tools, and resources to address patients' psychosocial health needs. Together, these services reduce patients' suffering, help them adhere to prescribed treatments, and support their return to health."

References

1 Institute of Medicine (2008) *Cancer Care for the Whole Patient: Meeting Psychosocial Health Needs*, National Academies Press, Washington, DC.

2 Kessler, R.C. & Wang, P.S. (2008) The descriptive epidemiology of commonly occurring mental disorders in the United States. *Annual Review of Public Health*, **29**, 115–129.

3 Hoffman, K.E., McCarthy, E.P., Recklitis, C.J. & Ng, A.K. (2009) Psychological distress in long-term survivors of adult onset cancer: results of a national survey. *Archives of Internal Medicine*, **169**, 1274–1281.

4 Dalton, S.O., Laursen, T.M., Ross, L., Mortensen, P.B. & Johansen, C. (2009) Risk for a depression hospitalization after a cancer diagnosis: a nationwide population-based study of cancer patients in Denmark from 1973 to 2003. *Journal of Clinical Oncology*, **27**, 1440–1445.

5 Polsky, D., Doshi, J.A., Marcus, S. *et al.* (2005) Long-term risk for depressive symptoms after a medical diagnosis. *Archives of Internal Medicine*, **165**, 1260–1266.

6 Stanton, A. (2006) Psychosocial concerns and interventions for cancer survivors. *Journal of Clinical Oncology*, **24**, 5132–5137.

7 Burgess, C., Cornelius, V., Love, S., Graham, J., Richards, M. & Ramirez, A. (2005) Depression and anxiety I women with early breast cancer: five year observational cohort study. *BMJ (Clinical Research Ed.)*, **330**, 704.

8 Kangas, M., Henry, J. & Bryant, R. (2002) Posttraumatic stress disorder following cancer: a conceptual and empirical review. *Clinical Psychology Review*, **22**, 499–524.

9 Misono, S., Weiss, N.S., Fann, J.R., Redman, M. & Yueh, B. (2008) Incidence of suicide in persons with cancer. *Journal of Clinical Oncology*, **26**, 4731–4738.

10 Miller, M., Mogun, H., Azrael, D., Hempstead, K. & Solomon, D.H. (2008) Cancer and the risk of suicide in older Americans. *Journal of Clinical Oncology*, **26**, 4720–4724.

11 Cella, D. (1995) Methods and problems in measuring quality of life. *Supportive Care in Cancer*, **3**, 11–22.

12 Fisher, D., Kwong, L., Chin, L. *et al.* (2008) Melanoma. In: V.T. DeVita Jr, S. Hellman & S.A. Rosenberg (eds), *Cancer: Principles and Practice of Oncology*, 8th ed., pp. 1889–1966. Lippincott Williams & Wilkins, Philadelphia, PA.

13 Kiebert, G.M., Jonas, D.L. & Middleton, M.R. (2003) Health-related quality of life in patients with advanced metastatic melanoma: results of a randomized phase III study comparing temozolomide with dacarbazine. *Cancer Investigation*, **21**, 821–829.

14 Revicki, D.A., Osoba, D., Fairclough, D. *et al.* (2001) Recommendations on health-related quality of life research to support labeling and promotional claims in the United States. *Quality of Life Research*, **9**, 887–900.

15 Cormier, J.N., Davidson, L., Xing, Y., Webster, K. & Cella, D. (2005) Measuring quality of life in patients with melanoma: development of the FACT-Melanoma subscale. *Journal of Supportive Oncology*, **3**, 139–145.

16 Chren, M.M., Sahay, A.P., Bertenthal, D., Sen, S. & Landefeld, C.D. (2007) Quality-of-life outcomes of treatments for cutaneous basal cell carcinoma and squamous cell carcinoma. *Journal of Investigative Dermatology*, **127**, 1351–1357.

17 Blackford, S., Roberts, D., Salek, M.S. & Finlay, A. (1996) Basal cell carcinomas cause little handicap. *Quality of Life Research*, **5**, 191–194.

18 Rhee, J.S., Matthews, B.A., Neuburg, M., Smith, T.L., Burzynski, M. & Nattinger, A.B. (2004) Quality of life and sun-protective behavior in skin cancer patients. *Archives of Otolaryngology Head and Neck Surgery*, **130**, 141–146.

19 Rhee, J.S., Matthews, B.A., Neuburg, M., Smith, T.L., Burzynski, M. & Nattinger, A.B. (2004) Skin cancer and quality of life: assessment with the Dermatology Life Quality Index. *Dermatologic Surgery*, **30**, 525–529.

20 Rhee, J.S., Matthews, B.A., Neuburg, M., Logan, B.R., Burzynski, M. & Nattinger, A.B. (2006) Validation of a quality-of-life instrument for patients with nonmelanoma skin cancer. *Archives of Facial Plastic Surgery*, **8**, 314–318.

21 Querfeld, C., Guitart, J., Kuzel, T.M. & Rosen, S.T. (2003) Primary cutaneous lymphomas: a review with current treatment options. *Blood Reviews*, **17**, 131–142.

22 Willemze, R., Jaffe, E.S., Burg, G. *et al.* (2005) WHO-EORTC classification for cutaneous lymphomas. *Blood*, **105**, 3768–3785.

23 Sampogna, F., Frontani, M., Baliva, G. *et al.* (2009) Quality of life and psychological distress in patients with cutaneous lymphoma. *British Journal of Dermatology*, **160**, 815–822.

24 Wagner, L.I., Berg, S.R., Gandhi, M., *et al.* (2013) The development of a Functional Assessment of Cancer Therapy (FACT) questionnaire to assess dermatologic symptoms associated with epidermal growth factor receptor inhibitors (FACT-EGFRI-18). *Journal of Supportive Care in Cancer*, **21**, 1033–1041.

25 Wagner, L., Zaluda, L., Guitart, J., Kuzel, T., Querfeld, C. & Rosen, S. (2010) Health-related quality of life among patients with cutaneous lymphoma: development of the Functional Assessment of Cancer Therapy – Cutaneous Lymphoma (FACT-CTCL). Oral presentation at the First World Congress of Cutaneous Lymphomas, September 2010, Chicago IL, USA.

26 Demierre, M.F., Tien, A. & Miller, D. (2005) Health-related quality-of-life assessment in patients with cutaneous T-cell lymphoma. *Archives of Dermatology*, **141**, 325–330.

27 Duvic, M., Kuzel, T.M., Olsen, E.A. *et al.* (2002) Quality-of-life improvements in cutaneous T-cell lymphoma patients treated with denileukin diftitox (Ontak®). *Clinical Lymphoma*, **2**, 222–228.

28 Aktan, S., Ozmen, E. & Sanli, B. (1998) Psychiatric disorders in patients attending a dermatology outpatient clinic. *Dermatology (Basel, Switzerland)*, **197**, 230–234.

29 Gupta, M.A. & Gupta, A.K. (1998) Depression and suicidal ideation in dermatology patients with acne, alopecia areata, atopic dermatitis and psoriasis. *British Journal of Dermatology*, **139**, 846–850.

30 Picardi, A. & Abeni, D. (2001) Stressful life events and skin diseases: disentangling evidence from myth. *Psychotherapy and Psychosomatics*, **70**, 118–136.

31 Picardi, A., Pasquini, P., Abeni, D., Fassone, G., Mazzotti, E. & Fava, G.A. (2005) Psychosomatic assessment of skin diseases in clinical practice. *Psychotherapy and Psychosomatics*, **74**, 315–322.

32 Picardi, A., Abeni, D., Renzi, C., Braga, M., Melchi, C.F. & Pasquini, P. (2003) Treatment outcome and incidence of psychiatric disorders in dermatological outpatients. *Journal of the European Academy of Dermatology and Venereology*, **17**, 155–159.

33 Chren, M.M., Lasek, R.J., Flocke, S.A. & Zyzanski, S.J. (1997) Improved discriminative and evaluative capability of a refined version of Skindex, a quality-of-life instrument for patients with skin diseases. *Archives of Dermatology*, **133**, 1433–1440.

34 Wagner, L.I. & Lacouture, M. (2007) Dermatologic toxicities associated with EGFR inhibitors: the clinical psychologist's perspective. *Oncology*, **21**, 34–36.

35 Motzer, R.J., Hutson, T.E., Tomczak, P. *et al.* (2007) Sunitinib versus interferon alfa in metastatic renal-cell carcinoma. *New England Journal of Medicine*, **356**, 115–124.

36 Huggins, R.H., Kuzel, T.M., Anderson, R.T. *et al.* (2008) Hand foot skin reaction (HFSR) by the multikinase inhibitors (MKIs) sorafenib and sunitinib: impact on quality of life (QoL). *Journal of Clinical Oncology*, **26**, Abstract 16122.

37 Gressett, S.M., Stanford, B.L. & Hardwicks, F. (2006) Management of hand-foot syndrome induced by capecitabine. *Journal of Oncology Pharmacy Practice*, **12**, 131–141.

38 Lacouture, M.E., Wu, S., Robert, C. *et al.* (2008) Evolving strategies for the management of hand-foot skin reaction associated with the multitargeted kinase inhibitors sorafenib and sunitinib. *The Oncologist*, **13**, 1001–1011.

39 Hackbarth, M., Haas, N., Fotopoulou, C., Lichtenegger, W. & Schouli, J. (2008) Chemotherapy-induced dermatological toxicity: frequencies and impact on quality of life in women's cancers: results of a prospective study. *Supportive Care in Cancer*, **16**, 267–273.

40 Lemieux, J., Maunsell, E. & Provencher, L. (2008) Chemotherapy-induced alopecia and effects on quality of life among women with breast cancer: a literature review. *Psycho-Oncology*, **17**, 317–328.

41 Hesketh, P.J., Batchelor, D., Golant, M., Lyman, G.H., Rhodes, N. & Yardley, D. (2004) Chemotherapy-induced alopecia: psychosocial impact and therapeutic approaches. *Supportive Care in Cancer*, **12**, 543–549.

42 Gandhi, M., Oishi, K., Zubal, B. & Lacouture, M.E. (2010) Unanticipated toxicities from anticancer therapies: survivors' perspectives. *Supportive Care in Cancer*, **18**, 1461–1468.

43 Kinahan, K., Gandhi, M., Lacouture, M.E. *et al.* (2009) Dermatologic issues in adult survivors of childhood cancer. *Journal of Cancer Survivorship*, **3**, 158–163.

44 Oeffinger, K.C., Mertens, A.C., Sklar, C.A. *et al.* (2006) Chronic health conditions in adult survivors of childhood cancer. *New England Journal of Medicine*, **355**, 1572–1582.

45 Spelten, E.R., Sprangers, M., Verbeek, J. (2002) Factors reported to influence the return to work of cancer survivors: A literature review. *Psycho-Oncology*, **11**, 124–131.

46 Valentine, A.D., Meyers, C.A., Kling, M.A., Richelson, E. & Hauser, P. (1998) Mood and cognitive side effects of interferon-alpha therapy. *Seminars in Oncology*, **25** (Suppl. 1), 39–47.

47 Musselman, D.L., Lawson, D.H., Gumnick, J.F. *et al.* (2001) Paroxetine for the prevention of depression induced by high-dose interferon alfa. *New England Journal of Medicine*, **344**, 961–966.

48 Quek, R., Morgan, J.A., George, S. *et al.* (2009) Small-molecule tyrosine kinase inhibitor and depression. *Journal of Clinical Oncology*, **27**, 312–313.

49 Pirl, W.F., Solis, J., Greer, J., Sequist, L., Temel, J.S. & Lynch, T.J. (2009) Epidermal growth factor receptor tyrosine kinase inhibitors and depression. *Journal of Clinical Oncology*, **27**, e49–e50.

50 Marqueling, A.L. & Zane, L.T. (2005) Depression and suicidal behavior in acne patients treated with isotretinoin: a systematic review. *Seminars in Cutaneous Medicine and Surgery*, **24**, 92–102.

51 Fallowfield, L., Ratcliffe, D., Jenkins, V. & Saul, J. (2001) Psychiatric morbidity and its recognition by doctors in patients with cancer. *British Journal of Cancer*, **84**, 1011–1015.

52 Keller, M., Sommerfeldt, S., Fischer, C. *et al.* (2004) Recognition of distress and psychiatric morbidity in cancer patients: a multi-method approach. *European Society for Medical Oncology*, **15**, 1243–1249.

53 Merckaert, I., Libert, Y., Delvaux, N. *et al.* (2005) Factors that influence physicians' detection of distress in patients with cancer: can a communication skills training program improve physicians' detection? *Cancer*, **104**, 411–421.

54 Detmar, S.B., Aaronson, N.K., Wever, L.D., *et al.* (2000) How are you feeling? Who wants to know? Patients' and oncologists' preferences for discussing health-related quality-of-life issues. *Journal of Clinical Oncology*, **18** (18), 2395–3301.

55 Holland, J.C., Andersen, B., Breitbart, W.S. *et al.* (2010) Distress management: clinical practice guidelines in oncology. *Journal of the National Comprehensive Cancer Network*, **8**, 448–485.

56 Mitchell, A.J. (2010) Short screening tools for cancer-related distress: a review and diagnostic validity meta-analysis. *Journal of the National Comprehensive Cancer Network*, **8**, 487–494.

57 Butt, Z., Wagner, L.I., Beaumont, J.L. *et al.* (2008) Use of a single-item screening tool to detect clinically significant fatigue, pain, distress, and anorexia in ambulatory cancer practice. *Journal of Pain and Symptom Management*, **35**, 20–30.

58 Chochinov, H.M., Wilson, K.G., Enns, M., Lander, S. (1997) Are you depressed? Screening for depression in the terminally ill. *American Journal of Psychiatry*, **154**, 674–676.

59 Carlson, L.E., Groff, S.L., Maciejewski, O., Bultz, B.D. (2010) Screening for Distress in Lung and Breast Cancer Outpatients: A Randomized Controlled Trial. *J. Clin. Oncol.* **28** (33), 4884–4891.

60 Both, H., Essink-Bot, M.L., Busschbach, J. & Nijsten, T. (2007) Critical review of generic and dermatology-specific health-related quality of life instruments. *Journal of Investigative Dermatology*, **127**, 2726–2739.

61 Haley, A.C., Calahan, C., Gandhi, M., West, D.P., Rademaker, A. & Lacouture, M.E. (2011) Skin care management in cancer patients: an evaluation of quality of life and tolerability. *Supportive Care in Cancer*, **19**, 545–554.

62 Frith, H., Harcourt, D. & Fussell, A. (2007) Anticipating an altered appearance: women undergoing chemotherapy treatment for breast cancer. *European Journal of Oncology Nursing*, **11**, 385–391.

63 Verhoeven, L., Kraaimaat, F., Duller, P., van de Kerkhof, P. & Evers, A. (2006) Cognitive, behavioral, and physiological reactivity to chronic itching: analogies to chronic pain. *International Journal of Behavioral Medicine*, **13**, 237–243.

7 Dermatopathology

Molly A. Hinshaw[1,2] and James L. Troy[2]
[1]University of Wisconsin School of Medicine and Public Health, Wisconsin, WI, USA
[2]Medical College of Wisconsin, Milwaukee, WI, USA

Introduction

A skin biopsy is simple to perform. Interpretation of that skin biopsy, particularly in the context of a patient with a skin eruption who is on multiple medications, has undergone or is undergoing chemotherapy or radiation, can be a challenge. Inflammatory skin diseases pass through stages of evolution and therefore the histologic findings in a skin biopsy vary with the stage of the disease. Disparate entities may share histologic features and the final diagnosis often rests with the clinical–pathologic correlation. At early stages some inflammatory conditions may not have evolved entirely diagnostic histologic features. Nonetheless, one may expect that an experienced dermatopathologist anticipates such issues and, in the context of a detailed clinical history, can compile a report that is diagnostically relevant and helps guide patient care.

This chapter details the dermatopathologic features, differential diagnoses, and distinguishing clues to neoplastic and inflammatory processes that frequently cause diagnostic dilemmas in the practice of oncology.

Mucocutaneous neoplasms

Solar (actinic) keratosis

Clinically, these are recognized as scaly, slightly erythematous macules. Histologically, one sees partial thickness cytologic atypia of intraepidermal keratinocytes with an altered cornified layer usually with parakeratosis. Solar keratoses may come to the attention of the oncologist when they acutely become inflamed during the early course of treatment with various chemotherapeutic agents including 5-fluorouracil, doxorubicin, epidermal growth factor receptor inhibitors, capecitabine, and sorafenib [1–3].

Squamous cell carcinoma

These malignant neoplasms occur on a histologic spectrum from well-differentiated with areas of keratinization to poorly differentiated requiring immunoperoxidase staining to confirm they are epithelial malignancies. They may arise in association with actinic keratosis or squamous cell carcinoma *in situ* or as *de novo* invasive malignancies.

One clinically and histologically distinct variant of squamous cell carcinoma (SCC) is keratoacanthoma. Clinically, keratoacanthoma presents as a rapidly evolving, variably tender, erythematous nodule often with a keratin-filled crateriform center. Histologically, it is a well-differentiated, endo-exophytic epithelial tumor arising from the epidermis composed of keratinocytes with abundant pale eosinophilic "glassy" cytoplasm containing aggregates of neutrophils and extending into the dermis with a relatively smooth base without an infiltrative pattern. There is sharp demarcation from adjacent uninvolved epidermis (Figure 7.1).

Features that have led to the conclusion that the keratoacanthoma is a distinct subset of SCC include the well-recognized eruptive variant with numerous widespread simultaneous lesions, the regressive stage where the epithelium is thinned with little cytologic atypia [4], and the frequent (but not wholly predictable) complete spontaneous involution even when incompletely excised.

One new observation in keratoacanthoma is their onset in patients on tyrosine kinase inhibitors, specifically inhibitors of the RAF–MEK pathway (e.g., vemurafenib, dabrafenib, sorafenib [5]). This association occurs in patients who may simultaneously develop other epithelial abnormalities including keratosis pilaris and verruca-like lesions. Indeed, many of the keratoacanthomas seen in these patients have verrucoid changes; research is ongoing as to the relevance of this observation.

Keratoacanthoma is therefore considered a less aggressive variant of SCC. Given the similar features of the upper portions

Dermatologic Principles and Practice in Oncology: Conditions of the Skin, Hair, and Nails in Cancer Patients, First Edition. Edited by Mario E. Lacouture.
© 2014 John Wiley & Sons, Inc. Published 2014 by John Wiley & Sons, Inc.

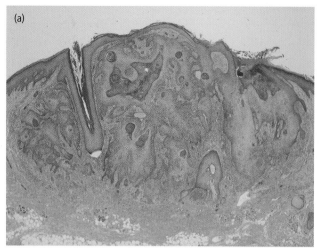

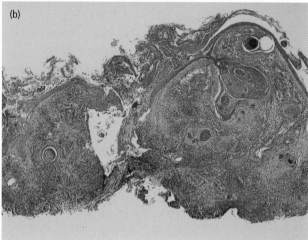

Figure 7.1 (a) Keratoacanthoma. Note the symmetric, endo-exophytic architecture and sharp cut off from uninvolved skin. (b) Nonkeratoacanthoma squamous cell carcinoma (SCC). Note the lack of circumscription and the infiltrative architecture.

Table 7.1 Histologic features of melanoma.

Architecture	
Asymmetric, broad (often >6 mm)	Poor circumscription
Epidermal	
Confluent growth	Irregular distribution nests
Predominance of single cells over nests	Epidermal pagetoid scatter of melanocytes
Dermal	
Sheet-like growth	Variability in size, shape nests
Lack of maturation with descent	Mitoses, esp. deep, atypical

of other variants of SCC and keratoacanthoma, a pathologist may diagnose these tumors as SCC without a comment about keratoacanthoma features. We note that there are cases in the literature of tumors diagnosed as keratoacanthoma that have had perineural invasion and/or metastasized [6], and best clinical management should be complete lesion removal. Molecular studies are underway to attempt to identify features that distinguish keratoacanthoma from nonkeratoacanthoma variants of SCC. In general, skin biopsies are often obtained by shave technique. While useful as a screening tool, if the shave biopsy does not remove the entire lesion then the architectural characteristics cannot be fully evaluated.

Melanocytic tumors

The majority of melanocytic tumors can be readily characterized as benign or malignant, particularly if the entire clinical lesion is completely removed by the initial biopsy. The nomenclature of

benign, but clinically unusual, nevi varies and includes Clark nevus, nevus with architectural disorder, and dysplastic nevus [7].

Well-established features of melanoma may be identified in partial biopsies (Table 7.1). However, when the key features of size, symmetry, and circumscription cannot be evaluated, a dermatopathologist may suggest the possibility of melanoma without making an unequivocal diagnosis until the entire lesion is re-excised and histologically evaluated.

Distinction between Spitz nevi and melanoma can also be difficult as they share some histologic features [8]. Both have at times spindled and epithelioid cytology and have extension of melanocytes above the epidermal basal layer (i.e., pagetoid scatter; Figure 7.2). Immunoperoxidase stains can be utilized to confirm a melanocytic origin but are otherwise of limited use in distinguishing a benign from a malignant melanocytic neoplasm (Table 7.2). At the time of this writing, fluorescence *in situ* hybridization (FISH) identifying several chromosomal aberrations is being utilized as a component of the evaluation of difficult melanocytic tumors that have overlapping histologic features. One commercially available FISH probe set was reported to have 86.7% sensitivity and 95.4% specificity in the diagnosis of melanoma and benign melanocytic tumors [9].

Inflammatory dermatoses

Interface (lichenoid) dermatitis
Interface dermatitis is the histologic pattern of an infiltrate of mostly lymphocytes obscuring the dermal–epidermal junction with associated necrotic keratinocytes within the epidermis or adjacent dermis. Some pathologists use the term "lichenoid" to describe similar changes, but in our view that term is best reserved for those band-like lymphohistiocytic eruptions close to the epidermis but with hardly any epidermal disruption. The terms interface dermatitis and lichenoid dermatitis suggest a differential diagnosis and additional histologic features may further aid in making a more specific diagnosis (Figure 7.3; Table 7.3).

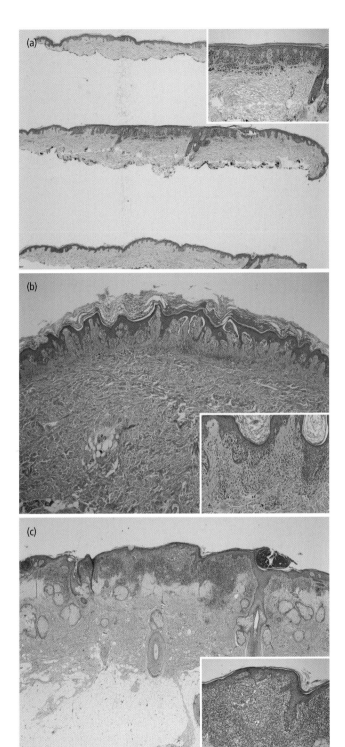

Figure 7.2 (a) Clark (dysplastic) nevus. Note slight asymmetry, architectural disorder. (b) Spitz nevus. Note relative symmetry, spindled and epithelioid cytology, dispersion of dermal melanocytes as single units and small nests, slight pagetoid scatter. (c) Melanoma. Note breadth, asymmetry, pagetoid scatter across lesion, lack of dermal melanocytic maturation.

Table 7.2 Immunoperoxidase and special stains commonly utilized in dermatopathology.

Immunoperoxidase/ special stain	Staining pattern	What it stains
Immunoperoxidase stain		
S100	Nucleus, cytoplasm	Melanocytes, Langerhans, nerves
MelanA/Mart-1*	Cytoplasm	Melanocytes
HMB-45*	Cytoplasm	Melanocytes
MITF	Nucleus	Melanocytes
AE1/3	Cytoplasm	Epithelia
Special stain		
PAS, PAS-D	Cell wall	Fungi (pink)
GMS (Gomori methinamine-silver)	Cell wall	Fungi (black)
Gram (Brown–Brenn)	Cell wall	Bacteria: G+ (purple);G– (pink)
AFB or Fite (acid-fast bacilli)	Cell wall	Atypical mycobacteria (red)
Verhoeff–van Gieson		Elastic fibers (black)
Fontana–Masson		Melanin-argentaffin (black)
Von Kossa		Calcium (black)
Giemsa		Mast cell granules (purple), leishmania (red)

G+, gram positive, G–, gram negative.
*Usually negative in spindle cell and desmoplastic melanoma.

Paraneoplastic pemphigus is a severe autoimmune bullous disease precipitated by an underlying occult or known malignancy [10]. Patients present with painful blisters on skin and mucosae. Histology shows a unique combination of interface dermatitis and acantholysis (e.g., keratinocytes lose their cohesion). Direct immunofluorescence shows intercellular and epidermal basement membrane staining usually with IgG and/or C3.

Acute graft versus host disease (AGVHD) is a systemic reaction often in the setting of allogeneic bone marrow transplantation. When it involves the skin, AGVHD manifests with a histologic pattern of interface alteration (Table 7.3). Chronic graft versus host disease (CGVHD) is the systemic reaction that develops months after transplantation and presents as a lichenoid or sclerodermoid variant (Table 7.3).

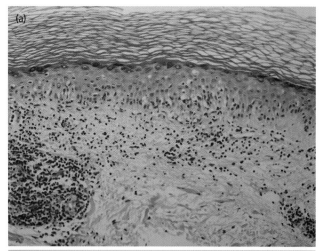

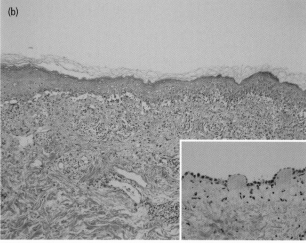

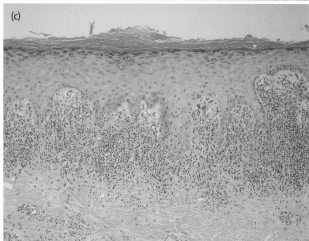

Figure 7.3 Patterns of interface dermatitis. (a) Erythema multiforme. Note vacuolar alteration of epidermal basal layer with dyskeratotic keratinocytes at all levels, little alteration in cornified layer. (b) Paraneoplastic pemphigus. Note vacuolar alteration of basal layer with associated acantholysis of keratinocytes. Direct immunofluorescence would show IgG and/or C3 along the dermal–epidermal junction and between keratinocytes (intercellular pattern). (c) Lichen planus. Note heavy, band-like distribution of inflammation along the dermal–epidermal junction in association with dyskeratotic keratinocytes mostly low in the epidermis, hyperkeratosis.

Table 7.3 Clinical entities with histologic interface dermatitis.

Clinical entity	Distinguishing features
Acute GVHD	Sparse inflammation, satellite cell necrosis (one or more lymphocyte in contiguity with necrotic keratinocyte), involvement of adnexal structures
Chronic GVHD	Varies: Alteration of the epidermal basal layer often with irregular epidermal hyperplasia simulating lichen planus; may resemble AGVHD; sclerodermoid form has subtle interface alteration and prominent dermal fibrosis often with atrophy of adnexae
EM/SJS/TEN*	Necrotic keratinocytes at all levels of the epidermis, no eosinophils, often papillary dermal edema in EM
Paraneoplastic pemphigus	Necrotic keratinocytes, suprabasal acantholysis, DIF of perilesional skin shows intercellular and basement membrane staining with C3 and/or IgG, IIF using pt serum on murine bladder epithelium has intercellular staining
Fixed drug eruption	Neutrophils and eosinophils in the dermal infiltrate, often a solitary lesion clinically
Lichen planus	Brisk lymphohistiocytic infiltrate along DEJ, hyperkeratosis, epidermal hyperplasia, hypergranulosis
Lichenoid drug eruption	Brisk lymphohistiocytic infiltrate along DEJ, parakeratosis, hypergranulosis, dermal eosinophils

DEJ, dermal–epidermal junction; DIF, direct immunofluorescence; EM, erythema multiforme; GVHD, graft versus host disease; IIF, indirect immunofluorescence; SJS, Stevens–Johnson syndrome; TEN, toxic epidermal necrolysis.

*These entities must be defined and distinguished based on established clinical criteria.

Given that interface dermatitis is, like any inflammatory condition, a process in evolution, histologic changes may be early or late in a given biopsy. In some cases, it is not possible to make a specific diagnosis and one may consider additional biopsies from lesions in other stages of evolution and/or from other anatomic locations.

Spongiotic dermatitis

Spongiotic dermatitis is a histologic descriptor of separation of intraepidermal keratinocytes by edema usually with associated superficial perivascular inflammation. This histologic pattern is most often seen in various eczematous dermatitides including atopic, nummular, allergic contact, seborrheic, hypersensitivity, and stasis dermatitis, each of which is usually readily defined based on clinical distribution.

Superficial or superficial and deep perivascular lymphohistiocytic inflammation

This pattern of inflammation is relatively nonspecific. Superficial and deep perivascular lymphohistiocytic inflammation may be

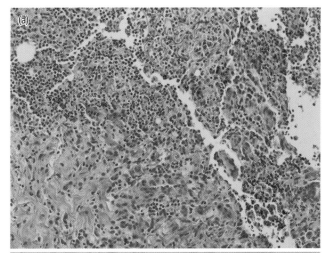
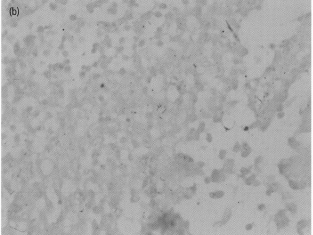

Table 7.4 Suppurative and granulomatous reaction pattern.

Clinical diagnosis	Secondary clues to making the diagnosis
Deep fungal infection	Often has pseudoepitheliomatous hyperplasia, PAS or GMS stain showing fungi (e.g. spores, hyphae, pseudohyphae)
Atypical mycobacterial infection	AFB stain showing short, slender rods
Ruptured folliculitis or follicular cyst	Cornified cells and/or benign epithelium in dermis
Foreign body	Polarizable or nonpolarizable foreign material
Interstitial granulomatous dermatitis	Inflammatory infiltrate in between collagen bundles with little palisading, little if any necrosis, ± leukocytoclastic vasculitis or interface dermatitis

AFB, acid-fast bacilli; GMS, Gomori methinamine-silver; PAS, periodic acid–Schiff.

Figure 7.4 (a) Suppurative and granulomatous dermatitis (20x) composed of lymphocytes, histiocytes including multinucleate forms and neutrophils. (b) Acid-fast bacilli stain positively decorating slender short organisms that subsequently were culture-proven *Mycobacterium marinum* (60x).

seen in a wide variety of clinical settings including morbilliform drug eruption, viral exanthem, arthropod bite, or as a manifestation of autoimmune connective tissue diseases. Other histologic clues may aid distinction between these and other entities including the presence or absence of eosinophils (may be seen in arthropod bite or response to drug) or dermal mucin (more frequent in autoimmune connective tissue disease). Inherent in making the diagnosis of superficial and deep perivascular inflammation is a biopsy that has been taken at a depth sufficient to evaluate the deep perivascular space (i.e., punch or deep saucerization biopsy).

Suppurative and granulomatous dermatitis

Suppurative and granulomatous dermatitis is a histologic reaction pattern that may be seen in a variety of clinical contexts (Figure 7.4; Table 7.4) including in the setting of various infections and indeed is a clue to the dermatopathologist to look for an infectious agent (Table 7.2). Histologically, one sees a mixed inflammatory

infiltrate of small lymphocytes, neutrophils, and histiocytes with multinucleate forms. It is generally prudent to evaluate for mycotic and mycobacterial infectious organisms by special stains and/or cultures. Tissue culture and molecular tests are more sensitive than tissue staining.

Conclusions

Clinical–pathologic correlation is critical to making accurate diagnoses in dermatology. Whether the primary process is a neoplasm or an inflammatory dermatosis, choosing the appropriate biopsy technique (i.e., shave, punch, incision, excision) will maximize the likelihood that the dermatopathologist views relevant diagnostic features. In context of the clinical setting, the oncologist should expect a biopsy interpretation that guides patient care.

References

1 Dubauskas, Z., Kunishige, J., Prieto, V.G., Jonasch, E., Hwu, P. & Tannir, N.M. (2009) Cutaneous squamous cell carcinoma and inflammation of actinic keratoses associated with sorafenib. *Clinical Genitourinary Cancer*, **7** (1), 20–23.
2 Serrao, V.V. & Feio, A.B. (2008) Inflammation of actinic keratoses with capecitabine therapy for colon cancer. *European Journal of Dermatology*, **18** (2), 200.
3 Lacouture, M.E., Desai, A., Soltani, K. *et al.* (2006) Inflammation of actinic keratoses subsequent to therapy with sorafenib, a multitargeted tyrosine-kinase inhibitor. *Clinical and Experimental Dermatology*, **31** (6), 783–785.

4 Weedon, D., Brooks, D., Malo, J. & Williamson, R. (2010) Abortive keratoacanthoma: a hitherto unrecognized variant. *Pathology*, **42** (7), 661–663.

5 Smith, K.J., Haley, H., Hamza, S. & Skelton, H.G. (2009) Eruptive keratoacanthoma-type squamous cell carcinomas in patients taking sorafenib for the treatment of solid tumors. *Dermatologic Surgery*, **35** (11), 1766–1770.

6 Piscioli, F., Boi, S., Zumiani, G. & Cristofolini, M. (1984) A gigantic, metastasizing keratoacanthoma: report of a case and discussion on classification. *American Journal of Dermatopathology*, **6** (2), 123–129.

7 Barnhill, R.L., Cerroni, L., Cook, M. *et al.* (2010) State of the art, nomenclature, and points of consensus and controversy concerning benign melanocytic lesions: outcome of an international workshop. *Advances in Anatomic Pathology*, **17** (2), 73–90.

8 Miteva, M. & Lazova, R. (2010) Spitz nevus and atypical spitzoid neoplasm. *Seminars in Cutaneous Medicine and Surgery*, **29** (3), 165–173.

9 Gerami, P., Jewell, S.S., Morrison, L.E. *et al.* (2009) Fluorescence in situ hybridization (FISH) as an ancillary diagnostic tool in the diagnosis of melanoma. *American Journal of Surgical Pathology*, **33** (8), 1146–1156.

10 Kaplan, I., Hodak, E., Ackerman, L., Mimouni, D., Anhalt, G.J. & Calderon, S. (2004) Neoplasms associated with paraneoplastic pemphigus: a review with emphasis on non-hematologic malignancy and oral mucosal manifestations. *Oral Oncology*, **40** (6), 553–562.

2 Cancer-Related Dermatologic Disorders

8 Paraneoplastic, Inherited Cancer Syndrome, and Environmental Carcinogen-Related Dermatoses

Cindy England Owen and Jeffrey P. Callen

University of Louisville School of Medicine, Louisville, KY, USA

Skin findings can serve both as a marker of internal malignancy and for inherited syndromes that carry an increased cancer risk. In paraneoplastic dermatoses, skin findings indicate a potential underlying neoplasia. In *Cancer of the Skin*, Curth [1] outlined criteria to determine the relationship between a dermatosis and an internal malignancy:

1. Concurrent onset;
2. Parallel course;
3. Uniform site or type of malignancy;
4. Statistical association; and
5. Genetic association (Table 8.1).

In most cases, few of these criteria are met, yet they serve as a guide in analyzing the relationship. Paraneoplastic dermatoses include a wide spectrum of inflammatory, proliferative, metabolic, and neoplastic disorders that do not directly involve tumor cells from the malignancy. Certainly, the skin can manifest direct involvement of visceral malignancy, by extension of the tumor to the skin or by tumor metastases. Direct involvement is not considered under the heading of paraneoplastic disorders and is covered in Chapter 3.

Paraneoplastic disorders

Skin changes from hormone-secreting tumors

Glucagonoma syndrome

Glucagonoma syndrome consists of a triad of findings:

1. Neoplastic proliferation of glucagon-secreting alpha cells of the pancreas;
2. Diabetes mellitus; and
3. An eruption known as necrolytic migratory erythema (NME).

NME presents as patches of intense erythema with superficial epidermal necrosis resulting in fragile superficial vesicles that unroof easily and crust. The patches spread centrifugally with central healing, producing an annular appearance with irregular outlines. Coalescence of patches leads to polycyclic configurations. The most frequently involved sites are the perioral and distal extremities, but the groin, abdomen, buttocks, and thighs may also be involved. Lesions can be induced by minor trauma. NME will develop during the course of all patients with glucagonoma, and is the presenting symptom in about 70% [2]. Anemia, weight loss, stomatitis, abdominal pain, diarrhea, and thromboembolic phenomena are also associated with glucagonoma syndrome.

Diagnosis is made by clinical features, an elevated serum glucagon, and evidence of a neuroendocrine tumor. NME follows a parallel course with glucagonoma. Treatment with octreotide controls NME effectively, but may not change the course of malignancy [2].

Carcinoid syndrome

Carcinoid tumors are neoplasms of peptide- and amine-producing neuroendocrine cells that secrete a variety of substances including serotonin, corticotropin, histamine, dopamine, prostagladins, and kallikrein. Carcinoid syndrome manifests as episodic flushing, diarrhea, abdominal pain, cramping, and occasionally wheezing and valvular heart disease. Flushing involves the upper half of the body and last 10–30 minutes. Eventually, a permanent flush with telangiectasia can develop, resembling rosacea, or a persistent edema and erythema leading to leonine facies. In some cases a pellagra-like dermatitis may result, caused by the shunting of tryptophan stores for nicotinic acid production to the 5-hydroxylation pathway to make the serotonin precursor, 5-hydroxytryptophan (5-HT). In the normal state, 1% of tryptophan goes to this pathway, whereas in carcinoid syndrome, an estimated 60% is used to make 5-HT [3].

Incidence of carcinoid syndrome is about 15% in localized disease, and up to 50% in extensive disease [3]. Tumors of the embryologic midgut (small intestine, appendix, and proximal

Table 8.1 Curth's postulates. Not all criteria need to be met to postulate a relationship between skin disease and underlying malignancy.

1. The malignancy and skin disease have a concurrent onset
2. The malignancy and skin disease follow a parallel course. If the malignancy is successfully treated the dermatosis resolves. Recurrence of the malignancy leads to reappearance of cutaneous signs
3. A uniform site or type of malignancy is associated with a specific dermatosis
4. A statistical association exists between the malignancy and a specific cutaneous eruption
5. A genetic association exists between the cutaneous disease and the malignancy

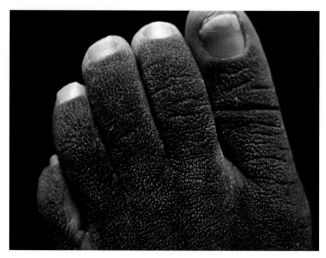

Figure 8.1 Hyperpigmented, verrucous plaque of the dorsal foot in a patient with generalized acanthosis nigricans. This patient had also presented with erythema gyratum repens (see Figure 8.5).

colon) are the most strongly associated with carcinoid syndrome, as are those with metastases to the liver or involving extraintestinal sites. Diagnosis of carcinoid syndrome is supported by elevated urinary 5-hydroxyindoleacetic acid (5-HIAA). Somatostatin analogs can be used to help relieve the symptoms of carcinoid syndrome.

Ectopic ACTH-producing tumors

ACTH (corticotropin) is derived from proopiomelanocortin (POMC), which is normally produced by the pituitary gland and is the major regulator of glucocorticoid and adrenal androgen secretion. Melanocyte stimulating hormone (MSH) is also derived from POMC. The ectopic corticotropin syndrome is a unique disorder of POMC production by nonendocrine tumors. The most striking clinical finding is hyperpigmentation, induced by MSH, in addition to a direct effect on melanogenesis by corticotropin [4,5]. Associated signs and symptoms include proximal weakness, truncal obesity, and moon facies. Hypertension, hypokalemic metabolic alkalosis, and abnormal glucose tolerance may also be seen. The latter two are highly suggestive of ectopic corticotropin syndrome, as they are rarely seen in patients with Cushing disease [4].

The lung is the most likely organ to harbor an ectopic POMC-secreting tumor. The most common lung tumor to secrete POMC is small cell carcinoma, followed by carcinoid tumors. POMC-secreting tumors in other locations include (in decreasing order of frequency): islet cell tumors of the pancreas, carcinoid tumors of the thymus, medullary thyroid tumors, adrenal pheochromocytomas, and ovarian, cervical, or prostate carcinomas [4].

In a patient with suspected ectopic ACTH production, assays may include include 24-hour urine for free cortisol, plasma corticotropin levels, and dexamethasone suppression testing.

Proliferative and inflammatory paraneoplastic dermatoses

Acanthosis nigricans

Acanthosis nigricans (AN) is a common disorder characterized by hyperpigmented velvety plaques in intertriginous areas and areas of trauma. AN is usually associated with insulin resistance. The sites involved most commonly are the posterior and lateral neck, axillae, and inguinal folds. Malignant AN may develop rapidly and become generalized (Figure 8.1), and lacks the characteristic predilection for black or Hispanic patients [6]. Histopathologic changes are identical to those seen in other type of AN. Other paraneoplastic dermatoses may occur simultaneously with malignant AN, such as tripe palms, florid cutaneous papillomatosis, or the sign of Leser–Trélat.

The most commonly associated malignancies are gastrointestinal (gastric) and genitourinary adenocarcinomas. Malignant AN may develop as a result of increased levels of epidermal growth factors, stimulating keratinocytes and dermal fibroblasts [6]. Because AN is common, work-up for underlying malignancy should be initiated only in cases with atypical distribution or with suspicious signs or symptoms. Unexplained weight loss in an older adult, for example, when associated with AN, should prompt a work-up of the gastrointestinal tract, in addition to cervical examination and mammography in women, and prostate specific antigen in men.

Tripe palms

Tripe palms are characterized by a ridged or rugose appearance of the palms (and occasionally the soles), so named because it resembles the bovine foregut (Figure 8.2). Some consider this to be a manifestation of AN on the palms. It is considered separately from AN, however, because the malignant association is different from that of AN. However, when AN and tripe palms coincide, the most commonly associated malignancies are gastric and pulmonary (about 25% each). When tripe palms present alone, pulmonary cancer accounts for over 50% of the associated neoplasms [7].

Sign of Leser–Trélat

The sign of Leser–Trélat is the abrupt appearance or rapid increase in size of multiple seborrheic keratoses (Figure 8.3). The lesions

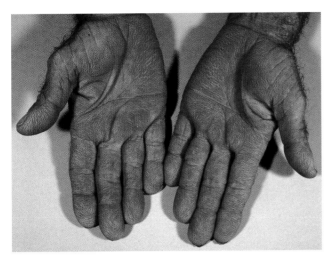

Figure 8.2 Rugose plaques of tripe palms.

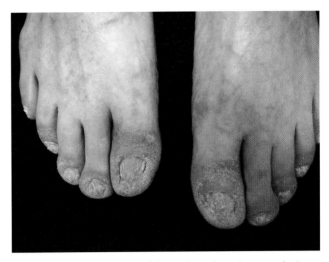

Figure 8.4 Psoriasiform plaques of the toes in acrokeratosis paraneoplastica (Bazex syndrome).

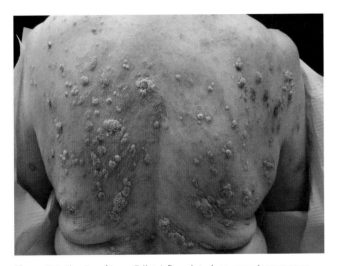

Figure 8.3 The sign of Leser–Trélat. Inflamed stuck-on appearing verrucous plaques of the trunk.

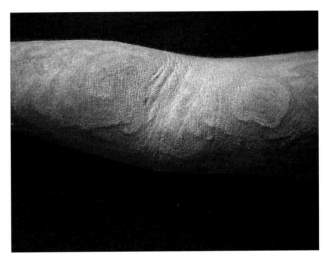

Figure 8.5 Parallel bands with a wood grain appearance in erythema gyratum repens (the patient also had generalized acanthosis nigricans).

themselves are indistinguishable from common seborrheic keratoses. This sign is most commonly associated with gastrointestinal adenocarcinoma [8]. Work-up for malignancy may be indicated if associated with AN, or in a patient complaining of weight loss or other symptoms. In addition to gastrointestinal adenocarcinoma, associated malignancies include breast carcinoma, lymphoma, and leukemia.

Acrokeratosis paraneoplastica (Bazex syndrome)
Bazex syndrome is rare but very strongly associated with carcinoma of the upper "aerodigestive" tract. This is a psoriasiform eruption that begins with erythema and fine scale of the fingers, toes, aural helices, and nasal tip. As it progresses, a violaceous keratoderma may develop on the palms and soles, with associated nail dystrophy (Figure 8.4). In a review of 93 cases by Bolognia *et al.* [9], an associated malignancy was detected in all cases.

Squamous cell carcinoma of the head and neck, and squamous cell carcinoma of unknown primary involving cervical lymph nodes were most the most common associated neoplasms. In 91% of patients, the rash improved significantly upon treatment of the neoplasm, but with persistence of nail dystrophy.

Erythema gyratum repens
Erythema gyratum repens (EGR) is a reactive erythema characterized by pruritic serpiginous scaly bands in a configuration that resembles wood grain (Figure 8.5). The parallel bands can be either macular or papular and migrate at a rapid rate. EGR usually involves the trunk and proximal extremities. Eighty percent of patients have an associated neoplasm, most commonly lung, followed by esophageal and breast cancer. The EGR develops, on average, 4–9 months prior to discovery of the internal malignancy [10].

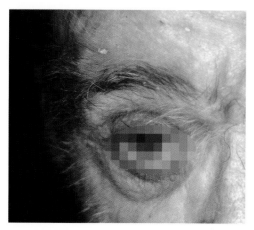

Figure 8.6 Nonpigmented, silky lanugo hairs of the face in hypertrichosis lanuginosa acquisita.

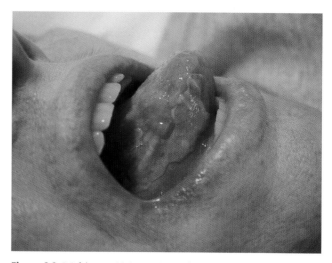

Figure 8.8 Painful stomatitis in a patient with paraneoplastic pemphigus.

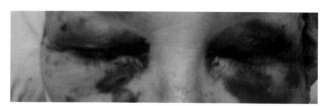

Figure 8.7 Pinch purpura of systemic amyloidosis in a hospitalized patient following chest compressions.

Hypertrichosis lanuginosa acquisita

Hypertrichosis lanuginose acquisita (also known as malignant down) is a rare syndrome in which excessive growth of lanugo hair develops on the forehead, ears, and nose (and less commonly the trunk or extremities). This differs from hirsutism which is the excess growth of terminal hairs. Lanugo hairs are nonpigmented and silky, and in this syndrome they grow to great length and are easily pulled out (Figure 8.6). The most common associations are lung and gastrointestinal cancer [11]. Painful glossitis, angular cheilitis, and enlarged red fungiform papillae of the anterior tongue may be associated with hypertrichosis lanuginosa acquisita.

Primary systemic amyloidosis

Amyloidosis refers to the extracellular deposition of insoluble fibrillar proteins. Primary systemic amyloidosis (AL type) occurs in the setting of plasma cell dyscrasias, especially multiple myeloma [12]. The most common mucocutaneous findings are purpura, petechiae, and ecchymoses following minor trauma ("pinch purpura"). A classic finding is periorbital purpura following Valsalva maneuvers or dependent positioning (Figure 8.7). Papules and plaques may also be seen, and are characteristically waxy in appearance. Macroglossia, enlarged shoulder pads, bullous lesions, and sclerodermatous changes have also been

reported. Diagnosis is confirmed by histology. Amyloid deposits appear as homogeneous eosinophilic masses with a fissured or "cracked pavement" appearance. If an AL type amyloidosis is confirmed, the patient must undergo work-up for plasma cell dyscrasia by serum protein electropheresis or immunofixation electropheresis.

Scleromyxedema

Scleromyxedema (generalized lichen myxedematosus) is a cutaneous mucinosis that presents with a widespread eruption of firm waxy papules arranged in a linear fashion, most commonly on the face, neck, forearms, and hands. When the lesions coalesce, a sclerodermoid induration may be noted. Associated findings include sparse eyebrow, axillary, and pubic hair, or leonine facies. The paraproteinemia associated with scleromyxedema is immunoglobulin G (IgG) lambda in most cases. To make the diagnosis of scleromyxedema, the following criteria must be met:
1. Generalized papular or sclerdermoid eruption;
2. Mucin deposition, fibrosis, and fibroblast proliferation on biopsy;
3. Monoclonal gammapathy; and
4. Absence of thyroid disease [13].

In a patient with the characteristic eruption and histologic findings, serum protein electrophoresis and/or immunofixation electrophoresis should be performed.

Paraneoplastic pemphigus

Paraneoplastic pemphigus (PNP) is an autoimmune mucocutaneous blistering condition with a variable presentation. The most consistent clinical feature is the development of painful stomatitis (Figure 8.8). Cutaneous lesions include tense blisters, erythema multiforme-like targetoid lesions, lichenoid lesions, and even confluent erosions resembling toxic epidermal necrolysis. Toxic epidermal necrolysis is the most common differential diagnosis. The diagnosis of PNP requires demonstration of antiplakin antibodies in the serum by indirect immunofluorescence. Histology and direct immunofluorescence findings are variable, but can assist in the differential diagnosis.

PNP-associated malignancies include non-Hodgkin's lymphoma (42%), chronic lymphocytic leukemia (29%), Castleman disease (10%), thymoma, sarcoma, and Waldenstrom macroglobulinemia [14]. Anhalt [14] has proposed four minimal criteria for diagnosing PNP:
1. Painful progressive stomatitis;
2. Histologic features of acantholysis, lichenoid, or interface dermatitis;
3. Demonstration of antiplakin antibodies (immunohisto-chemistry demonstrating antibodies against periplakin and envoplakin, at the least);
4. Demonstration of an underlying lymphoproliferative neoplasm.

Involvement of the bronchial and alveolar airways can lead to bronchiolitis obliterans, a severe life-threatening complication [15]. Treatment with oral corticosteroids and other immunosuppressive medications can lead to improvement of skin lesions, but bronchiolitis obliterans may still progress. PNP is generally progressive despite treatment of the underlying neoplasm.

Antiepiligrin cicatricial pemphigoid

Antiepiligrin cicatricial pemphigoid (AECP) is an autoimmune blistering condition characterized by severe painful lesions of the oral mucosa, and skin bullae and erosions on an erythematous base. AECP is a subset of cicatricial pemphigoid that shows IgG antibodies to laminin 5 (also known as laminin 332). Nearly all patients will have oral involvement, with involvement of other sites in decreasing order of frequency including ocular, laryngeal, nasal, pharyngeal, esophageal, genital, and anal [16]. Sequelae of these lesions can be severe and lead to gingival destruction, tooth loss, blindness, dysphagia, dysphonia, and airway compromise.

Diagnostic criteria for AECP require:
1. The presence of erosive and/or blistering lesions of mucous membranes;
2. *In situ* deposits of IgG autoantibodies in epidermal basement membranes, or circulating IgG autoantibodies that bind the dermal side of salt-split skin; and
3. Circulating IgG that immunoprecipitates laminin 5 on radiolabeled human keratinocytes [16].

Patients with AECP have a relative risk for cancer of 6.8 (95% CI 3.3–12.5) [17]. The cancer type varies but most are solid tumors. Immunosuppressive therapies are commonly utilized but AECP is often a progressive disease.

Sweet syndrome

Sweet syndrome (acute febrile neutrophilic dermatosis) consists of fever, neutrophilia, arthralgia, and tender plaques and nodules. The lesions typically appear on the upper extremities, face, and neck as erythematous to violaceous, sharply demarcated plaques, sometimes with a pseudovesicular appearance . Pathergy is often noted, with lesions developing at sites of trauma. Systemic corticosteroids result in prompt resolution of lesions and symptoms. Diagnosis is supported by the histologic findings of a dense infiltrate of mature neutrophils filling the mid to upper dermis.

Sweet syndrome is classically associated with upper respiratory infections, inflammatory bowel disease, and pregnancy. Less commonly, it can be paraneoplastic or drug-induced (usually secondary to granulocyte colony-stimulating factors). Hematologic malignancies are most common (accounting for 85% of associated malignancies), especially acute myeloid leukemia, but solid tumors are also reported [18]. The most commonly associated solid tumors are those of the genitourinary tract. In paraneoplastic Sweet syndrome, lesions tend to recur, and may involve areas such as the oral mucosa or lower extremities. While classic Sweet syndrome occurs more frequently in females, paraneoplastic Sweet syndrome does not have a female predominance [18].

Pyoderma gangrenosum

Pyoderma gangrenosum (PG) is a neutrophilic dermatosis characterized by painful ulcerations with dusky, violaceous overhanging borders. These typically occur on the lower extremities, and, like Sweet syndrome, can be pathergic. Unlike Sweet syndrome, PG usually heals with cribriform scars. The associations include inflammatory bowel disease, hematologic malignancy, monoclonal gammopathy (usually of IgA), and arthritis. Hematologic malignancy-associated PG may present as an atypical or bullous variant with superficial ulceration that is more common on the upper extremities and head [19]. Histologic findings are nonspecific, and other causes of similar histologic patterns must be ruled, especially infectious or vascular causes of ulceration. Systemic corticosteroids are often used to treat PG, usually followed by or in conjunction with dapsone or immunosuppressive steroid-sparing agents. Meticulous wound care should be provided, but with avoidance of debridement, as this can enlarge the ulcer. Diagnosis of PG that is unexplained by existing conditions should prompt a work-up to assess for underlying malignancy or inflammatory bowel disease.

Dermatomyositis

Dermatomyositis (DM) is a condition that presents with characteristic cutaneous findings and an associated inflammatory myopathy. The pathognomonic skin findings include scaly violaceous papules overlying the bony prominences of the hands (known as Gottron papules), and the so-called heliotrope rash characterized by a violaceous patches of the eyelids. Other cutaneous findings include poikilodermatous patches and plaques in a photodistribution, scaly plaques of the scalp and lateral thighs, periungual telangiectasia, and ragged cuticles. The myopathy usually presents with a progressive symmetric proximal weakness. Elevated creatine kinase, aldolase, abnormal elecromyogram, and findings on muscle biopsy can supplement the clinical examination in determining the extent of muscle involvement in DM.

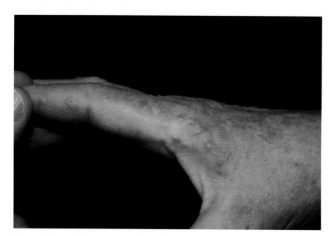

Figure 8.9 Lightly erythematous papules of the hand in multicentric reticulohistiocytosis.

Table 8.2 Diagnostic criteria for Muir–Torre syndrome. Diagnosis requires one criterion from groups A and B, or all three from group C, in the absence of predisposing factors.

Group A
Sebaceous adenoma
Sebaceous epithelioma
Sebaceous carcinoma
Keratoacanthoma with sebaceous differentiation

Group B
Visceral malignancy

Group C
Multiple keratoacanthomas
Multiple visceral malignancies
Family history of Muir–Torre syndrome

Source: Adapted from Schwartz and Torre [23] reproduced with permission from Elsevier.

The malignancies associated with DM include ovarian, breast, uterine, lung, gastric, colorectal, and pancreatic cancers. Associated malignancies are usually detected within 1 year of diagnosis. Malignancy work-up should be repeated yearly for at least 3 years, then subsequently according to age-based health maintenance guidelines. Many dermatologists will also add computed tomography (CT) scan of the chest, abdomen, and pelvis [20]. A recent study examined the use of positron emission tomography (PET) scanning in lieu of other malignancy screening that is traditionally performed and found that PET was as effective and perhaps less costly [21].

Multicentric reticulohistiocytosis

Multicentric reticulohistiocytosis (MRH) is a rare multisystem disease consisting of a cutaneous histiocytosis and destructive polyarthritis. Skin lesions are flesh-colored to yellow–brown papules and nodules with a predilection for the upper body, most frequently the face, hands, forearms, and ears (Figure 8.9). Lesions around the fingernails have a "coral bead" appearance. One-third of patients have a coexistent xanthelasma. Diagnosis of the reticulohistiocytosis is made by histopathology, with circumscribed dermal infiltrates of mononuclear and multinucleated giant cells containing eosinophilic "ground glass" cytoplasm. The cells of the dermal infiltrate stain most consistently with CD68. The arthritis of MRH varies by location and severity, but can be rapidly destructive and progress to arthritis mutilans in half of patients. Other associated symptoms include fever, weight loss, and weakness.

MRH is associated with underlying malignancy in 25% of patients. The associated malignancies vary widely in type but most common are breast, hematologic, and gastric cancers [22]. MRH tends to resolve spontaneously after an average of 8 years, but the arthritis can cause marked joint destruction during the course.

Inherited syndromes with increased cancer risk and skin effects

Muir–Torre syndrome

Muir–Torre syndrome (MTS) is an autosomal dominant syndrome of associated sebaceous neoplasms, keratoacanthomas, and internal malignancy. It is considered to be a subset of hereditary nonpolyposis colon cancer syndrome (HNPCCS). Schwartz and Torre's [23] criteria to define MTS include the diagnosis of a sebaceous neoplasm (adenoma, epithelioma, or carcinoma) or keratoacanthoma with sebaceous differentiation and the presence of an internal malignancy; or a family history of MTS with a personal history of keratoacanthomas and multiple visceral malignancies (Table 8.2). Solitary sebaceous neoplasms of the head and neck are common and often not associated with internal malignancy. The associated internal malignancies are most commonly colorectal, genitourinary, breast, and hematologic (in decreasing order of frequency).

In patients diagnosed with a sebaceous tumor, many advocate testing the lesion for microsatellite instability or by immunohistochemistry to demonstrate loss of staining for particular mismatch repair genes: MSH2 (most common), MLH1, and possibly MSH6 [24]. Patients diagnosed with MTS should undergo screening as published in recent guidelines [25].

Gardner syndrome

Gardner syndrome is an autosomal dominant disorder characterized by extensive polyposis of the gastrointestinal tract, bony tumors, and cutaneous lesions. Cutaneous lesions include epidermoid cysts, trichilemmomas, fibromas, lipomas, leiomyomas, and neurofibromas. Osteomas of the mandible, skull, or long bones are noted on radiographs. Congenital hypertrophy of the retinal pigment epithelium occurs in a

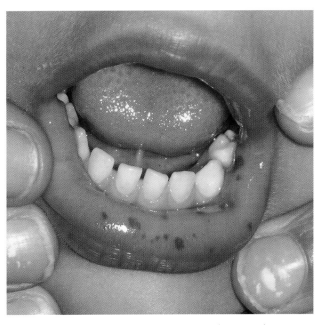

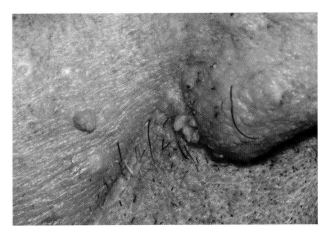

Figure 8.10 Facial trichelemmomas in a patient with Cowden syndrome.

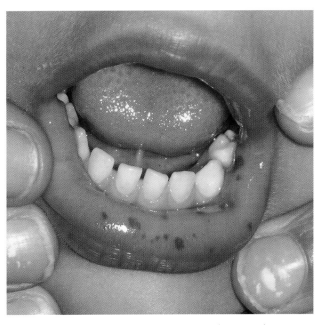

Figure 8.11 Pigmented labial macules in a patient with Peutz–Jeghers syndrome.

majority of patients. Patients with Gardner syndrome are at increased risk for desmoid tumors, which are invasive fibromatoses, most commonly found in the abdomen [26].

Gardner syndrome is best considered within the scope of familial adenomatous polyposis (FAP). FAP is caused by a germline mutation in the adenomatous polyposis coli (*APC*) tumor suppressor gene. Thyroid cancer (papillary type most commonly) is also reported in FAP, with increased risk in females [26].

Cowden syndrome

Cowden syndrome (CS), also known as multiple hamartoma syndrome, is an autosomal dominant condition characterized by facial trichelemmomas, acral keratoses, papillomas of the oral cavity (Figure 8.10), and macrocephaly. CS is caused by germline mutations resulting in loss of function of the *PTEN* gene (in 80% of cases) [27]. Patients with CS are at increased risk for thyroid, breast, and endometrial cancers. Hamartomas can be seen in the gastrointestinal tract, with asymptomatic polyps present in 60–90% of patients. Women with CS will develop benign breast disease and/or uterine leiomyomas or fibroids.

Peutz–Jeghers syndrome

Peutz–Jeghers syndrome (PJS) is an autosomal dominant disorder that presents with pigmented mucosal lesions and hamartomotous polyps in the gastrointestinal tract. Patients with PJS are at increased risk for various malignancies including pancreatic, lung, breast, uterine, ovarian, gastrointestinal, and testicular. Most cases appear to be caused by a mutation in *STK11* gene, which encodes for a serine–threonine kinase [28]. The pigmented lesions of PJS are noted on the lips (Figure 8.11), and around the mouth, eyes, nostrils, and buccal mucosa. These are typically macular and range in size 1–5 mm. Diagnosis is made by the presence of hamartomatous polyps plus family history or pigmented mucosal lesions.

Birt–Hogg–Dubé

Birt–Hogg–Dubé (BHD) is an autosomal dominant condition that presents with benign hair follicle tumors (fibrofolliculomas and/or trichodiscomas), and skin tags of the head and neck. These skin findings do not usually appear until after age 20. BHD carries an increased risk of renal cell cancer [29]. More than 80% of patients with BHD have multiple lung cysts [29]. Lung function is usually normal but there is an increased risk for spontaneous pneumothorax. BHD has been linked to truncating mutations of the *FLCN* gene, which encodes for the folliculin protein. Criteria for diagnosis include at least five fibrofolliculomas or trichodiscomas (at least one histologically confirmed) of adult onset, or known *FLCN* germline mutation. Diagnosis can also be made if two of the following criteria are present: multiple basally located lung cysts, renal cancer (early onset or multifocal/bilateral or mixed chromophobe/oncocytic histology), or first degree relative with BHD [29].

Howel–Evans syndrome

Howel–Evans syndrome (tylosis with esophageal cancer; TOC) is an autosomal dominant condition characterized by the presence of thickened skin of the palms and soles (tylosis) and esophageal cancer. The focal nonepidermolytic palmoplantar keratoderma usually develops in childhood and is worse over pressure sites. Another skin finding is oral leukoplakia. Patients with this syndrome are at high risk of squamous cell esophageal cancer. The genetic locus, known as TOC, has been mapped to a region of chromosome 17q25 [30]. Annual upper endoscopy is indicated in patients and affected family members.

Hereditary leiomyomatosis/renal cell cancer syndrome

Hereditary leiomyomatosis/renal cell cancer (HLRCC, or Reed) syndrome is an autosomal dominant condition caused by a germline mutation in the gene encoding for fumarate hydratase. Patients with HLRCC have cutaneous and uterine leiomyomas. The cutaneous leiomyomas present as grouped firm, sometimes tender, flesh-colored to brown papules of the trunk or extremities. The renal cancers associated with HLRCC often present with metastatic disease and carry a high mortality rate. Given this, screening of the kidneys by CT or magnetic resonance imaging (MRI) is indicated for patients suspected of having HLRCC [31].

Environmental carcinogens with increased cancer risk and skin effects

Arsenic

Cutaneous signs of arsenic ingestion include small keratoses of the palms, soles, and hyperpigmentation of the trunk. Arsenic is present in drinking water, especially in well water in certain geographic areas, but also may encountered in industrial products, and, in the past, as a component in medicinal solutions and tablets. Arsenic exposure leads to increased risk for skin cancers, especially Bowen disease, squamous cell carcinoma, and basal cell carcinoma. While the skin is the most frequent site for arsenic-induced malignancy, lung, bladder, kidney, prostate, liver, and uterine cancer have also been reported [32]. Arsenic exposure also increases the risk for peripheral vascular, cardiovascular, and cerebrovascular disease, and bronchitis. Arsenic exposure can be documented by analysis of water, hair, nails, or urine [33]. Patients should be educated regarding safe water sources, and followed with regular skin examinations.

Vinyl chloride

Exposure to vinyl chloride can occur by air pollution, intake of contaminated drinking water, ingestion of food or use of cosmetics packaged in polyvinyl chloride, or by occupational exposure. In workers with high levels of exposure to vinyl chloride, there is an increased risk for angiosarcoma of the liver, and a possible increased risk for brain tumors [34]. The skin effects of vinyl chloride may include scleroderma and Raynaud phenomenon [35].

Ionizing radiation

With high doses of radiation there is an increased risk for leukemia and malignancies of the lung, thyroid, and breast [35]. Skin findings include acute radiation effects, such as erythema, acute radiodermatitis (characterized by intense local inflammation), and chronic radiodermatitis. Chronic radiodermatitis is characterized by atrophy, telangiectasia, induration, and mottled hyper- and hypopigmentation. There is also an increased risk for skin cancers, usually squamous cell and basal cell carcinomas [36].

References

1 Curth, H.O. (1976) Skin lesions and internal carcinoma. In: R. Andrade, S.L. Gumport, G.L. Popkin, *et al.* (eds), *Cancer of the Skin*, pp. 1308–1309. W.B. Saunders, Philadelphia, PA.

2 Chastain, M.A. (2001) The glucagonoma syndrome: a review of its features and discussion of new perspectives. *American Journal of the Medical Sciences*, **321** (5), 306–320.

3 Schnirer, I.I., Yao, J.C. & Ajani, J.A. (2003) Carcinoid: a comprehensive review. *Acta Oncologica (Stockholm, Sweden)*, **42** (7), 672–692.

4 Beuschlein, F. & Hammer, G.D. (2002) Ectopic proopiomelanocortin syndrome. *Endocrinology and Metabolism Clinics of North America*, **31** (1), 191–234.

5 Wakamatsu, K., Graham, A., Cook, D. & Thody, A.J. (1997) Characterisation of ACTH peptides in human skin and their activation of the melanocortin-1 receptor. *Pigment Cell Research*, **10**, 288–297.

6 Schwartz, R.A. (1994) Acanthosis nigricans. *Journal of the American Academy of Dermatology*, **31**, 1–19.

7 Cohen, P.R., Grossman, M.E., Almeida, L. & Kurzrock, R. (1993) Tripe palms and cancer. *Clinics in Dermatology*, **11**, 165–173.

8 Schwartz, R.A. (1994) Sign of Leser–Trélat. *Journal of the American Academy of Dermatology*, **31**, 1–19.

9 Bolognia, J.L., Brewer, Y.P. & Cooper, D.L. (1991) Bazex syndrome (acrokeratosis paraneoplastica): an analytic review. *Medicine*, **70**, 269–280.

10 Boyd, A.S., Neldner, K.H. & Menter, A. (1992) Erythema gyratum repens: a paraneoplastic phenomenon. *Journal of the American Academy of Dermatology*, **26**, 757–762.

11 Hovenden, A.L. (1987) Acquired hypertrichosis lanuginosa associated with malignancy. *Archives of Internal Medicine*, **147**, 2013–2018.

12 Falk, R.H., Comenzo, R.L. & Skinner, M. (1997) The systemic amyloidosis. *New England Journal of Medicine*, **337**, 898–909.

13 Rongioletti, F. & Rebora, A. (2001) Updated classification of papular mucinosis, lichen myxedematosus, and scleromyxedema. *Journal of the American Academy of Dermatology*, **44** (2), 273–281.

14 Anhalt, G.J. (2004) Paraneoplastic pemphigus. *Journal of Investigative Dermatology. Symposium Proceedings*, **9**, 29–33.

15 Nousari, H.C., Deterding, R., Wojtczack, H., Aho, S., Uitto, J. & Hashimoto, T. (1999) The mechanism of respiratory failure in paraneoplastic pemphigus. *New England Journal of Medicine*, **340**, 1406–1410.

16 Egan, C.A., Lazarova, Z., Darling, T.N., Yee, C. & Yancey, K.B. (2003) Anti-epiligrin cicatricial pemphigoid: clinical findings, immunopathogenesis, and significant associations. *Medicine*, **82**, 177–186.

17 Egan, C.A., Lazarova, Z., Darling, T.N., Yee, C., Coté, T. & Yancey, K.B. (2001) Anti-epiligrin cicatricial pemphigoid and relative risk for cancer. *Lancet*, **57**, 1850–1851.

18 Cohen, P.R. & Kurzrock, R. (2000) Sweet's syndrome: a neutrophilic dermatosis classically associated with acute onset and fever. *Clinics in Dermatology*, **18**, 265–282.

19 Hensley, C.D. & Caughman, S.W. (2000) Neutrophilic dermatoses associated with hematologic disorders. *Clinics in Dermatology*, **18**, 355–367.

20 Callen, J.P. (2002) When and how should the patient with dermatomyositis and amyopathic dermatomyositis be assessed for possible cancer? *Archives of Dermatology*, **138**, 969–971.

21 Selva-O'Callaghan, A., Grau, J.M., Gámez-Cenzano, C. *et al.* (2010) Conventional cancer screening versus PET/CT in dermatomyositis/polymyositis. *American Journal of Medicine*, **123** (6), 558–562.

22 Snow, J.L. & Muller, S.A. (1995) Malignancy-associated multicentric histiocytosis: a clinical, histological, and immunophenotypic study. *British Journal of Dermatology*, **133**, 71–76.

23 Schwartz, R.A. & Torre, D.P. (1995) The Muir–Torre syndrome: a 25-year retrospective. *Journal of the American Academy of Dermatology*, **33**, 90–104.

24 Eisen, D.B. & Michael, D.J. (2009) Sebaceous lesions and their associated syndromes: part II. *Journal of the American Academy of Dermatology*, **61**, 563–578.

25 Levin, B., Lieberman, D.A., McFarland, B. *et al.* (2008) Screening and surveillance for the early detection of colorectal cancer and adenomatous polyps, 2008: a joint guideline from the American Cancer Society, the US Multisociety Task Force on Colorectal Cancer, and the American College of Radiology. *CA: A Cancer Journal for Clinicians*, **58**, 130–160.

26 Galiatsatos, P. & Foulkes, W.D. (2006) Familial adenomatous polyposis. *American Journal of Gastroenterology*, **101**, 385–398.

27 Blumenthal, G.M. & Dennis, P.A. (2008) PTEN hamartoma tumor syndromes. *European Journal of Human Genetics*, **16**, 1289–1300.

28 Kopacova, M., Tacheci, I., Rejchrt, S. & Bures, J. (2009) Peutz–Jeghers syndrome: diagnostic and therapeutic approach. *World Journal of Gastroenterology*, **15** (43), 5397–5408.

29 Menko, F.H., van Steensel, M.A.M., Giraud, S. *et al.* (2009) Birt–Hogg–Dubé syndrome: diagnosis and management. *Lancet Oncology*, **10**, 1199–1206.

30 McRonald, F.E., Liloglou, T., Xinarianos, G. *et al.* (2006) Down-regulation of the cytoglobin gene, located on 17q25, in tylosis with esophageal cancer (TOC): evidence for *trans*-allele expression. *Human Molecular Genetics*, **15**, 1271–1277.

31 Alam, N.A., Olpin, S. & Leigh, I.M. (2005) Fumarate hydratase mutations and predisposition to cutaneous leiomyomas, uterine leiomyomas, and renal cancer. *British Journal of Dermatology*, **153**, 11–17.

32 Sengupta, S.F., Das, N.K. & Datta, P.K. (2008) Pathogenesis, clinical features, and pathology of chronic arsenicosis. *Indian Journal of Dermatology, Venereology and Leprology*, **74**, 559–570.

33 Das, N.K. & Sengupta, S.R. (2008) Arsenicosis: diagnosis and treatment. *Indian Journal of Dermatology, Venereology and Leprology*, **74**, 571–581.

34 Kielhorn, J., Melber, C., Wahnschaffe, U., Aitio, A. & Mangelsdorf, I. (2000) Vinyl chloride: still a cause for concern. *Environmental Health Perspectives*, **108**, 579–588.

35 Haustein, U.F. & Ziegler, V. (1985) Environmentally induced systemic sclerosis-like disorders. *International Journal of Dermatology*, **24**, 147–151.

36 Goldschmidt, J. & Sherwin, W.K. (1980) Reactions to ionizing radiation. *Journal of the American Academy of Dermatology*, **3**, 551–579.

3 Dermatologic Conditions During Cancer Therapy

9 Oral Mucosal Complications of Cancer Therapy

Stephen T. Sonis

Brigham and Women's Hospital and the Dana-Farber Cancer Institute; Harvard School of Dental Medicine, Boston, MA, USA

Introduction

The oral mucosa is a common site for manifestations of toxicities associated with drug, therapeutic transplants, and radiation therapy used for the treatment of cancer. Mucosal manifestations of regimen-related toxicities vary in their biology, clinical course and presentation, impact on patients' health, and associated incremental health and economic cost.

Oral mucosal complications of cancer therapy can be placed into four major categories:
1. Lesions associated with cytotoxic drug and radiation therapy;
2. Lesions attributable to targeted agents;
3. Lesions as late sequelae to treatment (e.g., graft versus host disease; GVHD);
4. Lesions that are a consequence of infection (e.g., candidiasis or herpes).

This chapter focuses on the noninfectious oral mucosal complications.

Mucosal injury attributable to cytotoxic therapy

Mucosal injury has been reported as a toxicity of both radiation therapy and chemotherapy since the advent of each [1]. Although all segments of the gastrointestinal tract are susceptible to regimen-related injury, the tissues of the oral cavity have been the best studied. Importantly, oral mucositis is consistently reported as the most symptomatically significant complication of treatment by patients receiving head and neck radiation therapy or those undergoing myeloablative chemotherapy [2]. Historically, the term "stomatitis" was used to describe mouth sores induced by cancer therapy. However, because stomatitis is often associated with other etiologies, especially infection, "mucositis" is more accurate as it is specifically associated with cancer treatment etiology.

Oral mucositis (OM) is common. It occurs to some degree in virtually every patient who receives radiation therapy, with or without concomitant chemotherapy, for the treatment of cancers of the head and neck. Conditioning regimens prior to hematopoietic stem cell transplant are often stomatotoxic. In a recently reported multicenter study of 1315 patients, the overall incidence of all grades of OM was over 70% and ulcerative mucositis occurred with a frequency of about 40%. The incidence of severe mucositis, 98%, was even more dramatic when the conditioning regimen consisted of etoposide, cyclophosphamide, and total body irradiation [3].

In general, when a patient develops mucositis in one cycle, the risk of a recurrence goes up with subsequent chemotherapy. For example, among breast cancer patients being treated with standard therapy (doxorubicin/cyclophosphamide and paclitaxel), the reported frequency of ulcerative mucositis in the first cycle of treatment is about 20% and jumps to 70% in subsequent cycles [4].

Interestingly, the true incidence of mucositis (and probably most other toxicities) is not easy to ascertain from the literature and in the majority of cases is probably under-reported. It has become an accepted practice when describing regimen-related toxicities to report only those deemed "severe" (usually grades 3 and 4). This distinction is made based on clinician reporting. First, the choice of which toxicity scale is selected markedly impacts the severity description. Figure 9.1 demonstrates mucositis scoring in the same cohort of patients in which two scales were used. Scale 1, the Radiation Therapy Oncology Group (RTOG) scale, ranks mucositis severity based on clinician-described lesion size, while scale 2 scores mucositis using the World Health Organization (WHO) scale in which the severity of mucositis is attributable to a combination of clinical findings

Dermatologic Principles and Practice in Oncology: Conditions of the Skin, Hair, and Nails in Cancer Patients, First Edition. Edited by Mario E. Lacouture.
© 2014 John Wiley & Sons, Inc. Published 2014 by John Wiley & Sons, Inc.

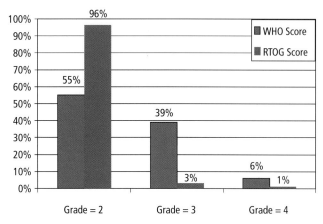

Figure 9.1 Comparison of mucositis scoring using RTOG or WHO criteria. Whereas WHO criteria combine functional (ability to eat) and objective (ulceration) outcomes, the RTOG scale used in this study was based solely on objective criteria. The disparity between the severity (grade) of mucositis between the two scales indicates the potential to underestimate the clinical impact of the condition in the absence of a functional or subjective component to a grading scale.

Table 9.1 Percentage area of ulceration of clinically significant mucositis.

Site	Ulceration (%)
Upper lip	4.7
Lower lip	7.0
Right cheek	16.6
Left cheek	16.9
Right ventral and lateral tongue	19.1
Left ventral and lateral tongue	18.7
Floor of mouth	10.0
Soft palate	6.9

(ulceration) and the impact of the lesion on patient's ability to function (eating). Second, the accuracy with which toxicities are described is inconsistent. Typically, the incidence of toxicity is higher (often significantly higher) when it is the focus of a study compared to its description as an adverse event. Finally, there tends to be a marked disconnect between clinician attributions of toxicity and those described by patients. When queried about symptoms of OM, a cohort of colorectal cancer patients treated with FOLFOX reported an incidence of over 70%, whereas the literature only reports 15% [5].

Clinical features and course of mucositis

The clinical presentation of chemotherapy-induced mucositis is similar to that induced by radiation, but the course is different [6]. The first clinical manifestations of OM include erythema, the appearance of thinned mucosa, and pain. The pain associated with early OM is similar to that described for a food burn. In the case of chemotherapy-induced mucositis, symptoms usually begin about 4 days following drug infusion, whereas symptoms of radiation-induced mucositis start between weeks 1 and 2 (cumulative radiation doses of 10–20 Gy).

The most clinically significant lesion of mucositis is ulceration and always confined to the movable mucosa of the lips, cheeks, ventral and lateral tongue, and soft palate (Table 9.1). While no area of the nonkeratinized mucosa is spared the risk of mucositis, it is most commonly seen on the buccal mucosa, floor of mouth, and lateral and ventral tongue. The keratinized mucosa is typically spared (e.g., gingiva, dorsal tongue, or hard palate). Consequently, ulcerative lesions of the gingiva, dorsal tongue, or hard palate are usually of infectious etiology (Figure 9.2).

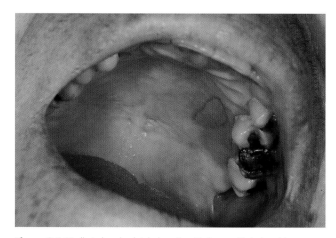

Figure 9.2 Virally-induced palatal ulceration. Oral mucositis induced by radiation or chemotherapy manifests itself on the movable oral mucosa, for example labial mucosa, buccal mucosa, ventral and lateral surfaces of the tongue, floor of the mouth and soft palate. It does not affect the more keratinized mucosa of the hard palate, gingiva or dorsal surface of the tongue.

Ulcerative lesions of mucositis may be focal or diffuse (Figure 9.3 and Figure 9.4). They are characterized by uneven borders, an inconsistency in the presence of peripheral erythema, their depth, and the presence of a necrotic psuedomembrane. The most consistent symptom associated with mucositis is pain – often requiring opiod therapy and, not infrequently, even breaking through this form of analgesia. Ulceration development usually peaks about a week after chemotherapy infusion and lasts for up to 7–10 days, although typically lesions begin to resolve in less time. Interestingly, in neutropenic patients, mucosal resolution usually begins a couple of days before white blood cell recovery. Ulceration begins at cumulative radiation doses of 30 Gy and typically persists for up to 4 weeks following the completion of treatment. While not a uniform finding, coincident mucosal bleeding may be noted. As a consequence of pain, oral and oropharyngeal function is adversely impacted and patients are often not able to tolerate a normal diet during the period of their injury.

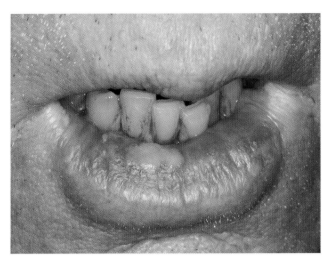

Figure 9.3 A focal lesion of oral mucositis involving the labial mucosa. Note that the outer aspect of the lip (the vermillion border) is spared.

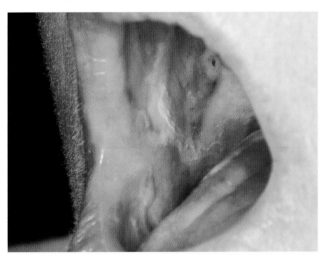

Figure 9.4 Confluent ulcerative oral mucositis of the right buccal mucosa and lateral tongue in a patient receiving radiation therapy for the treatment of a cancer of the head and neck.

In the majority of cases, mucositis resolves spontaneously. Healing occurs without scarring.

Mucositis scoring

Clinician-based scoring

Mucositis incidence and severity are most often assessed based on clinician-based scoring criteria. There are three major reasons to assess mucositis severity:

1. To determine the stomatotoxicity of a particular cancer-treatment regimen;

2. To evaluate and optimize patient management; and

3. As a research tool to evaluate the efficacy of a potential mucositis intervention.

Toxicity description and assessment

The most common scoring scales are those used to define the stomatotoxicity of a particular drug or radiation regimen. Among the most used are those developed by the National Cancer Institute Common Toxicity Criteria (NCI-CTC), the Radiation Therapy Oncology Group (RTOG), and the World Health Organization [7]. To a large degree, these scales are focused on clinician examination of the oral mucosa and the assignment of a score based on observed clinical changes such as erythema and ulceration. They may also have a component that is based on patient function or use of analgesics (Table 9.1).

Patient management scales

Patient management scales tend to be based on a holistic and composite evaluation of the patient's oral health, of which only one element is mucosal damage. They have been primarily developed by nurses for the daily care of their patients.

These instruments often include assessments of patient speech, salivary function and quality, gingival health, swallowing, lips, and oral hygiene. While of great value in formulating treatment plans that focus on overall oral cavity health, the evaluation of the oral mucosa is not the primary target of these scales. Examples are the Oral Assessment Guide (OAG) [8], the Western Consortium for Cancer Nursing Research (WCCNR) [9], and the MacDibbs scale [10].

Research-directed scales

Over the years scales have been developed to be used primarily in mucositis research studies. These tend to provide highly quantitative outputs that are based on a series of strictly defined parameters. The two most commonly cited scales of this type are the Oral Mucositis Index (OMI) [11] and the Oral Mucositis Assessment Scale (OMAS) [12]. The endpoints for both scales are dependent of clinician assessment. While the OMAS tends to be very focused on mucosal changes, the OMI has more broad criteria.

Variability between mucositis scales

The severity of mucositis is not evenly reflected across scales. What may be graded as severe in one scale, may be slight or moderate in another [13]. For example, two studies were conducted to evaluate the effect of a new antimucositis drug on the course of severe mucositis induced by a particular conditioning regimen prior to hematopoietic stem cell transplant (HSCT). Each study used a different scale to measure mucositis severity. In the first study, the duration of severe mucositis was the same among patients who received the test drug and those who received placebo [14]. In the second study, not only was the duration of mucositis in placebo patients almost 4 times that observed in the first study (16.6 vs. 4.4 days), but the duration in patients being treated with the interventional drug was 11.9 vs. 4.8 days in the first study [15]. The difference between the two studies was the scale that was used to measure mucositis.

Patient-reported instruments to assess mucositis severity

There are a number of patient-reported (PRO) instruments for mucositis. In general, these tools rely on categorical and visual analog outcomes.

Categorical scales, for example the Oral Mucositis Daily Questionnaire (OMDQ) [16], ask patients to grade mucositis symptoms by circling a prescribed hierarchical list of possible outcomes. For example, they might ask the patient to circle a description of their mouth pain in which the options are delineated or to circle a numerical indicator.

Visual analog scales (VAS) are less defined. Typically, they present patients with a 10-cm line with descriptors of extremes at either end, such as no pain on one end and worse possible pain on the other. Patients are then asked to put a mark at that position on the line that best describes their symptoms.

PRO scales for mucositis also vary in their specificity. Some are mucositis focused and seek patient input on symptoms and/or functional consequences related solely to mucositis. Among these are the OMAS [12], the Patient-Reported Oral Mucositis Symptom (PROMS) scale [16], and the OMDQ [17]. A second category gather more broad symptomatic input of which mucositis is one component of the overall scale. These scales are largely disease-based (e.g. head and neck cancer), and include the Functional Assessment of Cancer Therapy – Head and Neck (FACT-HN), the MD Anderson symptom inventory head and neck module [18], and the Vanderbilt Head and Neck Symptom Survey [19].

Minimizing inter-observer variability in mucositis assessment

A major challenge with any scale that depends on clinical judgement for scoring is to assure inter-observer consistency. For the assessment of OM a number of factors impact on grading accuracy and consistency:

1. *Training.* In many instances, clinicians receive little formal training on the performance of an examination of the mouth and oropharynx. Consequently, the rigor of an OM evaluation can vary widely relative to the inclusiveness of the structures observed and graded. Aggressive training in examination technique and scoring criteria helps minimize variability.

2. *Lighting.* It is virtually impossible to assess the condition of the oral mucosa if one can not see easily. Good lighting an essential element of providing an accurate examination. As both hands are optimal for an oral examination, a headlight is desirable. Those for campers work well and are relatively inexpensive.

3. *Clarity of outcome criteria.* The examiner(s) should be absolutely clear as to the criteria by which scoring is carried out.

4. *Standardization of clinical assessment technique* (see Chapter 6). All examiners should perform their evaluation in the same sequence.

Impact of mucositis

Mucositis impacts patients' quality of life, ability to tolerate treatment, and use of health resources [20]. Pain is a universal symptom associated with ulcerative mucositis. As a consequence, patients with mucositis use more analgesics, of greater strength and for longer periods of time than do patients without the condition. As food intake is often limited in patients with mucositis, the use of parenteral feeding alternatives is greater in patients with mucositis. For example, among HSCT patients with mucositis, both the frequency and duration of total parenteral nutrition use is increased [21]. Likewise, gastrostomy tube feeding is a common requirement among patients being treated for cancers of the head and neck. In fact, the anticipation of severe mucositis is so great in this population that prophylactic placement of feeding tubes is the norm at many sites. Mucositis is a frequent cause for unplanned physician office visits or visits to the emergency room. Ultimately, it is a cause for hospitalization for fluid support or pain management [20]. In the case of hospitalized patients, such as those receiving HSCT, the presence of mucositis is associated with extended length of hospital stay [21].

The increased resource use incurred by mucositis results in higher healthcare costs. Among patients being treated for head and neck or lung cancers, the incremental cost of mucositis is more than $17 000 [22]. Likewise, HSCT recipients who develop mucositis incur more costs than do patients without the condition [21].

Mucositis increases the risk of bacteremia and sepsis in granulocytopenic patients. The loss of the mucosal barrier provides a ready portal of entry for the numerous bacteria that habit the oral cavity [23].

Pathobiology of mucositis

The concept that radiation or chemotherapy causes mucositis (and other epithelial injury) solely by indiscriminate direct killing of rapidly dividing normal basal stem cells has been overturned by an accumulation of data that demonstrate that mucosal injury is the culmination of a series of complex events that ultimately target the epithelium (Figure 9.5). [6,24].

Three events characterize the *initiation phase*. Radiation and chemotherapy directly damage DNA, cause strand breaks, and induce clonogenic death of some basal epithelial cells. Injured cells in the submucosa release endogenous damage-associated pattern molecules (chemotherapy and radiation-associated molecular pattern molecules; CRAMPs) in a pulsatile way which have the potential to bind to pathogen recognition receptors (PRRs) , and reactive oxygen species (ROS) are generated [25].

During the *primary damage response phase* transduction pathways triggered by DNA strand breaks, PRRs and lipid

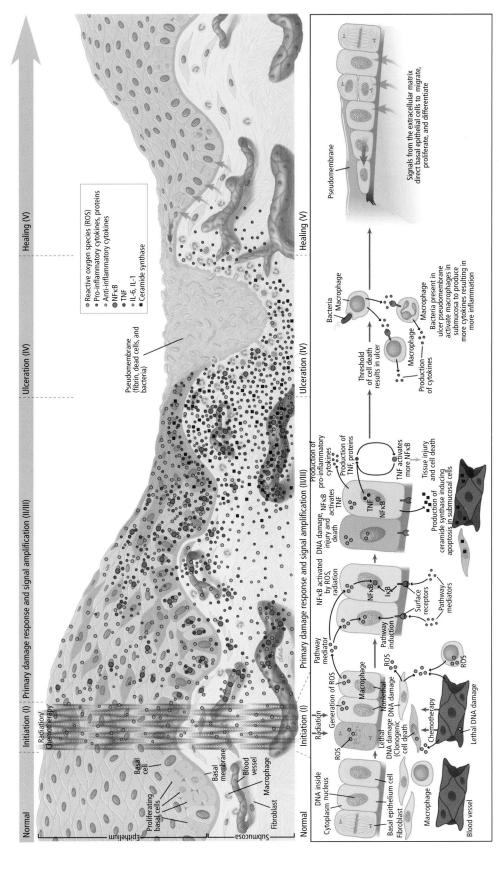

Figure 9.5 A diagramatic representation of the biological steps involved in the pathogenesis of mucositis. The biology is essentially the same for any epithelial tissue and consists of a series of phases which are the consequence of a cascade of events, typically initiated by reactive oxygen species, the innate immune response and selective activation of a number of transcription factors. At least fourteen canonical pathways are involved in process. Reproduced with permission from Sonis ST. A Biological Approach to Mucositis. J Support Oncol 2004; 2:21–36. Elsevier B. V.

peroxidation prompt the activation of a number of transcription factors, such as NF-κB, Wnt, p53, p38, and their associated canonical pathways. The NF-κB pathway appears to have a critical role in mucositis biology [26]. Chemotherapy and radiation can directly activate NF-κB. Indirectly, it can be activated by CRAMPs and ROS. Among the 200 genes whose expression is governed by NF-κB are those associated with the production of molecules that have demonstrated activity in the pathogenesis of mucositis including cytokines and cytokine modulators, stress responders (e.g. COX-2, inducible NO-synthase, superoxide dismutase), and cell adhesion molecules. Apoptosis is an important consequence of the effects of NF-κB in normal cells.

The initiation of the ceramide pathway through ceramide synthase and sphingomylinase activation has damaging consequences for the oral mucosa. Radiation and chemotherapy-mediated damage to the connective tissue results in fibrinolysis and consequent macrophage stimulation resulting in the production of matrix metalloproteinases.

Although the biologic hits noted above begin within seconds of the tissue being exposed to radiation or chemotherapy, the damage incurred to the most susceptible cells in the epithelium does not immediately translate into clinically detectable changes. Rather, while basal epithelial stem cells are the targeted drivers of mucositis, the time from their demise to ulceration takes about a week to be fully manifest.

Signal amplification

Many of the molecules induced by the primary response have the ability to positively or negatively feedback and alter the local tissue response. For example, tumor ncrosis factor (TNF) may positively feedback on NF-κB to amplify its response, and initiates mitogen-activated protein kinase (MAPK) signaling, leading to activation of JNK signaling which is associated with OM.

The most clinically significant stage in mucositis development is ulceration. Ulceration develops as a consequence of the direct and indirect mechanisms noted above causing damage and apoptotic changes to mucosal epithelium. Mucositis ulcers are deep and quickly colonized by oral bacteria. In animal models, the number of mucosal bacteria goes up over 300-fold in the transition between intact and ulcerated epithelium.

The bacteria on the ulcer surface are active contributors to the mucositis process. Cell wall products penetrate into the submucosa, now rich in macrophages, to stimulate those cells to secrete further proinflammatory cytokines. In granulocytopenic patients , there is a risk that bacteria may invade submucosal vessels to produce bacteremia or sepsis.

Most cases of OM heal spontaneously. Ulcer resolution is the result of an active biologic process in which signaling from the submucosa's extracellular matrix (ECM) guides the proliferation, migration, and differentiation of the epithelium bordering the ulcer. Disruption of the submucosal ECM is the likely initiator of cases in which healing is delayed or, in rare instances, does not occur at all.

Risk factors for mucositis

Of new patients who will be treated for noncutaneous cancers , approximately 8% will be at high risk (a greater than 50% chance) of developing ulcerative mucositis. Conversely, 43% (over 500 000) will be at little or no risk for the condition. These patients will be treated with curative surgery, peripheral radiation, or low dose chemotherapy. The majority of new cancer patients fall into an intermediate category of mucositis risk in which 20–49% will develop ulcerative mucositis at some time during their treatment.

Patients in the high risk group fall into the head and neck cancer population and those individuals being treated with high dose myeloablative chemotherapy. While the incidence of mucositis is significant in this group, it is by no means universal. For patients at "some risk," risk disparity is even more profound. This group is composed of individuals being treated for the most common solid tumors such as cancers of the breast, colon, rectum, and lung. Each cycle of therapy incurs mucositis risk. For patients who develop mucositis in one cycle, the risk of mucositis increases with subsequent cycles. For example, the likelihood that a patient being treated with a conventional regimen for breast cancer will develop ulcerative OM is about 20% during the first cycle of chemotherapy. If there is no change in drug dose going forward, the risk of OM jumps to about 70% in the second treatment cycle.

Historically, mucositis risk has been considered to be associated with the aggressiveness of therapy or the patient-related variables [1,27]. Treatment-related variables include those associated with the type of therapy (i.e., radiation or chemotherapy), dose, and route of administration. To a large extent, treatment type and dose can be overwhelming risk factors. Thus, for a patient with a tongue cancer who is receiving chemoradiation the likelihood of mucositis is close to 100%. On the other hand, a patient with a hypopharyngeal cancer, also receiving chemoradiation, may have a mucositis risk that is markedly less, around 50%, because the tissues of the oral cavity are not primarily included in the radiation field. Patients receiving conditioning regimens in preparation for HSCT have been considered to be at high risk of mucositis. This was true of many regimens, especially those includingtotal body irradiation and/or high doses of stomatotoxic drugs. In an attempt to ameliorate risk, transplanters have adopted less toxic protocols. As only 19% of the total annual OM cases occur in the head and neck cancer and HSCT populations, it is clear that other factors are critical in determining risk.

Among patient-associated risk factors, age, body mass, and gender have been particularly evaluated. For the most part these are poorly defined, although a reasonable amount of data supports that being female confers increased toxicity risk for 5-fluorouracil and methotrexate [28].

Comorbid medical conditions appear to influence mucositis risk in so far as common biologic mechanisms are involved. In a study of patients receiving induction therapy for leukemia, OM risk was found to be reduced in patients with psoriasis and higher in individuals who had precancer diagnoses of Addison disease

[29]. The results were attributed to the impact of psoriasis on epithelial proliferation and, conversely, the higher levels of proinflammatory cytokines in patients with Addison disease.

Genetic factors are likely to have a dominant role in determining mucositis risk. The most extensively studied genetic determinants of mucositis risk are of genes associated with chemotherapy metabolism. For example, Schwab *et al.* [30] assessed the predictive value of three polymorphisms associated with the metabolism of fluorouracil for toxicity risk. They found a significant association between dihydropyrimidine dehydrogenase (DPYD) variants and the development of OM, although the sensitivity of DPYD for mucositis was low (7.7%) [31]. Other investigators have demonstrated similar findings. However, the genes that impact drug metabolism are applicable to risk prediction of only a small group of patients – maybe 5%. The authors of a large recently completed randomized trial in patients being treated for advanced colorectal cancer reached a similar conclusion [31].

It seems more likely that differences in the expression of genes associated with OM pathogenesis are more likely to impact risk. For example, TNF-α appears to have a role in the development of OM, and a number of polymorphisms control individuals' TNF-α production. Bogunia-Kubik *et al.* [32] evaluated the role of the expression of TNFA*1,2 on toxicity risk, including mucositis, among patients undergoing allogeneic HSCT and found that its presence resulted in an odds ratio for toxicity that was more than twice that attributable to the use of aggressive conditioning regimens. The simultaneous expression of two deletion polymorphisms associated with glutathione S-transferase, an enzyme that modulates ROS levels, were shown to increase significantly the risk of OM in another transplant population [33]. A similar finding was shown when patient risk for radiation-induced dermatitis was studied [34].

The tumor itself is biologically active and might contribute to OM risk since tumor-derived peptides and protein products could directly modify normal cell response to radiation or chemotherapy, while others, such as matrix mellatoproteinases enhance the breakdown of the local tissue environment.

The oral environment and mucositis

The oral cavity is one of the most complex environments in the body. The mucosa is bathed in saliva containing a wide microbiota comprised of bacteria, fungi, and viruses. A number of studies have evaluated the role of saliva and microorganisms in the development and course of mucositis. Overwhelmingly, these investigations have concluded that while the course of mucositis might be influenced by the local environment, neither changes in saliva nor the microflora are significant in the primary etiology of OM [35,36].

When changes in numbers of colonizing bacteria in the mouth were studied in an established animal model of radiation-induced mucositis, while peak bacterial loads coincided with peak mucositis scores, colonization lagged behind the development of

ulcerative mucositis (N.G. Uzel *et al.*, personal communication). This finding contradicts a hypothesis that would suggest that increases in bacterial numbers drive OM, while the observation that the mean bacterial load increased by over 300% compared with baseline suggested that ulcerated mucosa represented a desirable colonization site. Bacterial numbers decreased as ulcers spontaneously resolved, indicating that the presence of large numbers of organisms was not enough to inhibit healing. Consistent with early studies, increases in Gram-negative organisms were seen during ulceration, but re-establishment of normal bacterial proportions was a requirement for spontaneous ulcer resolution, irrespective of bacterial numbers. Clinical trial results suggest that antibacterial strategies have been ineffective as OM interventions.

The impact of saliva on mucositis is unclear. However, treatment approaches directed at stimulating salivary flow as OM treatments have largely failed [37]. Molecules that have shown to affect mucosal response to injury, such as trefoil factor and epidermal growth factor, are present in saliva, but their role in mucositis requires more study [38,39].

Roles for fungi (*Candida*) and viruses (herpes simplex 1; HSV1) in the etiology of mucositis have been the subject of speculation for some time and remain marginally controversial [40–42]. Candidiasis is a common finding among patients receiving head and neck radiation or myeloablative chemotherapy so it is not unexpected that these organisms can be identified in patients with mucositis as a coincident condition, rather than causal. Antifungals as mucositis interventions have not been effective [43].

The hypothesis that mucositis might simply represent a manifestation of an HSV1 infection has been mentioned in the literature since the 1980s. Subsequently, data have emerged that rebut HSV as a primary driver of mucositis. Woo *et al.* [40] showed that OM development was unrelated to HSV antibody status or positive viral cultures, and acyclovir prophylaxis was ineffective in preventing OM in HSCT patients. A similar conclusion was reached by Djuric *et al.* [41] who reported that the rate of HSV1 reactivation was no different before or after chemotherapy. They also found that there was no relationship between the rate of viral reactivation and the presence or absence of OM.

Status of the development of therapies for mucositis

There have been three major changes in how toxicities associated with conventional cytotoxic therapy are viewed.

1. Toxicities are not simply the by-product of nonspecific cell death, but rather represent the clinical manifestation of a culmination of a complex series of interactive biologic events.

2. It is becoming increasingly clear that specific toxicities do not occur in isolation – patients who develop OM are likely to simultaneously manifest diarrhea, fatigue, cutaneous lesions, or other adverse events. It appears that the cohesive element in toxicity clusters is their similar pathogenesis.

3. Toxicity risk is multifactorial, predictable, quantifiable, and largely genetically determined. Our ability to develop effective risk prediction will be an important step in the development of customized patient interventions.

Normal cells and tumor cells do not respond in the same way to cytotoxic therapy, therefore pharmacologic toxicity prevention at the mechanistic level is a realistic goal without jeopardizing tumor response to treatment.

Finding an effective mucositis pharmacologic or biologic intervention has not been easy. There have been a number of false starts and disappointments. While some of these negative results can be attributed to a compound's lack of sufficient activity, it also seems that others are the consequence of poor study design or execution. The 2004 approval of palifermin as a first in class agent for mucositis is important therefore for a number of reasons [3]. This finding has been substantiated in patients being treated with sarcoma [43]. First, it is likely that palifermin's OM efficacy is a manifestation of its robust biologic activity. Second, the enabling study's primary endpoint was clinically meaningful, able to be achieved with minimal inter-site variability, and frames important trial design elements for new agents. Third, the impact of successful amelioration of clinically scored OM on patient-reported and overall health outcomes was demonstrated.

There will not be a single "magic bullet" to treat OM. Patients who develop burning erythema require a completely different level of treatment than do others who are at risk for diffuse ulcerative mucositis. It is more likely that our formularies will contain a range of options based on activity, formulation, and cost allowing us to make choices based on an individual's risk.

Mucosal changes associated with targeted therapies

New classes of antitumor agents continue to be developed. Targeted therapies include antibodies and small molecules that, mechanistically, are designed to interfere with key pathways in tumor growth or development. In general, the oral mucosal response to these agents is variable. For some agents, such as the mammalian target of rapamycin (mTOR) inhibitors, oral mucosal injury is the foremost dose-limiting toxicity. For others, it appears that concurrent administration of targeted and cytotoxic agents results in a synergistic effect that results in more mucosal damage than seen with either drug individually. Importantly, the mucosal injury that results from targeted therapies is not consistently the same – clinically or pathoetiologically – as is ascribed to cytotoxic drugs or radiation.

Mucosal injury associated with mTOR inhibitors

Because of its role as a central regulator of key pathways thought to be important in the proliferation of cancers, mTOR has emerged as a viable target for the generation of a new group of antitumor agents. Everolimus and temsirolimus both been approved for the management of renal cell carcinoma. The most common toxicity ascribed to mTOR inhibitors is mouth ulcers which occur in about 40% of patients. mTOR inhibitors have been used in an immunosuppressive role for managing solid organ transplants and GVHD for some time and ulceration of the oral mucosa has been reported to be a frequent and dose-limiting adverse event arising from mTOR inhibitors use in an anticancer setting.

The term "mucositis" has been erroneously assigned to describe these lesions. While criteria used to categorize adverse events (such as ICD-9 criteria, MedDRA, NCI-CTC) associate the diagnosis of mucositis with *cytotoxic* drug and radiation treatment regimens for cancer, mTOR inhibitors are *cytostatic*. Lesions associated with mTOR inhibitors (mTOR inhibitor associated stomatitis; mIAS) differ in their course and presentation from those of conventional mucositis [44].

The clinical presentation of mIAS closely resembles aphthous stomatitis. Lesions appear as distinct oval ulcers that have a central gray area surrounded by an erythematous band. mIAS ulcers are localized to the movable mucosa of the mouth and oropharynx, and are not present on the more keratinized mucosa of the palate, gingival and dorsal surface of the tongue, a fact that distinguishes them from lesions of viral etiology. In general, the lesions of mIAS have a more rapid onset than those of mucositis and resolve in approximately 1 week. Furthermore, whereas oral mucositis often occurs concurrent with damage to other areas of the gastrointestinal tract, mIAS rarely does so. In contrast, mIAS is associated with the presence of cutaneous lesions: the incidence of nonspecific rash is approximately three times higher in patients who experience mIAS compared with those who do not.

Small molecules and antibodies

Both antibodies and small molecules have been developed as therapies that interfere with specific (targeted) molecules expressed by tumor cells. Among these, HER2 directed therapies are probably the most common. Trastuzumab (Herceptin) is a monoclonal antibody that is currently used in the treatment of HER2-overexpressing breast cancers. Bevacizumab is a monoclonal antibody that targets VEGF that is used in conjunction with standard 5-FU regimens for the treatment of colorectal cancers. Lapatinib, sorafenib, and sunitinib are small molecule tyrosine kinase inhibitors. Sorefenib and sunitinib inhibit VEGF signaling and PDGF receptors as well. Lapatinib is used with capecitabine for the treatment of advanced breast cancer. Sunitinib, an orally administered multitargeted tyrosine kinase inhibitor, has been used for advanced renal cell cancers and gastrointestinal stromal tumors.

Mucosal injury is reported with relatively high frequency as a consequence of targeted therapy use [45]. However, two factors complicate our ability to determine the true incidence of mucosal toxicity: the mechanism(s) by which it arises, and its impact on treatment tolerability, outcomes, and cost. From the standpoint of toxicity definition, the synergistic use of targeted agents with conventional cytotoxic drugs or with each other is challenging and makes it difficult to discriminate which agent is the driver of mucosal damage. Second, the lack of robust sequential clear descriptions of the nature of mucosal injury associated with most forms of targeted therapies is lacking. Largely because of convenience, such injury is termed mucositis while, as is the case with the mTOR inhibitors, the condition fails to resemble conventional mucositis in its presentation or behavior. For example, mucosal changes associated with sunitinib use have been alternatively described as mucosal inflammation, mucositis, and stomatitis.

What does seem clear is that targeted therapies given alone or in combination are associated with mucosal injury. Among patients being treated for advanced renal cell cancer with either sunitimib or sorafinib in a small study (n = 48), 39.5% of patients developed low grades of mucositis [46]. Of the patients reported in the study, 28 patients were treated tyrosine kinase inhibitors alone. It was used as a second line treatment following failure of cytokine therapy for the remainder.

A reported incidence of 16–21% of patients being treated with sunitinib for gastrointestinal stromal tumors developed mucositis with symptoms of mouth pain, but not universal ulceration [47].

The potential mucosal toxicity synergism of agents is reflected by the results of a recent study in which paclitaxel, trastuzumab, and everolimus were used in combination to treat metastatic breast cancer [48]. In this small trial in which the dose of everolimus was increased, mucositis was the most common overall toxicity reported. Interestingly, the dose of everolimus impacted both the incidence and severity of the mucositis reported (5 mg/day – OM 50%; 10 mg/day – OM 94%, of which 18% was grade 3–4; 30 mg/day – OM 80%, of which 50% was grade 3–4). This percentage is not significantly different from that reported when mTOR inhibitors have been used alone. Oral mucosal injury is not consistently reported with trastuzumab, but pharyngitis has been described with the antibody alone or in combination with paclitaxel.

The mechanism by which HER2-directed agents might elicit mucosal injury has yet to be studied. Only limited data exist on the presence of *Her2/neu* gene expression in normal oral mucosa and that suggests that it is low (10%) [49]. A multicenter pharmacogenomic association study of 219 patients treated only with sunitinib which targeted 31 polymorphisms of 12 candidate genes found that an association with mucosal inflammation was increased in the presence of the G allele in *CYP1A12455A/G*. This cytochrome polymorphism is likely associated with sunitinib metabolism.

Oral manifestations of graft versus host disease

Oral mucosal lesions of GVHD occur with significant frequency in patients who have undergone allogeneic HSCT [50]. GVHD occurs in both acute and chronic manifestations.

Acute GVHD manifests within 100 days following transplantation. Its frequency is associated with the donor source of the transplant: about one-third of patients having matched related donors and about twice as high for patients with matched unrelated donors. Of patients with acute GVHD, oral manifestations are seen in close to half. The clinical manifestations are similar regardless of the donor source and consist of inflammatory-like changes of the movable mucosa, atrophy, and ulceration. In the majority of cases, patients complain of pain.

Chronic GVHD is about as frequent as the acute form and affects half of allogeneic transplant recipients. The oral changes associated with chronic GVHD are more consistent in frequency and presentation than those of the acute form. Approximately 80% of patients with chronic GVHD will have oral mucosal changes. The oral lesions of chronic GVHD are similar to those of oral erosive lichen planus. This observation is not surprising given the similarities in the immunopathogenesis of the two conditions. Patients present with reticulated keratotic lesions similar to Wickham striae, vesiculobullous lesions, and frank ulceration. Gingival atrophy, edema, and erythema are not uncommon. Lesions are associated with pain and increased sensitivity to spicy foods.

Aside from good hygiene practices, treatment of the oral lesions of GVHD is largely predicated on immunosuppression with topical or systemic steroids including fluocinonide, triamcinolone, or clobetasol, which can be used in a locally applied gel or cream formulation. For diffuse lesions or lesions of the posterior soft palate or oropharynx, dexamethasone elixir can be prescribed as a swish and gargle. Refractory or severe cases may be treated with a short but aggressive course of systemic steroids, followed by topical therapy. Phototherapy using psoralen has been used for the treatment of GVHD-associated skin lesions and may also have a role for managing oral lesions.

Conclusions

The oral mucosa is a frequent target of toxicities associated with cancer therapies. Aside from the pain and suffering associated with mucosal injury, it is a significant driver of increased morbidity and mortality, a common reason why patients are unable to receive optimum schedules or doses of treatment, and a major contributor to health and economic costs associated with added use of resources. Although it has been reported since the inception of drug and radiation cancer therapy, treatment options are currently limited. With the advent of new classes of cancer drugs, new forms of oral mucosal complications are being reported. Fortunately, better understanding of the pathobiology of oral mucosal injury has paved the way for the development of effective interventions. A range of new agents are currently in various stages of clinical development and it is hoped will reach the clinic in the next few years.

References

1 Sonis, S.T., Elting, L.S., Keefe, D. *et al.* (2004) Perspectives on cancer therapy-induced mucosal injury: pathogenesis, measurement,

epidemiology, and consequences for patients. *Cancer*, **100** (9 Suppl.), 1995–2025.

2 Bellm, L.A., Epstein, J.B., Rose-Ped, A., Martin, P. & Fuchs, H.J. (2000) Patient reports of complications of bone marrow transplantation. *Supportive Care in Cancer*, **8**, 33–39.

3 Speilberger, R., Stiff, P., Bensinger, W. *et al.* (2004) Palifermin for oral mucositis after intensive therapy for hematologic cancers. *New England Journal of Medicine*, **351**, 2590–2598.

4 Aprile, G., Ramoni, M., Keefe, D. & Sonis, S. (2009) Links between regimen-related toxicities in patients being treated for colorectal cancer. *Current Opinion in Supportive and Palliative Care*, **3**, 50–54.

5 Grunberg, S., Hesketh, P., Randolph-Jackson, P. *et al.* (2007) Risk and quality of life impact of mucosal injury among colorectal cancer patients receiving FOLFOX chemotherapy. *Supportive Care in Cancer*, **15**, 704.

6 Sonis, S.T. (2009) Mucositis: the impact, biology and therapeutic opportunities of oral mucositis. *Oral Oncology*, **45**, 1015–1020.

7 Keefe, D.M., Schubert, M.M., Elting, L.S. *et al.* (2007) Updated clinical practice guidelines for the prevention and treatment of mucositis. *Cancer*, **109**, 820–831.

8 Eilers, J., Berger, A.M. & Petersen, M.C. (1988) Development, testing, and application of the oral assessment guide. *Oncology Nursing Forum*, **15**, 325–330.

9 Dyck, S. (1991) Development of a staging system for chemotherapy-induced stomatitis. *Cancer Nursing*, **14**, 6–12.

10 Dibble, S.L., Shiba, G., MacPhail, L. & Dodd, MJ. (1996) MacDibbs Mouth Assessment: a new tool to evaluate mucositis in the radiation therapy patients. *Cancer Practice*, **4**, 135–140.

11 Sonis, S.T., Eilers, J.P., Epstein, J.B. *et al.* (1999) Validation of a new scoring system for assessment of clinical trial research of oral mucositis induced by radiation or chemotherapy: Mucositis Study Group. *Cancer*, **85**, 2103–2113.

12 McGuire, D.B., Peterson, D.E., Muller, S., Owen, D.C., Slemmons, M.F. & Schubert, M.M. (2002) The 20 item oral mucositis index: reliability and validity in bone marrow and stem cell transplant patients. *Cancer Investigation*, **20**, 893–903.

13 Sonis, S.T., Eilers, L.S., Keefe, D. *et al.* (2004) Perspectives on cancer therapy-induced mucosal injury: pathogenesis, measurement, epidemiology, and consequences for patients. *Cancer*, **100** (Suppl.), 1995–2025.

14 Dazzi, C., Cariello, A., Giovanis, P. *et al.* (2003) Prophylaxis with GM-CSF mouthwashes does not reduce frequency and duration of severe oral mucositis in patients with solid tumors undergoing high-dose chemotherapy with autologous blood stem cell transplantation rescue: a double blind, randomized, placebo-controlled study. *Annals of Oncology*, **14**, 559–563.

15 Bez, C., Demarosi, F., Sardella, A. *et al.* (1999) CGM-CSF mouthwashes in the treatment of severe oral mucositis: a pilot study. *Oral Surgery, Oral Medicine, and Oral Pathology*, **88**, 311–315.

16 Stiff, P.J., Erder, H., Bensinger, W.I. *et al.* (2006) Reliability and validity of a patient self-administered daily questionnaire to assess impact of oral mucositis (OM) on pain and daily function in patients undergoing autologous hematopoietic stem cell transplantation (HSCT). *Bone Marrow Transplantation*, **37**, 393–401.

17 Kushner, J.A., Lawrence, H.P., Shoval, I. *et al.* (2008) Development and validation of a patient-reported oral mucositis symptom (ROMS) scale. *Journal of the Canadian Dental Association*, **74**, 59.

18 Rosenthal, D.I., Mendoza, T.R., Chambers, M.S. *et al.* (2008) The M.D. Anderson symptom inventory-head and neck module, a patient-reported outcome instrument, accurately predicts the severity of radiation-induced mucositis. *International Journal of Radiation Oncology, Biology, Physics*, **72**, 1355–1361.

19 Murphy, B.A., Dietrich, M.S., Wells, N. *et al.* (2010) Reliability and validity of the Vanderbilt Head and Neck Symptom Survey: a tool to assess symptom burden in patients treated with chemoradiation. *Head and Neck*, **32**, 26–37.

20 Vera-Llonch, M., Oster, G., Hagiwara, M. & Sonis, S. (2006) Oral mucositis in patients undergoing radiation treatment for head and neck cancers. *Cancer*, **106**, 329–336;

21 Sonis, S.T., Oster, G., Fuchs, H. *et al.* (2001) Oral mucositis and the clinical and economic outcomes of hematopoietic stem-cell transplantation. *Journal of Clinical Oncology*, **19**, 2201–2205.

22 Nonzee, N.J., Dandade, N.A., Patel, U. *et al.* (2008) Evaluating the supportive costs of severe radiochemotherapy-induced mucositis and pharyngitis: results from a Northwestern University Cost of Cancer Program pilot study with head and neck and nonsmall cell lung cancer patients who received care at a county hospital, a veterans administration hospital, or a comprehensive cancer center. *Cancer*, **113**, 1446–1452.

23 Ruescher, T.J., Sodeifi, A., Scrivani, S.J., Kaban, L.B. & Sonis, S.T. (1998) The impact of mucositis on alpha-hemolytic streptococcal infection in patients undergoing autologous bone marrow transplantation for hematologic malignancies. *Cancer*, **82**, 2275–2281.

24 Sonis, S.T. (2004) The pathobiology of mucositis. *Nature Reviews Cancer*, **4**, 277–284.

25 Sonis, S.T. (2010) New thoughts on the initiation of mucositis. *Oral Diseases*, **16**, 597–600.

26 Logan, R.M., Gibson, R.J., Sonis, S.T. & Keefe, D.M. (2007) Nuclear factor-κB (NF-κB) and cyclooxygenase (COX-2) expression in the oral mucosa following administration of mucotoxic drugs. *Oral Oncology*, **43**, 395–401.

27 Barasch, A. & Peterson, D.E. (2003) Risk factors for ulcerative oral mucositis in cancer patients: unanswered questions. *Oral Oncology*, **39**, 91–100.

28 Chansky, K., Benedetti, J. & Macdonald, J.S. (2005) Differences in toxicity between men and women treated with 5-fluorouracil therapy for colorectal carcinoma. *Cancer*, **103**, 1165–1171.

29 Chen, E. (2004) Impact of pre-existing psoriasis and Addison's disease on chemotherapy-induced mucositis in patients hematological malignancies. Pre-doctoral thesis. Harvard School of Dental Medicine.

30 Schwab, M., Zanger, U.M., Marx, C. *et al.* (2008) Role of genetic and nongenetic factors for fluorouracil treatment-induced severe toxicity: a prospective clinical trial by the 5-FU toxicity study group. *Journal of Clinical Oncology*, **26**, 2131–2138.

31 Braun, M.S., Richman, S.D., Thompson, L. *et al.* (2009) Association of molecular markers with toxicity outcomes in a randomized trial of chemotherapy for advanced colorectal cancer: the FOCUS trial. *Journal of Clinical Oncology*, **27**, 5519–5528.

32 Bogunia-Kubik, K., Polak, M. & Lange, A. *et al.* (2003) TNF polymorphisms are associated with toxic but not aGVHD complications in the recipients of allogeneic sibling hematopoietic stem cell transplantation. *Bone Marrow Transplantation*, **32**, 617–622.

33 Hahn, T., Zhelnova, E., Sucheston, L. *et al.* (2010) A deletion polymorphism in glutathione-S-transferase mu (GSTM1) and/or theta (GSTT1) is associated with an increased risk of toxicity after

autologous blood and marrow transplantation. *Journal of the American Society for Blood and Marrow Transplantation*, **16**, 801–808.

34 Seruga, B., Zhang, H., Bernstein, L.J. & Tannock, I.F. (2008) Cytokines and their relationship to the symptoms and outcomes of cancer. *Nature Reviews Cancer*, **8**, 887–899.

35 Avivl, I., Avraham, S., Koren-Michowitz, M. *et al.* (2009) Oral integrity and salivary profile in myeloma patients undergoing high-dose therapy followed by autologous SCT. *Bone Marrow Transplantation*, **43**, 801–806.

36 Donnelly, J.P., Bellm, L.A., Epstein, J.B., Sonis, S.T. & Symonds, R.P. (2003) Antimicrobial therapy to prevent or treat oral mucositis. *Lancet Infectious Diseases*, **3**, 405–412.

37 Lockhart, P.B., Brennan, M.T., Kent, M.L. *et al.* (2005) Randomized controlled trial of pilocarpine hydrochloride for the moderation of oral mucositis during autologous stem cell transplantation. *Bone Marrow Transplantation*, **35**, 713–720.

38 Storesund, T., Schreurs, O., Messelt, E.B., Kolltveit, K.M. & Schenck, K. (2009) Trefoil factor family 3 expression in the oral cavity. *European Journal of Oral Sciences*, **117**, 636–643.

39 Peterson, D.E., Barker, N.P., Akhmadullina, L.I. *et al.* (2009) Phase II, randomized, double-blind, placebo-controlled study of recombinant human intestinal trefoil factor oral spray for prevention of oral mucositis in patients with colorectal cancer who are receiving florouracil-based chemotherapy. *Journal of Clinical Oncology*, **27**, 4333–4338.

40 Woo, S.B., Sonis, S.T. & Sonis, A.L. (1990) The role of herpes simplex virus in the development of oral mucositis in bone marrow transplant patients. *Cancer*, **66**, 2375–2379.

41 Djuric, M., Jankovic, L., Jovanovic, T. *et al.* (2009) Prevalence of oral herpes simplex virus reactivation in cancer patients: a comparison of different techniques of viral detection. *Journal of Oral Pathology and Medicine*, **38**, 167–173.

42 El-Sayed, S., Nabid, A., Shelley, W. *et al.* (2002) Prophylaxis of radiation-associated mucositis in conventionally treated patients with head and neck cancer: a double-blind, phase III, randomized, controlled trial evaluating the clinical efficacy of an antimicrobial lozenge using a validated mucositis scoring system. *Journal of Clinical Oncology*, **20**, 3956–3963.

43 Deng, Z., Kiyuna, A., Hasegawa, M., Nakasone, I., Hosokawa, A. & Suzuki, M. (2010) Oral candidiasis in patients receiving radiation therapy for head and neck cancer. *Otolaryngology and Head and Neck Surgery*, **143** (2), 242–247.

44 Sonis, S., Treister, N., Chawla, S., Demetri, G. & Haluska, F. (2010) Preliminary characterization of oral lesions associated with inhibitors of mammalian target of rapamycin in cancer patients. *Cancer*, **116**, 210–215.

45 Keefe, D.M. & Gibson, R.J. (2007) Mucosal injury from targeted anti-cancer therapy. *Supportive Care in Cancer*, **15**, 483–490.

46 Muriel, C., Esteban, E., Corral, N. *et al.* (2010) Impact of incorporation of tyrosine kinase inhibitor agents on the treatment of patients with a diagnosis of advanced renal cell carcinoma: study based on experience at the Hospital Universitario Central de Asturias. *Clinical and Translational Oncology*, **12**, 562–567.

47 Joensuu, H., Trent, J.C. & Reichardt, P. (2011) Practical management of tyrosine kinase inhibitor-associated side effects in GIST. *Cancer Treatment Reviews*, **37**, 75–88.

48 Andre, F., Campone, M., O'Regan, R. *et al.* (2010) Phase I study of everolimus plus weekly paclitaxel and trastuzumab in patients with metastatic breast cancer pretreated with trastuzumab. *Journal of Clinical Oncology*, **28**, 5110–5115.

49 Fong, Y., Chou, S.J., Hung, K.F., Wu, H.T. & Kao, S.Y. (2008) An investigation of the differential expression of Her2/neu gene expression in normal oral mucosa, epithelial dysplasia, and oral squamous cell carcinoma in Taiwan. *Journal of the Chinese Medical Association*, **71**, 123–127.

50 Couriel, D., Carpenter, P.A., Cutler, C. *et al.* (2006) Ancillary therapy and supportive care of chronic graft-versus-host disease: National Institutes of Health consensus development project on criteria for clinical trials in chronic graft-versus-host disease V. Ancillary therapy and Supportive Care Working Group Report. *Journal of the American Society for Blood and Marrow Transplantation*, **12**, 375–396.

10 Hair Disorders Associated with Anticancer Agents

Caroline Yeager and Elise A. Olsen

Department of Dermatology, Duke University Medical Center, Durham, NC, USA

Introduction

Hair loss is a common adverse effect of cytotoxic agents, monoclonal antibodies, epidermal growth factor inhibitors (EGFRIs), and multikinase inhibitors (MKIs). For each agent, or combination of agents that causes chemotherapy-induced hair loss/alopecia (CIA), alopecia may be of different types, assume a different degree of loss, and have a different potential or time course for regrowth after therapy. Although alopecia is not a life-threatening adverse event (AE) and in most cases is temporary, it has great psychologic significance, and may even impact on the decision to choose a particular type of chemotherapy. Forty-seven percent of female cancer patients considered alopecia the most traumatic aspect of chemotherapy, and 8% would even decline chemotherapy because of this fear of hair loss [1, 2]. Study participants relate their distress to the alopecia being a visible reminder of their cancer that both identifies them as a cancer patient and confronts them as individuals with the seriousness of disease [3–6]. In school-age children and teenagers, hair loss may also result in reduced social interactions [7]. Interestingly, several studies have also noted that less severe hair loss does not necessarily correlate with less distress; patients noted to have only partial hair loss have found the side effect just as troublesome as those patients with total alopecia [8–10].

For the purpose of counseling and supporting patients, it is important for physicians to be aware of the amount of alopecia patients may experience at a given dosage or regimen of chemotherapy and the usual time course for regrowth after completion of treatment. For those agents being studied in clinical trials, it is important to be able to track and document the amount and type of hair loss that patients experience. At the present time, there are no US Food and Drug Administration (FDA) approved medications that affect the amount of hair loss seen with chemotherapy, but there are some agents showing benefits in preclinical models.

This chapter reviews the types and amounts of hair loss seen with various anticancer agents, newer methods of tracking and defining the amount of hair loss and the severity of the psychosocial impact, and potential measures to prevent or hasten the regrowth seen with CIA.

Basic hair anatomy and function

There are approximately 100 000 hair follicles on the scalp, 150 hair follicles on each eyebrow, 90–160 eyelashes on the upper eyelid, and 75–80 eyelashes on the lower eyelid [11, 12]. Each mature hair follicle consists of a hair shaft of fused bundles of keratin, two surrounding root sheaths, and a germinative bulb. The germinative bulb at the base surrounds the dermal papilla and contains the matrix cells that proliferate to form the shaft. The inner and outer root sheaths help to protect and shape the growing hair. Vertically, the hair follicle consists of four distinct layers, the bulb at the base of the follicle, the suprabulbar region which extends to the insertion of the arrector pili muscle, the isthmus from the insertion of the arrector pili muscle to the opening of the sebaceous gland duct, and the infundibulum from the opening of the sebaceous gland duct to the surface of the skin [13].

Hair grows in a three-part cycle, consisting of anagen, or the growth phase; catagen, a brief involution phase; and telogen, an inactive phase before recapitulation of hair regrowth. About 85–90% of scalp hair are in anagen, normally for 3–6 years. Catagen follows as a 2–4 week transition period, where the bulb matrix and root sheaths below the arrector pili muscle undergo apoptosis causing cessation of cellular proliferation. The other 10% of scalp hair is in the telogen phase, which lasts approximately 3–4 months, at the conclusion of which the hair is shed. About

Dermatologic Principles and Practice in Oncology: Conditions of the Skin, Hair, and Nails in Cancer Patients, First Edition. Edited by Mario E. Lacouture.
© 2014 John Wiley & Sons, Inc. Published 2014 by John Wiley & Sons, Inc.

50–100 hairs are shed each day. Anagen is reinitiated when signals from the dermal papilla stimulate stem cells in the bulge region of the follicle which then migrate down along the previous tract to form a new bulb matrix and root sheath. Scalp hair grows about 1 cm per month, though this rate of hair growth will slow as people age.

Types of chemotherapy-induced hair loss/alopecia

There are three main types of hair abnormalities seen with CIA: telogen effluvium, anagen effluvium, and abnormal hair growth. Cytotoxic chemotherapy traditionally causes either a telogen or anagen effluvium whereas targeted therapies can also cause abnormal hair growth.

Telogen effluvium

Telogen effluvium is characterized by an increased proportion of hairs in telogen and subsequent shedding of these hairs which are now poorly anchored. The increase in hair shedding in chemotherapy-related telogen effluvium may begin sooner than the typical 3 months post exposure to inciting agents that is generally seen with endocrine disorders, nonchemotherapy drugs, dietary issues, post surgery, severe illness, or stress. Clinically, this telogen effluvium presents as a marked increase in hair shedding upon combing, brushing, showering, or any mild tension on the hair and is confirmed by performing a gentle "hair pull" of 25–50 hairs in multiple areas of the scalp: a normal hair pull will only produce 1–2 telogen hairs on multiple pulls, whereas in a telogen effluvium it is common to generate 3–10 hairs on a simple hair pull at all areas of the scalp (Figure 10.1). It may not be readily apparent to the physician that a telogen effluvium has occurred because usually 50% hair loss must occur before it is obvious to others and this percentage may be greater or lesser depending on

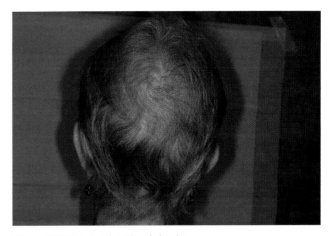

Figure 10.2 Patient with 50% scalp hair loss.

whether hair was very dense or fine or thin at baseline (Figure 10.2). Chemotherapeutic agents that cause this type of hair loss are generally monoclonal antibodies, immunomodulatory agents, and enzyme inhibitors. Typical agents that cause a telogen effluvium are methotrexate, 5-fluorouracil and retinoids. Telogen effluvium is generally fully reversible although it may take 6–12 months off the offending drug to see full regrowth.

Anagen effluvium

Anagen effluvium is also characterized clinically by increased shedding upon tension on scalp hairs but, on closer inspection, there is also generally an associated breakage of hairs. In this situation, the hair matrix and its progeny [including the inner root sheath that anchors the anagen (growing) hair shaft to the scalp and the anagen hair shaft itself] are adversely affected, leading to poorly anchored hair and distorted or weak shafts that break off close to the scalp surface as they grow out. The hair loss affects 90% of all hair on the scalp because usually that is the percentage of hair that is in the growth phase at any given time (Figure 10.3). Clinically, one can distinguish this from telogen effluvium by the much greater quantity of hair that is being lost and more specifically by examination of proximal ends of hair obtained by hair pull which may show some telogen hairs but also distorted hairs that break off on pulling (Figure 10.4), "bayonet" hairs (Figure 10.5). Examination of the distal ends of short hairs also confirms the major trauma at the matrix level that results in hairs breaking off beyond the scalp surface at the weakened site of the shaft. Common chemotherapeutic agents that cause an anagen effluvium include cyclophosphamide, doxorubicin, etoposide, topotecan, docetaxel, and paclitaxel. Those agents that cause at least 50% hair loss are shown in Table 10.1. Anagen effluvium caused by single agent chemotherapy is usually reversible but the hair that grows in may be of a different texture, color, or density than pretreatment. The multikinase inhibitor sorafenib and the EGFRIs can also cause mild alopecia with new hair growth curlier than prior to treatment [14–17].

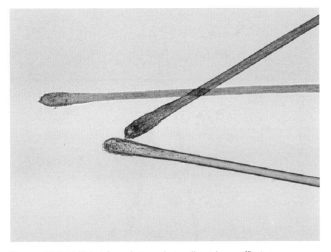

Figure 10.1 Multiple telogen hairs on hair pull in telogen effluvium.

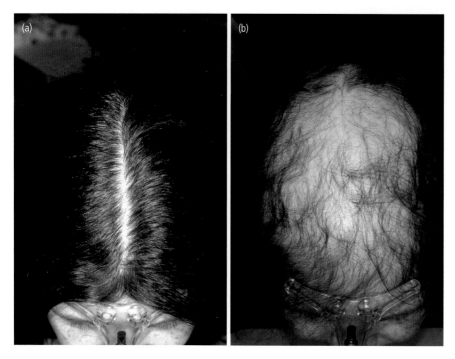

Figure 10.3 Anagen effluvium: (a) baseline pre-chemotherapy; (b) 32 days after starting chemotherapy with cyclophosphamide, docetaxel, and doxorubicin HCl.

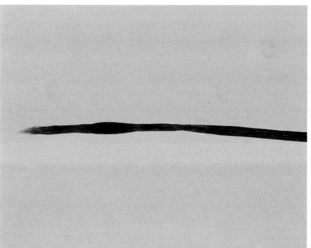

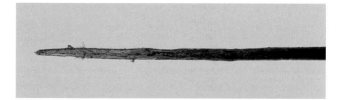

Figure 10.5 Bayonet hair.

Figure 10.4 Distorted anagen hairs typical of anagen effluvium. Reprinted with permission from Olsen E.A. in Olsen [13]. Reproduced with permission.

Table 10.1 Chemotherapeutic agents that cause at least 50% hair loss.

Chemotherapy agent	Trade name(s)	FDA indications for use	Patients reporting alopecia	Type of alopecia reported	References
Daunorubicin	Cerubidine	Acute lymphocytic leukemia, acute myelogenous leukemia	Approx. 100%	Total to near total alopecia	[99–101]
Doxorubicin	Adriamycin, Rubex	Acute lymphocytic leukemia, acute myelogenous leukemia, bladder cancer, breast cancer, gastric cancer, lymphomas (incl. Hodgkin), lung cancer, neuroblastoma, sarcomas, thyroid cancer, Wilms tumor	80–100%	Approximately two-thirds of patients report severe (total) alopecia	[102–104]

Table 10.1 (*Continued*)

Chemotherapy agent	Trade name(s)	FDA indications for use	Patients reporting alopecia	Type of alopecia reported	References
Paclitaxel	Onxol, Taxol	Breast cancer, Kaposi sarcoma, lung cancer, ovarian cancer	62–100%	Approximately three-quarters of patients report severe (total) alopecia, though milder hair loss is also reported	[105–110]
Docetaxel	Taxotere	Breast cancer, gastric cancer, head and neck cancer, lung cancer, prostate cancer	35.5–95%	Hair thinning – complete hair loss reported (44–75% of patients report severe alopecia with total to near total hair loss)	[111–115]
Idarubicin	Idamycin	Acute myelogenous leukemia	31–77%	In trial with 77% reporting alopecia [74], 40% of patients reported total alopecia, and 37% had milder alopecia	[116–118]
Cyclophosphamide	Cytoxan, Neosar	Lymphoma, leukemias, multiple myeloma, neuroblastoma, retinoblastoma, adenocarcinoma of the ovary, breast cancer	30–70%, more commonly around 70% in the literature	Diffuse thinning to total alopecia reported; approx. 50% of patients develop total alopecia	[37, 119–125]
Irinotecan	Camptosar	Colorectal cancer	46.1–70%	Reports vary, but approximately half of patients with hair loss have mild alopecia and the other half report moderate–total hair loss	[126–131]
Etoposide (VP-16)	Etopophos, Toposar, VePesid	Lung cancer (incl. small cell) and testicular cancer	8–66%	Severity of alopecia reported ranges from mild to total alopecia	[132–134]
Topotecan	Hycamtin	Cervical cancer, lung cancer (incl. small cell), ovarian cancer	49% in those who receive intravenous infusion; 20% reported in a trial of those receiving the drug orally	Total alopecia was reported in 31% of those receiving the drug through IV infusion	[135–138]
Vincristine	Oncovin, Vincasar, VCR	Acute lymphoblastic leukemia, lymphomas (incl. Hodgkin), malignant glioma, neuroblastoma, rhabdomyosarcoma, soft tissue sarcoma, Wilms tumor	20%	May be partial or total, but usually at least 25% of hair lost	[139]
Teniposide (VM-26)	Vumon	Acute lymphocytic leukemia	9%	Usually mild, but sometimes total	[140]
Gefitinib	Iressa	Lung cancer (incl. nonsmall cell lung cancer)	3.2%	CTCAE grades 1–2	[17, 141–143]

CTCAE, Common Terminology Criteria for Adverse Events; FDA, US Food and Drug adminstration.

Abnormal hair growth

It has long been recognized that conditions with total hair loss such as radiation, alopecia areata, and certain chemotherapeutic agents can lead to a different texture or hair color in the hair regrowing post treatment. However, targeted therapies (including EGFRIs, BRAF inhibitors, and MKIs) can lead to abnormal hair growth while on treatment [14–17]. With EGFRIs, abnormalities have been recorded in all parts of the body and include increased length and thickness of eyebrows and eyelashes (Figure 10.6), and increased periocular, chin, beard hair, and chest hair [18–24]. Hair on the scalp during EGFRI treatment has been reported to be finer, more brittle, curlier, and more slow growing than pretreatment (Figure 10.7) [25–27]. Both patchy hair growth on the central scalp as well as a mild diffuse scalp hair loss have also been reported with EGFRI use [17, 28]. In contrast, small vellus hairs of the face and female lip may show hypertrichosis [29]. Anticancer treatments can result in hypertrichosis, a disorder characterized by hair density or length beyond the accepted limits

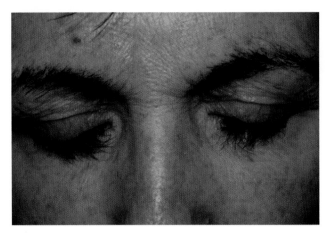

Figure 10.6 Increased thickness and length of eyelashes in patient on an EGFR inhibitor. Reprinted from [20]. Reproduced with permission.

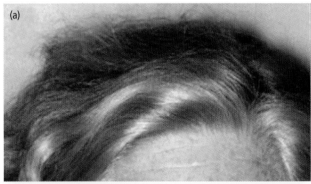

(a)

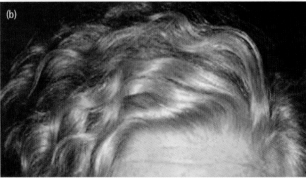

(b)

Figure 10.7 Change in hair texture and curl post EGFR inhibitor: (a) pre-EGFR inhibitor treatment; (b) post-EGFR inhibitor treatment. Reprinted from [26]. Reproduced with permission from Elsevier.

of normal in a particular body region, for a particular age or race, or hirsutism, a disorder characterized by the presence of excessive hair growth in women in anatomic sites where growth is considered to be a secondary male characteristic and where hair growth is under androgen control, such as beard, moustache, chest, or abdomen. Agents used in oncology patients that are

associated with hirsutism or hypertrichosis include cyclosporine, antiretrovirals, corticosteroids, and EGFRIs. When patients are on EGFRIs for longer than 3–6 months, 87.5% experience hair changes including trichomegaly of the eyelashes and hirsutism and/or hypertrichosis on the face [30].

Permanent chemotherapy-induced alopecia

Permanent alopecia following anagen effluvium, although rare, is a possibility that generates a great amount of anxiety among patients. In general, literature reports have associated chemotherapy-induced permanent alopecia with high-dose chemotherapy regimens preceding bone marrow transplantation (BMT) [31–38]. A study in 2007 by Machado *et al.* [32] found that the incidence of permanent alopecia among patients who underwent hematopoietic stem cell transplantation (HSCT) was 0.8%. Of the reports of permanent alopecia associated with high-dose chemotherapy conditioning regimens, almost all regimens included the agent busulfan, usually in combination with cyclophosphamide. Eight cases of permanent alopecia resulting from a high-dose cyclophosphamide, thiotepa, and carboplatin combination regimen followed by peripheral blood progenitor cell transplantation have also been reported [34]. A case of permanent alopecia following a high-dose cyclophosphamide and etoposide regimen was also reported; the patient in question also received total body irradiation, which in itself may cause permanent alopecia [32]. Among children, chronic graft versus host disease, older age, and prior cranial irradiation were all significant risk factors for subsequent development of permanent alopecia following high-dose chemotherapy for bone marrow transplantation [38].

Reports have also documented permanent CIA, outside of the BMT conditioning regimens, such as the three cases of severe irreversible nonscarring alopecia that developed following docetaxel/letrozole, or paclitaxel [39], and a case of a 72-year-old woman who had no hair regrowth 13 months following adjuvant docetaxel, carboplatin, and trastuzumab for breast cancer [31]. In a report of over 10 years of breast cancer treatment at St. Louis University, 13 women treated with standard breast cancer chemotherapy regimens developed permanent nonscarring alopecia [40]. Eleven woman had received anthracycline-cyclophosphamide (AC) followed by (AC-Taxol regimen) and the other two had AC alone. The 13 women were of a diverse age range (28–78 years), but the authors did note a slightly higher prevalence of permanent alopecia in African-American women, which was the ethnic background for 10 of the 13 patients reported. Masidonski and Mahon [40] identified no confounding reasons for these women's permanent alopecia other than that six of the women were placed on an aromatase inhibitor following their chemotherapy. Carlini *et al.* [41] previously reported a case of temporary alopecia in a premenopausal woman on letrozole and triptorelin where androgenization of the patient's hair follicles and a male pattern-type hair loss was appreciated. In general, all the case reports above suggest that, while still rare, permanent CIA outside of the bone marrow transplantation setting may be more common than initially thought.

Radiation-induced alopecia

Almost from the beginning of radiation technology alopecia has been recognized as a potential AE, with the first literature report of radiation-induced alopecia dating back to 1896, 1 year after Roentgen's original discovery of X-rays [42]. Forty years after this first report, in 1936 Borak [43] determined the lethal radiation doses required for the various components of the skin. In his studies, Borak found that 1600 roentgen (radiation doses in air) destroyed hair follicles. Translated into gray units (radiation doses in tissue), Severs et al. [44] determined that approximately 16 Gy (grays) is lethal for hair follicles. In a more recently developed dose–response relationship analysis, Lawenda et al. [45] concluded that a follicle dose of 25 Gy in 30 fractions is associated with <20% risk of permanent radiation-induced alopecia, while 10 Gy in 30 fractions has a <10% risk of permanent alopecia.

With the ability to focus the delivery of radiation, the most common current cancers with indication for direct radiation to the scalp are primary and metastatic brain tumors. McCarthy [46] described three grades of the severity of skin response to radiation. Because of the sensitivity of hair follicles compared with other skin features, as noted above, even a first grade skin reaction involves loss of scalp hair. With only a first grade reaction, however, hair will typically regrow within 2–4 months. For both the second and third grade reactions described by McCarthy, hair loss is permanent; moreover, in the third grade reaction, hair loss is accompanied by scarring. In general, this cicatricial form of induced alopecia is primarily seen secondary to radiation therapy and not other types of anticancer therapies such as chemotherapy. Of note, although hair follicles in general are relatively sensitive to the effects of radiation, the 1950 studies of Geary [47] and Van Scott and Reinertson [48] determined that hairs in the anagen phase are more susceptible than those in telogen, as is also seen with chemotherapy. Patients exposed to cranial radiation consequently often will initially experience less than total hair loss, with the sparing of hair follicles resting in the telogen phase.

Radiation-induced alopecia has been ameliorated by the advent in the late 1950s of megavoltage radiation sources. Megavoltage radiation involves energy in the 2–40 MeV range instead of the 90–500 keV range of historically used orthovoltage radiotherapy [44]. As a result of its greater voltage, megavoltage radiation generally targets deeper tissue and is relatively sparing of the skin, in turn helping to prevent skin-related AEs. However, the use of such megavoltage radiation does not completely eliminate adverse skin reactions . Fajardo [49] noted that even with optimal megavoltage irradiation conditions, 25% of patients still have observable skin reactions.

Grading scales utilized for determining degree of hair loss or regrowth

There is limited information on the degree and type of hair loss seen with the various chemotherapeutic agents and less on the course of regrowth. This is partly because the methods previously used to determine hair loss as an AE during clinical trials were not quantitative or inconsistently documented. Regrowth was either poorly defined, not tracked for a sufficient period of time (minimum of 6–12 months) after completion of therapy, or not tracked at all. Methods utilized to identify CIA prior to 2007 were as follows:

1. The World Health Organization (WHO) classification of CIA, introduced in 1981, has five categories of hair loss: Grade 0, none; Grade 1, minimal; Grade 2, moderate patchy; Grade 3, complete but reversible; and Grade 4, complete and irreversible. It is unclear why patchy was utilized as a descriptor because the hair loss with CIA is always diffuse. It is also unclear how long patients were followed to determine whether the hair loss was reversible and why the potential for regrowth was introduced into a scale looking at hair loss and only for those patients with complete hair loss.

2. In 1986 Perez et al. utilized a three-point scale for CIA: Grade 1, no hair loss; Grade 2, minor hair loss not requiring the use of a wig; and Grade 3, hair loss requiring the use of a wig. The problem with utilizing the patient's use of a wig to determine severity of hair loss is that the threshold to cover up the hair loss with a wig varies with the patient and with the amount of hair present at baseline and underestimates hair loss that does not reach at least 50%.

3. In 1996 Sredni et al. [50] utilized a five-point scale. Grade 0, no detectable alopecia; Grade 1+, mild alopecia defined as less than 50% hair loss; Grade 2+, moderately severe alopecia defined as more than 50% hair loss; and Grade 3+, total or virtually total alopecia (>90% hair loss).

4. The Common Terminology Criteria for Adverse Events (CTCAE) v3.0 from 2006 had only two grades of alopecia: Grade 1, thinning or patchy; and Grade 2, complete.

In 2007, Olsen developed a quantitative CIA scale that would extend the ability to capture the amount of hair loss and regrowth in a given patient treated with chemotherapy or radiation therapy to the scalp. This scale utilized terminology that also allowed the scale to be interpreted qualitatively. Olsen combined some of the categories for the Multinational Association of Supportive Care in Cancer (MASCC) scale published in 2010 (Table 10.2) and for the CTCAE v4.0 (Table 10.3) published in 2010, each of which addressed whether either an intervention or psychosocial impact occurred in keeping with the definition of these scales. A comparison of all methods for grading CIA is shown in Table 10.4. The hair loss in one patient is quantified over time, using the Olsen CIA scale, in Figure 10.8.

Because hair may also be abnormal either during therapy with chemotherapeutic agents or after extensive hair loss that affects

Table 10.2 Multinational Association of Supportive Care in Cancer (MASCC) epidermal growth factor inhibitorskin toxicity tool: scalp hair loss or alopecia.

Grades			
Mild: asymptomatic or mild symptoms; intervention not indicated	Moderate: minimal, local or noninvasive intervention indicated; limiting age-appropriate instrumental ADL		Severe: severe or medically significant but not immediately life-threatening; hospitalization or prolongation of hospitalization indicated; disabling; limiting of self-care ADL.
1	2A	2B	3/4
Hair loss <50% of normal for that individual that may or may not be noticeable to others but is associated with increased shedding and overall feeling of less volume. May require different hair style to cover but does not require hair piece to camouflage	Hair loss associated with marked increase in shedding and 50–74% loss compared to normal for that individual. Hair loss is apparent to others, may be difficult to camouflage with change in hair style and may require hairpiece	Marked loss of at least 75% of hair compared to normal for that individual with inability to camouflage except with a full wig or new cicatricial hair loss documented by biopsy that covers at least 5% scalp surface area. May impact on functioning in social, personal, or professional situations	

ADL, activities of daily living.

Table 10.3 Common Terminology Criteria for Adverse Events (CTCAE) hair loss and increased hair growth. Alopecia: a disorder characterized by decreased density of hair compared to normal for a given individual at a given age and body location. Hypertrichosis: a disorder characterized by hair density or length beyond the accepted limits of normal in a particular body region, for a particular age or race. Hirsutism: a disorder characterized by the presence of excessive hair growth in women in anatomic sites where growth is considered to be a secondary male characteristic (beard, moustache, chest, abdomen), where hair growth is under androgen control.

CTCAE Version	Description of hair change	Grades		
		1 Mild: asymptomatic or mild symptoms; clinical or diagnostic observations only; intervention not indicated	2 Moderate: minimal, local or noninvasive intervention indicated; limiting age-appropriate instrumental ADLs	3–5 Severe: hospitalization or prolongation of hospitalization indicated to death related to AE
V3.0	Hair loss alopecia scalp or body	Thinning or patchy	Complete	
V4.0	Alopecia	Hair loss up to 50% of normal for that individual that is not obvious from a distance but only on close inspection: a different hair style may be required to cover hair loss, but it does not require a wig or hair piece to camouflage	Hair loss of ≥50% normal for that individual that is readily apparent to others; a wig or hair piece is necessary if the patient desires to completely camouflage the hair loss: associated with psychosocial impact	
V4.0	Hirsutism	In women, increase in length, thickness or density of hair in a male distribution that the patient is able to camouflage by periodic shaving, bleaching, or removal of hair	In women, increase in length, thickness or density of hair in a male distribution that requires daily shaving or consistent destructive means of hair removal to camouflage; associated with psychosocial impact	
V4.0	Hypertrichosis	Increase in length, thickness or density of hair that the patient is either able to camouflage by periodic shaving or removal of hairs or is not concerned enough about the overgrowth to use any form of hair removal	Increase in length, thickness or density of hair at least on the usual exposed areas of the body [face (not limited to beard/moustache area) plus/minus arms] that requiresfrequent shaving or use of destructive means of hair removal to camouflage; associated with psychosocial impact	

Table 10.4 Comparison of chemotherapy-induced alopecia grading scales.

	Minimal	Moderate		Extensive	Complete
WHO classification 1981	Grade 1: minimal	Grade 2: moderate			Grade 3: complete but reversible
CTCAE V3.0 2006	Grade 1: thinning or patchy				Grade 2: complete
Olsen CIA Scale 2007*	Minimal	Moderate		Extensive	Complete
	Grade 1: 1–24% loss	Grade 2: 25–49% loss	Grade 3: 50–74% loss	Grade 4: 75–99% loss	Grade 5: 100% loss
MASCC 2010	Grade 1: no intervention		Grade 2: local or noninvasive intervention		
	<50% loss		Grade 2A: 50–74% loss	Grade 2B: ≥75% loss; full wig required; psychosocial impact	
CTCAE V4.0 2010	Grade 1: <50% loss		Grade 2: >50% loss; psychosocial impact		

Source: E.A. Olsen, unpublished information.

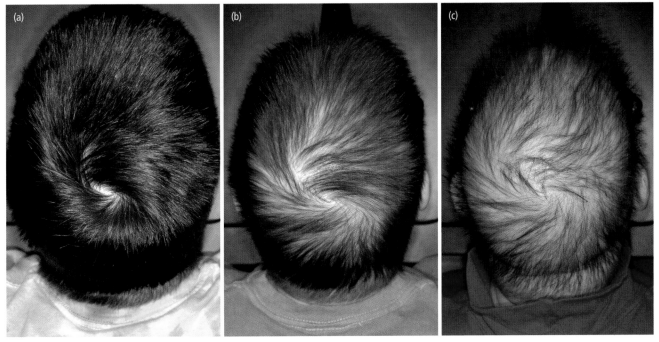

Figure 10.8 Hair loss from carboplatin and paclitaxel chemotherapy quantified and categorized according to Olsen and Common Terminology Criteria Adverse Events Version 4 (CTCAE V4.0): (a) baseline; (b) 50% loss (Olsen CIA Grade 3, CTCAE Grade 2); (c) 75% loss (Olsen CIA Grade 4A, CTCAE Grade 2).

Table 10.5 MASCC EGFR inhibitor skin toxicity tool – abnormal and increased hair growth.

Adverse event	Grade			
	Mild: no intervention	**Moderate: minimal, local, or noninvasive intervention**		
	1	**2A**	**2B**	**3–4**
Increased hair growth Specify all body areas that apply: • Facial hair (diffuse, not just in beard or mustache areas) • Eyelashes • Eyebrows • Body hair • Moustache and/or beard areas only	Increase in length, thickness, and/or density of hair that the patient is able to camouflage by periodic shaving, bleaching, or removal of individual hairs	Increase in length, thickness, and/or density of hair that is very noticeable and requires regular shaving or removal of hairs in order to camouflage. May cause mild symptoms related to hair overgrowth	Marked increase in hair density, thickness, and/or length of hair that requires either frequent shaving or destruction of the hair to camouflage. May cause symptoms related to hair overgrowth. Without hair removal, inability to function normally in social, personal, or professional situations	
Hair changes: disruption of normal hair growth Specify: • Facial hair (diffuse, not just in male beard/mustache areas) • Eyelashes • Eyebrows • Body hair • Beard and moustache hair (hirsutism)	Some distortion of hair growth but does not cause symptoms or require intervention	Distortion of hair growth in many hairs in a given area that cause discomfort or symptoms that may require individual hairs to be removed	Distortion of hair growth of most hairs in a given area with symptoms or resultant problems requiring removal of multiple hairs	

the anagen hairs, Olsen developed a separate scale for this type of hair abnormality. This has now been published in the CTCAE v4.0 guidelines and is shown in Table 10.5.

Potential treatments for chemotherapy-induced alopecia

Prevention of hair loss
Human trials
Physical measures
Some of the earliest approaches to preventing CIA were nonpharmaceutical. In a set of letters to the *British Medical Journal* in 1966, two English physicians discussed their independent use of a sphygmomanometer cuff worn as a headband to cut blood supply to the cranial skin from 5 minutes before to 5 minutes after chemotherapy injection [51, 52]. Both physicians found that scalp tourniquet use minimized or eliminated chemotherapy-induced hair loss. Scalp tourniquets continued to be discussed as an option for preventing CIA in a series of letters published in the *New England Journal of Medicine* in the 1970s [53–56]. Few new mentions of scalp tourniquets are made in the literature from 1980 onward, however, and few practitioners currently seem to use this as a method of preventing chemotherapy hair loss.

Another nonpharmaceutical approach, scalp cooling, is by far the most extensively used and discussed treatment method for CIA. Scalp hypothermia is hypothesized to prevent chemotherapy-associated hair loss either through slowing down scalp cellular metabolism or by reducing perfusion, and therefore chemotherapy delivery to the scalp, much like the scalp tourniquet [57]. Notably, although much has been published concerning the use of scalp cooling, most of the discussion has involved patient case series; an excellent review of the literature on scalp cooling from 1973 to 2003 found only seven randomized trials among the 53 articles published [58]. No further randomized controlled trials have been published since 2003. The seven trials are difficult to compare, as different chemotherapy regimens, patient populations, hair loss evaluation methods, and even cooling mechanisms were used. Nevertheless, six of the seven randomized controlled trials found a significant advantage in the amount of hair preserved during chemotherapy [59–65]. A recent systematic review of nonpharmacologic methods for dealing with common chemotherapy AEs also found that despite the variability in the baseline populations studied and the outcome parameters of the various trials, a tentative recommendation could be made for the use of scalp cooling to prevent CIA [66].

Recently, more attention has been paid to which particular cooling techniques are most effective in preventing hair loss. Along with articles evaluating specific cooling caps that have been developed, a series of articles from a group at Eindhoven

University of Technology in the Netherlands has also examined the effective temperature range for scalp cooling [67–71]. In an examination of keratinocytes exposed to doxorubicin *in vitro*, Janssen *et al.* [71] found that cells cooled to 22°C had a significantly higher rate of survival than those that remained at 37°C. Interestingly, further cooling the cells to 10°C provided no significant survival advantage over the keratinocytes at 22°C. The same group also demonstrated a similarly plateauing effectiveness to temperature cooling on reduction in scalp perfusion [70]. In their study examining nine patients, Janssen *et al.* found that a reduction of 10°C in scalp temperature correlated with a scalp perfusion decrease to below 40% of normal. The group was unable to lower scalp perfusion much below 30% of normal even with further temperature reduction, however, and found reductions in temperature of 12°C to be an unnecessary discomfort for the patient. The group's findings correlate well with a 1982 study that found that scalp temperature had to be reduced to at least 22°C to prevent hair loss in a group of breast cancer patients receiving 40 mg/m² doxorubicin and 2 mg vincristine [72].

Despite the evidence that scalp cooling may have some beneficial effect on minimizing hair loss due to chemotherapy, the technique has not been commonly used in American oncology clinics and nearly all of the published reports regarding its use have come from European medical centers. Some of the hesitancy in the use of scalp cooling may be attributed to several publications that have suggested that cooling could be associated with the occurrence of scalp metastases. Several of the randomized trials evaluating scalp cooling first expressed concern that the cooling could provide a protective effect for micrometastases to the scalp skin [58, 61–63]. Witman *et al.* [73] and Forsberg [74] published reports on patients with mycosis fungoides and acute myeloblastic leukemia, respectively, that each believed developed scalp metastases secondary to cooling cap use. A series of more recent studies looking at breast cancer patients suggests that scalp cooling is a safe technique for this patient population, and perhaps more generally for all patients with solid malignancies [68, 75–77]. In particular, Lemieux *et al.* [76] followed 553 women who received scalp cooling and 87 women who did not for approximately 5.5 years and did not see a significant difference in scalp metastases between the two groups; there was a 1.1% incidence in those receiving the scalp cooling versus a 1.2% incidence in those who did not. At this time, however, hematologic malignancy remains a contraindication to receiving scalp cooling [57].

Topical agents

Although several pharmaceutical agents have been suggested in the literature to ameliorate CIA, few of these interventions have been tested in human populations. Of those pharmaceutical agents that have been looked at in human beings, minoxidil is currently the most well studied. Notably, however, two trials examining use of 2% topical minoxidil (one randomized controlled, the other prospective) both found that minoxidil failed to protect against the development of CIA [78, 79].

The immunomodulator AS101 is the only pharmaceutical treatment shown to protect against chemotherapy hair loss in humans [50]. AS101 is the tellurium compound ammonium trichloro(dioxoethylene-O,O-)tellurate and is thought to exert its effect partially through its upregulation of interleukin 1 (IL-1) or through its ras-dependent upregulation of keratinocyte growth factor. This study noticed a significant decrease in the severity of hair loss with this agent, although it did not completely prevent alopecia.

Vitamin D3 has also been looked at in humans as a potential preventative agent for CIA, likely through its effects on inhibiting DNA synthesis, arresting the cell cycle at the G0/G1 interphase, and inducing differentiation. A single trial examined 0.0025% and 0.005% topical topitriol (calcitriol, 1,25-dihydroxyvitamin D3) to prevent hair loss among women receiving 5-fluorouracil, nonliposomal doxorubicin, and cyclophosphamide [80]. The trial failed to show any protection from chemotherapy-induced hair loss, and a phase I trial is underway.

Tempol, a nitroxide radioprotector, has been shown to be protective against radiation-induced alopecia in both an animal and human models [81, 82]. In a phase Ib study, 11 human patients receiving whole brain radiation were treated with tempol starting 15 minutes before radiation and then washed off. In the first four patients, hair retention was localized to the base of the scalp where the tempol solution pooled after application. Subsequently, full scalp hair retention was seen in three of the final five evaluable patients after gauze was wrapped around the head to hold the tempol solution against the scalp. A phase II study of tempol is currently ongoing.

Animal studies

All other proposed pharmaceutical treatment methods have only been tested on one of the commonly used experimental animal models of CAI. The first model uses neonatal rats that have spontaneous anagen hair growth [83]; the second uses depilation to synchronize all hair follicles in adult mice in the anagen growth phase [84].

Importantly, several of these animal studies found drugs that were effective in preventing or minimizing the alopecia caused by some chemotherapeutic agents but not others. For instance, topical application of ImuVert, a biologic response modifier consisting of natural membrane vesicles and ribosomes derived from the bacterium *Serratia marcescens* and thought to impact hair follicles through upregulation of IL-1, protected against cytarabine-induced alopecia but not cyclophosphamide-induced alopecia [83]. Likewise, injections of IL-1, epithelial growth factors, fibroblast growth factors, and keratinocyte growth factor all failed to protect against cyclophosphamide-induced alopecia even though they successfully minimized cytarabine-induced alopecia [85–89].

In contrast, other animal model trials found topical and oral *N*-acetylcysteine and parathyroid hormone receptor antagonists were successful in diminishing the amount of hair loss with cyclophosphamide chemotherapy [90–92]. Botchkarev *et al.* [93]

also found that p53 knockout mice failed to lose their fur when injected with cyclophosphamide. These animal models suggest that rather than one preventive drug for CIA, several different treatment options may need to be developed to address the underlying mechanisms of the different chemotherapy agents. One particularly interesting example of such individualized alopecia prevention is demonstrated by the topical dox monoclonal antibody developed by Balsari *et al.* [94] that prevented doxorubicin-induced alopecia in the majority of treated rats. Because the antibody is given as a topical application, the drug is thought to be able to protect scalp hair without interfering with systemic treatment of the cancer.

Acceleration of regrowth after chemotherapy

The majority of trials looking at intervention in CIA have focused on prevention of hair loss rather than acceleration of hair regrowth following completion of chemotherapy. However, minoxidil, cyclosporine, and 17-beta-estradiol, known hair growth cycle modulators, have all been considered as possible means of facilitating hair recovery after chemotherapy completion. Duvic *et al.* [95] demonstrated in a double-blind randomized trial of 22 women that use of a 2% topical minoxidil solution significantly decreased the time required for hair regrowth following maximal chemotherapy hair loss. Patients applied 1 mL twice daily to the entire scalp throughout chemotherapy and up to 4 months post-chemotherapy resulting in shortened length of time between the womens' maximal hair loss and first regrowth by about 50.2 days, from a mean of 136.9 days in the placebo group to a mean of 86.7 days in the minoxidil group. Cyclosporine injections and topical 17-beta-estradiol have so far only been studied in the rat and mouse CIA models, but both agents accelerated post-chemotherapy hair regrowth in these animal models [84, 96–98].

Conclusions

Although not life-threatening, hair loss and hair growth alterations continue to be one of the most distressing and troublesome AEs of chemotherapy. Chemotherapeutic agents that are prone to causing more extensive hair loss in nearly all patients receiving them include cyclophosphamide and the anthracycline antibiotics daunorubicin, doxorubicin, and idarubicin. Another chemotherapy drug class with high associated rates of alopecia are the plant alkaloid agents: the taxanes (paclitaxel, docetaxel); the camptothecins (topotecan, irinotecan), the podophyllotoxins (etoposide, teniposide); and the vinca alkaloids (vinblastine, vincristine, vinorelbine). Traditional cytotoxic forms of chemotherapy generally cause an anagen or telogen effluvium pattern of hair loss. Notably, EGFRIs can cause hypertrichosis of the eyebrows, eyelashes, and vellus hairs of the face as well as an abnormally slow growth of scalp hair that is curlier, finer, and more brittle than the patient's normal pretreatment hair.

The recent development of quantitative grading scales for CIA should aid in the evaluation of possible interventions. Of the prophylactic treatment options already in use, scalp cooling has shown benefit in preventing hair loss. Furthermore, recent data suggest that patients with solid tumors who receive scalp cooling should be at no greater risk for scalp metastases, although hematologic malignancy remains a contraindication to the use of scalp cooling. Topical minoxidil is an additional option to help with hair regrowth following the end of chemotherapy.

References

1 McGarvey, E.L., Baum, L.D., Pinkerton, R.C. & Rogers, L.M. (2001) Psychological sequelae and alopecia among women with cancer. *Cancer Practice*, **9**, 283–289.

2 Tierney, A.J., Taylor, J. & Closs, S.J. (1992) Knowledge, expectations, and experiences of patients receiving chemotherapy for breast cancer. *Scandinavian Journal of Caring Sciences*, **6** (2), 75–80.

3 Freedman, T.G. (1994) Social and cultural dimensions of hair loss in women treated for breast cancer. *Cancer Nursing*, **17** (4), 334–341.

4 Maunsell, E., Brisson, C., Dubois, L., Lauzier, S. & Fraser, A. (1999) Work problems after breast cancer: an exploratory qualitative study. *Psycho-Oncology*, **8** (6), 467–473.

5 Richer, M.C. & Ezer, H. (2002) Living in it, living with it, and moving on: dimensions of meaning during chemotherapy. *Oncology Nursing Forum*, **29** (1), 113–119.

6 Rosman, S. (2004) Cancer and stigma: experience of patients with chemotherapy-induced alopecia. *Patient Education and Counseling*, **52** (3), 333–339.

7 Harrison, S. & Sinclair, R. (2003) Optimal management of hair loss (alopecia) in children. *American Journal of Clinical Dermatology*, **4**, 757–770.

8 Sitzia, J. & Dikken, C. (1997) Survey of the incidence and severity of side-effects reported by patients receiving six cycles of FEC chemotherapy. *Journal of Cancer Nursing*, **1** (2), 61–73.

9 Sitzia, J. & Huggins, L. (1998) Side effects of cyclophosphamide, methotrexate, and 5-fluorouracil (CMF) chemotherapy for breast cancer. *Cancer Practice*, **6** (1), 13–21.

10 Land, S.R., Kopec, J.A., Yothers, G. et al. (2004) Health-related quality of life in axillary node-negative, estrogen receptor-negative breast cancer patients undergoing AC versus CMF chemotherapy: findings from the National Surgical Adjuvant Breast and Bowel Project B-23. *Breast Cancer Research and Treatment*, **86** (2), 153–164.

11 Gandelman, M. (2005) A technique for reconstruction of eyebrows and eyelashes. *Seminars in Plastic Surgery*, **19** (2), 153–158.

12 Thibaut, S., De Becker, E., Caisey, L. et al. (2010) Human eyelash characterization. *British Journal of Dermatology*, **162** (2), 304–310.

13 Olsen, E.A. (ed.) (2003) *Disorders of Hair Growth: Diagnosis and Treatment.* New York, McGraw-Hill.

14 Gomberg-Maitland, M., Maitland, M.L., Barst, R.J. et al. (2010) A dosing/cross-development study of the multikinase inhibitor sorafenib in patients with pulmonary arterial hypertension. *Clinical Pharmacology and Therapeutics*, **87** (3), 303–310.

15 Hutson, T.E., Bellmunt, J., Porta, C. *et al.* (2010) Long-term safety of sorafenib in advanced renal cell carcinoma: follow-up of patients from phase III TARGET. *European Journal of Cancer*, **46** (13), 2432–2440.

16 Pongpudpunth, M., Demierre, M.F. & Goldberg, L.J. (2009) A case report of inflammatory nonscarring alopecia associated with the epidermal growth factor receptor inhibitor erlotinib. *Journal of Cutaneous Pathology*, **36** (12), 1303–1307.

17 Graves, J.E., Jones, B.F., Lind, A.C. & Heffernan, M.P. (2006) Nonscarring inflammatory alopecia associated with the epidermal growth factor receptor inhibitor gefitinib. *Journal of the American Academy of Dermatology*, **55** (2), 349–353.

18 Dueland, S., Sauer, T., Lund-Johansen, F., Ostenstad, B. & Tveit, K.M. (2003) Epidermal growth factor receptor inhibition induces trichomegaly. *Acta Oncologica (Stockholm, Sweden)*, **42** (4), 345–346.

19 Bouche, O., Brixi-Benmansour, H., Bertin, A., Perceau, G. & Lagarde, S. (2005) Trichomegaly of the eyelashes following treatment with cetuximab. *Annals of Oncology*, **16** (10), 1711–1712.

20 Pascual, J.C., Banuls, J., Belinchon, I., Blanes, M. & Massuti, B. (2004) Trichomegaly following treatment with gefitinib (ZD1839). *British Journal of Dermatology*, **151** (5), 1111–1112.

21 Roé, E., Garca Muret, M.P., Marcuello, E., Capdevila, J., Pallarés, C. & Alomar, A. (2006) Description and management of cutaneous side effects during cetuximab or erlotinib treatments: a prospective study of 30 patients. *Journal of the American Academy of Dermatology*, **55** (3), 429–437.

22 Kerob, D., Dupuy, A., Reygagne, P. *et al.* (2006) Facial hypertrichosis induced by cetuximab, an anti-EGFR monoclonal antibody. *Archives of Dermatology*, **142** (12), 1656–1657.

23 Montagut, C., Grau, J.J., Grimalt, R., Codony, J., Ferrando, J. & Albanell, J. (2005) Abnormal hair growth in a patient with head and neck cancer treated with the anti-epidermal growth factor receptor monoclonal antibody cetuximab. *Journal of Clinical Oncology*, **23** (22), 5273–5275.

24 Lacouture, M.E., Maitland, M.L., Segaert, S. *et al.* (2010) A proposed EGFR inhibitor dermatologic adverse event-specific grading scale from the MASCC skin toxicity study group. *Supportive Care in Cancer*, **18** (4), 509–522.

25 Van Doorn, R., Kirtschig, G., Scheffer, E., Stoof, T.J. & Giaccone, G. (2002) Follicular and epidermal alterations in patients treated with ZD1839 (Iressa), an inhibitor of the epidermal growth factor receptor. *British Journal of Dermatology*, **147** (3), 598–601.

26 Agero, A.L., Dusza, S.W., Benvenuto-Andrade, C., Busam, K.J., Myskowski, P. & Halpern, A.C. (2006) Dermatologic side effects associated with the epidermal growth factor receptor inhibitors. *Journal of the American Academy of Dermatology*, **55** (4), 657–670.

27 Robert, C., Soria, J.C., Spatz, A. *et al.* (2005) Cutaneous side-effects of kinase inhibitors and blocking antibodies. *Lancet Oncology*, **6** (7), 491–500.

28 Lacouture, M.E., Basti, S., Patel, J. & Benson, A. 3rd. (2006) The SERIES clinic: an interdisciplinary approach to the management of toxicities of EGFR inhibitors. *Journal of Supportive Oncology*, **4** (5), 236–238.

29 Segaert, S. & Van Cutsen, E. (2005) Clinical signs, pathophysiology, and management of skin toxicity during therapy with epidermal growth factor receptor inhibitors. *Annals of Oncology*, **16** (9), 1425–1433.

30 Osio, A., Mateus, C., Soria, J.C. *et al.* (2009) Cutaneous side-effects in patients on long-term treatment with epidermal growth factor receptor inhibitors. *British Journal of Dermatology*, **161** (3), 515–521.

31 Tallon, B., Blanchard, E. & Goldberg, L.J. (2010) Permanent chemotherapy-induced alopecia: case report and review of the literature. *Journal of the American Academy of Dermatology*, **63** (2), 333–336.

32 Machado, M., Moreb, J.S. & Khan, S.A. (2007) Six cases of permanent alopecia after various conditioning regimens commonly used in hematopoietic stem cell transplantation. *Bone Marrow Transplantation*, **40** (10), 979–982.

33 Tosti, A., Piraccini, B.M., Vincenzi, C. & Misciali, C. (2005) Permanent alopecia after busulfan chemotherapy. *British Journal of Dermatology*, **152** (5), 1056–1058.

34 de Jonge, M.E., Mathot, R.A., Dalesio, O., Huitema, A.D., Rodenhuis, S. & Beijnen, J.H. (2002) Relationship between irreversible alopecia and exposure to cyclophosphamide, thiotepa and carboplatin (CTC) in high-dose chemotherapy. *Bone Marrow Transplantation*, **30** (9), 593–597.

35 Tran, D., Sinclair, R.D., Schwarer, A.P. & Chow, C.W. (2000) Permanent alopecia following chemotherapy and bone marrow transplantation. *Australasian Journal of Dermatology*, **41** (2), 106–108.

36 Ljungman, P., Hassan, M., Bekássy, A.N., Ringdén, O. & Oberg, G. (1995) Busulfan concentration in relation to permanent alopecia in recipients of bone marrow transplants. *Bone Marrow Transplantation*, **15** (6), 869–871.

37 Baker, B.W., Wilson, C.L., Davis, A.L. *et al.* (1991) Busulphan/cyclophosphamide conditioning for bone marrow transplantation may lead to failure of hair re-growth. *Bone Marrow Transplantation*, **7** (1), 43–47.

38 Vowels, M., Chan, L.L., Giri, N., Russell, S. & Lam-Po-Tang, R. (1993) Factors affecting hair regrowth after bone marrow transplantation. *Bone Marrow Transplantation*, **12** (4), 347–350.

39 Prevezas, C., Matard, B., Pinquier, L. & Reygagne, P. (2009) Irreversible and severe alopecia following docetaxel or paclitaxel cytotoxic therapy for breast cancer. *British Journal of Dermatology*, **160** (4), 883–885.

40 Masidonski, P. & Mahon, S.M. (2009) Permanent alopecia in women being treated for breast cancer. *Clinical Journal of Oncology Nursing*, **13** (1), 13–14.

41 Carlini, P., Di Cosimo, S., Ferretti, G. *et al.* (2003) Alopecia in a premenopausal breast cancer woman treated with letrozole and triptorelin. *Annals of Oncology*, **14** (11), 1689–1690.

42 Daniel, J. (1896) The x-rays. *Science*, **3**, 562–563.

43 Borak, J. (1936) The radiation biology of the cutaneous glands. *Radiology*, **27**, 651–655.

44 Severs, G.A., Griffin, T. & Werner-Wasik, M. (2008) Cicatricial alopecia secondary to radiation therapy: case report and review of the literature. *Cutis; Cutaneous Medicine for the Practitioner*, **81** (2), 147–153.

45 Lawenda, B.D., Gagne, H.M., Gierga, D.P. *et al.* (2004) Permanent alopecia after cranial irradiation: dose–response relationship. *International Journal of Radiation Oncology, Biology, Physics*, **60** (3), 879–887.

46 McCarthy, L. (1940) *Diagnosis and Treatment of Diseases of the Hair*, CV Mosby, St. Louis, MO.

47 Geary, J.R. (1952) Effect of roentgen rays during various phases of the hair cycle of the albino rat. *American Journal of Anatomy*, **91** (1), 51–105.

48 Van Scott, E.J. & Reinertson, R.P. (1957) Detection of radiation effects on hair roots of the human scalp. *Journal of Investigative Dermatology*, **29** (3), 205–212.

49 Fajardo, L.F. (1983) *Pathology of Radiation Injury*, Mosby, New York, NY.

50 Sredni, B., Xu, R., Albeck, M. *et al.* (1996) The protective role of the immunomodulator AS101 against chemotherapy-induced alopecia studies on human and animal models. *International Journal of Cancer*, **65** (1), 97–103.

51 Simister, J.M. (1966) Letter: alopecia and cytotoxic drugs. *British Medical Journal*, **2** (5522), 1138.

52 Hennessy, J.D. (1966) Letter: alopecia and cytotoxic drugs. *British Medical Journal*, **2** (5522), 1138.

53 Pesce, A., Cassuto, J.P. & Audoly, P. (1978) Letter: scalp tourniquets in the prevention of chemotherapy-induced alopecia. *New England Journal of Medicine*, **298** (21), 1204–1205.

54 Soukop, M., Campbell, A., Gray, M.M. *et al.* (1978) Letter: scalp tourniquet in cancer therapy. *New England Journal of Medicine*, **299** (11), 605–606.

55 Helson, L. & Prager, D. (1971) Letter: vincristine and alopecia. *New England Journal of Medicine*, **284** (6), 336.

56 O'Brien, R., Zelson, J.H., Schwartz, A.D. & Pearson, H.A. (1970) Letter: scalp tourniquet to lessen alopecia after vincristine. *New England Journal of Medicine*, **283** (26), 1489.

57 Trueb, R.M. (2009) Chemotherapy-induced alopecia. *Seminars in Cutaneous Medicine and Surgery*, **28** (1), 11–14.

58 Grevelman, E.G. & Breed, W.P.M. (2005) Prevention of chemotherapy-induced hair loss by scalp-cooling. *Annals of Oncology*, **16**, 352–358.

59 Edelstyn, G.A., MacDonald, M. & MacRae, K.D. (1977) Doxorubicin-induced hair loss and possible modification by scalp cooling. *Lancet*, **2** (8031), 253–254.

60 Kennedy, M., Packard, R., Grant, M., Padilla, G., Presant, C. & Chillar, R. (1983) The effect of using Chemocap on occurrence of chemotherapy-induced alopecia. *Oncology Nursing Forum*, **10** (1), 19–24.

61 Satterwhite, B. & Zimm, S. (1984) The use of scalp hypothermia in the prevention of doxorubicin-induced hair loss. *Cancer*, **54** (1), 34–37.

62 Parker, R. (1987) The effectiveness of scalp hypothermia in preventing cyclophosphamide-induced alopecia. *Oncology Nursing Forum*, **14** (6), 49–53.

63 Giaccone, G., Di Gulio, F., Morandini, M.P. & Calciati, A. (1988) Scalp hypothermia in the prevention of doxorubicin-induced hair loss. *Cancer Nursing*, **11** (3), 170–173.

64 Ron, I.G., Kalmus, Y., Kalmus, Z., Inbar, M. & Chaitchik, S. (1997) Scalp cooling in the prevention of alopecia in patients receiving depilating chemotherapy. *Supportive Care in Cancer*, **5**, 136–138.

65 Macduff, C., Mackenzie, T., Hutcheon, A., Melville, L. & Archibald, H. (2003) The effectiveness of scalp cooling in preventing alopecia for patients receiving epirubicin and docetaxel. *European Journal of Cancer Care*, **12** (2), 154–161.

66 Lofti-Jam, K., Carey, M., Jefford, M., Schofield, P., Charleson, C. & Aranda, S. (2008) Nonpharmacologic strategies for managing common chemotherapy adverse effects: a systematic review. *Journal of Clinical Oncology*, **26** (34), 5618–5629.

67 Peck, H.J., Mitchell, H. & Stewart, A.L. (2000) Evaluating the efficacy of scalp cooling using the Penguin cold cap system to reduce alopecia in patients undergoing chemotherapy for breast cancer. *European Journal of Oncology Nursing*, **4** (4), 246–248.

68 Ridderheim, M., Bjurberg, M. & Gustavsson, A. (2003) Scalp hypothermia to prevent chemotherapy-induced alopecia is effective and safe: a pilot study of a new digitalized scalp-cooling system used in 74 patients. *Supportive Care in Cancer*, **11** (6), 371–377.

69 Massey, C.S. (2004) A multicentre study to determine the efficacy and patient acceptability of the Paxman Scalp cooler to prevent hair loss in patients receiving chemotherapy. *European Journal of Oncology Nursing*, **8** (2), 121–130.

70 Janssen, F.P., Rajan, V., Steenbergen, W., van Leeuwen, G.M. & van Steenhoven, A.A. (2007) The relationship between local scalp temperature and cutaneous perfusion during scalp cooling. *Physiological Measurement*, **28** (8), 829–839.

71 Janssen, F.P., Bouten, C.V., van Leeuwen, G.M. & van Steenhoven, A.A. (2008) Effects of temperature and doxorubicin exposure on keratinocyte damage in vitro. *In Vitro Cellular & Developmental Biology – Animal*, **44** (3–4), 81–86.

72 Gregory, R.P., Cooke, T., Middleton, J., Buchanan, R.B. & Williams, C.J. (1982) Prevention of doxorubicin-induced alopecia by scalp hypothermia: relation to degree of cooling. *British Medical Journal (Clinical Research Ed.)*, **284** (6330), 1674.

73 Witman, G., Cadman, E. & Chen, M. (1981) Letter: misuse of scalp hypothermia. *Cancer Treatment Reports*, **65**, 507–508.

74 Forsberg, S. (2001) Letter: scalp cooling therapy and cytotoxic treatment. *Lancet*, **357**, 1134.

75 Lemenager, M., Lecomte, S., Bonneterre, M.E., Bessa, E., Dauba, J. & Bonneterre, J. (1997) Effectiveness of Cold Cap in the prevention of docetaxel-induced alopecia. *European Journal of Cancer*, **33**, 297–300.

76 Lemieux, J., Amireault, C., Provencher, L. & Maunsell, E. (2009) Incidence of scalp metastases in breast cancer: a retrospective cohort study in women who were offered scalp cooling. *Breast Cancer Research and Treatment*, **118** (3), 547–552.

77 van de Sande, M.A., van den Hurk, C.J., Breed, W.P. & Nortier, J.W. (2010) Allow scalp cooling during adjuvant chemotherapy in patients with breast cancer; scalp metastases rarely occur. *Nederlands Tijdschrift voor Geneeskunde*, **154** (33), A2134.

78 Granai, C.O., Frederickson, H., Gajewski, W., Goodman, A., Goldstein, A. & Baden, H. (1991) The use of minoxidil to attempt to prevent alopecia during chemotherapy for gynecologic malignancies. *European Journal of Gynaecological Oncology*, **12** (2), 129–132.

79 Rodriguez, R., Machiavelli, M., Leone, B. *et al.* (1994) Minoxidil (Mx) as a prophylaxis of doxorubicin-induced alopecia. *Annals of Oncology*, **5** (8), 769–770.

80 Hidalgo, M., Rinaldi, D., Medina, G., Griffin, T., Turner, J. & Von Hoff, D.D. (1999) A phase 1 trial of topical topitriol (calcitriol, 1, 25-dihydroxyvitamin D3) to prevent chemotherapy-induced alopecia. *Anti-Cancer Drugs*, **10** (4), 393–395.

81 Cuscela, D., Coffin, D., Lupton, G.P. *et al.* (1996) Protection from radiation-induced alopecia with topical application of nitroxides: fractionated studies. *Cancer Journal From Scientific American*, **2** (5), 273–278.

82 Metz, J.M., Smith, D., Mick, R. *et al.* (2004) A phase I study of topical Tempol for the prevention of alopecia induced by whole brain radiography. *Clinical Cancer Research*, **10** (19), 6411–6417.

83 Hussein, A.M., Jimenez, J.J., McCall, C.A. & Yunis, A.A. (1990) Protection from chemotherapy-induced alopecia in a rat model. *Science*, **249** (4976), 1564–1566.

84 Paus, R., Handjiski, B., Eichmuller, S. & Czarnetzki, B.M. (1994) Chemotherapy-induced alopecia in mice: induction by cyclophosphamide, inhibition by cyclosporine-A, and modulation by dexamethasone. *American Journal of Pathology*, **144** (4), 719–734.

85 Hussein, A.M. (1993) Chemotherapy-induced alopecia: new developments. *Southern Medical Journal*, **86** (5), 489–496.

86 Jimenez, J.J., Wong, G.H.W. & Yunis, A.A. (1991) Interleukin 1 protects from cytosine arabinoside-induced alopecia in a rat model. *FASEB Journal*, **5** (10), 2456–2458.

87 Hussein, A.M. (1991) Interleukin 1 protects against 1-beta-D-arabinofuranosylcytosine-induced alopecia in the newborn rat model. *Cancer Research*, **51** (12), 3329–3330.

88 Jimenez, J.J. & Yunis, A.A. (1992) Protection from 1-beta-D-arabinofuranosylcytosine-induced alopecia by epidermal growth factor and fibroblast growth factor in the rat model. *Cancer Research*, **52** (2), 413–415.

89 Danilenko, D.M., Ring, B.D., Yanagihara, D. *et al.* (1995) Keratinocyte growth factor is an important endogenous mediator of hair follicle growth, development, and differentiation: normalization of the *nu/nu* follicular differentiation defect and amelioration of chemotherapy-induced alopecia. *American Journal of Pathology*, **147** (1), 145–154.

90 Jimenez, J.J., Haung, H.S. & Yunis, A.A. (1992) Treatment with ImuVert/*N*-acetylcysteine protects rats from cyclophosphamide/cytarabine-induced alopecia. *Cancer Investigation*, **10** (4), 271–276.

91 D'Agostini, F., Bagnasco, M., Giunciuglio, D., Albini, A. & De Flora, S. (1998) Inhibition by oral *N*-acetylcysteine of doxorubicin-induced clastogenicity and alopecia, and prevention of primary tumors and lung micrometastases in mice. *International Journal of Oncology*, **13** (2), 217–224.

92 Peters, E.M., Foitzik, K., Paus, R., Ray, S. & Holick, M.F. (2001) A new strategy for modulating chemotherapy-induced alopecia, using PTH/PTHrP receptor agonist and antagonist. *Journal of Investigative Dermatology*, **117** (2), 173–178.

93 Botchkarev, V.A., Komarova, E.A., Siebenhaar, F. *et al.* (2000) p53 is essential for chemotherapy-induced hair loss. *Cancer Research*, **60** (18), 5002–5006.

94 Balsari, A.L., Morelli, D., Menard, S., Veronesi, U. & Colnaghi, M.I. (1994) Protection against doxorubicin-induced alopecia in rats by liposome-entrapped monoclonal antibodies. *FASEB Journal*, **8** (2), 226–230.

95 Duvic, M., Lemak, N.A., Valero, V., Hymes, S.R., Farmer, K.L. & Hortobagyi, G.N. *et al.* (1996) A randomized trial of minoxidil in chemotherapy-induced alopecia. *Journal of the American Academy of Dermatology*, **35** (1), 74–78.

96 Hussein, A.M., Stuart, A. & Peters, W.P. (1995) Protection against chemotherapy-induced alopecia by cyclosporine A in the newborn rat model. *Dermatology (Basel, Switzerland)*, **190** (3), 192–196.

97 Shirai, A., Tsunoda, H., Tamaoki, T. & Kamiya, T. (2001) Topical application of cyclosporin A induces rapid-remodeling of damaged anagen hair follicles produced in cyclophosphamide administered mice. *Journal of Dermatological Science*, **27** (1), 7–13.

98 Ohnemus, U., Unalan, M., Handjiski, B. & Paus, R. (2004) Topical estrogen accelerates hair regrowth in mice after chemotherapy-induced alopecia by favoring the dystrophic catagen response pathway to damage. *Journal of Investigative Dermatology*, **122** (1), 7–13.

99 *Cerubidine (package insert)*. (2004) Ben Venue Laboratories, Inc., Bedford, OH.

100 Wiernik, P.H. & Serpick, A.A. (1972) A randomized clinical trial of daunorubicin and a combination of prednisone, vincristine, 6-mercaptopurine, and methotrexate in adult acute nonlymphocytic leukemia. *Cancer Research*, **32** (10), 2023–2026.

101 Weil, M., Glidewell, O.J., Jacquillat, C. *et al.* (1973) Daunorubicin in the therapy of acute granulocytic leukemia. *Cancer Research*, **33** (5), 921–928.

102 *Doxorubicin hydrochloride (package insert)*. (2006) Pharmacia & Upjohn Co, New York, NY.

103 Henderson, I.C., Allegra, J.C., Woodcock, T. *et al.* (1989) Randomized controlled trial comparing mitoxantrone to doxorubicin in previously treated patients with metastatic breast cancer. *Journal of Clinical Oncology*, **7** (5), 560–571.

104 Lawton, P.A., Spittle, M.F., Ostrowski, M.J. *et al.* (1993) A comparison of doxorubicin, epirubicin, and mitozantrone as single agents in advanced breast carcinoma. *Clinical Oncology (Royal College of Radiologists (Great Britain))*, **5** (2), 80–84.

105 *Taxol (package insert)*. (2008), Bristol-Myers Squibb Co., Princeton, NJ.

106 *Onxol (package insert)*. (2005) IVAX Pharmaceuticals, Inc., Miami, FL.

107 Ranson, M., Davidson, N., Nicolson, M. *et al.* (2000) Randomized trial of paclitaxel plus supportive care versus supportive care for patients with advanced non-small-cell lung cancer. *Journal of the National Cancer Institute*, **92** (13), 1074–1080.

108 Gill, P.S., Tulpule, A., Espina, B.M. *et al.* (1999) Paclitaxel is safe and effective in the treatment of advanced AIDS-related Kaposi's sarcoma. *Journal of Clinical Oncology*, **17** (6), 1876–1883.

109 Curtin, J.P., Blessing, J.A., Webster, K.D. *et al.* (2001) Paclitaxel, an active agent in nonsquamous carcinomas of the uterine cervix: a gynecologic oncology group study. *Journal of Clinical Oncology*, **19** (5), 1275–1278.

110 Di Leo, A., Gomez, H.L., Aziz, Z. *et al.* (2008) Phase III, double-blind, randomized study comparing lapatinib plus paclitaxel with placebo plus paclitaxel as first-line treatment for metastatic breast cancer. *Journal of Clinical Oncology*, **26** (34), 5544–5552.

111 *Taxotere (package insert)*. (2008) Sanofi-Aventis U.S. LLC, Bridgewater, NJ.

112 Hanna, N., Shepherd, F.A., Fossella, F.V. *et al.* (2004) Randomized phase III trial of pemetrexed versus docetaxel in patients with non-small-cell lung cancer previously treated with chemotherapy. *Journal of Clinical Oncology*, **22** (9), 1589–1597.

113 Sjöström, J., Blomqvist, C., Mouridsen, H. *et al.* (1999) Docetaxel compared with sequential methotrexate and 5-fluorouracil in patients with advanced breast cancer after anthracycline failure: a randomized phase III study with crossover on progression by the Scandinavian breast group. *European Journal of Cancer*, **35** (8), 1194–1201.

114 Bonneterre, J., Roche, H., Monnier, A. *et al.* (2002) Docetaxel vs 5-fluorouracil plus vinorelbine in metastatic breast cancer after anthracycline therapy failure. *British Journal of Cancer*, **87** (11), 1210–1215.

115 Cortes, J.E. & Pazdur, R. (1995) Docetaxel. *Journal of Clinical Oncology*, **13** (10), 2643–2655.

116 *Idamycin (package insert)*. (2006) Pharmacia & Upjohn Co., New York, NY.

117 Vogler, W.R., Velez-Garcia, E., Weiner, R.S. *et al.* (1992) A phase III trial comparing idarubicin and daunorubicin in combination with cytarabine in acute myelogenous leukemia: a southeastern cancer study group study. *Journal of Clinical Oncology*, **10** (7), 1103–1111.

118 Lopez, M., Contegiacomo, A., Vici, P. *et al.* (1989) A prospective randomized trial of doxorubicin versus idarubicin in the treatment of advanced breast cancer. *Cancer*, **64** (12), 2431–2436.

119 *Cytoxan (package insert)*. (2005) Bristol-Myers Squibb Co., Princeton, NJ.

120 Ahmed, A.R. & Hombal, S.M. (1984) Cyclophosphamide (Cytoxan): a review on relevant pharmacology and clinical uses. *Journal of the American Academy of Dermatology*, **11** (6), 1115–1126.

121 Mendelson, D., Block, J. & Serpick, A. (1970) Effect of large intermittent intravenous doses of cyclophosphamide in lymphoma. *Cancer*, **25** (3), 715–720.

122 Coggins, P.R., Ravdin, R.G. & Eisman, S.H. (1960) Clinical evaluation of a new alkylating agent: cytoxan (cyclophosphamide). *Cancer*, **13**, 1254–1260.

123 Sweeney, M.J., Tuttle, A.H., Etteldorf, J.N. & Whittington, G.L. (1962) Cyclophosphamide in the treatment of common neoplastic diseases of childhood. *Journal of Pediatrics*, **61** (5), 702–708.

124 Brincker, H., Mouridsen, H.T. & Andersen, K.W. (1983) Adjuvant chemotherapy with cyclophosphamide or CMF in premenopausal women with stage II breast cancer. *Breast Cancer Research and Treatment*, **3** (1), 91–95.

125 McLean, R.D.W. (1965) Cyclophosphamide in the management of advanced bronchial carcinoma. *Thorax*, **20** (6), 555–561.

126 *Camptosar (package insert)*. (2008) Pharmacia & Upjohn Co., New York, NY.

127 Armand, J.P., Ducreux, M., Mahjoubi, M., Abigerges, D., Bugat, R. & Chabot, G. (1995) CPT-11 (irinotecan) in the treatment of colorectal cancer. *European Journal of Cancer*, **31A** (7/8), 1283–1287.

128 Ychou, M., Raoul, J.L., Douillard, J.Y. *et al.* (2009) A phase III randomized trial of LV5FU2 + irinotecan versus LV5FU2 alone in adjuvant high-risk colon cancer (FNCLCC Accord02/FFCD9802). *Annals of Oncology*, **20** (4), 674–680.

129 Duffour, J., Gourgou, S., Desseigne, F., Debrigode, C., Mineur, L. & Pinguet, F. (2007) Multicentre phase II study using increasing doses of irinotecan combined with a simplified LV5FU2 regimen in metastatic colorectal cancer. *Cancer Chemotherapy and Pharmacology*, **60** (3), 383–389.

130 Andre, T., Louvet, C., Maindrault-Goebel, F., Couteau, C., Mabro, M. & Lotz, J.P. (1999) CPT-11 (irinotecan) addition to bimonthly, high-dose leucovorin and bolus and continuous infusion 5-fluorouracil (FOLFIRI) for pretreated metastatic colorectal cancer. *European Journal of Cancer*, **35** (9), 1343–1347.

131 Pitot, H.C., Wender, D.B., O'Connell, M.J., Schroeder, G., Goldberg, R.M. & Rubin, J. (1997) Phase II trial of irinotecan in patients with metastatic colorectal carcinoma. *Journal of Clinical Oncology*, **15** (8), 2910–2919.

132 *Etopophos (package insert)*. (2005) Bristol-Myers Squibb Co., Princeton, NJ.

133 *Vepesid (package insert)*. (2006) Bristol-Myers Squibb Co., Princeton, NJ.

134 Fleming, R.A., Miller, A.A. & Stewart, C.F. (1989) Etoposide: an update. *Clinical Pharmacy*, **8** (4), 274–293.

135 *Hycamtin (package insert)*. (2008) GlaxoSmithKline, Research Triangle Park, NC.

136 ten Bokkel Huinink, W., Gore, M., Carmichael, J. *et al.* (1997) Topotecan versus paclitaxel for treatment of recurrent epithelial ovarian cancer. *Journal of Clinical Oncology*, **15** (6), 2183–2193.

137 Ramlau, R., Gervais, R., Krzakowski, M. *et al.* (2006) Phase III study comparing oral topotecan to intravenous docetaxel in patients with pretreated advanced non-small-cell lung cancer. *Journal of Clinical Oncology*, **24** (18), 2800–2807.

138 Gordon, A.N., Tonda, M., Sun, S. & Rackoff, W. (2004) Long-term survival advantage for women treated with pegylated liposomal doxorubicin compared with topotecan in a phase 3 randomized study of recurrent and refractory epithelial ovarian cancer. *Gynecologic Oncology*, **95** (1), 1–8.

139 *Vincristine sulfate (package insert)*. (2007) Hospira, Inc., Lake Forest, IL.

140 *Vumon (package insert)*. (2009) Bristol-Myers Squibb Co., Princeton, NJ.

141 *Iressa (package insert)*. (2006) AstraZeneca Pharmaceuticals LP, Wilmington, DE.

142 Donovan, J.C., Ghazarian, D.M. & Shaw, J.C. (2008) Scarring alopecia associated with use of the epidermal growth factor receptor inhibitor gefitinib. *Archives of Dermatology*, **144** (11), 1524–1525.

143 Kim, E.S., Hirsh, V., Mok, T., Socinski, M.A., Gervais, R. & Wu, Y.L. (2008) Gefitinib versus docetaxel in previously treated non-small-cell lung cancer (INTEREST): a randomized phase III trial. *Lancet*, **372** (9652), 1809–1818.

11 Nail Abnormalities in Oncology Practice

Robert Baran[1,2], Bernard Fouilloux[3] and Caroline Robert[2]

[1]Nail Disease Center, Cannes, France
[2]Dermatology Department, Cancer Institute Gustave Roussy, Villejuif, France
[3]Dermatology Department, Hôpital Nord, Saint-Etienne, France

Introduction

The purpose of this chapter is to show how frequently cytotoxic and targeted anticancer agents produce nail abnormalities. For a better understanding of these skin manifestations, the nail anatomy is reviewed here. The nail unit is made of four epithelial structures and the distal bony phalanx. The nail comes from an invagination that has a roof, the proximal nail fold and a floor, the matrix producing the nail plate. The only visible portion of the distal nail matrix is characteristic on the thumb, sometimes on the second fingernail and less often on the third one as an opaque half moon area involving the base of the nail plate. At this location, adherence of nail keratin and subungual tissue is weak [1].

In front of the lunula the nail bed arranged in longitudinal ridges adheres tightly to the nail. Anterior to the nail bed, the hyponychium is the region where the nail plate separates from the nail bed. The nail grows continuously. A full regrowth takes 5–6 months for normal fingernails while 12–18 months are necessary for toenails. Melanocytes are less numerous in the nail matrix than in the skin. They are rare in the nail bed. Most of them are dormant but may be activated.

Antimitotic nail adverse events (AEs) usually develop several weeks after the treatment has begun and they more often involve fingers than toes, probably because fingernails grow faster [2].

Some definitions of nail terms are needed :
• *Beau's line:* transverse linear depression emerging from beneath the proximal nail fold.
• *Onycholysis:* distal and/or lateral detachment of the nail from the subungual tissue.
• *Onychomadesis:* proximal nail plate–subungual tissue separation. It remains latent for a long time before nail shedding.

• *Nail brittleness:* soft, breakable, or friable nail.
• *Paronychia:* swelling, redness, and pain of the proximal nail fold.
• *Pitting:* usually small depressions on the dorsum of the nail plate. They emerge from under the proximal nail fold. At the base of the nail they may be covered with loose parakeratotic cells.
• *Koilonychia:* spoon-shaped nail plate.

The most frequent reasons for patient consultation on anticancer therapies for nail AEs are summarized in Table 11.1.

Drugs

Classic cytotoxic drugs
Among the cytotoxic drugs, the taxanes docetaxel (Taxotere®) and paclitaxel (Taxol®), which are widely used in different types of cancers, are the greatest culprtis of nail modifications. The incidence of patients developing nail changes is about 80% with docetaxel [3] and 20% with paclitaxel [4]. Nail dystrophies were reported in up to 88.5% of patients receiving more than seven cycles [3] of combined trastuzumab and docetaxel [5]. Taxanes are mainly known for inducing onycholysis (sometimes acute) [6] as well as subungual hemorrhages which can cause severe pain due to the high pressure or to the appearance of abscesses in the subungual areas [7]. Development of a typical orange discoloration of the nail plate and exudative painful paronychia are frequent. Pyogenic granulomas may also occur [8]. Interestingly, subungual hyperkeratosis can result from previous exudative paronychia [9]. A neurogenic mechanism has been suggested because of unilateral nail changes in the unaffected side of a patient with a denervated hand [10]. The effects of the traditional cytotoxic agents are directly proportional to the dose intensity of the treatment.

Dermatologic Principles and Practice in Oncology: Conditions of the Skin, Hair, and Nails in Cancer Patients, First Edition. Edited by Mario E. Lacouture.
© 2014 John Wiley & Sons, Inc. Published 2014 by John Wiley & Sons, Inc.

Table 11.1 Reasons for consultation of the patient on anticancer therapy.

Beau's lines, onychomadesis

Nail fragility (brittle nails); sometimes nail thickness

Painful nails mainly at the tip of the digit (xerosis, fissures) with predilection for the big toenail

Hot red foot, occasionally edematous

Periungual redness

Pins and needles, stinging painful swelling of the palms and soles sometimes associated with erythema (neuropathy, hand-foot syndrome)

Nail dyschromia with or without hemorrhages

Infection presenting as vesicles, ulcerations on the soles

Troubles of motricity with muscular and articular patterns

Onycholysis with or without pyogenic granuloma or hemorrhage

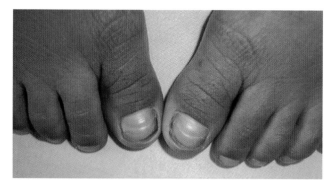

Figure 11.1 Beau's lines (Courtesy P. Chang, Guatemala).

Table 11.2 Anti-human epidermal growth-factor receptor (anti HER1) agents.

Anti-HER type	Molecules	Targets
Tyrosine kinase inhibitors	Erlotinib	EGFR
	Gefitinib	
	Lapatinib	EGFR + HER2
	Canertinib	EGFR + HER2
	Vandetanib	EGFR + VEGFR
Monoclonal antibodies	Cetuximab	EGFR
	Panitumumab	EGFR
	Matuzumab	EGFR
	Pertuzumab	EGFR + HER2
	Nimotuzumab	EGFR

Source: After Wasner *et al.* [10] with kind permission from Springer Science and Business Media.

Epidermal growth factor receptor inhibitors

A new category of anticancer drugs, targeted agents, can be monoclonal antibodies or small-molecule kinase inhibitors (Table 11.2). These targeted agents specifically inhibit proteins that are involved in the tumoral process. Unfortunately, these new agents are not devoid of AEs even if their safety profile is radically different from that of classic cytotoxic drugs. Among them, the inhibitors of the epidermal growth factor receptor (EGFR), used for treating lung, colon, head and neck, and pancreatic cancers, have a predilection for toxicity of the nail unit.

There are four types of HER receptors (HER1–4). HER1/EGFR and HER2 are the most studied because they are involved in growth and cellular differentiation. HER1/EGFR is expressed by 30–100% of solid tumors and its overexpression and/or activation by mutations is associated with a poor prognosis [11].

Other targeted agents such as imatinib and similar agents blocking the kinase function of c-Kit, PGDFR-ß, and the Bcr-Abl fusion protein found in chronic myeloid leukemia can induce nail hyperpigmentation and onychodystrophy.

Antiangiogenic multikinase inhibitors such as sorafenib and sunitinib induce subungual hemorrhages in approximately 30% of patients [12].

Symptoms

Nail matrix and nail plate alterations

A decrease in linear nail growth is common. The surface of the nail may appear ridged but pitting is rare and might be brought about by an associated psoriasiform condition. Transverse pitting can be present as grooves characteristic of Beau's lines (Figure 11.1). Onychomadesis is caused when the nail matrix stops its activity for 2–4 weeks (proximal nail plate shedding). Brittle nails with onychorrhexis (longitudinal striations of the nail plate) are often associated with distal fissuring. Trachyonychia (rough nails), thinning or thickening of the nail, and onychoschizia can be observed. These alterations can be seen with many cytotoxic agents and after hematopoietic transplants, and are not related to one specific drug.

Nail dyschromia is frequent, especially melanonychia (Figure 11.2), and may result from treatment with doxorubicin, bleomycin, busulfan, capecitabine, cetuximab, cyclophosphamide, docetaxel, hydroxyurea, imatinib, methotrexate, paclitaxel, and 5-fluorouracil [11]. Electron beam radiation treatment for lymphoma can result in transverse melanonychia [13]; however, a case has been published of a patient with transient leuconychia [14]. Transverse, true leukonychia (horizontal white bands that do not fade with pressure) (Figure 11.3) may be observed with any drug (e.g., cyclophosphamide, doxorubicin, vincristine) [15]. Apparent leukonychia (a white discoloration of the nail that fades when pressure is applied) is mainly seen in children [16].

Nail fold involvement

Among periungual and nail toxicity (Figure 11.4), ingrown nails (Figure 11.5), paronychia (Figure 11.6), and pyogenic granuloma

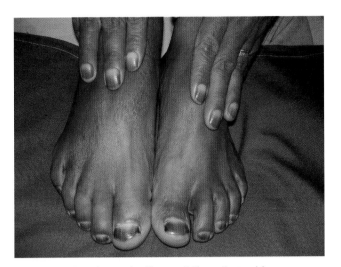

Figure 11.2 Hyperpigmentation (Courtesy P. Chang, Guatemala).

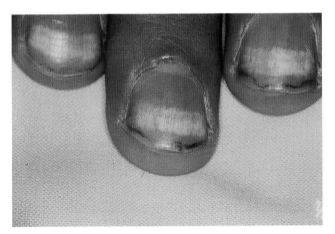

Figure 11.3 Transverse leuconychia.

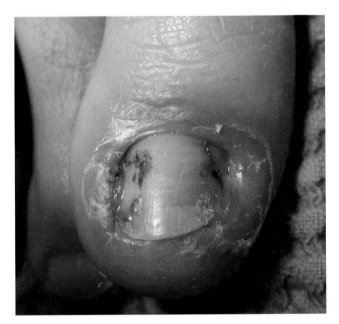

Figure 11.4 Exsudative painful paronychia.

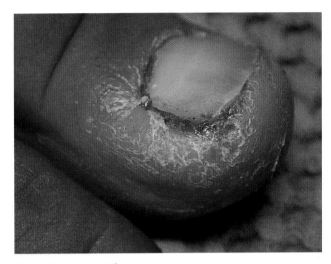

Figure 11.5 Ingrown nail.

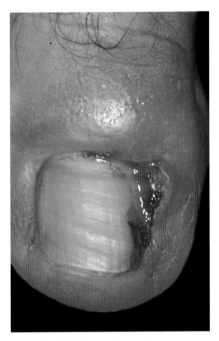

Figure 11.6 Paronychia with tiny pyogenic granuloma.

lesions (Figure 11.7) are frequent [17], especially with EGFR-targeted agents. Fissuring of distal fingers can be seen in 6–12% of patients.

Disruption or absence of cuticle or periungual erythema is followed by tenderness and pain. Pyogenic granuloma presents with excess granulation tissue, easy bleeding, and finally becomes covered by the skin.

All EGFR inhibitors can give rise to paronychia [17–19], but classic chemotherapies such as doxorubicin, capecitabine and docetaxel can also induce paronychial inflammation. Periungual abscesses are common but should receive treatment.

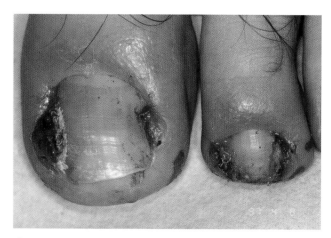

Figure 11.7 Ingrown nail with excess granulation tissue.

A correlation between nail toxicity and clinical benefit to therapy has not been determined [20]. In early lesions, periungual and nail lesions are not infected. Initial cultures are negative for bacteria and for *Candida* spp; however, superinfections often occur in persistent lesions with over 20 different species, including positive cultures of *Staphylococcus aureus* and other Gram-positive bacteria in 72%, Gram-negative bacteria in 23%, and *Candida* in 5% [21].

As these lesions are rather "well-tolerated" according to the literature, they rarely require cessation of therapy. Nevertheless, they can be severely painful and interfere with activities of daily living (ADLs).

Nail bed involvement

Splinter hemorrhages, sometimes pronounced, are observed with sunitinib (30%), sorafenib (60%), and other antiangiogenic inhibitors of vascular endothelial growth factors (VEGF) receptors [12]. Targeting receptors of VEGF might be the direct cause for subungual splinter hemorrhages, by blocking a physiologic repair process [12]. Onycholysis, with or without hemorrhages (Figure 11.8a,b), may raise the nail plate by pressure (mitoxantrone, doxorubicin, taxanes) [22]. Epothilones (e.g., ixabepilone) treatment induces nail modifications similar to those induced by taxanes [23].

Digit tip xerosis

Xerosis and/or erythema can be asymptomatic but fissures of the fingertips are frequent and may interfere with "instrumental" or with "self-care" ADLs. Most common culprit are EGFRIs.

Classification

Unlike the papulopustular reaction that occurs early within the first 1–4 weeks of EGFR inhibitor initiation, nail abnormalities occur later during the course of the treatment, after weeks 6–8.

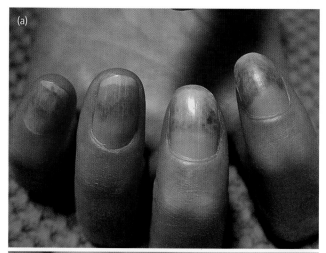
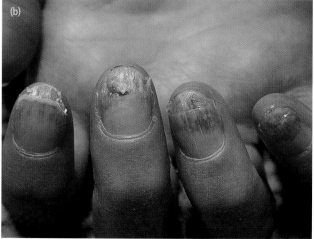

Figure 11.8 (a) Onycholysis (b) Oozing and subungual abcess (same patient).

Periungual and ungual AEs including paronychia and xerosis with desquamation of the digit tips are reported to occur in up to 58% of patients treated with EGFR inhibitors (EGFRIs). Although EGFRI-induced nail abnormalities are generally mild to moderate in severity, if they are not adequately managed they can result in significant pain, interfere with ADLs, and lead to EGFRI dose modification or interruption. Previously, all graded nail abnormalities were contained within one single category. The new version (4.0) of the Common Terminology Criteria for Adverse Events (CTCAE) has divided these events for greater specificity (Table 11.3). However, this classification was not designed optimal for grading modifications induced by EGFRIs and may result in underreporting and poor grading scale of distinctive AEs. Therefore, the Multinational Association of Supportive Care in Cancer (MASCC) proposed a scale more consistent with dermatologists' terminology as it divides nail abnormalities into those of the nail plate, folds, and digit tips, and implements classification as done for nail psoriasis modifications (Table 11.4) [24–26]. This class-specific grading scale has been

Table 11.3 Common Terminology Criteria for Adverse Events (CTCAE) Version 4.0: Terms in the dermatology/skin section relevant to nail adverse events (AEs).

Adverse event	Grade 1	Grade 2	Grade 3	Grade 4	Grade 5
Name and description	**Mild**	**Moderate**	**Severe**	**Life-threatening or disabling**	**Death related to AE**
Paronychia A disorder characterized by an infectious process involving the soft tissues around the nail	Nail fold edema or erythema, disruption of the cuticle	Localilized intervention indicated oral intervention indicated (e.g., antibiotic, antifungal, antiviral); nail fold edema or erythema with pain; associated with discharge or nail plate separation; limiting instrumental ADL[a]	Surgical intervention or IV antibiotics indicated; limiting self-care ADL[b]		
Nail loss A disorder chracterized by loss of all or a portion of the nail	Asymptomatic separation	Symptomatic separation of the nail bed from the nail plate or nai loss; limiting instrumental ADL[a]			
Nail ridging A disorder characterize by vertical or horizontal ridges on the nails	Asymptomatic clinical or diagnostic observations only; intervention not indicated				
Nail discoloration A disorder characterized by a change in the color of the nail plate	Asymptomatic; clinical or diagnostic observations only; intervention not indicated				
Dry skin	Covering <10% BSA and no associated erythema or pruritus	Covering 10–30% BSA and associated with erythema or pruritus; limiting instrumental ADL[a]M	Covering >30% BSA and associated with erythema or pruritus; limiting self-care ADL[b]		

ADL, activity of daily living; BSA, body surface area.
[a]Instrumental ADL refers to preparing meals, shopping for groceries or clothes, using the telephone, managing money etc.
[b]Self-care ADL refers to bathing, dressing and undressing, feeding self, using the toilet, taking medications, and not bedridden.
A semi-colon indicates "or" within the description of the grade. Not all grades are appropriate for all AEs. Therefore, some AEs are listed with fewer than five options for grade selection (Grades 1–5).
Source: After Eames *et al.* [21].

Table 11.4 Proposed Multinational Association of Supportive Care in Cancer (MASCC) Study Group epidermal growth factor receptor inhibitor(EGFRI) dermatologic adverse event (AE) grading scale for nail changes.

Adverse event	Grade 1	Grade 2	Grade 3	Grade 4	Grade 5
Changes of the nail plate	Onycholysis or ridging without pain	Onycholysis with mild–moderate pain, any nail plate lesion interfering with instrumental ADL	Nail plate changes interfering with self-care ADL		
Changes of the nail fold	Disruption or absence of cuticle; *or* erythema	Erythematous/tender/painful; *or* pyogenic granuloma; *or* crusted lesions *or* any fold lesion interfering on instrumental ADL	Periungual abscess; *or* fold changes interfering with self-care ADL		
Changes of the digit tip	Xerosis *and/or* erythema without pain	Xerosis *and/or* erythema with mild–moderate pain or stinging; *or* any digit tip lesion interfering with instrumental ADL	Digit tip lesions interfering with self-care ADL		

ADL, activities of daily living.
A semi-colon indicates "or" within the description of the grade. Instrumental ADL refer to preparing meals, shopping for groceries or clothes, using the telephone, managing money, etc. Self-care ADL refer to bathing, dressing and undressing, feeding self, using the toilet, taking medications, and not bedridden. Not all grades are appropriate for all AEs. Therefore, some AEs are listed with fewer than five options for grade selection.
Source: Lacouture *et al.* [24].

proposed to help standardize assessment and to improve reporting of EGFRI-associated dermatologic AEs [24].

Treatment

Management strategies for nail changes are set forth in the following section.

1. *Nail fragility syndrome.* Patients should wear cotton gloves underneath plastic gloves for any wet work. Oral intake of biotin or silicium is based on anecdotal evidence. Dark nail varnish may be useful in case of phototoxicity drugs.

2. *Onycholysis.* Trimming or debridement of the nail plate is necessary, followed by gentle cleaning with 3% peroxide, then rubbing of the nail bed with mupirocin ointment. Treat nail plate lesions interfering with instrumental or self-care ADLs.

3. *Hematomas.* There is no treatment for splinter hemorrhages in contrast to painful "pressure" hematomas. Partial or total avulsion is carried out to control the bleeding and clean the nail bed. Sometimes, a periungual abscess is discovered after avulsion; its removal with gauze should be followed by antiseptic baths, then gentle rubbing with mupirocin ointment.

4. *Nail fold lesions.* Disruption or absence of cuticle can be improved by applications of petrolatum ointment. Erythema, tenderness, or pain, especially if associated with pyogenic granuloma, crusted lesion, or any fold lesion interfering with instrumental or self-care ADLs are usually accompanied by an ingrown nail, with or without periungual abscess. As the early lesions are not infections, intralesional long-acting corticosteroids may stop inflammation. In persistent lesions that do not respond to 200 mg doxycycline daily for 6 weeks [27,28], a 3–4 mm crescent-shaped piece of the proximal nail fold tissue should be excised [1]. Under local anesthesia, pyogenic granuloma should be curetted: after detachment of the proximal nail fold to the nail bed, one-fifth of the lateral edge of the nail is removed allowing the cauterization of the lateral horn of the matrix and the base of the excess of granulation tissue with phenol (88%) in a bloodless field (Figure 11.9) [1].

Prevention

In a preventive manner, the use of frozen gloves (−30°C) protected 89% of patients compared with 49% of patients with unprotected hands in a study of docetaxel administered every 3 weeks for a median number of six cycles [29]. A specialized device has given the same good result on the feet. Ice packs can provide similar benefit.

Conclusions

Nail changes in the cancer patient are frequent, especially with the use of taxanes, EGFRIs, anthracyclines, and antimetabolites. Whereas most of these events are mild to moderate in severity, the

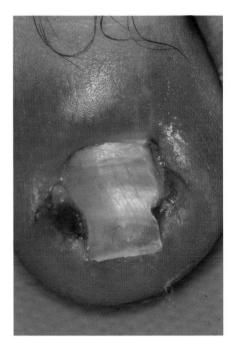

Figure 11.9 Ingrown toenail with excess granulation tissue, before cauterization of the matrix horns with phenol.

associated pain, interference with instrumental or self-care ADLs, and potential for secondary infections render nail changes to therapy as conditions that command attention. A high suspicion for infection should arise in settings where nail changes are associated with discharge, pain, odor, or color changes. Moreover, because of the slow growth of the nail plate, effective treatment of these conditions does not usually result in rapid improvement, and dose interruptions need to be lengthy (i.e., >2–4 weeks) to provide relief. Therefore, early prophylactic and management strategies are essential in order to minimize the impact that nail changes can have on ADLs and dose intensity of antineoplastic therapy.

References

1 Baran, R. (2008) Nail surgery. Chapter 246. In: K. Wolff, L.A. Goldsmith, S.I. Katz, *et al.* (eds), *Fitzpatrick's Dermatology in General Medicine*, pp. 2320–2330. Mc GrawHill, New York.

2 Piraccini, B.M. & Iorizzo, M. (2007) Drug reactions affecting the nail unit: diagnosis and management. *Dermatologic Clinics*, **25**, 215–221.

3 Winther, D., Saunte, D.M., Knap, M., Haahr, V. & Jensen, A.B. (2007) Nail changes due to docetaxel, a neglected side effect and nuisance for the patient. *Supportive Care in Cancer*, **15**, 1191–1197.

4 Hackbarth, M., Hass, N., Fotopoulou, C., Lichtenegger, W. & Sehouli, J. (2008) Chemotherapy-induced dermatological toxicity: frequencies and impact on quality of life in women's cancers: results of a prospective study. *Supportive Care in Cancer*, **16**, 267–273.

5 Alexandrescu, D.T., Vaillant, J. & Wiernik, P.H. (2006) Trastuzumab/docetaxel-induced nail dystrophy. *International Journal of Dermatology*, **45**, 1334–1336.

6 Rall, S., Lohmeyer, J.A., Machens, H.G. & Mailander, P. (2008) Acute onycholysis during chemotherapy with docetaxel. *Journal of Hand Surgery (European Volume)*, **33**, 214–215.

7 Minisini, A.M., Tosti, A., Sobrero, A.F. *et al.* (2003) Taxane-induced nail changes: incidence, clinical presentation and outcome. *Annals of Oncology*, **14**, 333–337.

8 Devillers, C., Vanhooteghem, O., Henrijean, A., Ramaut, M. & de la Brassinne, M. (2009) Subungual abscesses and pyogenic granuloma secondary to docetaxel therapy. *Clinical and Experimental Dermatology*, **34**, 251–252.

9 Correia, O., Azevedo, C., Pinto Ferreira, E., Braga Cruz, F. & Polónia, J. (1999) Nail changes secondary to docetaxel (taxotere). *Dermatology (Basel, Switzerland)*, **198**, 288–290.

10 Wasner, G., Hilpert, F., Schattschneider, J., Binder, A., Pfisterer, J. & Baron, R. (2002) Docetaxel-induced nail changes – a neurogenic mechanism: a case report. *Journal of Neuro-Oncology*, **58**, 167–174.

11 Mateus, C. & Robert, C. (2009) Effets cutanés des nouvelles molécules utilisées en cancérologie. *Revue de Medecine Interne*, **30**, 401–410.

12 Robert, C., Faivre, S., Raymond, E. *et al.* (2005) Subungual splinter hemorrhages: a clinical window to inhibition of vascular endothelial growth factor receptors? *Annals of Internal Medicine*, **143**, 313–314.

13 Quinlan, K.E., Janiga, J.J., Baran, R. & Lim, H.W. (2005) Transverse melanonychia secondary to electron beam therapy: a report of 3 cases. *Journal of the American Academy of Dermatology*, **53**, S112–S114.

14 Erös, N., Marschalkó, M., Bajcsay, A., Polgár, C., Fodor, J. & Kárpáti, S. (2011) Transient leukonychia after total skin electron beam irradiation. *Journal of the European Academy of Dermatology and Venereology*, **25**, 115–116.

15 Chapman, S. & Cohen, P.R. (1997) Transverse leukonychia in patients receiving cancer chemotherapy. *Southern Medical Journal*, **90**, 395–398.

16 Chen, W., Yu, Y.S., Liu, Y.H., Sheen, J.M. & Hsiao, C.C. (2007) Nail changes associated with chemotherapy in children. *Journal of the European Academy of Dermatology and Venereology*, **21**, 186–190.

17 Robert, C., Soria, J.C., Spatz, A. *et al.* (2005) Cutaneous side-effect of kinase inhibitors and blocking antibodies. *Lancet Oncology*, **6**, 491–500.

18 Busam, K.J., Capodieci, P., Motzer, R., Kiehn, T., Phelan, D. & Halpern, A.C.. (2001) Cutaneous side-effects in cancer patients treated with the antiepidermal growth factor receptor antibody C225. *British Journal of Dermatology*, **144**, 1169–1176.

19 Lee, M.W., Seo, C.W., Kim, S.W. *et al.* (2004) Cutaneous side effects in non-small cell lung cancer patients treated with Iressa (ZD1839), an inhibitor of epidermal growth factor. *Acta Dermato-Venereologica*, **84**, 23–26.

20 Hu, J.C., Sadeghi, P., Pinter-Brown, L.C., Yashar, S. & Chiu, M.W. (2007) Cutaneous side effects of epidermal growth factor receptor inhibitors: clinical presentation, pathogenesis, and management. *Journal of the American Academy of Dermatology*, **56**, 317–326.

21 Eames, T., Grabein, B., Kroth, J. & Wollenberg, A. (2010) Microbiological analysis of epidermal growth factor receptor inhibitor therapy-associated paronychia. *Journal of the European Academy of Dermatology and Venereology*, **24**, 958–960.

22 Creamer, J.D., Mortimer, P.S. & Powles, T.J. (1995) Mitozantrone-induced onycholysis: a series of five cases. *Clinical and Experimental Dermatology*, **20**, 469–461.

23 Alimonti, A., Nardoni, C., Papaldo, P. *et al.* (2005) Nail disorders in a woman treated with ixabepilone for metastatic breast cancer. *Anticancer Research*, **25**, 3531–3532.

24 Lacouture, M.E., Maitland, M.L., Segaert, S. *et al.* (2010) A proposed EGFR inhibitor dermatologic adverse event-specific grading scale from the MASCC skin toxicity study group. *Supportive Care in Cancer*, **18**, 509–522.

25 Fox, L.P. (2007) Nail toxicity associated with epidermal growth factor receptor inhibitor therapy. *Journal of the American Academy of Dermatology*, **56**, 460–465.

26 Baran, R. (2004) A nail psoriasis severity index. *British Journal of Dermatology*, **150**, 568–569.

27 Suh, K.Y., Kindler, H.L., Medenica, M. & Lacouture, M. (2006) Doxycycline for the treatment of paronychia induced by the EGFRI cetuximab. *British Journal of Dermatology*, **154**, 191–192.

28 Geyer, C.E., Forster, J., Lindquist, D. *et al.* (2006) Lapatinib plus capecitabine for HER2-positive advanced breast cancer. *New England Journal of Medicine*, **355**, 2733–2743.

29 Scotté, F., Tourani, J.M., Banu, E. *et al.* (2005) Multicenter study of frozen glove to prevent docetaxel-induced onycholysis and cutaneous toxicity of the hand. *Journal of Clinical Oncology*, **23**, 4424–4429.

12 Pruritus

Tejesh Patel[1] and Gil Yosipovitch[2]

[1]Department of Dermatology, University of Tennessee Health Science Center, Memphis, TN, USA
[2]Department of Dermatology, Temple University School of Medicine, Philadelphia, PA, USA

Introduction

Pruritus is defined as an unpleasant sensation that leads to a desire to scratch. This distressing symptom is not only common but is often overlooked in cancer patients where other symptoms may take precedence. In patients who may already have a compromised lifestyle, pruritus may have a profound impact on quality of life and is even associated with a poor prognosis in certain malignancies (e.g., Hodgkin disease) [1]. Pruritus has a profound impact on quality of life through disturbances related to sleep, attention, and sexual function. In the oncologic setting, pruritus may be attributable to a primary cutaneous disease, a concurrent systemic or psychiatric disease, therapy, or the cancer itself. In a study of 700 solid and hematologic cancer patients, generalized pruritus was present in 12.9% of patients with dermatologic conditions, even prior to anticancer therapies [2]. A survey of 379 cancer survivors showed that 36% experienced pruritus during their oncologic treatment and, of these, 44% indicated that this adverse event (AE) had a negative impact on their lives [3].

Cutaneous diseases

Although the same pruritic cutaneous diseases can affect both patients with and without malignancy, certain diseases may be more prevalent in the former. Xerosis (dry skin) is the most common cause of pruritus in cancer patients [4]. Factors that may lead to xerosis in the oncologic setting include cachexia, radiation therapy, and chemotherapy (Table 12.1). Notably, infectious etiologies of pruritus may be more common in patients with cancer, especially if they are immunosuppressed or within institutionalized care settings. Pruritus may also occur as part of a primary pruritic cutaneous disease associated with malignancy such as erythroderma, transient acantholytic dermatosis, generalized granuloma annulare, acrokeratosis paraneoplastica, and dermatomyositis [5].

Systemic and psychiatric diseases

A number of systemic diseases can be associated with pruritus such as chronic kidney disease, chronic liver disease, diabetes, thyroid disorders, and iron deficiency anemia. In addition, pruritus may be affected by psychologic stress and depression, conditions that may be particularly prevalent in patients with cancer [6].

Malignancy

Although the underlying pathophysiology is poorly understood, it is important to note that pruritus may be the presenting sign of malignancy. In small studies, underlying malignancy was found to be the cause of generalized pruritus in less than 10% of patients [7]. Although pruritus may be associated with any type of malignancy, hematologic malignancies have the greatest incidence: it can be present in polycythemia vera and Hodgkin disease in up to 50% and 30% of cases, respectively, and patients with Sezary syndrome, leukemia, multiple myeloma, Waldenstrom macroglobulinemia, and cutaneous T-cell lymphomas are also affected [8]. Of note, pruritus has been associated with a poor prognosis in Hodgkin disease [1]. In addition, pruritus may be secondary to a systemic disease caused by the malignancy itself, such as biliary obstruction.

Therapy

In patients with cancer, pruritus may be attributable to chemotherapeutic agents, radiation therapy or other medications, especially those used for palliation of symptoms. Each major class of chemotherapeutic agent includes medications that may lead to pruritus, frequently as a result of xerosis thought to be related to effects on sebaceous and sweat glands (Table 12.2) [9,10].

Dermatologic Principles and Practice in Oncology: Conditions of the Skin, Hair, and Nails in Cancer Patients, First Edition. Edited by Mario E. Lacouture.
© 2014 John Wiley & Sons, Inc. Published 2014 by John Wiley & Sons, Inc.

Table 12.1 Chemotherapeutic agents that cause xerosis [70].

Aldesleukin	Daunorubicin	Nilotinib
Azacitidine	Docetaxel	Nilutamide
Axitinib	Enzalutamide	Panitumumab
Bendamustine	Erlotinib	PEG-Interferon
Bevacizumab	Estramustine	Pertuzumab
Bexarotene	Floxuridine	Pomalidomide
Bleomycin	Fluorouracil	Ponatinib
Brentuximab vedotin	Gefitinib	Sorafenib
Busulfan	GoserelinHydroxyurea	Sunitinib
Cabozantinib	Imatinib	Tamoxifen
Capecitabine	Interferon Alfa	Temsirolimus
Cetuximab	Lapatinib	Vandetanib
Clofarabine	Lenalidomide	Vemurafenib
Dasatinib	Mechlorethamine	

Table 12.2 Chemotherapeutic agents that cause pruritus [70,71].

Aldesleukin	Denileukin	Nilotinib
Abarelix	Docetaxel	Nilutamide
Aldesleukin	Epirubicin	Omacetaxine
Alemtuzumab	Erlotinib	mepesuccinate
Altretamine	Estramustine	Oxaliplatin
Anagrelide	Etoposide	Panitumumab
Axitinib	Floxuridine	Paclitaxel
Azacitidine	Fludarabine	PEG-Interferon
Bendamustine	Fluorouracil	Pemetrexed
Bevacizumab	Gefitinib	Pertuzumab
Bexarotene	Gemcitabine	Pomalidomide
Bicalutamide	Goserelin	Pralatrexate
Bleomycin	Hydroxyurea	Procarbazine
Bortezomib	Ibritumomab	Raltitrexed
Bosutinib	Imatinib	Rituximab
Brentuximab vedotin	Ipilimumab	Sorafenib
Capecitabine	Irinotecan	Streptozocin
Carboplatin	Lenalidomide	Sunitinib
Cetuximab	Letrozole	Tamoxifen
Cetuximab	Leuprolide	Temozolomide
Cisplatin	Levamisole	Temsirolimus
Cladribine	Levoleucovorin	Thioguanine
Clofarabine	Mechlorethamine	ThiotepaTrastuzumab
Cyclophosphamide	Melphalan	Valrubicin
Cytarabine	Mercaptopurine	Vandetanib
Dactinomycin	Melphalan	Vemurafenib
Dasatinib	Methotrexate	Vincristine
Daunorubicin	Mitomycin	Vinorelbine
Decitabine	Mitotane	

Epidermal growth factor receptor (EGFR) inhibitors have a particularly high rate of xerosis and pruritus. This skin toxicity is most likely related to the inhibition of EGFR in the skin, which is crucial for the normal development and physiology of the epidermis. In addition, a recent preliminary study has suggested a role for mast cells in EGFR-induced pruritus [11]. Hypersensitivity reactions to chemotherapeutic agents may induce skin toxicity that includes pruritus, although this is rare. Furthermore, in patients who have undergone bone marrow transplantation, xerosis and pruritus may be associated with cutaneous changes related to graft versus host disease.

Radiation therapy frequently causes xerosis, pruritus, and dry desquamation within the treatment field. The severity of the reaction has been attributed to treatment-related factors, such as beam energy, dose per fraction, treatment duration, use of bolus, treatment site, as well as patient-specific factors such as skin type and diabetes [12]. Xerosis and pruritus typically occur early during radiation therapy and may be the result of an impairment in the skin barrier leading to increased transepidermal water loss [13]. Later during therapy, basal layer stem cells become depleted in the treatment field resulting in the stimulation of nonproliferating basal cells with shortened cell cycles which manifests as cutaneous peeling and is defined as dry desquamation. Moist desquamation results if all stem cells are eradicated from the basal layer, and is characterized by serous oozing and exposure of the dermis [14].

Many medications used in the oncologic setting, whether employed as part of the primary treatment plan or for palliation of symptoms, can lead to pruritus. The most notable such class is the opioid derived analgesics. Interestingly, an imbalance of the endogenous opioidergic system may have a role in the pathophysiology of pruritus. Itch is induced by both μ-opioid receptor agonists and κ-opioid receptor antagonists, while μ-receptor antagonists and κ-receptor agonists can reduce it.

Clinical findings

Chronic pruritus may be the presenting sign of malignancy and may even be a symptom for several years before the tumor becomes clinically detectable. Signs of primary cutaneous disease may be remarkably subtle or nonspecific in patients with malignancy, especially if immunosuppressed. Patients with pruritus in the absence of a primary cutaneous disease frequently present with secondary skin lesions which include excoriations, lichenification, and cutaneous pigmentary alteration (Table 12.3. Lichenification results from continuous rubbing or scratching and consists of well-developed thickened plaques with marked accentuation of skin creases (Figure 12.1). Cutaneous pigmentary alteration is common in patients with darker skin types. Lichenified plaques most commonly occur in areas the patient can easily scratch or rub (i.e., nape of neck, below the elbow, ankle, buttock, and genitalia). The butterfly sign consists of normal-appearing skin in the middle of the back in the shape of spread butterfly wings. Other clues include shiny fingernails which may result from prolonged rubbing. Prurigo nodularis are

Table 12.3 Skin findings secondary to pruritus and scratching.

Lichenification	Thickened plaques with marked accentuation of skin creases
Pigmentary alteration	Especially in patients with darker skin
Prurigo nodularis	Nodules that form as a result of chronic scratching and are often found on extensor aspects of limbs

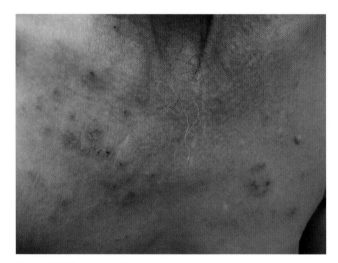

Figure 12.2 Prurigo nodularis.

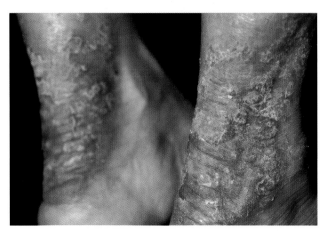

Figure 12.1 Lichenification secondary to chronic rubbing and scratching.

nodules that form as a result of chronic scratching and are often found on extensor aspects of limbs (Figure 12.2).

Specific clinical patterns of pruritus may be associated with certain malignancies. Pruritus with ichthyosis of the extremities or new onset dermatitis may be associated with Hodgkin disease [15–17]. In addition, severe intractable pruritus is frequently seen with lymphoma. Pruritus that develops minutes after contact with water of any temperature with no visible skin rash or urticaria is termed aquagenic pruritus. It is more commonly known to be associated with polycythemia vera; however, several reports demonstrate an association with other lymphoproliferative diseases [15,18]. Specific tumors are sometimes associated with localized itch such as scrotal itch with prostate cancer, itch in the nostrils with brain tumors which infiltrate the floor of the fourth ventricle, vulval itch with cervical cancer, and perianal itch with cancers of the sigmoid colon and rectum [8]. Pruritus may also occur as part of a primary pruritic cutaneous disease associated with malignancy (Table 12.4).

Visual analog scale for pruritus

No itching ——————————————— Very severe itching

The visual analog scale is a continuous measurement instrument that can be used to measure pruritus. It is a horizontal line,

100 mm in length, with descriptive anchors at the two extremes. The patient marks on the line what they feel represents their perception of their pruritus. The visual analog scale score is then determined by measuring in millimeters from the left-hand side.

Management

General principles

If an underlying cause is discovered it should be treated, as pruritus frequently improves when the underlying etiology is addressed. In cancer patients, physical impairments may make application of topical treatments impossible and compliance may become an issue. Comorbid conditions, especially kidney and liver, as well as the frequent polypharmacy in this patient group means that adverse drug reactions are more likely. Management of pruritus in patients with malignancy takes on an individually tailored approach. Some of the treatments discussed are not registered for use in pruritus and should be administered under specialist supervision.

There are a number of general measures that may be useful in the management of pruritus in patients with cancer, irrespective of the underlying cause:
• Regular use of moisturizers or barrier creams, ideally with low pH (e.g., ammonium lactate, urea 5–20%);
• Application of moisturizers immediately following bathing ensures a high retention of moisture;
• Keeping finger nails short;
• Wearing light and loose clothing;
• Using a humidifier at home, especially in winter;
• Restricting time in the shower or bathtub to 15 minutes;
• Shower/bathe in cool or lukewarm water as hot water can be drying;
• Avoid cleansers with a high pH or containing alcohol.

Table 12.4 Common Terminology Criteria for Adverse Events (CTCAE) Version 4.0: grading of pruritus.

Adverse event	Grade 1	Grade 2	Grade 3	Grade 4	Grade 5
Pruritus	Mild or localized; topical intervention indicated	Intense or widespread; intermittent; skin changes from scratching (e.g., edema, papulation, excoriations, lichenification, oozing/crusts); oral intervention indicated; limiting instrumental ADL	Intense or widespread; constant; limiting self-care ADL or sleep; oral corticosteroid or immunosuppressive therapy indicated	–	–

A semi-colon indicates "or" within the description of the grade. A single dash (–) indicates a grade is not available. Instrumental activities of daily living (ADL) refer to preparing meals, shopping for groceries or clothes, using the telephone, managing money, etc. Self-care ADL refer to bathing, dressing and undressing, feeding self, using the toilet, taking medications, and not bedridden. Not all grades are appropriate for all adverse events (AEs). Therefore, some AEs are listed with fewer than five options for grade selection (Grades 1–5).

Table 12.5 Topical treatments.

Drug class	Medication and suggested dose	Notes/adverse events
Emollients and moisturizers	Various including petroleum	Especially useful for xerosis, low pH products may be particularly useful
Salicylic acid	2–6%	Useful in lichen simplex chronicus, may cause stinging
Topical calcineurin inhibitors	Tacrolimus 0.03% and 0.1% ointment Pimecrolimus 1% cream	Particularly useful inflammatory skin dermatoses, no skin atrophy, may experience transient burning and stinging
Topical corticosteroids	Variable	Not directly antipruritic, useful in inflammatory skin dermatoses, risk of skin atrophy and adrenal suppression
Doxepin	5% cream	20–25 % risk of sedation, risk of allergic contact dermatitis
Menthol	1–3 % cream or lotion	Useful in patients who report cooling as an alleviating factor
Capsaicin	0.025–0.1% cream	Particularly useful in neuropathic itch, may experience initial transient burning
Local anesthetics	Pramoxine 1.0–2.5% Lidocaine patch 5% Eutectic mixture of lidocaine 2.5% and prilocaine 2.5% 5% urea + 3% polidocanol (laurylmacrogol)	Both moisturizing and anesthetic properties
Cannabinoids	Creams containing *N*-palmitoylethanolamine	

Patient education is central to the management of pruritus [19]. Identifying and removing aggravating factors is often the initial step in effective treatment for pruritus. Breaking the itch–scratch cycle is critical and patients should be informed of the increased cutaneous inflammation that scratching causes. Simple measures such as keeping fingernails short may help to interrupt this vicious cycle. The sensation of pruritus is often heightened by warmth, thus measures such as tepid showering, light clothing, and use of air conditioning should be undertaken to keep the skin cool where appropriate. Simple topical regimens are preferable wherever possible in order to maximize adherence and avoid potential adverse drug reactions.

Topical treatments
Moisturizers and emollients
Moisturizers and emollients form the cornerstone of pruritus treatment in cancer patients, especially in cases associated with xerosis (Table 12.5). They reduce pruritus through improved barrier function helping to prevent transepidermal water loss and possibly preventing entry of irritants and itch-causing agents. Topical therapies with a low pH may be especially useful in optimizing the skin barrier function through their maintenance of the normal acidic pH of the skin surface. In addition, low pH topical therapies may be of further benefit through their reduction in activity of serine proteases such as mast cell tryptase which is

known to activate protease-activating receptor 2 (PAR2) on skin nerve fibers. This notion stems from recent studies suggesting serine proteases, via PAR2 located on C fiber terminals, may have an important role in mediating pruritus [20,21].

Topical corticosteroids

Topical corticosteroids are not directly antipruritic and exert a beneficial effect on pruritus through a reduction in skin inflammation. Therefore they should only be used to provide relief of itching associated with inflammatory skin diseases. Topical corticosteroids should not be used to treat generalized chronic itch or for prolonged periods. Although higher strengths of corticosteroid have greater efficacies, there is also an increased risk of AEs (e.g., skin atrophy, telangiectasia, and hypothalamus–pituitary axis suppression). Of note, recent data have shown that topical steroids not only reduce radiation dermatitis and the associated pruritus, but may also be preventative [22,23].

Topical immunomodulators

The topical calcineurin inhibitors, tacrolimus and pimecrolimus, have been shown to be effective in reducing pruritus in a number of conditions including graft versus host disease and prurigo nodularis [24]. The antipruritic effects of topical calcineurin inhibitors may be mediated via TRPV1, a member of the transient receptor potential (TRP) family of excitatory ion channels, located on nerve fibers. Although recognized AEs of these agents include transient burning and stinging sensations, they may be particularly useful as sites of radiation as there is no associated risk of skin atrophy. These agents may also be a better option in darkly pigmented individuals, as they are not associated with hypopigmentation that occurs as an AE to topical steroids.

Topical antihistamines

Doxepin, a tricyclic antidepressant, is a potent H1 and H2 antagonist. Doxepin 5% cream has been shown to reduce pruritus significantly in patients with varying conditions including lichen simplex chronicus [25,26]. However, drowsiness, through systemic absorption of doxepin, occurs in approximately 20–25% of patients, which may limit its use, especially in patients with cancer. In order to minimize this AE it should not be used on more than 10% of the body surface area. Other common AE of this treatment include localized cutaneous burning and allergic contact dermatitis [25,26].

Menthol

Menthol, a naturally occurring cyclic terpene alcohol of plant origin, is frequently used as a topical antipruritic at concentrations of 1–3%. It has been shown that menthol elicits the same cool sensation as low temperature through the TRPM8 receptor and cooling the skin and menthol both result in the relief of experimentally induced itch, although the latter is not associated

with a decrease in skin temperature. Of note, patients with cancer who report a reduction in pruritus with cooling may especially benefit from topical therapies containing menthol [27].

Capsaicin

Capsaicin has been reported to have a beneficial effects in chronic localized pruritic disorders, particularly those of neuropathic origin, such as notalgia paresthetica and brachioradial pruritus as well as other pruritic conditions (e.g., prurigo nodularis, aquagenic pruritus, and pruritus associated with chronic kidney disease) [28–32]. The TRPV1 receptor has recently been implicated in the pathogenesis of pruritus and may be the target through which capsaicin exerts its antipruritic effect [33]. A recognized AE is an initial intense transient burning sensation at the application site which may lead to poor adherence.

Topical salicylic acid

Topical salicylic acid, a cyclooxygenase inhibitor, has been shown to reduce pruritus significantly in patients with lichen simplex chronicus, possibly by its inhibitory effects on prostanoids [34,35]. Of note, oral aspirin has been shown to relieve pruritus in polycythemia vera [36].

Local anesthetics

Topical local anesthetics such as pramoxine 1–2.5%, lidocaine 5%, and the eutectic mixture of lidocaine 2.5% and prilocaine 2.5%, have all been shown to have antipruritic properties [37–39]. Pramoxine, a local anesthetic, reduces itch by interfering with transmission of impulses along sensory nerve fibers and has been shown to reduce pruritus in adult hemodialysis patients in double-blinded study [40]. Interestingly, intravenous lidocaine has recently been reported to ameliorate the severity of pruritus in a case series of patients with chronic cholestatic liver diseases [41]. Polidocanol is a nonionic surfactant with both local anesthetic properties and moisturizing effects.

Topical cannabinoids

The cannabinoid receptor CB2 agonist, N-palmitoylethanolamine, has been incorporated into creams and reduced pruritus reported in patients with lichen simplex, prurigo nodularis, and chronic kidney disease-associated pruritus [42–44].

Systemic treatments
Antihistamines

With the exception of chronic urticaria, antihistamines have little effect on conditions with associated pruritus. Sedating (first generation) antihistamines may have a role via their soporific effects but in patients with cancer caution must be taken not to cause excessive drowsiness given such patients may already be on other sedating medication, and the risk of falls may increase (Table 12.6) [45].

Table 12.6 Systemic treatments.

Drug class	Medication and suggested dose	Notes/adverse events
Antihistamines	Hydroxyzine: start at 25 mg/day and taper up to 75 mg/day as tolerated	No direct effect on pruritus except in urticaria, sedating antihistamines useful through their soporific effects, may cause excessive drowsiness
Antidepressants		Recommend starting at low doses and tapering up to avoid side effects
SNRIs	Mirtazapine 7.5–15 mg PO qhs	Associated with increased weight, appetite and somnolence
SSRIs	Paroxetine 10–40 mg PO qd Fluvoxamine 25–150 mg PO qd	May be useful in pruritus in cancer patients with symptoms of anxiety and depression, associated with increased weight gain, associated with central nervous system (e.g., drowsiness) and gastrointestinal (e.g., nausea and vomiting) side effects
µ-opioid receptor antagonists	Naltrexone 25–50 mg PO qd	May reverse effects of analgesia, may cause nausea, vomiting and drowsiness, recommend use under specialist supervision
κ-opioid receptor agonists	Butorphanol 1–4 mg intranasally qd	Useful in nocturnal and intractable pruritus, may cause nausea and vomiting as well as drowsiness, recommend use under specialist supervision
	Nalfurafine 2.5–5 µg PO qd	May cause insomnia, recommend use under specialist supervision
Neuroleptics	Gabapentin 100–2400 mg/day PO in three divided doses	Useful in neuropathic pruritus, start at low doses and taper up, may cause drowsiness, weight gain and leg swelling, avoid in patients with cholestasis
	Pregablin 25–150 mg/day PO in two divided doses	Start at low doses and taper up in the elderly, should not be stopped abruptly due to the risk of withdrawal symptoms
Substance P antagonist	Aprepitan 80 mg PO qd	Benefical in pruritus associated with the Sézary syndrome, expensive
Thalidomide	100 mg PO qd	Useful for patients with pruritus in multiple myeloma and lymphoproliferative disease, teratogenic, peripheral neuropathy, drowsiness
Aspirin	300 mg qd	Useful in pruritus associated with polycythemia vera only

PO, orally (per os); qhs, every night at bedtime; qd, every day; SNRI, selective neuroepinephrine reuptake inhibitor.

Antidepressants

The selective neuroepinephrine reuptake inhibitor, mirtazapine, has been reported to relieve itch in patients with advanced cancer, leukemia, and lymphoma (including cutaneous lymphoma) as well as chronic kidney disease and cholestasis [46–48]. Mirtazapine may also improve insomnia, anorexia, and depression, all of which are common in cancer patients [47]. In addition, it is associated with weight gain, which can be another advantage in cachectic patients [46].

Selective serotonin reuptake inhibitors (SSRIs) may also have antipruritic effects. The SSRI paroxetine has been shown to reduce pruritus in patients with lymphoma and solid carcinoma as well as reduce aquagenic pruritus from polycythaemia vera and cholestatic pruritus due to gastrointestinal malignancy [49–51]. The SSRI fluvoxamine has also been shown to reduce pruritus in patients with lymphoma and solid carcinoma. The associated weight gain with these agents may be beneficial in cachectic patients. On the other hand, central nervous system (e.g., drowsiness) and gastrointestinal (e.g., nausea and vomiting) AEs may limit the use of these agents in cancer patients.

Although the antipruritic mechanism of antidepressants is unclear, medications interfering with neuronal reuptake of neurotransmitters such as serotonin and norepinephrine may act through the cerebral cortex to reduce the perception of pruritus [52]. Antidepressants may be particularly useful in patients with malignancy who have symptoms of anxiety and depression. Of note, it may be prudent to start with lower doses of antidepressants in patients with cancer and then taper up cautiously to avoid the significant AEs associated with these medications.

Opioid agonists and antagonists

An imbalance of the endogenous opioidergic system may have a role in the pathophysiology of pruritus with µ-receptor antagonists and κ-receptor agonists leading to a reduction in pruritus. Studies have shown antipruritic effects of µ-opioid receptor antagonists such as naltrexone (in patients with cholestasis, end-stage renal disease, burns, and atopic dermatitis) and nalmefene (in patients with cholestasis, atopic dermatitis, and urticaria) [53–57]. The κ-opioid receptor agonists butorphanol and nalfurafine appear to have an antipruritic effect in patients with chronic intractable itch including lymphoma and chronic kidney disease, respectively [58,59]. Importantly, opioid antagonists may be of limited value in patients with cancer as they may reverse analgesic effects used in cancer-associated pain. Because of the potential AEs associated with opioid agonists and antagonists, treatment is advised under specialist supervision and at lower initial doses, especially in patients with malignancy.

Neuroleptics

The neuroleptics gabapentin and pregabalin are structural analogs of the neurotransmitter γ-aminobutyric acid (GABA). The exact mechanisms of their antipruritic effects are not clear but may be related inhibition of central itch pathways. Neuroleptics may be particularly useful in cancer patients for neuropathic pruritus such as brachioradial pruritus, postherpetic neuralgia, and nostalgia paresthetica [6,54,60]. Gabapentin has been shown to reduce pruritus in patients with lymphoma as well as chronic kidney disease but actually worsened pruritus in patients with cholestasis [48,61]. Of note, it has been suggested that using a lower dose of gabapentin with slow upward titration may reduce the risk of gabapentin-induced neurotoxicity and/or coma in patients with reduced renal function, a problem that may be more prevalent in the patients with cancer [62]. Additionally, treatment with pregabalin should not be stopped abruptly because of the risk of withdrawal symptoms [63]. Pregabalin has also been found to be effective in the management of pruritus induced by the EGFR, cetuximab, in a case report [64].

Substance P antagonist

Aprepitant, an oral antiemetic drug that antagonizes the effect of substance P on neurokinin type 1 receptor, has recently been shown to be effective against pruritus associated with the Sézary syndrome in a case series of three patients [65]. A recent study in patients with therapy-resistant chronic itch showed a 80% response rate to 1 week of therapy with aprepitant [66]. Aprepitant has also been reported to be effective in the management of pruritus induced by the EGFR inhibitor, erlotinib, in two patients[67]. A major drawback for its current use in the United States is that it is expensive.

Thalidomide

The antipruritic activity of thalidomide could be related to several mechanisms, including inhibition of tumor necrosis factor α (TNF-α) synthesis, CNS and PNS depression. The beneficial effects are seen after approximately 2–3 weeks. The major AEs with thalidomide are peripheral neuropathy and its high teratogenic effect that requires mandatory monitoring in women of reproductive potential. In the past 5 years, thalidomide became an important part of therapy for hematologic malignancies including myeloma, lymphoma, and solid tumors. Interestingly, the less neurotoxic derivative of thalidomide, lenalidomide, which has been recently approved, has been reported to induce pruritus [68].

Physical treatments

Phototherapy

Ultraviolet A (UVA), broadband ultraviolet B (BB-UVB) and narrowband UVB (NB-UVB) based phototherapy has been used for over three decades to treat various pruritic conditions. This treatment option avoids the risk of adverse drug reactions (although the risk of phototoxicity is increased) but may not be feasible in severely ill patients or in patients receiving photosensitizing drugs (e.g., voriconazole, vandetanib, 5-fluorouracil, vinblastine, dacarbazine, EGFR inhibitors, quinonolones, tetracyclines, sulfonamides, isotretinoin, hydrochlorothiazide, or furosemide).

Bio-behavioral therapy

Stress, anxiety and depression are common in cancer patients and are important factors in aggravating chronic itch. Patients with pruritic symptoms were documented to experience a higher psychologic stress than those without pruritic symptoms [69]. Several studies have shown that behavioral therapy for stress reduction reduces itch perception intensity.

Conclusions

Pruritus in patients with malignancy is common and poses a diagnostic and therapeutic challenge. In the oncologic setting, pruritus may be attributable to a primary cutaneous disease, a concurrent systemic or psychiatric disease, therapy, or the cancer itself. Physical limitations, multiple comorbid conditions, and polypharmacy are some aspects that can influence choice of treatment in this patient group. Currently, management of pruritus in patients with malignancy takes an individually tailored approach.

References

1 Gobbi, P.G., Cavalli, C., Gendarini, A. et al. (1985) Reevaluation of prognostic significance of symptoms in Hodgkin's disease. *Cancer*, **56**, 2874–2880.

2 Kilic, A., Gul, U. & Soylu, S. (2007) Skin findings in internal malignant diseases. *International Journal of Dermatology*, **46**, 1055–1060.

3 Gandhi, M., Oishi, K., Zubal, B. & Lacouture, M.E. (2010) Unanticipated toxicities from anticancer therapies: survivors' perspectives. *Supportive Care in Cancer*, **18**, 1461–1468.

4 Dangel, R.B. (1986) Pruritus and cancer. *Oncology Nursing Forum*, **13**, 17–21.

5 Yosipovitch, G. (2010) Chronic pruritus: a paraneoplastic sign. *Dermatologic Therapy*, **23**, 590–596.

6 Yosipovitch, G. & Samuel, L.S. (2008) Neuropathic and psychogenic itch. *Dermatologic Therapy*, **21**, 32–41.

7 Cohen, P.R. (1994) Cutaneous paraneoplastic syndromes. *American Family Physician*, **50**, 1273–1282.

8 Twycross, R., Greaves, M.W., Handwerker, H. *et al.* (2003) Itch: scratching more than the surface. *QJM: Monthly Journal of the Association of Physicians*, **96**, 7–26.

9 Hood, A.F. (1986) Cutaneous side effects of cancer chemotherapy. *Medical Clinics of North America*, **70**, 187–209.

10 Dunagin, W.G. (1982) Clinical toxicity of chemotherapeutic agents: dermatologic toxicity. *Seminars in Oncology*, **9**, 14–22.

11 Gerber, P.A., Buhren, B.A., Cevikbas, F., Bolke, E., Steinhoff, M. & Homey, B. (2010) Preliminary evidence for a role of mast cells in epidermal growth factor receptor inhibitor-induced pruritus. *Journal of the American Academy of Dermatology*, **63**, 163–165.

12 Kumar, S., Juresic, E., Barton, M. & Shafiq, J. (2010) Management of skin toxicity during radiation therapy: a review of the evidence. *Journal of Medical Imaging and Radiation Oncology*, **54**, 264–279.

13 Schmuth, M., Sztankay, A., Weinlich, G. *et al.* (2001) Permeability barrier function of skin exposed to ionizing radiation. *Archives of Dermatology*, **137**, 1019–1023.

14 Harper, J.L., Franklin, L.E., Jenrette, J.M. & Aguero, E.G. (2004) Skin toxicity during breast irradiation: pathophysiology and management. *Southern Medical Journal*, **97**, 989–993.

15 Khalifa, N., Singer, C.R. & Black, A.K. (2002) Aquagenic pruritus in a patient associated with myelodysplasia and T-cell non-Hodgkin's lymphoma. *Journal of the American Academy of Dermatology*, **46**, 144–145.

16 Rubenstein, M. & Duvic, M. (2006) Cutaneous manifestations of Hodgkin's disease. *International Journal of Dermatology*, **45**, 251–256.

17 Wang, H. & Yosipovitch, G. (2010) New insights into the pathophysiology and treatment of chronic itch in patients with end-stage renal disease, chronic liver disease, and lymphoma. *International Journal of Dermatology*, **49**, 1–11.

18 Ratnaval, R.C., Burrows, N.P., Marcus, R.E. & Norris, P.G. (1993) Aquagenic pruritus and acute lymphoblastic leukaemia. *British Journal of Dermatology*, **129**, 348–349.

19 van Os-Medendorp, H., Ros, W.J., Eland-de Kok, P.C. *et al.* (2007) Effectiveness of the nursing programme "Coping with itch": a randomized controlled study in adults with chronic pruritic skin disease. *British Journal of Dermatology*, **156**, 1235–1244.

20 Steinhoff, M., Neisius, U., Ikoma, A. *et al.* (2003) Proteinase-activated receptor-2 mediates itch: a novel pathway for pruritus in human skin. *Journal of Neuroscience*, **23**, 6176–6180.

21 Yosipovitch, G. & Papoiu, A.D. (2008) What causes itch in atopic dermatitis? *Current Allergy and Asthma Reports*, **8**, 306–311.

22 Miller, R.C., Schwartz, D.J., Sloan, J.A. *et al.* (2011) Mometasone furoate effect on acute skin toxicity in breast cancer patients receiving radiotherapy: a phase III double-blind, randomized trial from the North Central Cancer Treatment Group N06C4. *International Journal of Radiation Oncology, Biology, Physics*, **79**, 1460–1466.

23 Neben-Wittich, M.A., Atherton, P.J., Schwartz, D.J. *et al.* (2011) Comparison of provider-assessed and patient-reported outcome measures of acute skin toxicity during a phase III trial of mometasone cream versus placebo during breast radiotherapy: the North Central Cancer Treatment Group (N06C4). *International Journal of Radiation Oncology, Biology, Physics*, **81**, 397–402.

24 Stander, S., Schurmeyer-Horst, F., Luger, T.A. & Weisshaar, E. (2006) Treatment of pruritic diseases with topical calcineurin inhibitors. *Journal of Therapeutics and Clinical Risk Management*, **2**, 213–218.

25 Drake, L.A., Fallon, J.D. & Sober, A. (1994) Relief of pruritus in patients with atopic dermatitis after treatment with topical doxepin cream. The Doxepin Study Group. *Journal of the American Academy of Dermatology*, **31**, 613–616.

26 Drake, L.A. & Millikan, L.E. (1995) The antipruritic effect of 5% doxepin cream in patients with eczematous dermatitis. Doxepin Study Group. *Archives of Dermatology*, **131**, 1403–1408.

27 Patel, T., Ishiuji, Y. & Yosipovitch, G. (2007) Menthol: a refreshing look at this ancient compound. *Journal of the American Academy of Dermatology*, **57**, 873–878.

28 Stander, S., Luger, T. & Metze, D. (2001) Treatment of prurigo nodularis with topical capsaicin. *Journal of the American Academy of Dermatology*, **44**, 471–478.

29 Leibsohn, E. (1992) Treatment of notalgia paresthetica with capsaicin. *Cutis; Cutaneous Medicine for the Practitioner*, **49**, 335–336.

30 Breneman, D.L., Cardone, J.S., Blumsack, R.F., Lather, R.M., Searle, E.A. & Pollack, V.E. (1992) Topical capsaicin for treatment of hemodialysis-related pruritus. *Journal of the American Academy of Dermatology*, **26**, 91–94.

31 Goodless, D.R. & Eaglstein, W.H. (1993) Brachioradial pruritus: treatment with topical capsaicin. *Journal of the American Academy of Dermatology*, **29**, 783–784.

32 Lotti, T., Teofoli, P. & Tsampau, D. (1994) Treatment of aquagenic pruritus with topical capsaicin cream. *Journal of the American Academy of Dermatology*, **30**, 232–235.

33 Imamachi, N., Park, G.H., Lee, H. *et al.* (2009) TRPV1-expressing primary afferents generate behavioral responses to pruritogens via multiple mechanisms. *Proceedings of the National Academy of Sciences of the United States of America*, **106**, 11330–11335.

34 Yosipovitch, G., Sugeng, M.W., Chan, Y.H., Goon, A., Ngim, S. & Goh, C.L. (2001) The effect of topically applied aspirin on localized circumscribed neurodermatitis. *Journal of the American Academy of Dermatology*, **45**, 910–913.

35 Andoh, T., Nishikawa, Y., Yamaguchi-Miyamoto, T., Nojima, H., Narumiya, S. & Kuraishi, Y. (2007) Thromboxane A2 induces itch-associated responses through TP receptors in the skin in mice. *Journal of Investigative Dermatology*, **127**, 2042–2047.

36 Jackson, N., Burt, D., Crocker, J. & Boughton, B. (1987) Skin mast cells in polycythaemia vera: relationship to the pathogenesis and treatment of pruritus. *British Journal of Dermatology*, **116**, 21–29.

37 Yosipovitch, G. & Maibach, H.I. (1997) Effect of topical pramoxine on experimentally induced pruritus in humans. *Journal of the American Academy of Dermatology*, **37**, 278–280.

38 Shuttleworth, D., Hill, S., Marks, R. & Connelly, D.M. (1988) Relief of experimentally induced pruritus with a novel eutectic mixture of local anaesthetic agents. *British Journal of Dermatology*, **119**, 535–540.

39 Sandroni, P. (2002) Central neuropathic itch: a new treatment option? *Neurology*, **59**, 778–779.

40 Young, T.A., Patel, T.S., Camacho, F. *et al.* (2009) A pramoxine-based anti-itch lotion is more effective than a control lotion for the treatment of uremic pruritus in adult hemodialysis patients. *Journal of Dermatological Treatment*, **20**, 76–81.

41 Villamil, A.G., Bandi, J.C., Galdame, O.A., Gerona, S. & Gadano, A.C. (2005) Efficacy of lidocaine in the treatment of pruritus in patients with chronic cholestatic liver diseases. *American Journal of Medicine*, **118**, 1160–1163.

42 Szepietowski, J.C., Szepietowski, T. & Reich, A. (2005) Efficacy and tolerance of the cream containing structured physiological lipids with

endocannabinoids in the treatment of uremic pruritus: a preliminary study. *Acta Dermatovenerologica Croatica*, **13**, 97–103.

43 Eberlein, B., Eicke, C., Reinhardt, H.W. & Ring, J. (2008) Adjuvant treatment of atopic eczema: assessment of an emollient containing N-palmitoylethanolamine (ATOPA study). *Journal of the European Academy of Dermatology and Venereology*, **22**, 73–82.

44 Stander, S., Reinhardt, H.W. & Luger, T.A. (2006) [Topical cannabinoid agonists. An effective new possibility for treating chronic pruritus]. *Der Hautarzt; Zeitschrift fur Dermatologie, Venerologie, Und Verwandte Gebiete*, **57**, 801–807.

45 Patel, T., Ishiuji, Y. & Yosipovitch, G. (2007) Nocturnal itch: why do we itch at night? *Acta Dermato-Venereologica*, **87**, 295–298.

46 Davis, M.P., Frandsen, J.L., Walsh, D., Andresen, S. & Taylor, S. (2003) Mirtazapine for pruritus. *Journal of Pain and Symptom Management*, **25**, 288–291.

47 Hundley, J.L. & Yosipovitch, G. (2004) Mirtazapine for reducing nocturnal itch in patients with chronic pruritus: a pilot study. *Journal of the American Academy of Dermatology*, **50**, 889–891.

48 Demierre, M.F. & Taverna, J. (2006) Mirtazapine and gabapentin for reducing pruritus in cutaneous T-cell lymphoma. *Journal of the American Academy of Dermatology*, **55**, 543–544.

49 Kumler, T., Hedlund, D., Hast, R. & Hasselbalch, H.C. (2008) [Aquagenic pruritus from polycythaemia vera–treatment with paroxetine, a selective serotonin reuptake inhibitor]. *Ugeskrift for Laeger*, **170**, 2981.

50 Stander, S., Bockenholt, B., Schurmeyer-Horst, F. *et al.* (2009) Treatment of chronic pruritus with the selective serotonin re-uptake inhibitors paroxetine and fluvoxamine: results of an open-labelled, two-arm proof-of-concept study. *Acta Dermato-Venereologica*, **89**, 45–51.

51 Unotoro, J., Nonaka, E., Takita, N. & Suzuki, Y. (2010) [Paroxetine treatment of 3 cases of cholestatic pruritus due to gastrointestinal malignancy]. *Nippon Shokakibyo Gakkai Zasshi the Japanese Journal of Gastro-Enterology*, **107**, 257–262.

52 Stander, S., Weisshaar, E. & Luger, T.A. (2008) Neurophysiological and neurochemical basis of modern pruritus treatment. *Experimental Dermatology*, **17**, 161–169.

53 Bergasa, N.V., Alling, D.W., Talbot, T.L., Wells, M.C. & Jones, E.A. (1999) Oral nalmefene therapy reduces scratching activity due to the pruritus of cholestasis: a controlled study. *Journal of the American Academy of Dermatology*, **41**, 431–434.

54 Monroe, E.W. (1989) Efficacy and safety of nalmefene in patients with severe pruritus caused by chronic urticaria and atopic dermatitis. *Journal of the American Academy of Dermatology*, **21**, 135–136.

55 Patel, T. & Yosipovitch, G. (2010) Therapy of pruritus. *Expert Opinion on Pharmacotherapy*, **11**, 1673–1682.

56 Peer, G., Kivity, S., Agami, O., Fireman, E., Silverberg, D. & Blum, M. (1996) Iaina A: randomised crossover trial of naltrexone in uraemic pruritus. *Lancet*, **348**, 1552–1554.

57 Phan, N.Q., Bernhard, J.D., Luger, T.A. & Stander, S. (2010) Antipruritic treatment with systemic mu-opioid receptor antagonists: a review. *Journal of the American Academy of Dermatology*, **63**, 680–688.

58 Dawn, A.G. & Yosipovitch, G. (2006) Butorphanol for treatment of intractable pruritus. *Journal of the American Academy of Dermatology*, **54**, 527–531.

59 Kumagai, H., Ebata, T., Takamori, K., Muramatsu, T., Nakamoto, H. & Suzuki, H. (2010) Effect of a novel kappa-receptor agonist, nalfurafine hydrochloride, on severe itch in 337 haemodialysis patients: a phase III, randomized, double-blind, placebo-controlled study. *Nephrology, Dialysis, Transplantation*, **25**, 1251–1257.

60 Wood, G.J., Akiyama, T., Carstens, E., Oaklander, A.L. & Yosipovitch, G. (2009) An insatiable itch. *Journal of Pain*, **10**, 792–797.

61 Bergasa, N.V., McGee, M., Ginsburg, I.H. & Engler, D. (2006) Gabapentin in patients with the pruritus of cholestasis: a double-blind, randomized, placebo-controlled trial. *Hepatology (Baltimore, Md.)*, **44**, 1317–1323.

62 Manenti, L. & Vaglio, A. (2005) Gabapentin for uraemic pruritus. *Nephrology, Dialysis, Transplantation*, **20**, 1278–1279.

63 Ehrchen, J. & Stander, S. (2008) Pregabalin in the treatment of chronic pruritus. *Journal of the American Academy of Dermatology*, **58**, S36–S37.

64 Porzio, G., Aielli, F., Verna, L. *et al.* (2006) Efficacy of pregabalin in the management of cetuximab-related itch. *Journal of Pain and Symptom Management*, **32**, 397–398.

65 Duval, A. & Dubertret, L. (2009) Aprepitant as an antipruritic agent? *New England Journal of Medicine*, **361**, 1415–1416.

66 Stander, S., Siepmann, D., Herrgott, I., Sunderkotter, C. & Luger, T.A. (2010) Targeting the neurokinin receptor 1 with aprepitant: a novel antipruritic strategy. *PLoS ONE*, **5**, e10968.

67 Vincenzi, B., Tonini, G. & Santini, D. (2010) Aprepitant for erlotinib-induced pruritus. *New England Journal of Medicine*, **363**, 397–398.

68 Bonkowski, J.J., Vermeulen, L.C. & Kolesar, J.M. (2010) The clinical utility of lenalidomide in multiple myeloma and myelodysplastic syndromes. *Journal of Oncology Pharmacy Practice*, **16**, 223–232.

69 Yamamoto, Y., Yamazaki, S., Hayashino, Y. *et al.* (2009) Association between frequency of pruritic symptoms and perceived psychological stress: a Japanese population-based study. *Archives of Dermatology*, **145**, 1384–1388.

70 Litt's DERM Database. Available from: www.drugeruptiondata.com (accessed 14 April 2013).

71 Fischer, A., Rosen, A.C., Ensslin, C.J., Wu, S. & Lacouture, M.E. (2013) Pruritus to anticancer agents targeting the EGFR, BRAF, and CTLA-4. *Dermatologic Therapy*, **26**(2), 135–148.

13 Management Options for Hot Flashes in Cancer Patients

Amanda R. Moraska[1] and Charles L. Loprinzi[2]

[1]Anesthesiology Institute, Cleveland Clinic, Cleveland, OH, USA
[2]Mayo Clinic, Rochester, MN, USA

Introduction

Hot flashes are a common and distressing symptom experienced by nearly three-quarters of women during menopause [1,2]. They are usually described as intense heat starting in the chest, neck, and face; often accompanied by flushing, profuse sweating, red blotching, palpitations, and anxiety [1,3]. Episodes typically last 2–4 minutes but vary greatly in frequency, from several times a day to monthly, beginning before menopause and continuing for 5 years or more [4]. Many studies indicate that hot flashes have significant detrimental effects on work, recreation, sleep, and overall perception of quality of life [4].

In addition to affecting natural menopausal women, hot flashes are also a significant problem in some cancer patients. Premenopausal women with breast cancer and other gynecologic malignancies commonly undergo chemotherapy, radiation, oophorectomy, or anti-estrogenic therapy, precipitating an abrupt onset of menopausal symptoms such as hot flashes [5,6]. Unfortunately, these tend to be more frequent and severe than those reported with natural menopause [7,8]. Discontinuation of estrogen replacement therapy and use of aromatase inhibitors and tamoxifen, choice drugs for treatment of breast cancer, are also associated with an increased occurrence of hot flashes [5,9].

Additionally, hot flashes are problematic for many men with prostate cancer, affecting nearly 75% of men receiving androgen deprivation therapy [10,11]. More specifically, hot flashes have been reported in 70% of men after orchiectomy, 80% of those receiving neoadjuvant hormonal therapy before prostatectomy, and 70–80% of men who receive long-term androgen deprivation therapy [10,12,13]. In addition to the physical symptoms attributed to hot flashes, men describe accompanying feelings of anxiety, irritability, and being out of control, significantly affecting their perception of quality of life [14].

There are a number of options, nonpharmacologic and pharmacologic, available for treatment of hot flashes, each with varying degrees of efficacy. This chapter outlines evidence for and against several of these interventions.

Grading of hot flashes

In oncology clinical trials, the severity of hot flashes is sometimes graded using the Common Terminology Criteria for Adverse Events (CTCAE) Version 4.0 (Table 13.1). However, in clinical trials investigating agents for the management of hot flashes, a score reported by each individual patient is usually used, which is based on frequency and severity. In addition to the number of events, one point is given for every mild hot flash, two for a moderate hot flash, three for a severe hot flash, and four for a very severe hot flash (Figure 13.1). These are all added together to make the hot flash score. Patients can not only accurately report the level of hot flash activity, but they do it in a remarkably complete and consistent manner (Figure 13.2) [15].

Treatment of hot flashes

Pharmacologic interventions
Hormonal therapy
Estrogen
Estrogen, a primary hot flash treatment for many years, continues to be the most effective option, reducing hot flash symptoms by 80–90% [16–18]. However, use of estrogen is controversial because of long-term health risks, including coronary artery disease, stroke, pulmonary embolism, venous thrombosis, and invasive breast cancer [18,19]. Thus, estrogen is contraindicated in patients with a history of these events, and avoided in those with breast cancer.

Table 13.1 Common Terminology Criteria for Adverse Events (CTCAE) Version 4.0: vascular disorders, a disorder characterized by an uncomfortable and temporary sensation of intense body warmth, flushing, sometimes accompanied by sweating upon cooling.

Adverse event	Grade				
	1	2	3	4	5
Hot flashes	Mild symptoms; intervention not indicated	Moderate symptoms; limiting instrumental ADL	Severe symptoms; limiting self-care ADL	–	–

AE, adverse event.
A semi-colon indicates "or" within the description of the grade. A single dash (–) indicates a grade is not available. Instrumental ADL refer to preparing meals, shopping for groceries or clothes, using the telephone, managing money, etc. Self-care ADL refer to bathing, dressing and undressing, feeding self, using the toilet, taking medications, and not bedridden. Not all grades are appropriate for all AEs.

Some studies suggest certain subsets of breast cancer survivors may be safely treated with estrogen [6,20]. However, a randomized trial of estrogen in breast cancer survivors was stopped when increased recurrence was observed [21]. Thus, most physicians avoid estrogen in these patients [18,22], and use the lowest possible dose for the shortest effective length of time in all patients [18,23].

Recent investigations regarding short-term and low-dose estrogen have shown promise. In one randomized double-blinded trial, micro-dose transdermal estrogen patches showed significant reductions in hot flashes compared with placebo [24]. Another study demonstrated similar results with low-dose estradiol gel [25]. Additionally, research suggests a decreased risk of serious complications with low-dose estrogen [23,24].

Estrogen therapy in men with hot flashes has also shown significant efficacy. A randomized double-blind placebo-controlled trial demonstrated approximately 75% reduction in hot flashes with estrogen [26]. However, estrogen has been avoided in these patients because of undesirable adverse events (AEs), including breast tenderness and enlargement.

Progesterone analogs
Since the 1970s, progesterone analogs have showed potential for hot flash control. One study of breast and prostate cancer survivors found megestrol acetate (40 mg/day) effectively reduced hot flashes 75–80%, compared with 20–25% with placebo [27]. After 3 years, one-third of patients continued use of megestrol acetate for hot flash relief [28]. More recently, a study demonstrated that 20 mg/day megestrol acetate is just as effective as 40 mg/day [29].

Intramuscular depomedroxyprogesterone acetate (DMPA) also showed efficacy in several trials [30–32]. A recent study compared DMPA with megestrol acetate in postmenopausal women, finding similar efficacy in each group, with an 80–90% average hot flash reduction [33]. It also suggested compliance benefits with DMPA injections versus oral daily megestrol acetate. An observational study of DMPA in breast cancer survivors found hot flashes decreased by 90% [34]. Additionally, a randomized trial demonstrated equivalent efficacy for hot flash reduction between DMPA and conjugated-equine estrogen [35].

Progesterone creams have also been studied, with controversial results. One trial demonstrated an 83% decrease in hot flashes with the cream, compared with 19% with placebo [36]. However, a 2009 study showed no statistically significant benefit [37].

Use of progestational agents in breast or prostate cancer survivors is controversial. Some evidence indicates that they are active against breast cancer [38], while *in vitro* studies show they increase epithelial cell proliferation, which may stimulate tumor growth [39]. However, an epidemiologic study could not find an increased breast cancer risk in women who used progesterone alone [40]. For men with prostate cancer, megestrol treatment was found to cause undesirable increases in prostate-specific antigen levels [41,42]. Given these data, it is important that patients with a history of breast or prostate cancer be counseled about potential risks before beginning treatment.

Nonhormonal therapies
The potential for serious AEs described with hormonal therapies, particularly in patients with a history of breast or prostate cancer, has sparked investigations into nonhormonal therapeutic options for hot flash management.

Newer antidepressants
During the 1990s, reductions in hot flash severity and frequency were noted amongst women after they started some antidepressants. A pooled analysis examined published randomized trials before December 2007 that evaluated newer antidepressants for hot flashes [43]. This supported that select antidepressants effectively decrease hot flashes.

Venlafaxine
Venlafaxine acts by selectively inhibiting serotonin, norepinephrine, and dopamine reuptake. It was first studied as an agent for hot flash treatment in a 1998 pilot trial involving breast and prostate cancer survivors. Patients reported a 55% decrease in hot flashes after taking 12.5 mg venlafaxine twice daily for 4 weeks [44]. Patients also reported improvements in associated symptoms, such as fatigue, sweating, and difficulty sleeping. At study completion, 64% of study patients elected to continue venlafaxine.

Following the success of this pilot study, a randomized trial compared placebo with venlafaxine [45]. After 4 weeks, there was a 27%, 37%, 61%, and 61% decrease in hot flashes in the placebo, 37.5, 75, and 150 mg/day venlafaxine arms, respectively. Patients taking venlafaxine reported improvements in depression scores and overall quality of life. Although the 75 mg/day dose was superior to 37.5 mg/day, there was no further benefit with

FIRST STUDY WEEK (BASELINE)

DAILY PATIENT QUESTIONNAIRE: DOUBLE-BLIND PHASE

No tablets this week

Date week started: __ __ / __ __ / __ __ __ __
m m d d y y y y

	Day 1	Day 2	Day 3	Day 4	Day 5	Day 6	Day 7**
Number of today's hot flashes that were mild, moderate, severe, or very severe?	__mild __moderate __severe __very severe	__mild __moderate __severe __very severe	__mild __moderate __severe __very severe	__mild __moderate __severe __very severe	__mild __moderate __severe __very severe	__mild __moderate __severe __very severe	__mild __moderate __severe __very severe
Total number of hot flashes today*							

* One day should be considered to be a 24 hour period (i.e. 7:00 a.m. to 7:00 a.m. or midnight to midnight).

Date week stopped: __ __ / __ __ / __ __ __ __
m m d d y y y y

Do you have any of the following symptoms?:

appetite loss	__ no	__ yes	abnormal sweating	__ no	__ yes
sleepiness	__ no	__ yes	constipation	__ no	__ yes
nausea	__ no	__ yes	trouble sleeping	__ no	__ yes
dizziness	__ no	__ yes	nervousness	__ no	__ yes
tiredness (fatigue)	__ no	__ yes	mood changes	__ no	__ yes
dry mouth	__ no	__ yes			
other	__ no	__ yes, please describe ______			

Comments: ____________________

Blood Pressure ______ / ______ Date blood pressure obtained: __ __ / __ __ / __ __ __ __
m m d d y y y y

**Please complete the next 3 pages on Day 7

Figure 13.1 Daily patient hot flash questionnaire used in supportive care trials. From Sloan *et al.* [15]. Reproduced with permission.

150 mg/day. Rather, patients in the 150 mg/day arm experienced increased toxicities including dry mouth, constipation, nausea, and decreased appetite.

At study completion, many women elected to remain on or start venlafaxine for an 8-week continuation study [46]. Results of the continuation study supported longer term venlafaxine efficacy for hot flash relief without additional toxicity. Another randomized placebo-controlled trial confirmed these findings, demonstrating improved hot flash symptoms and quality of life in those women taking 75 mg/day venlafaxine for 12 weeks [47].

More recently, a randomized trial compared venlafaxine with DMPA [48]. After 6 study weeks, patients having received the single DMPA injection reported a 79% decrease in hot flash frequency while those in the venlafaxine group reported a 55% reduction, with no significant difference in toxicities.

Venlafaxine has also been evaluated for hot flash control in men. In a pilot study, men taking 12.5 mg venlafaxine twice daily experienced a 54% reduction in hot flashes without significant toxicities [49]. Another small study found most men taking 37.5 mg/day venlafaxine had at least a 50% reduction in hot flash scores, with 75% of men electing to continue venlafaxine [50].

(a)

PATIENT INFORMATION SHEET

HOT FLASH DEFINITIONS FOR THE FEMALE PATIENT

Please refer to these examples of hot flashes that have been given by cancer survivors in previous studies when describing their hot flash severity. One or more of these descriptions may help to categorize your hot flash as mild, moderate, severe, or very severe.

MILD

    Duration: Lasting less than 5 minutes
    Physical symptoms: Warmth, felt uncomfortable, red face
    Emotional symptoms: Not expected
    Action needed: Usually no action taken

MODERATE

    Duration: Lasting up to 15 minutes
    Physical symptoms: Head, neck, ears, or whole body felt warm; tense, tight muscles; clammy (wet skin;
    a change in heart rate or rhythm (heart speeds up or changes beat); some sweating; dry mouth
    Emotional symptoms: Felt irritated, felt agitated (restless), felt as though energy was drained out, felt
    embarrassed when having a hot flash in front of others, felt tired, felt annoyed
    Action needed: Needed to use a fan, awakened sometimes at night, needed to uncover, took off layers
    of clothing, drank water, opened the windows even when cold outside, wore lighter clothing

SEVERE

    Duration: Lasting up to 20 minutes
    Physical symptoms: Warmth, sometimes described as a raging furnace or burning up; a change in heart
    rate or rhythm (heart speeds up or changes beat); felt faint; headache; severe sweating; weakness, a
    pricking, stinging sensation over skin; chest heaviness
    Emotional symptoms: Embarrassment, anxiety, feelings of having a panic attack
    Action needed: Needed to stop what was being done at that time, usually awakened at night and
    removed covers, needed to remove clothes, opened windows, kept the house a cooler temperature,
    frequently used fans

VERY SEVERE

    Duration: Lasting up to 45 minutes
    Physical symptoms: Boiling heat, rolling sweat, difficulty breathing, felt faint, felt dizzy, feel and/or legs
    cramping, a change in the heart rate or rhythm (heart speeds up or changes beat), felt slightly sick to
    stomach
    Emotional symptoms: Felt distressed, had the urge to escape, had difficulty functioning
    Action needed: Awakened frequently at night, needed to change sheets and pajamas, needed to take a
    cold shower, needed to hold ice on skin

Figure 13.2 Definition of hot flash severity information sheets for: (a) female and (b) male patients. From Sloan *et al.* [15]. Reproduced with permission.

Taking all of these study results in summary, it would appear that although venlafaxine does not offer the same degree of hot flash reduction achieved with hormonal treatments, it is still a viable option to alleviate hot flash related symptoms.

Desvenlafaxine

Desvenlafaxine is a succinate salt of the active metabolite in venlafaxine, and thus has the same mechanism of action [51]. Two published clinical trials support that this drug decreases hot flashes similarly to venlafaxine [52,53].

Paroxetine

Paroxetine is a selective serotonin reuptake inhibitor (SSRI). Two pilot trials supported that this drug decreased hot flashes [54,55]. Following these, two randomized double-blinded trials were performed. One trial investigated 10 and 20 mg/day paroxetine in breast cancer survivors [56]. After 4 weeks, patients in both

paroxetine treatment arms reported significant hot flash reductions (41% and 52%) compared with placebo (14%), with no statistically significant difference between the paroxetine arms. Another trial paralleled these results [57].

Paroxetine has also been investigated as an option for prostate cancer survivors with hot flashes. A pilot study indicated a 50% reduction in hot flash frequency when men started 12.5 mg/day paroxetine increasing it to 37.5 mg/day over 4 weeks [58]. There are no randomized trials to date examining paroxetine for male hot flashes.

Fluoxetine

The efficacy of fluoxetine, another SSRI, for hot flash reduction was examined in an 8-week phase III crossover study [59]. During the first 4-week treatment period, patients on fluoxetine reported a 50% decrease in hot flash score, compared with 36% with

(b)

```
┌─────────────────────────────────────────────────────────────────────────┐
│                                                                           │
│                       PATIENT INFORMATION SHEET                           │
│                                                                           │
│             HOT FLASH DEFINITIONS FOR THE MALE PATIENT                    │
│             ──────────────────────────────────────────                   │
│                                                                           │
│   Please refer to these examples of hot flashes that have been given by   │
│   cancer survivors in previous studies when describing their hot flash    │
│   severity. One or more of these descriptions may help to categorize your │
│   hot flash as mild, moderate, severe, or very severe.                    │
│                                                                           │
│   MILD                                                                     │
│                                                                           │
│       Duration: Lasting less than 3 minutes                               │
│       Physical symptoms: Very light perspiration, generalized warmth, or  │
│       a flushed sensation                                                  │
│       Emotional symptoms: None or rare                                    │
│       Action needed: Usually no action taken                              │
│                                                                           │
│   MODERATE                                                                 │
│                                                                           │
│       Duration: Lasting up to 5 minutes                                   │
│       Physical symptoms: Light-to-moderate perspiration, moderate warmth  │
│       and/or perspiration                                                  │
│       Emotional symptoms: Mild anxiety, some irritability, loss of        │
│       concentration                                                        │
│       Action needed: Needed to use a fan, needed to loosen clothing,      │
│       needed to remove clothing, needed to remove bedding                 │
│                                                                           │
│   SEVERE                                                                   │
│                                                                           │
│       Duration: Lasting up to 10 minutes                                  │
│       Physical symptoms: Described as feeling "hotter" or "very hot",     │
│       heavy perspiration, dizziness, nausea, shortness of breath,         │
│       weakness, extreme discomfort                                        │
│       Emotional symptoms: Moderate anxiety, moderate irritability         │
│       Action needed: Needed to loosen clothing, needed to change          │
│       clothing, needed to change bedding                                  │
│                                                                           │
│   VERY SEVERE                                                              │
│                                                                           │
│       Duration: Lasting up to 30 minutes                                  │
│       Physical symptoms: Described as feeling "very hot", drenching       │
│       perspiration, dizziness, nausea, shortness of breath, weakness,     │
│       chest discomfort, extreme discomfort                                │
│       Emotional symptoms: Severe anxiety, severe irritability,            │
│       restlessness, totally out of control                                │
│       Action needed: Needed to change clothing, needed to towel off,      │
│       needed to change bedding, used wet towels, took a bath or shower,   │
│       needed a rest                                                        │
│                                                                           │
└─────────────────────────────────────────────────────────────────────────┘
```

Figure 13.2 (*Continued*)

placebo. This difference was not statistically significant. However, a crossover analysis did demonstrate a significant improvement in hot flash score with fluoxetine compared with placebo ($p = 0.02$). There was no difference between groups in reported toxicities. Although fluoxetine shows mild improvements in hot flashes it is rarely used for this indication as other antidepressants and therapies appear to work better.

Citalopram

Based on data from two pilot trials supporting decreased hot flashes with citalopram [60,61], a randomized trial divided women into four groups: placebo, versus citalopram 10, 20, or 30 mg/day. Hot flash frequency was significantly reduced in all active treatment arms with a 46%, 43%, and 50% decreases in the 10, 20, and 30 mg/day citalopram groups, respectively, compared with only 20% with placebo [62]. Thus, citalopram can be considered for hot flash treatment.

Sertraline

Based on anecdotal information suggesting efficacy, there have been three double-blinded placebo-controlled clinical trials examining the utility of sertraline for treating hot flashes in women [43]. Despite suggestion that this drug slightly decreases hot flashes, none of these trials revealed statistically significant hot flash reductions.

Other antidepressants

Fewer data exist on the potential of other antidepressants for hot flash management. Mirtazapine enhances central noradrenergic and serotonergic activity. It does this by blocking alpha2 receptors and antagonizing, selectively, 5-HT2 and 5-HT3 receptors. In a pilot study of women with hot flashes and a history of breast cancer or apprehension about estrogen use, 15 or 30 mg mirtazapine taken before bedtime reduced hot flash scores by 53% and 60%, respectively [63]. Patients also reported improved sleep and only minor AEs including decreased appetite and dry mouth.

In contrast, a pilot trial of bupropion, which selectively inhibits reuptake of norepinephrine and dopamine but has no serotonergic activity, showed no benefit for hot flashes over placebo [64]. Similarly, a pilot trial examining desipramine, an older tricyclic antidepressant which works primarily through inhibiting norepinephrine reuptake with only minimal serotoninergic effects [65], did support that this drug could decrease hot flashes either. These two trials support the idea that increased serotonin activity appears to be an important means for antidepressants to decrease hot flashes.

Important interactions: Tamoxifen and newer antidepressants

When considering treatments that are appropriate for hot flashes in cancer patients it is important to consider drug interactions. Tamoxifen is a selective estrogen receptor modulator and appears to be dependent upon metabolism to its active endoxifen form by CYP2D6 [66,67]. It is known that many older SSRIs inhibit CYP2D6, which lowers endoxifen levels and thus efficacy of tamoxifen [68]. Some newer antidepressants such as paroxetine and fluoxetine are strong inhibitors of this enzyme and decrease endoxifen. Venlafaxine is a weaker inhibitor and shows no significant effect on plasma endoxifen levels [66,69]. No clear evidence exists for the effects of citalopram on plasma endoxifen levels, although it appears to not be clinically significant. Given the current knowledge, venlafaxine appears to be the best antidepressant for hot flash relief in patients taking tamoxifen.

Anticonvulsants

Gabapentin

Gabapentin is widely used as an anticonvulsant and for neuropathic pain. Although structurally related to the neurotransmitter γ-aminobutyric acid (GABA), its exact mechanism remains unknown. This drug first came to attention as a possible treatment for hot flashes following a case series of six patients who reported an 89% hot flash reduction while taking gabapentin [70]. Following a positive pilot trial [71], multiple randomized trials evaluated the efficacy of gabapentin. One trial demonstrated significant reductions in hot flash frequency and score, compared with placebo, after 12 weeks of 900 mg/day gabapentin [72]. Another trial, involving breast cancer survivors, yielded similar results, with both 300 and 900 mg/day gabapentin resulting in hot flash improvement compared with placebo [73].

A randomized controlled trial then compared high dose gabapentin, conjugated estrogens, and placebo [74]. Patients were given either 0.625 mg/day conjugated estrogens, placebo, or gabapentin, titrated to 2400 mg/day, for 12 weeks. Women reported 71% and 72% decreases in hot flashes with gabapentin and estrogen, respectively, compared with 54% with placebo. Although the results of this study would imply that high dose gabapentin was comparable to estrogen therapy for hot flashes, each arm had only 20 patients and thus is subject to type 2 error. This study brings to light a dose–response question with gabapentin and hot flash management that needs further investigation.

Gabapentin has also been explored as a nonhormonal option for hot flashes in men. A randomized study divided 214 men into four arms: placebo, versus gabapentin 300, 600, or 900 mg/day [75]. After 4 weeks, only the patients taking 900 mg/day gabapentin had a statistically significant improvement over placebo, similar to results seen in trials of gabapentin for hot flashes in women.

All of these studies support that gabapentin is moderately effective at reducing hot flashes. Additionally, gabapentin is not known to interfere with CYP2D6. Thus, it should be considered as a viable option for alleviating hot flashes, especially in patients taking tamoxifen [43].

Pregabalin

Pregabalin is a newer anticonvulsant, similar to gabapentin. However, its longer half-life made it attractive for hot flash treatment. A pilot trial demonstrated a 65% hot flash reduction with pregabalin [76]. These results were confirmed in a randomized double-blinded trial, which showed significant decreases in hot flashes compared with placebo with 75 or 150 mg pregabalin twice daily [77]. With the results of this study, it appears that pregabalin is an effective option for the treatment of hot flashes.

Clonidine

Clonidine, an α2-adrenergic agonist, was proposed for hot flash treatment in the 1970s [78–80]. It was thought that clonidine increases the threshold for hot flashes by decreasing norepinephrine release [81]. Transdermal clonidine (0.1 mg) was tested in a double-blind trial of breast cancer survivors and found to reduce hot flashes significantly compared with placebo [82]. However, participants experienced significant toxicities, including dry mouth, pruritus, constipation, and drowsiness that outweighed the benefits in many patients.

In another randomized trial, oral clonidine was evaluated in postmenopausal women receiving tamoxifen [83]. Although there was a reduction in hot flashes with clonidine (38%) compared with the placebo (24%), participants again reported significant toxicities. Transdermal clonidine was also evaluated in a randomized double-blind study for hot flashes in post-orchiectomy men and was not found to cause any significant reduction compared with placebo [84]. A 2006 meta-analysis of 10 trials involving clonidine for hot flashes found inconsistent results, with only half demonstrating efficacy [85]. Thus, clonidine is not an often used treatment for hot flash management because of its inconsistency, its significant AE profile, and the availability of other more active drugs.

Complementary agents

Vitamin E

Commonly taken for its antioxidant properties, vitamin E has been recommended in women's health journals since the 1940s to aid in relief of menopausal symptoms [86,87]. The only randomized controlled study to evaluate vitamin E objectively yielded only a little evidence for efficacy in decreasing hot flashes [88]. Thus, vitamin E, at 400 IU twice daily, is an inexpensive option that may decrease hot flashes a little.

Black cohosh

Black cohosh has long been used by American Indians as a remedy for "female ailments" [89]. Several small-scale trials in Europe and the United States reported improved vasomotor symptoms with use of this herb [90–94]. However, several randomized trials failed to show any significant improvement in hot flashes with black cohosh over placebo [95–98].

Phytoestrogens

Following the observation that hot flashes are significantly less common among Asians [99], with a prevalence of only 10–20% compared to 80–90% in the United States [100,101], some hypothesized that this was a result of high phytoestrogens in Asian diets. Phytoestrogens compete for estrogen receptor binding, making them an attractive potential hot flash treatment [102,103]. Many trials have been performed evaluating isoflavones like soy and red clover extract for hot flash relief, with most showing no significant benefit over placebo [85,93,104–107]. However, there are ongoing studies to investigate lignans, like flaxseed, as a therapeutic option [103,108–110].

Dehydroepiandrosterone

Dehydroepiandrosterone (DHEA), a proandrogen, is thought to decrease as women age. Thus, it was proposed that replacement of DHEA might help control hot flashes [111,112]. In a pilot trial, DHEA supplementation in postmenopausal women over 6 months was associated with significantly decreased vasomotor symptoms [113]. More recently, a study demonstrated 50% reduction in hot flash score after 4 weeks of DHEA [112]. This study also reported improved quality of life. These promising results have yet to be investigated in large randomized controlled trials.

Nonpharmacologic interventions

Over the last 20 years, the desire to find effective nonhormonal agents for the treatment of hot flashes fueled investigation of the many pharmacologic options already explored in this chapter. However, it also led to evaluation of several nonpharmacologic approaches to hot flash management.

Acupuncture

Acupuncture, an ancient medicinal tradition in Asia for over 2500 years, has recently been found effective and safe for treatment of chronic pain and chemotherapy-induced nausea [114]. Several pilot studies indicated that acupuncture might also be an effective hot flash treatment, with minimal AEs [115–117]. However, in several randomized, sham-controlled trials, acupuncture has failed to provide evidence of efficacy [118,119]. A recent review of 11 trials, showed no significant benefit for hot flash relief with acupuncture [120]. Thus, it is not recommended for the treatment of hot flashes.

Stellate ganglion block

Stellate ganglion blocks (SGB), commonly used to alleviate pain syndromes and treat vascular insufficiency [121], were reported in a case series to decrease hot flashes markedly [122]. Pilot studies involving breast cancer survivors also demonstrated significant hot flash improvement [123,124]. No studies reported

significant adverse events related to the procedure. Although SGB have yet to be evaluated in large randomized controlled trials, these preliminary studies give promising evidence for their efficacy in hot flash management.

Behavioral therapies

Relaxation techniques

Several relaxation techniques have been evaluated for hot flash treatment. Paced respiration, or slow rhythmic diaphragmatic breathing, has demonstrated some success for vasomotor symptoms in small randomized trials [125,126]. Relaxation training tapes have also been evaluated in breast cancer survivors, finding significant reduction in hot flashes after 1 month of the tapes but no significant difference compared with no intervention after 3 months [127]. Large randomized controlled trials are needed to further delineate the efficacy of these techniques.

Hypnosis

Hypnosis has been useful in management of pain, anxiety, and insomnia [128–131], and effective in reducing anxiety and distress among breast cancer patients [132,133]. A pilot study reported a 59% decrease in hot flash frequency with hypnosis [134]. Recently, a randomized trial found similar results [135]. These positive preliminary data suggest hypnosis as an effective nonpharmacologic therapy for hot flashes, although further randomized controlled trials are needed.

Physical measures

Despite many pharmacologic options for hot flash management, the North American Menopause Society still recommends lifestyle changes as first line therapy [136]. These measures can take many forms including simple techniques to reduce core body temperature such as sipping cold drinks, avoiding alcohol and spicy food, wearing loose clothing, using a fan, and keeping the thermostat cooler [136–138]. Aerobic exercise, although good for overall health, has not been found helpful in randomized trials for hot flashes [139,140].

Conclusions and recommendations

Hot flashes have long been acknowledged as one of the most common and distressing symptoms associated with menopause. However, in recent decades, these problematic vasomotor symptoms have also been observed in breast cancer survivors and men undergoing androgen deprivation for prostate cancer. Treatment of hot flashes in these patients can be particularly challenging as the most effective known therapy, estrogen or hormone replacement, is typically contraindicated. This dilemma sparked the extensive research presented in this chapter, investigating nonhormonal therapeutic options for hot flash control.

Patients with cancer experiencing hot flashes should first be educated on behavioral modifications, such as dressing in layers and having circulating air available. With mild hot flashes, patients may wish to try 400 IU vitamin E twice daily. With moderate to severe hot flashes use of one of the newer antidepressants, such as venlafaxine, paroxetine, or citalopram would be an appropriate option. Alternatively, gabapentin or pregabalin would be reasonable to try. If the initially chosen therapy does not control hot flashes, then trial of an alternative one of these agents would be reasonable. If hot flashes are persistent, then a progesterone analog, either a one-time intramuscular DMPA injection or oral megestrol acetate may be considered. However, the potential risks of progesterone analogs on breast and prostate cancer recurrence should be discussed in detail with the patient. Table 13.2 lists the recommended nonestrogenic agents for treating hot flashes while an algorithm for how to approach hot flash treatment in women is provided as Figure 13.3.

This algorithm could also be used for men undergoing androgen deprivation therapy. Although limited trials exist evaluating potential treatment options for men with hot flashes, a recent editorial suggests more similarities between male and female hot flashes than differences [141].

Table 13.2 Recommended non-estrogenic agents for hot flash management.

	Efficacy for hot flashes	Comments
Antidepressants		
Venlafaxine	Moderate	
Desvenlafaxine	Moderate	
Paroxetine	Moderate	Do not use with tamoxifen
Citalopram	Moderate	
Anticonvulsants		
Gabapentin	Moderate	
Pregabalin	Moderate	
Clonidine	Mild	Often more toxicities than benefit
Vitamin E	Minimal	
Progesterone analogs		
DMPA	Marked	Single intramuscular dose
Megestrol acetate	Marked	

DMPA, depomedroxyprogesterone acetate.

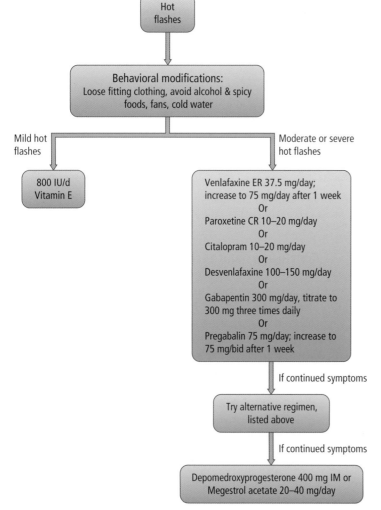

Figure 13.3 Algorithm for the management of hot flashes.

There are now many safe and efficacious nonhormonal therapeutic options for patients suffering from hot flashes, either resulting from natural menopause or cancer treatment. The number of these therapies is likely to grow as new discoveries are made to improve understanding of the pathophysiology of hot flashes.

References

1 Kronenberg, F. (1990) Hot flashes: epidemiology and physiology. *Annals of the New York Academy of Sciences*, **592**, 52–86; discussion 123–133.

2 Couzi, R.J., Helzlsouer, K.J. & Fetting, J.H. (1995) Prevalence of menopausal symptoms among women with a history of breast cancer and attitudes toward estrogen replacement therapy. *Journal of Clinical Oncology*, **13**, 2737–2744.

3 McKinlay, S.M. & Jefferys, M. (1974) The menopausal syndrome. *British Journal of Preventive and Social Medicine*, **28**, 108–115.

4 Daly, E., Gray, A., Barlow, D., McPherson, K., Roche, M. & Vessey, M. (1993) Measuring the impact of menopausal symptoms on quality of life. *British Medical Journal (Clinical Research Ed.)*, **307**, 836–840.

5 Love, R.R., Cameron, L., Connell, B.L. & Leventhal, H. (1991) Symptoms associated with tamoxifen treatment in postmenopausal women. *Archives of Internal Medicine*, **151**, 1842–1847.

6 Loprinzi, C.L., Barton, D.L. & Rhodes, D. (2001) Management of hot flashes in breast-cancer survivors. *Lancet Oncology*, **2**, 199–204.

7 Carpenter, J.S., Andrykowski, M.A., Cordova, M., Cunningham, L., Studts, J., McGrath, P. *et al.* (1998) Hot flashes in postmenopausal women treated for breast carcinoma: prevalence, severity, correlates, management, and relation to quality of life. *Cancer*, **82**, 1682–1691.

8 Carpenter, J.S. & Andrykowski, M.A. (1999) Menopausal symptoms in breast cancer survivors. *Oncology Nursing Forum*, **26**, 1311–1317.

9 Nabholtz, J.M. (2008) Long-term safety of aromatase inhibitors in the treatment of breast cancer. *Therapeutics and Clinical Risk Management*, **4**, 189–204.

10 Schow, D.A., Renfer, L.G., Rozanski, T.A. & Thompson, I.M. (1998) Prevalence of hot flushes during and after neoadjuvant hormonal therapy for localized prostate cancer. *Southern Medical Journal*, **91**, 855–857.

11 Charig, C.R. & Rundle, J.S. (1989) Flushing: long-term side effect of orchiectomy in treatment of prostatic carcinoma. *Urology*, **33**, 175–178.

12 Buchholz, N.P., Mattarelli, G. & Buchholz, M.M. (1994) Post-orchiectomy hot flushes. *European Urology*, **26**, 120–122.

13 Lanfrey, P., Mottet, N., Dagues, F. *et al.* (1996) Hot flashes and hormonal treatment of prostate cancer [in French]. *Progres en Urologie*, **6**, 17–22.

14 Clark, J.A., Wray, N., Brody, B., Ashton, C., Giesler, B. & Watkins, H. (1997) Dimensions of quality of life expressed by men treated for metastatic prostate cancer. *Social Science and Medicine*, **45**, 1299–1309.

15 Sloan, J.A., Loprinzi, C.L., Novotny, P.J., Barton, D.L., Lavasseur, B.I. & Windschitl, H. (2001) Methodologic lessons learned from hot flash studies. *Journal of Clinical Oncology*, **19**, 4280–4290.

16 Notelovitz, M., Lenihan, J.P., McDermott, M., Kerber, I.J., Nanavati, N. & Arce, J. (2000) Initial 17beta-estradiol dose for treating vasomotor symptoms. *Obstetrics and Gynecology*, **95**, 726–731.

17 Maclennan, A.H., Broadbent, J.L., Lester, S. & Moore, V. (2004) Oral oestrogen and combined oestrogen/progestogen therapy versus placebo for hot flushes. *Cochrane Database of Systematic Reviews*, **18** (4), CD002978.

18 Utian, W.H., Archer, D.F., Bachmann, G.A. *et al.* (2008) Estrogen and progestogen use in postmenopausal women: July 2008 position statement of the North American Menopause Society. *Menopause*, **15**, 584–602.

19 Rossouw, J.E., Anderson, G.L., Prentice, R.L. *et al.* (2002) Risks and benefits of estrogen plus progestin in healthy postmenopausal women: principal results From the Women's Health Initiative randomized controlled trial. *Journal of the American Medical Association*, **288**, 321–333.

20 Col, N.F., Hirota, L.K., Orr, R.K., Erban, J.K., Wong, J.B. & Lau, J. (2001) Hormone replacement therapy after breast cancer: a systematic review and quantitative assessment of risk. *Journal of Clinical Oncology*, **19**, 2357–2363.

21 Holmberg, L. & Anderson, H. (2004) HABITS (hormonal replacement therapy after breast cancer–is it safe?), a randomised comparison: trial stopped. *Lancet*, **363**, 453–455.

22 Hoda, D., Perez, D.G. & Loprinzi, C.L. (2003) Hot flashes in breast cancer survivors. *Breast Journal*, **9**, 431–438.

23 NIH (2005) National Institutes of Health State-of-the-Science Conference statement: management of menopause-related symptoms. *Annals of Internal Medicine*, **142**, 1003–1013.

24 Bachmann, G.A., Schaefers, M., Uddin, A. & Utian, W.H. (2007) Lowest effective transdermal 17beta-estradiol dose for relief of hot flushes in postmenopausal women: a randomized controlled trial. *Obstetrics and Gynecology*, **110**, 771–779.

25 Hedrick, R.E., Ackerman, R.T., Koltun, W.D., Halvorsen, M.B. & Lambrecht, L.J. (2009) Transdermal estradiol gel 0.1% for the treatment of vasomotor symptoms in postmenopausal women. *Menopause*, **16**, 132–140.

26 Atala, A., Amin, M. & Harty, J.I. (1992) Diethylstilbestrol in treatment of postorchiectomy vasomotor symptoms and its relationship with serum follicle-stimulating hormone, luteinizing hormone, and testosterone. *Urology*, **39**, 108–110.

27 Loprinzi, C.L., Michalak, J.C., Quella, S.K. *et al.* (1994) Megestrol acetate for the prevention of hot flashes. *New England Journal of Medicine*, **331**, 347–352.

28 Quella, S.K., Loprinzi, C.L., Sloan, J.A. *et al.* (1998) Long term use of megestrol acetate by cancer survivors for the treatment of hot flashes. *Cancer*, **82**, 1784–1788.

29 Goodwin, J.W., Green, S.J., Moinpour, C.M. *et al.* (2008) Phase III randomized placebo-controlled trial of two doses of megestrol acetate as treatment for menopausal symptoms in women with breast cancer: Southwest Oncology Group Study 9626. *Journal of Clinical Oncology*, **26**, 1650–1656.

30 Morrison, J.C., Martin, D.C., Blair, R.A. *et al.* (1980) The use of medroxyprogesterone acetate for relief of climacteric symptoms. *American Journal of Obstetrics and Gynecology*, **138**, 99–104.

31 Bullock, J.L., Massey, F.M. & Gambrell, R.D. Jr (1975) Use of medroxyprogesterone acetate to prevent menopausal symptoms. *Obstetrics and Gynecology*, **46**, 165–168.

32 Lobo, R.A., McCormick, W., Singer, F. & Roy, S. (1984) Depo-medroxyprogesterone acetate compared with conjugated estrogens

for the treatment of postmenopausal women. *Obstetrics and Gynecology*, **63**, 1–5.

33 Bertelli, G., Venturini, M., Del Mastro, L. *et al.* (2002) Intramuscular depot medroxyprogesterone versus oral megestrol for the control of postmenopausal hot flashes in breast cancer patients: a randomized study. *Annals of Oncology*, **13**, 883–888.

34 Barton, D., Loprinzi, C., Quella, S., Sloan, J., Pruthi, S. & Novotny, P. (2002) Depomedroxyprogesterone acetate for hot flashes. *Journal of Pain and Symptom Management*, **24**, 603–607.

35 Prior, J.C., Nielsen, J.D., Hitchcock, C.L., Williams, L.A., Vigna, Y.M. & Dean, C.B. (2007) Medroxyprogesterone and conjugated oestrogen are equivalent for hot flushes: a 1-year randomized double-blind trial following premenopausal ovariectomy. *Clinical Science (London)*, **112**, 517–525.

36 Leonetti, H.B., Longo, S. & Anasti, J.N. (1999) Transdermal progesterone cream for vasomotor symptoms and postmenopausal bone loss. *Obstetrics and Gynecology*, **94**, 225–228.

37 Benster, B., Carey, A., Wadsworth, F., Vashisht, A., Domoney, C. & Studd, J. (2009) A double-blind placebo-controlled study to evaluate the effect of progestelle progesterone cream on postmenopausal women. *Menopause International*, **15**, 63–69.

38 Dixon, A.R., Jackson, L., Chan, S., Haybittle, J. & Blamey, R.W. (1992) A randomised trial of second-line hormone vs single agent chemotherapy in tamoxifen resistant advanced breast cancer. *British Journal of Cancer*, **66**, 402–404.

39 Hofseth, L.J., Raafat, A.M., Osuch, J.R., Pathak, D.R., Slomski, C.A. & Haslam, S.Z. (1999) Hormone replacement therapy with estrogen or estrogen plus medroxyprogesterone acetate is associated with increased epithelial proliferation in the normal postmenopausal breast. *Journal of Clinical Endocrinology and Metabolism*, **84**, 4559–4565.

40 Schairer, C., Lubin, J., Troisi, R. (2000) Menopausal estrogen and estrogen-progestin replacement therapy and breast cancer risk. *Journal of the American Medical Association*, **283**, 485–491.

41 Sartor, O. & Eastham, J.A. (1999) Progressive prostate cancer associated with use of megestrol acetate administered for control of hot flashes. *Southern Medical Journal*, **92**, 415–416.

42 Burch, P.A. & Loprinzi, C.L. (1999) Prostate-specific antigen decline after withdrawal of low-dose megestrol acetate. *Journal of Clinical Oncology*, **17**, 1087–1088.

43 Loprinzi, C.L., Sloan, J., Stearns, V. *et al.* (2009) Newer antidepressants and gabapentin for hot flashes: an individual patient pooled analysis. *Journal of Clinical Oncology*, **27**, 2831–2837.

44 Loprinzi, C.L., Pisansky, T.M., Fonseca, R. *et al.* (1998) Pilot evaluation of venlafaxine hydrochloride for the therapy of hot flashes in cancer survivors. *Journal of Clinical Oncology*, **16**, 2377–2381.

45 Loprinzi, C.L., Kugler, J.W., Sloan, J.A. *et al.* (2000) Venlafaxine in management of hot flashes in survivors of breast cancer: a randomised controlled trial. *Lancet*, **356**, 2059–2063.

46 Barton, D., La, V.B., Loprinzi, C., Novotny, P., Wilwerding, M.B. & Sloan, J. (2002) Venlafaxine for the control of hot flashes: results of a longitudinal continuation study. *Oncology Nursing Forum*, **29**, 33–40.

47 Evans, M.L., Pritts, E., Vittinghoff, E., McClish, K., Morgan, K.S. & Jaffe, R.B. (2005) Management of postmenopausal hot flushes with venlafaxine hydrochloride: a randomized, controlled trial. *Obstetrics and Gynecology*, **105**, 161–166.

48 Loprinzi, C.L., Levitt, R., Barton, D. *et al.* (2006) Phase III comparison of depomedroxyprogesterone acetate to venlafaxine for managing hot flashes: North Central Cancer Treatment Group Trial N99C7. *Journal of Clinical Oncology*, **24**, 1409–1414.

49 Quella, S.K., Loprinzi, C.L., Sloan, J. *et al.* (1999) Pilot evaluation of venlafaxine for the treatment of hot flashes in men undergoing androgen ablation therapy for prostate cancer. *Journal of Urology*, **162**, 98–102.

50 Shafgat, A. (2004) A phase II study of venlafaxine for the treatment of hot flashes in men undergoing androgen deprivation for prostate cancer. 2004 Annual Meeting of the American Society of Clinical Oncology.

51 Deecher, D.C., Alfinito, P.D., Leventhal, L. *et al.* (2007) Alleviation of thermoregulatory dysfunction with the new serotonin and norepinephrine reuptake inhibitor desvenlafaxine succinate in ovariectomized rodent models. *Endocrinology*, **148**, 1376–1383.

52 Speroff, L., Gass, M., Constantine, G., Olivier, S. & Study 315 Investigators. (2008) Efficacy and tolerability of desvenlafaxine succinate treatment for menopausal vasomotor symptoms: a randomized controlled trial. *Obstetrics and Gynecology*, **111**, 77–87.

53 Archer, D.F., Dupont, C.M., Constantine, G.D., Pickar, J.H., Olivier, S. & Study 319 Investigators. (2009) Desvenlafaxine for the treatment of vasomotor symptoms associated with menopause: a double-blind, randomized, placebo-controlled trial of efficacy and safety. *American Journal of Obstetrics and Gynecology*, **200**, 238 e1–238 e10.

54 Stearns, V., Isaacs, C., Rowland, J. *et al.* (2000) A pilot trial assessing the efficacy of paroxetine hydrochloride (Paxil) in controlling hot flashes in breast cancer survivors. *Annals of Oncology*, **11**, 17–22.

55 Weitzner, M.A., Moncello, J., Jacobsen, P.B. & Minton, S. (2002) A pilot trial of paroxetine for the treatment of hot flashes and associated symptoms in women with breast cancer. *Journal of Pain and Symptom Management*, **23**, 337–345.

56 Stearns, V., Slack, R., Greep, N. *et al.* (2005) Paroxetine is an effective treatment for hot flashes: results from a prospective randomized clinical trial. *Journal of Clinical Oncology*, **23**, 6919–6930.

57 Stearns, V., Beebe, K.L., Iyengar, M. & Dube, E. (2003) Paroxetine controlled release in the treatment of menopausal hot flashes: a randomized controlled trial. *Journal of the American Medical Association*, **289**, 2827–2834.

58 Loprinzi, C.L., Barton, D.L., Carpenter, L.A. *et al.* (2004) Pilot evaluation of paroxetine for treating hot flashes in men. *Mayo Clinic Proceedings*, **79**, 1247–1251.

59 Loprinzi, C.L., Sloan, J.A., Perez, E.A. *et al.* (2002) Phase III evaluation of fluoxetine for treatment of hot flashes. *Journal of Clinical Oncology*, **20**, 1578–1583.

60 Barton, D.L., Loprinzi, C.L., Novotny, P. *et al.* (2003) Pilot evaluation of citalopram for the relief of hot flashes. *Journal of Supportive Oncology*, **1**, 47–51.

61 Loprinzi, C.L., Flynn, P.J., Carpenter, L.A. *et al.* (2005) Pilot evaluation of citalopram for the treatment of hot flashes in women with inadequate benefit from venlafaxine. *Journal of Palliative Medicine*, **8**, 924–930.

62 Barton, D.L.B., Sloan, J.A., Stella, P.J. *et al.* (2009) A phase III trial evaluating three doses of citalopram for hot flashes: NCCTG trial N05C9. *Journal of Clinical Oncology*, **26**, abstract 9538.

63 Perez, D.G., Loprinzi, C.L., Barton, D.L. *et al.* (2004) Pilot evaluation of mirtazapine for the treatment of hot flashes. *Journal of Supportive Oncology*, **2**, 50–56.

64 Stahl, S.M., Pradko, J.F., Haight, B.R., Modell, J.G., Rockett, C.B. & Learned-Coughlin, S. (2004) A review of the neuropharmacology of bupropion, a dual norepinephrine and dopamine reuptake inhibitor. *Primary Care Companion to the Journal of Clinical Psychiatry*, **6**, 159–166.

65 Barton, D.L., Loprinzi, C.L., Atherton, P. *et al.* (2007) Phase II evaluation of desipramine for the treatment of hot flashes. *Supportive Cancer Therapy*, **4**, 219–224.

66 Jin, Y., Desta, Z., Stearns, V. *et al.* (2005) CYP2D6 genotype, antidepressant use, and tamoxifen metabolism during adjuvant breast cancer treatment. *Journal of the National Cancer Institute*, **97**, 30–39.

67 Dehal, S.S. & Kupfer, D. (1997) CYP2D6 catalyzes tamoxifen 4-hydroxylation in human liver. *Cancer Research*, **57**, 3402–3406.

68 Stearns, V., Johnson, M.D., Rae, J.M. *et al.* (2003) Active tamoxifen metabolite plasma concentrations after coadministration of tamoxifen and the selective serotonin reuptake inhibitor paroxetine. *Journal of the National Cancer Institute*, **95**, 1758–1764.

69 Otton, S.V., Ball, S.E., Cheung, S.W., Inaba, T., Rudolph, R.L. & Sellers, E.M. (1996) Venlafaxine oxidation in vitro is catalysed by CYP2D6. *British Journal of Clinical Pharmacology*, **41**, 149–156.

70 Guttuso, T.J. Jr. (2000) Gabapentin's effects on hot flashes and hypothermia. *Neurology*, **54**, 2161–2163.

71 Loprinzi, L., Barton, D.L., Sloan, J.A. *et al.* (2002) Pilot evaluation of gabapentin for treating hot flashes. *Mayo Clinic Proceedings*, **77**, 1159–1163.

72 Guttuso, T. Jr., Kurlan, R., McDermott, M.P. & Kieburtz, K. (2003) Gabapentin's effects on hot flashes in postmenopausal women: a randomized controlled trial. *Obstetrics and Gynecology*, **101**, 337–345.

73 Pandya, K.J., Morrow, G.R., Roscoe, J.A. *et al.* (2005) Gabapentin for hot flashes in 420 women with breast cancer: a randomised double-blind placebo-controlled trial. *Lancet*, **366**, 818–824.

74 Reddy, S.Y., Warner, H., Guttuso, T. Jr. *et al.* (2006) Gabapentin, estrogen, and placebo for treating hot flushes: a randomized controlled trial. *Obstetrics and Gynecology*, **108**, 41–48.

75 Loprinzi, C.L., Dueck, A.C., Khoyratty, B.S. *et al.* (2009) A phase III randomized, double-blind, placebo-controlled trial of gabapentin in the management of hot flashes in men (N00CB). *Annals of Oncology*, **20**, 542–549.

76 Presant, C.A.K. (2007) Palliation of vasomotor instability (hot flashes) using pregabalin. *Community Oncology*, **4**, 83–84.

77 Loprinzi, C.L., Qin, R., Baclueva, E.P. *et al.* (2010) Phase III, randomized, double-blind, placebo-controlled evaluation of pregabalin for alleviating hot flashes, N07C1. *Journal of Clinical Oncology*, **28**, 641–647.

78 Laufer, L.R., Erlik, Y., Meldrum, D.R. & Judd, H.L. (1982) Effect of clonidine on hot flashes in postmenopausal women. *Obstetrics and Gynecology*, **60**, 583–586.

79 Schindler, A.E., Muller, D., Keller, E., Göser, R. & Runkel, F. (1979) Studies with clonidine (dixarit) in menopausal women. *Archives of Gynecology*, **227**, 341–347.

80 Clayden, J.R., Bell, J.W. & Pollard, P. (1974) Menopausal flushing: double-blind trial of a non-hormonal medication. *British Medical Journal*, **1**, 409–412.

81 Freedman, R.R. & Dinsay, R. (2000) Clonidine raises the sweating threshold in symptomatic but not in asymptomatic postmenopausal women. *Fertility and Sterility*, **74**, 20–23.

82 Goldberg, R.M., Loprinzi, C.L., O'Fallon, J.R. *et al.* (1994) Transdermal clonidine for ameliorating tamoxifen-induced hot flashes. *Journal of Clinical Oncology*, **12**, 155–158.

83 Pandya, K.J., Raubertas, R.F., Flynn, P.J. *et al.* (2000) Oral clonidine in postmenopausal patients with breast cancer experiencing tamoxifen-induced hot flashes: a University of Rochester Cancer Center Community Clinical Oncology Program study. *Annals of Internal Medicine*, **132**, 788–793.

84 Loprinzi, C.L., Goldberg, R.M., O'Fallon, J.R. *et al.* (1994) Transdermal clonidine for ameliorating post-orchiectomy hot flashes. *Journal of Urology*, **151**, 634–636.

85 Nelson, H.D., Vesco, K.K., Haney, E. *et al.* (2006) Nonhormonal therapies for menopausal hot flashes: systematic review and meta-analysis. *Journal of the American Medical Association*, **295**, 2057–2071.

86 Christy, C. (1945) Vitamin E in menopause. *American Journal of Obstetrics and Gynecology*, **50**, 84–87.

87 Finkler, R.S. (1949) The effect of vitamin E in the menopause. *Journal of Clinical Endocrinology and Metabolism*, **9**, 89–94.

88 Barton, D.L., Loprinzi, C.L., Quella, S.K. *et al.* (1998) Prospective evaluation of vitamin E for hot flashes in breast cancer survivors. *Journal of Clinical Oncology*, **16**, 495–500.

89 Wade, C.K.F., Kelly, A. & Murphy, P.A. (1999) Hormone-modulating herbs: implications for women's health. *Journal of the American Medical Women's Association*, **54**, 181–183.

90 Lieberman, S. (1998) A review of the effectiveness of Cimicifuga racemosa (black cohosh) for the symptoms of menopause. *Journal of Women's Health*, **7**, 525–529.

91 Liske EaW, P. (1998) Therapy of climacteric complaints with cimicguga racemosa: herbal medicine with clinically proven evidence. *Menopause (New York, NY)*, **5**, 250.

92 Pepping, J. (1999) Black cohosh: cimicifuga racemosa. *American Journal of Health-System Pharmacy*, **56**, 1400–1402.

93 Kronenberg, F. & Fugh-Berman, A. (2002) Complementary and alternative medicine for menopausal symptoms: a review of randomized, controlled trials. *Annals of Internal Medicine*, **137**, 805–813.

94 Pockaj, B.A., Loprinzi, C.L., Sloan, J.A. *et al.* (2004) Pilot evaluation of black cohosh for the treatment of hot flashes in women. *Cancer Investigation*, **22**, 515–521.

95 Pockaj, B.A., Gallagher, J.G., Loprinzi, C.L. *et al.* (2006) Phase III double-blind, randomized, placebo-controlled crossover trial of black cohosh in the management of hot flashes: NCCTG Trial N01CC1. *Journal of Clinical Oncology*, **24**, 2836–2841.

96 Reed, S.D., Newton, K.M., LaCroix, A.Z., Grothaus, L.C., Grieco, V.S. & Ehrlich, K. (2008) Vaginal, endometrial, and reproductive hormone findings: randomized, placebo-controlled trial of black cohosh, multibotanical herbs, and dietary soy for vasomotor symptoms: the Herbal Alternatives for Menopause (HALT) Study. *Menopause (New York, NY)*, **15**, 51–58.

97 Newton, K.M., Reed, S.D., LaCroix, A.Z., Grothaus, L.C., Ehrlich, K. & Guiltinan, J. (2006) Treatment of vasomotor symptoms of menopause with black cohosh, multibotanicals, soy, hormone therapy, or placebo: a randomized trial. *Annals of Internal Medicine*, **145**, 869–879.

98 Geller, S.E., Shulman, L.P., van Breemen, R.B. *et al.* (2009) Safety and efficacy of black cohosh and red clover for the management of vasomotor symptoms: a randomized controlled trial. *Menopause (New York, NY)*, **16**, 1156–1166.

99 Haines, C.J., Chung, T.K. & Leung, D.H. (1994) A prospective study of the frequency of acute menopausal symptoms in Hong Kong Chinese women. *Maturitas*, **18**, 175–181.

100 Oddens, B.J. (1994) The climacteric cross-culturally: the International Health Foundation South-East Asia study. *Maturitas*, **19**, 155–156.

101 Freeman, E.W. & Sherif, K. (2007) Prevalence of hot flushes and night sweats around the world: a systematic review. *Climacteric: Journal of the International Menopause Society*, **10**, 197–214.

102 Adlercreutz, H., Mousavi, Y., Clark, J. *et al.* (1992) Dietary phytoestrogens and cancer: in vitro and in vivo studies. *Journal of Steroid Biochemistry and Molecular Biology*, **41**, 331–337.

103 Tham, D.M., Gardner, C.D. & Haskell, W.L. (1998) Clinical review 97: potential health benefits of dietary phytoestrogens: a review of the clinical, epidemiological, and mechanistic evidence. *Journal of Clinical Endocrinology and Metabolism*, **83**, 2223–2235.

104 Quella, S.K., Loprinzi, C.L., Barton, D.L. *et al.* (2000) Evaluation of soy phytoestrogens for the treatment of hot flashes in breast cancer survivors: a North Central Cancer Treatment Group Trial. *Journal of Clinical Oncology*, **18**, 1068–1074.

105 Secreto, G., Chiechi, L.M., Amadori, A. *et al.* (2004) Soy isoflavones and melatonin for the relief of climacteric symptoms: a multicenter, double-blind, randomized study. *Maturitas*, **47**, 11–20.

106 MacGregor, C.A., Canney, P.A., Patterson, G., McDonald, R. & Paul, J. (2005) A randomised double-blind controlled trial of oral soy supplements versus placebo for treatment of menopausal symptoms in patients with early breast cancer. *European Journal of Cancer*, **41**, 708–714.

107 Nikander, E., Kilkkinen, A., Metsa-Heikkila, M. *et al.* (2003) A randomized placebo-controlled crossover trial with phytoestrogens in treatment of menopause in breast cancer patients. *Obstetrics and Gynecology*, **101**, 1213–1220.

108 Lewis, J.E., Nickell, L.A., Thompson, L.U., Szalai, J.P., Kiss, A. & Hilditch, J.R. (2006) A randomized controlled trial of the effect of dietary soy and flaxseed muffins on quality of life and hot flashes during menopause. *Menopause (New York, NY)*, **13**, 631–642.

109 Pruthi, S., Thompson, S.L., Novotny, P.J. *et al.* (2007) Pilot evaluation of flaxseed for the management of hot flashes. *Journal of the Society for Integrative Oncology*, **5**, 106–112.

110 Chen, J., Hui, E., Ip, T. & Thompson, L.U. (2004) Dietary flaxseed enhances the inhibitory effect of tamoxifen on the growth of estrogen-dependent human breast cancer (mcf-7) in nude mice. *Clinical Cancer Research*, **10**, 7703–7711.

111 Lasley, B.L., Santoro, N., Randolf, J.F.. *et al.* (2002) The relationship of circulating dehydroepiandrosterone, testosterone, and estradiol to stages of the menopausal transition and ethnicity. *Journal of Clinical Endocrinology and Metabolism*, **87**, 3760–3767.

112 Barton, D.L., Loprinzi, C., Atherton, P.J. *et al.* (2006) Dehydroepiandrosterone for the treatment of hot flashes: a pilot study. *Supportive Cancer Therapy*, **3**, 91–97.

113 Stomati, M., Monteleone, P., Casarosa, E. *et al.* (2000) Six-month oral dehydroepiandrosterone supplementation in early and late postmenopause. *Gynecological Endocrinology*, **14**, 342–363.

114 Conference, N. (1998) Acupuncture. *Journal of the American Medical Association*, **280**, 1518–1524.

115 Dong, H., Ludicke, F., Comte, I., Campana, A., Graff, P. & Bischof, P. (2001) An exploratory pilot study of acupuncture on the quality of life and reproductive hormone secretion in menopausal women. *Journal of Alternative and Complementary Medicine (New York, NY)*, **7**, 651–658.

116 Porzio, G., Trapasso, T., Martelli, S. *et al.* (2002) Acupuncture in the treatment of menopause-related symptoms in women taking tamoxifen. *Tumori*, **88**, 128–130.

117 Wyon, Y., Lindgren, R., Lundeberg, T. *et al.* (1995) Effects of acupuncture on climacteric vasomotor symptoms, quality of life, and urinary excretion of neuropeptides among postmenopausal women. *Menopause: Journal of the North American Menopause Society*, **2**, 3–12.

118 Vincent, A., Barton, D.L., Mandrekar, J.N. *et al.* (2007) Acupuncture for hot flashes: a randomized, sham-controlled clinical study. *Menopause (New York, NY)*, **14**, 45–52.

119 Lee, M.S., Kim, K.H., Choi, S.M. & Ernst, E. (2009) Acupuncture for treating hot flashes in breast cancer patients: a systematic review. *Breast Cancer Research and Treatment*, **115**, 497–503.

120 Cho, S.H. & Whang, W.W. (2009) Acupuncture for vasomotor menopausal symptoms: a systematic review. *Menopause (New York, NY)*, **16**, 1065–1073.

121 Elias, M. (2000) Cervical sympathetic and stellate ganglion blocks. *Pain Physician*, **3**, 294–304.

122 Lipov, E., Lipov, S. & Stark, J.T. (2005) Stellate ganglion blockade provides relief from menopausal hot flashes: a case report series. *Journal of Women's Health*, **14**, 737–741.

123 Lipov, E.G., Joshi, J.R., Sanders, S. *et al.* (2008) Effects of stellate-ganglion block on hot flushes and night awakenings in survivors of breast cancer: a pilot study. *Lancet Oncology*, **9**, 523–532.

124 Pachman, D., Barton, D., Carns, P. *et al.* (2011) Pilot evaluation of a stellate ganglion block for the treatment of hot flashes. *Supportive Care in Cancer*, **18**, 941–947.

125 Germaine, L.M. & Freedman, R.R. (1984) Behavioral treatment of menopausal hot flashes: evaluation by objective methods. *Journal of Consulting and Clinical Psychology*, **52**, 1072–1079.

126 Freedman, R.R. & Woodward, S. (1992) Behavioral treatment of menopausal hot flushes: evaluation by ambulatory monitoring. *American Journal of Obstetrics and Gynecology*, **167**, 436–439.

127 Fenlon, D.R., Corner, J.L. & Haviland, J.S. (2008) A randomized controlled trial of relaxation training to reduce hot flashes in women with primary breast cancer. *Journal of Pain and Symptom Management*, **35**, 397–405.

128 Borkovec, T.D. & Fowles, D.C. (1973) Controlled investigation of the effects of progressive and hypnotic relaxation on insomnia. *Journal of Abnormal Psychology*, **82**, 153–158.

129 Wadden, T.A. & Anderton, C.H. (1982) The clinical use of hypnosis. *Psychological Bulletin*, **91**, 215–243.

130 Stern, J.A., Brown, M., Ulett, G.A. & Sletten, I. (1977) A comparison of hypnosis, acupuncture, morphine, valium, aspirin, and placebo in the management of experimentally induced pain. *Annals of the New York Academy of Sciences*, **296**, 175–193.

131 Elkins, G. (1997) *Current Thinking and Research in Brief Therapy*, Brunner/Mazel, New York.

132 Gruber, B.L., Hersh, S.P., Hall, N.R. *et al.* (1993) Immunological responses of breast cancer patients to behavioral interventions. *Biofeedback and Self-Regulation*, **18**, 1–22.

133 Bridge, L.R., Benson, P., Pietroni, P.C. & Priest, R.G. (1988) Relaxation and imagery in the treatment of breast cancer. *British Medical Journal (Clinical Research Ed.)*, **297**, 1169–1172.

134 Elkins, G., Marcus, J., Stearns, V. & Hasan Rajab, M. (2007) Pilot evaluation of hypnosis for the treatment of hot flashes in breast cancer survivors. *Psycho-Oncology*, **16**, 487–492.

135 Elkins, G., Marcus, J., Stearns, V. *et al.* (2008) Randomized trial of a hypnosis intervention for treatment of hot flashes among breast cancer survivors. *Journal of Clinical Oncology*, **26**, 5022–5026.

136 north American Menopause Society. (2004) Treatment of menopause-associated vasomotor symptoms: position statement of The North American Menopause Society. *Menopause (New York, NY)*, **11**, 11–33.

137 Barton, D., Loprinzi, C. & Wahner-Roedler, D. (2001) Hot flashes: aetiology and management. *Drugs and Aging*, **18**, 597–606.

138 Casper, R.F. & Yen, S.S. (1985) Neuroendocrinology of menopausal flushes: an hypothesis of flush mechanism. *Clinical Endocrinology*, **22**, 293–312.

139 Daley, A., Stokes-Lampard, H. & Macarthur, C. (2011) Exercise for vasomotor menopausal symptoms. *Cochrane Database of Systematic Reviews*, **11** (5), CD006108.

140 Daley, A.J., Stokes-Lampard, H.J. & Macarthur, C. (2009) Exercise to reduce vasomotor and other menopausal symptoms: a review. *Maturitas*, **63**, 176–180.

141 Loprinzi, C.L. & Wolf, S.L. (2010) Hot flushes: mostly sex neutral? *Lancet Oncology*, **11**, 107–108.

4 Skin Toxicities to Chemotherapy

14 Alkylating Agents

Elisabeth Livingstone, Lisa Zimmer, Larissa Leister and Dirk Schadendorf

Department of Dermatology, University Hospital Essen, Essen, Germany

Introduction

The use of alkylating agents as chemotherapy dates from 1946, the year that nitrogen mustard was introduced [1]. Sulfur mustard was used as a warfare agent because of its vesicant effect on the skin and mucous membranes. The observation of its additional effect of hematopoietic and lymphoid system depression [2] led to the use of the less volatile nitrogen mustards in studies. In these studies, the regression of lymphomas could be demonstrated [3,4].

The alkylating agents react with (or "alkylate") many electron rich atoms in DNA bases, to form covalent bonds (Table 14.1) [5]. Monofunctional alkylating agents react with only one strand of DNA, which is recognized by the cell and leads to lethal reactions. Bifunctional agents react with two strands of DNA and produce a "cross-link" that, unless repaired, will prevent cell replication.

The main dermatologic adverse events (AEs) of alkylating agents are hyperpigmentation, mucositis, alopecia, hypersensitivity reactions, and xerosis with pruritus (Figure 14.1). Table 14.2 gives an overview of the incidences of specific dermatologic AEs of the different agents.

Nitrogen mustards

Nitrogen mustards produce cytotoxicity by forming covalent interstrand cross-links in DNA [5]. The main AEs are bone marrow suppression and neurologic toxicity.

Mustargen (mechlorethamine)

Mustargen is available as an intravenous preparation that can also be used topically for cutaneous malignancies. It is currently used in the MOPP regime (mustargen, vincristine, procarbazine, prednisone) for Hodgkin disease and topically for early stages of mycosis fungoides.

Dermatologic AEs after IV administration of mustargen include chemical cellulitis and phlebitis [6] (see Chapter 28). Alopecia is reported to occur often [7]. Angioedema and pruritus have been reported twice [8,9] but are otherwise exceedingly rare.

The mechanism of action of mustargen in topical administration may also be mediated by immune mechanisms (e.g., immunostimulation) or by interaction with the keratinocyte–Langerhans cell–T-cell axis [10]. Topical formulations of mustargen are either aqueous or ointment based methods in concentrations of 10–20% [10].

The most common acute complication to topical mechlorethamine is irritant (in 25% of patients using the ointment formulation) or allergic (delayed-type hypersensitivity) contact dermatitis [10], more commonly in areas such as the face or skin folds [10]. It is generally mild, and therapy can usually be continued with decreased frequency of application or with additional topical steroids. Patients using the aqueous solution seem to experience true allergic hypersensitivity reactions more often than those using the ointment (28–75% and <10%, respectively) [7,10–12]. The majority of the patients can be desensitized by reduction in the concentration of mustargen to 0.1–10 mg/L, followed by gradual escalation over several months.

Hyperpigmentation without preceding inflammation [11–15], due to an increased number of melanosomes in the keratinocytes of patients with Caucasian skin after topical application has been described [15]. Other rare AEs include urticaria [16,17] and erythema multiforme-like dermatitis [16,18,19].

Development of nonmelanoma skin cancers in patients treated with topical mustargen has been reported [20–22], especially when the aqueous solution was used. The overall risk is low, but

Table 14.1 Classifications of alkylating agents.

Sulfur mustards	Sulfur mustard
Nitrogen mustards	Mustargen (mechlorethamine)
	Cyclophosphamide
	Ifosfamide
	Melphalan
	Chlorambucil
Aziridines and epoxides	ThioTEPA
	Mitomycin
Alkyl sulfonates	Busulfan
Nitrosoureas	Carmustine (BCNU, bischloroethylnitrosourea)
	Streptozocin
Hydrazines and triazine derivatives	Procarbazine
	Dacarbazine
	Temozolomide
Ribonucleotide reductase inhibitor	Hydroxyurea

is problematic for patients treated with multiple skin-damaging therapies (e.g., phototherapy or radiation) or those who used mustargen on the genitals.

Cyclophosphamide

Cyclophosphamide is used for the treatment of various cancers. High doses of cyclophosphamide are frequently used in conjunction with bone marrow transplantation and for the treatment of autoimmune diseases. A unique toxicity of cyclophosphamide and other oxaphosphorines is a characteristic hemorrhagic cystitis [23,24] caused by irritation primarily by acrolein [25]. Cyclophosphamide is a non-vesicant [26], but redness, swelling, and pain can appear at the injection site [27,28]. Alopecia commonly occurs (40–60%) and begins 3–6 weeks after start of therapy [28,29]. Mucositis is another frequent AE of cyclophosphamide [13,30–32].

Cutaneous hyperpigmentation may be widespread [33,34] or localized to palms, soles, or nails. It generally appear between months 5 and 6 and fades 6 months to a year after completion of therapy [6]. The pattern of nail hyperpigmentation varies from diffuse to longitudinal (pigment from nail matrix) or transverse (pigment in nail plate) streaks (Figure 14.2) [6,13,34–37]. Oral mucosal hyperpigmentation occurs commonly [38]; rarely, the appearance of a brown discoloration above the gum line has been reported which does not disappear when therapy is stopped [39]. In general, however, hyperpigmentation produced by

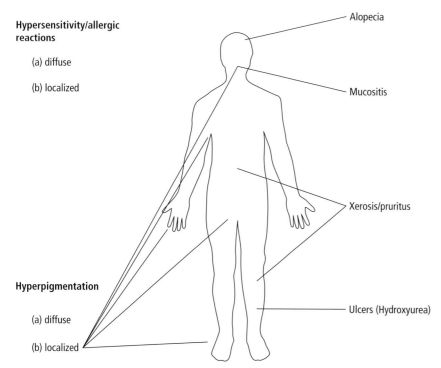

Hypersensitivity/allergic reactions

(a) diffuse

(b) localized

Alopecia

Mucositis

Xerosis/pruritus

Ulcers (Hydroxyurea)

Hyperpigmentation

(a) diffuse

(b) localized

Figure 14.1 Location of alkylating-agent induced dermatologic toxicities.

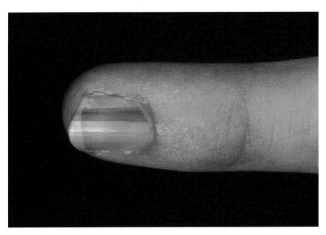

Figure 14.2 Longitudinal hyperpigmentation due to long-term treatment with cyclophosphamide.

cyclophosphamide is reversible, usually within 6–12 months after discontinuation of the drug [13].

Facial flushing following IV administration is reported in 1–10% of patients [27,28], other rare AEs are rash, hives, or itching (1–5%) [27,28], hand-foot syndrome [6], and type I hypersensitivity reactions [7,8,40–43]. A negative skin test to the parent compound is only of small assurance as the drug must be metabolized in the liver before it demonstrates appreciable chemical reactivity [43]. Therefore, skin testing with the parent compound as well as its metabolites may be necessary to find the true antigenic determinant of cyclophosphamide. There is a single case report in the literature assuming an association of cyclophosphamide and doxorubicin treatment for breast cancer with the appearance of a subacute lupus erythematosus [44].

Ifosfamide
Ifosfamide is a structural isomer of cyclophosphamide that is often used in the treatment of solid tumors, lymphomas, sarcomas, and pediatric tumors [5]. Extravasation can lead to local cellulitis; however, it is sometimes also classified as nonirritating. No specific measures need to be taken. Alopecia occurs commonly [7].

Hyperpigmentation is common [45], often occurring localized especially on the hands and feet [7] or in areas of occlusion such as areas under electrocardiogram pads, tape, or dressings [46]. Ifosfamide in combination with agents such as gemcitabine and etoposide has resulted in a characteristic eruption consisting of severe oral mucositis and extensive sunburn-like erythema with accentuation of the intertriginous and genitoanal areas [47–50]. Type 1 hypersensitivity reactions rarely occur with ifosfamide [7].

Melphalan
Melphalan is principally used for the treatment of multiple myeloma, for high-dose myeloablative therapy preceding stem

cell transplantation, and for the isolated limb perfusion of localized tumors [5,51], especially melanoma and sarcomas.

Melphalan is a vesicant and does not induce cellulitis. It can cause radiation sensitization and recall [6,7]. Hyperpigmented banding of the nails has been reported after systemic treatment [52]. Type I hypersensitivity reactions have been noted to occur in 2–5% of patients after systemic therapy [7,53,54], a higher incidence in patients with IgA kappa myeloma is suspected [54].

The majority of patients undergoing isolated limb perfusion (ILP) experience mild erythema or edema [55] which may be associated with pain. Blistering is noted in 50% of patients in the extremity 1–19 days after ILP. Delayed palmoplantar blistering can start up to 14 days after ILP. Temporary loss of nails and inhibition of hair growth on the perfused extremity can also be noticed. Localized scleroderma as a complication of ILP with melphalan and tumor necrosis factor α (TNF-α) have been reported in two patients and were attributed to the combined effects [56].

Chlorambucil
Chlorambucil is used for the treatment of B-cell chronic lymphocitic leukemia (CLL) and lymphomas. It is available orally and generally well tolerated with less mucositis than other alkylating agents [57].

Hypersensitivity reactions to chlorambucil are rare [58] and are usually type I. Allergic reactions have been associated with urticaria and angioedema [59–61], erythematous rashes and toxic epidermal necrolysis (TEN) [62,63], drug fever [64], and one case of immune hemolytic anemia [65]. A rare type of allergic reaction occurred in two patients on a single course of chlorambucil for CLL who demonstrated fever, chills, and rapidly progressing lymphadenopathy without evidence of disease progression or infection [66]. Rechallenge of chlorambucil led to the same symptoms; however, other alkylating agents were tolerated. TEN and drug rash with eosinophilia and systemic symptoms (DRESS) are uncommon but severe reactions to chlorambucil may require the use of systemic steroids [63,67–70].

Aziridines and epoxides

ThioTEPA
ThioTEPA is used as a conditioning treatment prior to stem cell transplantation, for controlling intracavitary malignant effusions, and treatment of adenocarcinoma of the breast and ovary, and papillary bladder carcinoma.

Alopecia has infrequently been associated with thioTEPA [6,7], whereas mucositis can be a dose-limiting toxicity of high doses [71]. Pruritus [72] and allergic/hypersensitivity reactions consisting of urticaria [6,73] have been described. Five of 164 (3%) patients receiving intravesical thioTEPA for bladder carcinoma developed urticaria, angioedema, pruritus, and fever [74].

Table 14.2 Incidence of dermatologic adverse events to alkylating agents

Drug name		Dermatologic toxicities								
Mustargen	Systemic treatment	Extravasation cellulitis, phlebitis [6]	Alopecia often [7]	Angioedema rare [8]	Rash rare [8]					
	Topical treatment	Contact dermatitis 25% [10]	Hyperpigmentation frequently [11,12,14,15]	Urticaria seldom [20–22]		Nonmelanoma skin cancer relationship possible [20–22]	Erythema multiforme-like dermatitis seldom [16,18–19]			
Cyclophosphamide	Systemic treatment	Extravasation only redness, swelling, pain [27,28]	Alopecia 40–60% [28,29]	Mucositis frequently [13, 30–32]	Hyperpigmentations (frequently)	Skin: widespread/localized [33,34]	Nail: diffuse longitudinal or vertical [6,13,34–37]	Mucosal: orally common [38]	Facial flushing 1–10% [27,28]	Rash, hives, itching 1–5% [27,28] · Hand-foot syndrome, Type I hypersensitivity rare [7,8,40–43]
Ifosfamide	Systemic treatment	Extravasation cellulitis	Alopecia common [7]		Hyperpigmentations (frequently) [45]	Skin: localized esp. hands and feet and under areas of occlusion	Mucositis in combination with gemcitabine/etoposid severe mucositis and sunburn-like erythema in intertriginous/genitanal areas [47–50]			Hypersensitivity Type I rare [7]
Melphalan	Systemic treatment	Extravasation no vesicant/cellulitis			Radiation sensitization/recall associated [6,7]	Hyperpigmentation nail: hyperpigmented banding [6,7]	Hypersensitivity 2–5% [7,53,54] higher incidence in patients with IgA kappa myeloma [54]			
	Isolated limb perfusion	Extravasation not applicable	Erythema/edema majority [55]	Blistering 50%		Localized scleroderma (single reports) after combination of melphalan and TNF [56]				
Chlorambucil	Systemic treatment	Extravasation not applicable	Mucositis less frequent		Hypersensitivity (rare) [58]: usually type I cutaneous reactions, urticaria, angioedema, rashes, TEN [59–61]	Toxic epidermal necrolysis rare [63,67,68]	DRESS single report [69]			
ThioTEPA	Systemic treatment	Extravasation local irritation	Alopecia infrequently [6,7]	Mucositis frequently [71]	Hypersensitivity urticaria, also with angioedema, pruritus, fever [6,73,74]	Pruritus associated [72]	Hyperpigmentation common, with exfoliation and desquamation less frequently especially hands/feet, occluded areas [75–81]			

Drug	Treatment	Extravasation					Other rare events
Mitomycin	Systemic treatment	Extravasation tissue injury [89,90], ulcers [91]	Mucositis frequently [6]	Hypersensitivity [6]: exfoliative dermatitis of palms and soles, generalized itch or localized predominantly type IV, also type III, 34% of patients treated topical for ocular neoplasias developed allergic reaction			pruritus, vasculitis, EEM
Busulfan	Systemic treatment	Extravasation inflammation	Alopecia possibly permanent [96] after high dose	Mucositis common	Hypersensitivity associated	Hyperpigmentation (after long-term treatment) [97–100] diffuse bronze hyperpigmentation of skin, can be associated weakness, weight loss and diarrhea	Porphyria cutanea tarda single reports [13, 103] hyperpigmentation, elevated urine uroporphyrin
Carmustine	Systemic treatment	Extravasation local irritation [104]	Hyperpigmentation not common [105]				
	Topical treatment	Extravasation not applicable	Erythema frequently [106], often with burning sensation esp. intertriginous areas	Hyperpigmentation [105,107,108] primarily in dark complexioned skin following primary irritant dermatitis	Teleangiectasia [106] in areas of erythema often spares lesions sites	Allergic reactions <10% [106,107], case reports with severe erosive inflammation [106–108]	
Streptozocin	Systemic treatment	Extravasation local inflammation [6,7]	Alopecia associated	Mucositis associated			
Procarbazine	Systemic treatment	Extravasation not applicable	Alopecia associated [6,7]	Flush syndrome or antabus effect [7,105] after alcohol ingestion due to inhibition of alcohol dehydrogenase	Hypersensitivity (common) [110,111] type I and III reactions with pulmonary and cutaneous reactions	Fixed drug eruption single case report [115]	
Dacarbazine	Systemic treatment	Extravasation chemical cellulitis, phlebitis [6]	Hypersensitivity (20%) [117] rash, fever, chills severe form with fever, hypereosinophilia, liver dysfunction and delayed medullar aplasia	Photosensitivity [13,119–121] common maculo-urticarial exanthema with stinging pain	Radiation recall single case report [122]	Inflammation of actinic keratoses single case report [123]	
Temozolomide	Systemic treatment	Extravasation not applicable	Alopecia 55% [154]	Rash and pruritus 8% [154]	Hypersensitivity rash, pruritus, swelling, dizziness, trouble breathing	Erythema multiforme Rare [154] / Stevens–Johnson syndrome Rare [154]	Erythema 1% [154]
Hydroxyurea	Systemic treatment	Extravasation not applicable	Alopecia rare [127]	Mucositis associated	Xerosis cutis frequently [125]	Hyperpigmentation — Skin (frequent) [125–128]: localized or generalized; Nail (rare) [125, 128,129, 132–139]: transverse/longitundinal bands; Mucosa (rare): bucchal dyschromia [128,129,132] / Ulcerations (common) [141] feet and lower legs / Dermatmyositis-like [145] skin changes: Gottron-like papules, streaky erythema dorsum of fingers	Non-melanoma skin cancer [149–152]: common

EEM, ; DRESS, drug rash with eosinophilia and systemic symptoms; TNF, tumor necrosis factor.

High-dose thioTEPA given alone or in combination commonly results in hyperpigmentation and erythema [75–81]; with exfoliation and desquamation reported less frequently [76,79–81]. In adults, acute erythroderma of the palmo-plantar surfaces [82] and hyperpigmentation of occluded skin [75] have been described. Pediatric patients receiving a combination therapy are commonly affected by dermatologic AEs (80–90%), predominantly erythema progressing to desquamation and hyperpigmentation [76,83], which likely results from a direct toxic effect, supported by the finding that intertriginous or occluded skin is most commonly affected [75,76,79]. Local factors such as friction, skin temperature, and eccrine gland distribution may contribute to toxicity of the skin [84].

Mitomycin C

Mitomycin is used for the treatment of upper gastrointestinal, anal, and breast cancer, topically for the treatment of ocular surface neoplasia [85], and for bladder instillation in superficial tumors. Topical mitomycin C has been investigated for the treatment of full-thickness burns [86], as an adjunctive in airway surgery [87] and in otolaryngeal surgery to reduce complications from postoperative scarring [88]. In general, it could not show to improve wound healing but may even worsen clinical appearance and scarring as well as prolong wound healing.

Extravasation of mitomycin can lead to tissue injury [89,90] resulting in extravasation ulcers [91]. Dimethyl sulfoxide (DMSO) should be applied topically; ulcers might require surgical treatment. Mitomycin has been associated with mucositis and hypersensitivity reactions [6]. Contact allergy to mitomycin C presenting as exfoliative dermatitis of the palms and soles or generalized itch has occurred with intravesical or topical administration [92–94]. Patch tests for mitomycin were positive, suggesting a type IV hypersensitivity reaction. However, type III reactions have also been described [92]. Of patients treated topically for ocular neoplasias, 34% developed an allergic reaction to mitomycin C [85].

Alkyl sulfonates

Busulfan

Busulfan (1,4-butandiol-bis(methansulfonate)) is a bi-functional alkylating agent with two labile methanesulfonates attached to opposite ends of a four-carbon alkyl chain. In aqueous solution, busulfan hydrolyzes and releases the methanesulfonate groups, resulting in reactive carbonium ions that alkylate DNA [95]. Busulfan is a component of many myeloablative conditioning regimens before infusion of an autologous or allogeneic graft and can also be used in the chronic phase of chronic myeloid leukemia (CML).

High doses of busulfan followed by stem cell transplantation have resulted in permanent alopecia [96]. Busulfan has also been associated with hypersensitivity reactions, inflammation at injection site, rash, pruritus, erythema multiforme, and vasculitis.

The most striking cutaneous AE of busulfan is a "dusky" hyperpigmentation [97–100], which can mimic Addison disease after long-term treatment [30,100]. The diffuse bronze hyperpigmentation is most prominent on the neck, upper portion of the trunk, nipples, abdomen and palmar creases; the buccal mucosa can be spared [13]. The mechanism of hyperpigmentation is thought to be secondary to a toxic effect on the melanocytes; histology showing increased melanin in the basal layer but no change in the number of melanocytes [101]. The incidence of hyperpigmentation is higher in darker individuals [102]. Hyperpigmentation can be managed with topical retinoids, hydroquinone, and corticosteroids, along with sun avoidance. Porphyria cutanea tarda, with hyperpigmentation and elevated urine uroporphyrin, hirsutism, and hyperpigmentation, has also been described [13,103].

Nitrosoureas

The members of the nitrosourea group of therapeutic alkylating agents are related to the alkylnitrosamines and similar compounds that have long been known to be carcinogenic.

Carmustine (bischloroethylnitrosourea)

Carmustine is used systemically for the treatment of lymphomas, brain tumors, and myeloma and locally for cutaneous T-cell lymphoma and melanoma.

When administered systemically, cutaneous complications are uncommon; local venous irritation [104] and hyperpigmentation has been infrequently reported [105]. Topical administration of bischloroethylnitrosourea (BCNU) may lead to erythema, especially with the BCNU solution, in the majority of patients [106]. This is often accompanied by a burning sensation, similar to sunburn. The erythema is frequent in the body folds, groins, and axillae and appears after 4–8 weeks. In black people, the inflammatory reaction is manifest by hyperpigmentation. In medium complexioned subjects, both erythema and hyperpigmentation can be observed [105,107,108]. Hyperpigmentation after topical application has been shown to be post-inflammatory pigmentation, following primary irritant contact dermatitis [13,109]. Erythema is commonly accompanied by skin tenderness, which can persist for several months if not treated with topical corticosteroids, cool compresses, cool baths, and emollients [106].

Severe, and occasionally moderate, erythematous reactions may be followed by telangiectasia [106], which can persist from months to years. Telangiectasias are benign, and in some cases spare the lesion site, thereby leaving a pale center surrounded by erythema [108].

Irritant or allergic dermatitis occurs in less than 10% of patients [106,107], with reports of allergic contact dermatitis with severe erosive inflammation at the treatment site [106–108]. A 0.1% aqueous solution of BCNU is recommended for patch testing, and desensitization with increasing concentrations is feasible.

Streptozocin

Streptozocin is used for the treatment of surgically incurable insulinomas (islet cell carcinomas) and malignant carcinoid tumors. Extravasation leads to local inflammation (i.e., edema, erythema, burning, tenderness, chemical cellulitis) [6,7], which generally resolves with supportive care the same day or within a few days. Streptozocin is also associated with allergic reactions and alopecia.

Hydrazines and triazine derivatives

The hydrazine and triazine derivatives compounds are analogous to the nitrosoureas in that they decompose spontaneously or are metabolized to produce an alkyl carbonium ion, which alkylates DNA [5].

Procarbazine

Procarbazine is used in the MOPP regimen for the treatment of Hodgkin disease, in the treatment of brain tumors and bronchogenic carcinoma [5].

Alopecia has been associated with procarbazine [6,7]. Secondary to the inhibition of the enzyme alcohol dehydrogenase by procarbazine, an antabuse effect characterized by flushing, headache, and diaphoresis after alcohol ingestion can occur [7,105].

Hypersensitivity reactions to procarbazine are common [110,111]. Procarbazine reactions can be immunoglobulin E (IgE) mediated but are also associated with a type III reaction manifested by pulmonary toxicity and cutaneous reactions [112]. Clinical features of hypersensitivity reactions are maculopapular rash, fever, reversible abnormal liver function test results, and pulmonary toxicity [113]. Concomitant exposure to anticonvulsants has been noted to increase hypersensitivity reactions, possibly through a reactive intermediate generated by CYP3A isoform induction [114]. There is a single case of a fixed drug eruption due to procarbazine in the literature; skin testing was negative, but rechallenge led to a flare-up of the lesion [115].

Dacarbazine

Dacarbazine (DTIC) is used for the treatment of melanoma [116], soft tissue sarcomas, neuroblastoma, rhabodmyosarcoma, and medullary thyroid carcinoma.

After IV administration of DTIC, especially after extravasation into the soft tissues, local reactions have been observed with chemical cellulitis and phlebitis [6] associated with pain. Treatment includes aspirating the extravasated drug, immobilization, and avoidance of sunlight [6,7]. DTIC has been associated with mild alopecia [6].

Hypersensitivity reactions to DTIC have been reported in up to 20% of patients [117]. Hypersensitivity most often occurs after the first or second course, with no dose dependency. Common

findings are erythematous and urticarial rashes, fevers, chills, malaise, and myalgia [118]. A few patients experience severe forms of hypersensitivity with fever, hypereosinophilia, liver dysfunction, and delayed medullar aplasia [117]. Antihistamines and glucocorticosteroids have been beneficial for pruritic hypersensitivity reactions with eosinophilia [6,7,89]. In case of fever and hypereosinophilia without liver dysfunction, DTIC may be continued together with symptomatic treatment. In the event of hepatic dysfunction and severe hematologic disorders (Budd–Chiari syndrome), potentially fatal complications can occur [117].

Exposure to sunlight following infusion of DTIC results in pruritic maculo-urticarial erythemas in exposed areas [13, 119–121]. Phototoxic reactions usually occur after the third and subsequent DTIC administration [121]. Phototesting demonstrated a lowered minimal erythema dose to ultraviolet B (UVB) [120]. In another study, Treudler et al. [121] demonstrated a clear clinical association between the onset of phototoxic skin reactions and the administration of DTIC, all of which resolved after drug discontinuation. Phototesting in five of these patients demonstrated an increased sensitivity mainly to UVA. Six patients were patch-tested 2–10 weeks after the eruption had cleared by using a strong dilution of DTIC; no positive reactions were seen confirming that the reaction is of a phototoxic rather than an allergic nature [121]. Phototoxic reactions are reported to be mainly due to 2-azahypoxanthine. It is unclear whether there is an accumulation of phototoxic products in the skin, or an ongoing decrease of enzymes that metabolize DTIC to MTIC, resulting in higher levels of DTIC for in vivo photodegradation. Patients receiving DTIC should be cautioned to avoid sun exposure and to use protective sunscreen agents [13]. Additionally, DTIC infusion bags have to be protected from light [121]. Skin reactions can be treated with topical corticosteroids and dose modifications, as the eruptions can become intolerable with increasing number of sessions and the phototoxic metabolite 2-azahypoxanthine may lack anticancer activity [121]. Patients may be switched to its sister compound temozolomide which does not induce phototoxic eruptions.

Radiation recall dermatitis has been described with DTIC monotherapy [122]. Mechanisms include an anamnestic inflammatory response or induction of heritable mutations within the surviving cells [89]. Treatment includes oral or topical corticosteroids and may be prevented in subsequent cycles with prior corticosteroid treatment [122].

There is a single case report of inflammation of actinic keratoses in a 44-year-old white person who received systemic chemotherapy with dactinomycin, vincristine, and dacarbazine [123]. The increased quantity of UV-induced DNA damage in dysplastic keratinocytes is assumed to make them susceptible to inflammation from cytotoxic agents. Inflammation of actinic keratosis is therapeutic because destruction of premalignant skin lesions results [89]. Topical corticosteroids may be given for symptomatic relief, but therapy discontinuation is not needed [7,89,123].

Temozolomide

In contrast to DTIC, temozolomide spontaneously decomposes to MTIC at all sites, which results in a more homogeneous systemic distribution. It is given orally for the treatment of brain tumors and melanoma.

Few reports have described dermatologic AEs such as rash and pruritus (8%). Hypersensitivity reactions can occur; serious reactions are rare. Symptoms may include rash, itching, swelling, severe dizziness, or trouble breathing. Alopecia (55%), dry skin, erythema (1%) and erythema multiforme and Stevens–Johnson syndrome have also been associated with temozolomide (see http://www.drugs.com/ppa/temozolomide.html).

Hydroxurea

Hydroxyurea is an oral drug used for the treatment of myeloproliferative disorders, including CML, polycythemia vera, essential thrombocytosis, and osteomyelofibrosis. Its action is specific for the S-phase of the cell cycle [124].

Cutaneous AEs of hydroxyurea occur commonly and are dose dependent. Xerosis is the most common dermatologic AE [125]; hyperpigmentations, either localized or generalized, are frequent [125–128] and develop after 1–3 years of therapy [129], and may fade or persist [128,130]. Hyperpigmentation is more frequent in black patients [128,131]. Buccal dyschromia is infrequent [128,129,132]. Discoloration of nails with transverse and longitudinal bands has been reported frequently [125,128,129,133–140]. The pathomechanism for hyperpigmentation is unknown; a direct toxic effect on the nail matrix [135], and/or focal deposition of melanin in the nail [135], or in the basal layer of the epidermis [132] have been proposed.

Painful cutaneous ulcerations can occur, predominantly over sites predisposed to trauma such as the malleoli, dorsa of the feet, the toes, and shins (Figure 14.3) [141, 142]. The pathophysiology is uncertain, but a direct cumulative and cytotoxic effect on basal keratinocytes causing cutaneous atrophy with delayed wound repair has been proposed [143]. As hydroxurea causes macrocytosis, erythrocytes are less susceptible to deformation, thus an impaired blood flow in the microcirculation might lead to anoxia and ulceration after trauma [144]. Treatment with hydroxyurea should be stopped and moist wound dressings applied to improve wound healing.

Dermatomyositis-like skin changes have been described after long-term use of hydroxyurea. Changes include Gottron-like papules and streaky erythema over the dorsal aspects of the fingers without muscle tenderness or weakness [145] and may result from inhibition of DNA synthesis in the basal epidermal layer [146]. Lesions are similar to graft versus host disease both clinically and histologically [147]. Symptoms are generally mild and no systemic therapy is required. Resolution of symptoms has been reported between 10 days to 18 months after discontinuation [148].

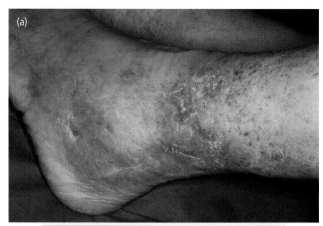

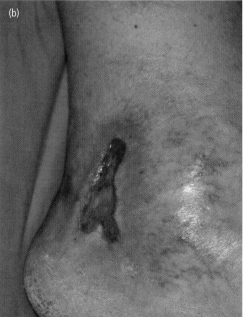

Figure 14.3 Hydroxyurea-induced ulcers on lower leg.

The eruption of nonmelanocytic skin cancers in photodistributed areas but also on mucosa is another well-known AE of long-term treatment with hydroxyurea [149–152]. Hydroxyurea has an intrinsic mutagenic activity and thus exerts a carcinogenic action [151,153]. Patients have to be informed on UV avoidance and regular dermatologic examinations with long-term treatment.

Other reported AEs include cutaneous atrophy [127], cutaneous vasculitis, fixed drug eruption, and mucositis.

References

1 Maanen, M.J., Smeets, C.J. & Beijnen, J.H. (2000) Chemistry, pharmacology and pharmacokinetics of N,N',N''-triethylenethio-phosphoramide (ThioTEPA). *Cancer Treatment Reviews*, **26** (4), 257–268.

2 Adair, F.E. & Bagg, H.J. (1931) Experimental and clinical studies on the treatment of cancer by dichlorethylsulphide (mustard gas). *Annals of Surgery*, **93** (1), 190–199.

3 Rhoads, C. (1946) Nitrogen mustards in the treatment of neoplastic disease. *Journal of the American Medical Society*, **131**, 6568.

4 Jacobson, L.O., Spurr, C.L. *et al.* (1946) Studies on the effect of methyl bis (beta-chloroethyl) amine hydrochloride on diseases of the hemopoietic system. *Journal of Clinical Investigation*, **25** (6), 909.

5 DeVita, V.T., Hellman, S. & Rosenberg, S.A. (2005) *Cancer: Principles and Practice of Oncology*, 7th ed., J. Pine, J. Murphy & S. Sebring (eds). Lippincott Wiliams & Wilkins, Philadelphia, PA, USA.

6 Koppel, R.A. & Boh, E.E. (2001) Cutaneous reactions to chemotherapeutic agents. *American Journal of the Medical Sciences*, **321** (5), 327–335.

7 Alley, E., Green, R. & Schuchter, L. (2002) Cutaneous toxicities of cancer therapy. *Current Opinion in Oncology*, **14** (2), 212–216.

8 Ross, W.E. & Chabner, B.A. (1977) Allergic reaction to cyclophosphamide in a mechlorethamine-sensitive patient. *Cancer Treatment Reports*, **61** (3), 495–496.

9 Wilson, K.S. & Alexander, S. (1981) Hypersensitivity to mechlorethamine. *Annals of Internal Medicine*, **94** (6), 823.

10 Kim, Y.H. (2003) Management with topical nitrogen mustard in mycosis fungoides. *Dermatologic Therapy*, **16** (4), 288–298.

11 Van Scott, E.J. & Winters, P.L. (1970) Responses of mycosis fungoides to intensive external treatment with nitrogen mustard. *Archives of Dermatology*, **102** (5), 507–514.

12 Epstein, E. Jr. & Ugel, A.R. (1970) Effects of topical mechlorethamine on skin lesions of psoriasis. *Archives of Dermatology*, **102** (5), 504–506.

13 Bronner, A.K. & Hood, A.F. (1983) Cutaneous complications of chemotherapeutic agents. *Journal of the American Academy of Dermatology*, **9** (5), 645–663.

14 Mandy, S., Taylor, J.R. & Halprin, K. (1971) Topically applied mechlorethamine in the treatment of psoriasis. *Archives of Dermatology*, **103** (3), 272–276.

15 Flaxman, B.A., Sosis, A.C. & Van Scott, E.J. (1973) Changes in melanosome distribution in Caucasoid skin following topical application of nitrogen mustard. *Journal of Investigative Dermatology*, **60** (5), 321–326.

16 Fitzpatrick, J.E. & Hood, A.F. (1988) Histopathologic reactions to chemotherapeutic agents. *Advances in Dermatology*, **3**, 161–183.

17 Van Scott, E.J. & Kalmanson, J.D. (1973) Complete remissions of mycosis fungoides lymphoma induced by topical nitrogen mustard (HN2): control of delayed hypersensitivity to HN2 by desensitization and by induction of specific immunologic tolerance. *Cancer*, **32** (1), 18–30.

18 Leshaw, S., Simon, R.S. & Bear, R.L. (1977) Failure to induce tolerance to mechlorethamine hydrochloride. *Archives of Dermatology*, **113** (10), 1406–1408.

19 Waldorf, D.S., Haynes, H.A. & Van Scott, E.J. (1967) Cutaneous hypersensitivity and desensitization to mechlorethamine in patients with mycosis fungoides lymphoma. *Annals of Internal Medicine*, **67** (2), 282–290.

20 Vonderheid, E.C., Tan, E.T., Kantor, A.F., Shrager, L., Micaily, B. & Van Scott, E.J. (1989) Long-term efficacy, curative potential, and carcinogenicity of topical mechlorethamine chemotherapy in cutaneous T cell lymphoma. *Journal of the American Academy of Dermatology*, **20** (3), 416–428.

21 Abel, E.A., Sendagorta, E. & Hoppe, R.T. (1986) Cutaneous malignancies and metastatic squamous cell carcinoma following topical therapies for mycosis fungoides. *Journal of the American Academy of Dermatology*, **14** (6), 1029–1038.

22 Lee, L.A., Fritz, K.A., Golitz, L., Fritz, T.J. & Weston, W.L. (1982) Second cutaneous malignancies in patients with mycosis fungoides treated with topical nitrogen mustard. *Journal of the American Academy of Dermatology*, **7** (5), 590–598.

23 Philips, F.S., Sternberg, S.S., Cronin, A.P. & Vidal, P.M. (1961) Cyclophosphamide and urinary bladder toxicity. *Cancer Research*, **21**, 1577–1589.

24 Forni, A.M., Koss, L.G. & Geller, W. (1964) Cytological study of the effect of cyclophosphamide on the epithelium of the urinary bladder in man. *Cancer*, **17**, 1348–1355.

25 Cox, P.J. (1979) Cyclophosphamide cystitis: identification of acrolein as the causative agent. *Biochemical Pharmacology*, **28** (13), 2045–2049.

26 British Columbia Cancer Agency. (2004) Provincial System Therapy Program Policy III-20: Prevention and management of extravasation of chemotherapy. Available from: http://www.bccancer.bc.ca/NR/rdonlyres/B10C0DC3-D799-45E8-8A61-A93F00906737/59243/III_20_ExtravasationManagement_1Jun2013.pdf (accessed 16 May 2013).

27 USP DI. (2002) Cyclophosphamide. In: *Drug Information for the Health Care Professional*, 20th ed. Vol 1. Englewood, CO: Micromedex, Inc.

28 Rose, B.D. (ed.) (2005) *Cyclophosphamide: Drug information*, UpToDate, Wellesley, MA.

29 Balis, F.M., Holcenberg, J.S. & Bleyer, W.A. (1983) Clinical pharmacokinetics of commonly used anticancer drugs. *Clinical Pharmacokinetics*, **8** (3), 202–232.

30 DeSpain, J.D. (1992) Dermatologic toxicity of chemotherapy. *Seminars in Oncology*, **19** (5), 501–507.

31 Hood, A.F. & Haynes, H.A. (1983) Mucocutaneous complication of cancer chemotherapy. In: T. Fitzpatrick, A. Eisen & K. Wolff (eds), *Update: Dermatology in General Medicine*, pp. 80–97. McGraw-Hill, New York.

32 Hood, A.F. (1986) Cutaneous side effects of cancer chemotherapy. *Medical Clinics of North America*, **70** (1), 187–209.

33 Solidoro, A. & Saenz, R. (1966) Effects of cyclophosphamide (NSC-26271) on 127 patients with malignant lymphoma. *Cancer Chemotherapy Reports. Part 1*, **50** (5), 265–270.

34 Romankiewicz, J.A. (1974) Cyclophosphamide and pigmentation. *American Journal of Hospital Pharmacy*, **31** (11), 1074–1075.

35 Inalsingh, C.H. (1972) Melanonychia after treatment of malignant disease with radiation and cyclophosphamide. *Archives of Dermatology*, **106** (5), 765–766.

36 Shah, P.C., Rao, K.R. & Patel, A.R. (1975) Letter: cyclophosphamide-induced nail pigmentation. *Lancet*, **2** (7934), 548–549.

37 O'Doherty, C.S. (1975) Letter: hyperpigmentation after cancer chemotherapy. *Lancet*, **2** (7930), 365–366.

38 Susser, W.S., Whitaker-Worth, D.L. & Grant-Kels, J.M. (1999) Mucocutaneous reactions to chemotherapy. *Journal of the American Academy of Dermatology*, **40** (3), 367–398; quiz 399–400.

39 Harrison, B.M. & Wood, C.B. (1972) Cyclophosphamide and pigmentation. *British Medical Journal*, **2** (5809), 352.

40 Lakin, J.D. & Cahill, R.A. (1976) Generalized urticaria to cyclophosphamide: type I hypersensitivity to an immunosuppressive agent. *Journal of Allergy and Clinical Immunology*, **58** (1 Pt 2), 160–171.

41 Krutchik, A.N., Buzdar, A.U. & Tashima, C.K. (1978) Cyclophosphamide-induced urticaria: occurrence in a patient with no cross-sensitivity to chlorambucil. *Archives of Internal Medicine*, **138** (11), 1725–1726.

42 Legha, S.S. & Hall, S. (1978) Acute cyclophosphamide hypersensitivity reaction: possible lack of cross-sensitivity to mechlorethamine and isophosphamide. *Cancer Treatment Reports*, **62** (1), 180–181.

43 Kim, H.C., Kesarwala, H.H., Colvin, M. & Saidi, P. (1985) Hypersensitivity reaction to a metabolite of cyclophosphamide. *Journal of Allergy and Clinical Immunology*, **76** (4), 591–594.

44 Guhl, G., Diaz-Ley, B., García-García, C., Fraga, J. & Garcia-Diez, A. (2009) Chemotherapy-induced subacute lupus erythematosus. *Lupus*, **18** (9), 859–860.

45 Branzan, A.L., Landthaler, M. & Szeimies, R.M. (2005) Skin changes with chemotherapy. *Der Hautarzt; Zeitschrift fur Dermatologie, Venerologie, und Verwandte Gebiete*, **56** (6), 591–602; quiz 603.

46 Burgin, S. (2005) New drugs, new rashes: update on cutaneous drug reactions. *Advances in Dermatology*, **21**, 279–302.

47 Prussick, R., Horn, T.D., Wilson, W.H. & Turner, M.C. (1996) A characteristic eruption associated with ifosfamide, carboplatin, and etoposide chemotherapy after pretreatment with recombinant interleukin-1 alpha. *Journal of the American Academy of Dermatology*, **35** (5 Pt 1), 705–709.

48 Linassier, C., Colombat, P., Reisenleiter, M. et al. (1990) Cutaneous toxicity of autologous bone marrow transplantation in nonseminomatous germ cell tumors. *Cancer*, **65** (5), 1143–1145.

49 Singal, R., Tunnessen, W.W. Jr., Wiley, J.M. & Hood, A.F. (1991) Discrete pigmentation after chemotherapy. *Pediatric Dermatology*, **8** (3), 231–235.

50 Beyer, J., Grabbe, J., Lenz, K. et al. (1992) Cutaneous toxicity of high-dose carboplatin, etoposide and ifosfamide followed by autologous stem cell reinfusion. *Bone Marrow Transplantation*, **10** (6), 491–494.

51 Norda, A., Loos, U., Sastry, M., Goehl, J. & Hohenberger, W. (1999) Pharmacokinetics of melphalan in isolated limb perfusion. *Cancer Chemotherapy and Pharmacology*, **43** (1), 35–42.

52 Malacarne, P. & Zavagli, G. (1977) Melphalan-induced melanonychia striata. *Archives of Dermatological Research*, **258** (1), 81–83.

53 Lawrence, B.V. (1980) Anaphylaxis due to oral melphalan. *Cancer Treatment Reports*, **64** (4–5), 731–732.

54 Cornwell, G.G. 3rd, Pajak, T.F. & McIntyre, O.R. (1979) Hypersensitivity reactions to IV melphalan during treatment of multiple myeloma: Cancer and Leukemia Group B experience. *Cancer Treatment Reports*, **63** (3), 399–403.

55 Vrouenraets, B.C., Kroon, B.B., Klaase, J.M., Nieweg, O.E., van Slooten, G.W. & van Dongen, J.A. (1995) Severe acute regional toxicity after normothermic or 'mild' hyperthermic isolated limb perfusion with melphalan for melanoma. *Melanoma Research*, **5** (6), 425–431.

56 Landau, M., Brenner, S., Gat, A., Klausner, J.M. & Gutman, M. (1998) Reticulate scleroderma after isolated limb perfusion with melphalan. *Journal of the American Academy of Dermatology*, **39** (6), 1011–1012.

57 Branten, A.J., Reichert, L.J., Koene, R.A. & Wetzels, J.F. (1998) Oral cyclophosphamide versus chlorambucil in the treatment of patients with membranous nephropathy and renal insufficiency. *QJM: Monthly Journal of the Association of Physicians*, **91** (5), 359–366.

58 Weiss, R.B. (1992) Hypersensitivity reactions. *Seminars in Oncology*, **19** (5), 458–477.

59 Knisley, R.E., Settipane, G.A. & Albala, M.M. (1971) Unusual reaction to chlorambucil in a patient with chronic lymphocytic leukemia. *Archives of Dermatology*, **104** (1), 77–79.

60 Millard, L.G. & Rajah, S.M. (1977) Cutaneous reaction to chlorambucil. *Archives of Dermatology*, **113** (9), 1298.

61 Peterman, A. & Braunstein, B. (1986) Cutaneous reaction to chlorambucil therapy. *Archives of Dermatology*, **122** (12), 1358–1360.

62 Hitchins, R.N., Hocker, G.A. & Thomson, D.B. (1987) Chlorambucil allergy: a series of three cases. *Australian and New Zealand Journal of Medicine*, **17** (6), 600–602.

63 Pietrantonio, F., Moriconi, L., Torino, F., Romano, A. & Gargovich, A. (1990) Unusual reaction to chlorambucil: a case report. *Cancer Letters*, **54** (3), 109–111.

64 Zervas, J., Karkantaris, C., Kapiri, E., Theocharis, S. & Konstantopoulos, K. (1992) Allergic reaction to chlorambucil in chronic lymphocytic leukaemia: case report. *Leukemia Research*, **16** (3), 329–330.

65 Thompson-Moya, L., Martin, T., Heuft, H.G., Neubauer, A. & Herrmann, R. (1989) Allergic reaction with immune hemolytic anemia resulting from chlorambucil. *American Journal of Hematology*, **32** (3), 230–231.

66 Levin, M. & Libster, D. (2005) Allergic reaction to chlorambucil in chronic lymphocytic leukemia presenting with fever and lymphadenopathy. *Leukemia and Lymphoma*, **46** (8), 1195–1197.

67 Barone, C., Cassano, A. & Astone, A. (1990) Toxic epidermal necrolysis during chlorambucil therapy in chronic lymphocytic leukaemia. *European Journal of Cancer*, **26** (11–12), 1262.

68 Torricelli, R., Kurer, S.B., Kroner, T. & Wüthrich, B. (1995) Delayed allergic reaction to Chlorambucil (Leukeran): case report and literature review. *Schweizerische Medizinische Wochenschrift*, **125** (40), 1870–1873.

69 Vaida, I., Roszkiewicz, F., Gruson, B., Makdassi, R. & Damaj, G. (2009) Drug rash with eosinophilia and systemic symptoms after chlorambucil treatment in chronic lymphocytic leukaemia. *Pharmacology*, **83** (3), 148–149.

70 Tas, S. & Simonart, T. (2003) Management of drug rash with eosinophilia and systemic symptoms (DRESS syndrome): an update. *Dermatology (Basel, Switzerland)*, **206** (4), 353–356.

71 Antman, K., Eder, J.P., Elias, A. et al. (1990) High-dose thiotepa alone and in combination regimens with bone marrow support. *Seminars in Oncology*, **17** (1 Suppl. 3), 33–38.

72 Dimopoulos, M.A., Alexanian, R., Przepiorka, D. et al. (1993) Thiotepa, busulfan, and cyclophosphamide: a new preparative regimen for autologous marrow or blood stem cell transplantation in high-risk multiple myeloma. *Blood*, **82** (8), 2324–2328.

73 Greenspan, E.M., Jaffrey, I. & Bruckner, H. (1977) Thiotepa, cutaneous reactions, and efficacy. *Journal of the American Medical Association*, **237** (21), 2288.

74 Veenema, R.J., Dean, A.L. Jr., Uson, A.C., Roberts, M. & Longo, F. (1969) Thiotepa bladder instillations: therapy and prophylaxis for superficial bladder tumors. *Journal of Urology*, **101** (5), 711–715.

75 Horn, T.D., Beveridge, R.A., Egorin, M.J., Abeloff, M.D. & Hood, A.F. (1989) Observations and proposed mechanism of N,N′,N″-triethylenethiophosphoramide (thiotepa)-induced hyperpigmentation. *Archives of Dermatology*, **125** (4), 524–527.

76 Saarinen, U.M., Hovi, L., Mäkipernaa, A. & Riikonen, P. (1991) High-dose thiotepa with autologous bone marrow rescue in pediatric solid tumors. *Bone Marrow Transplantation*, **8** (5), 369–376.

77 Lucidarme, N., Valteau-Couanet, D., Oberlin, O. *et al.* (1998) Phase II study of high-dose thiotepa and hematopoietic stem cell transplantation in children with solid tumors. *Bone Marrow Transplantation*, **22** (6), 535–540.

78 Finlay, J.L., Goldman, S., Wong, M.C. *et al.* (1996) Pilot study of high-dose thiotepa and etoposide with autologous bone marrow rescue in children and young adults with recurrent CNS tumors. The Children's Cancer Group. *Journal of Clinical Oncology*, **14** (9), 2495–2503.

79 Przepiorka, D., Dimopoulos, M., Smith, T. *et al.* (1994) Thiotepa, busulfan, and cyclophosphamide as a preparative regimen for marrow transplantation: risk factors for early regimen-related toxicity. *Annals of Hematology*, **68** (4), 183–188.

80 Finlay, J.L., August, C., Packer, R. *et al.* (1990) High-dose multi-agent chemotherapy followed by bone marrow 'rescue' for malignant astrocytomas of childhood and adolescence. *Journal of Neuro-Oncology*, **9** (3), 239–248.

81 Dunkel, I.J. & Finlay, J.L. (1996) High dose chemotherapy with autologous stem cell rescue for patients with medulloblastoma. *Journal of Neuro-Oncology*, **29** (1), 69–74.

82 Wolff, S.N., Herzig, R.H., Fay, J.W. *et al.* (1990) High-dose N,N′,N″-triethylenethiophosphoramide (thiotepa) with autologous bone marrow transplantation: phase I studies. *Seminars in Oncology*, **17** (1 Suppl. 3), 2–6.

83 Rosman, I.S., Lloyd, B.M., Hayashi, R.J. & Bayliss, S.J. (2008) Cutaneous effects of thiotepa in pediatric patients receiving high-dose chemotherapy with autologous stem cell transplantation. *Journal of the American Academy of Dermatology*, **58** (4), 575–578.

84 Horn, T.D. (1997) Antineoplastic chemotherapy, sweat, and the skin. *Archives of Dermatology*, **133** (7), 905–906.

85 Khong, J.J. & Muecke, J. (2006) Complications of mitomycin C therapy in 100 eyes with ocular surface neoplasia. *British Journal of Ophthalmology*, **90** (7), 819–822.

86 Tennyson, H., Helling, E.R., Wiseman, J., Dick, E. & Lyons, R.C. (2007) The effect of topical mitomycin C on full-thickness burns. *Plastic and Reconstructive Surgery*, **120** (4), 879–886.

87 Warner, D. & Brietzke, S.E. (2008) Mitomycin C and airway surgery: how well does it work? *Otolaryngology and Head and Neck Surgery*, **138** (6), 700–709.

88 Roh, J.L., Koo, B.S., Yoon, Y.H., Rha, K.S. & Park, C.I. (2005) Effect of topical mitomycin C on the healing of surgical and laser wounds: a hint on clinical application. *Otolaryngology and Head and Neck Surgery*, **133** (6), 851–856.

89 Wyatt, A.J., Leonard, G.D. & Sachs, D.L. (2006) Cutaneous reactions to chemotherapy and their management. *American Journal of Clinical Dermatology*, **7** (1), 45–63.

90 Rentschler, R. & Wilbur, D. (1988) Pyridoxine: a potential local antidote for Mitomycin-C extravasation. *Journal of Surgical Oncology*, **37** (4), 269–271.

91 Khanna, A.K., Khanna, A., Asthana, A.K. & Misra, M.K. (1985) Mitomycin C extravasation ulcers. *Journal of Surgical Oncology*, **28** (2), 108–110.

92 Kunkeler, L., Nieboer, C. & Bruynzeel, D.P. (2000) Type III and type IV hypersensitivity reactions due to mitomycin C. *Contact Dermatitis*, **42** (2), 74–76.

93 Colver, G.B., Inglis, J.A., McVittie, E., Spencer, M.J., Tolley, D.A. & Hunter, J.A. (1990) Dermatitis due to intravesical mitomycin C: a delayed-type hypersensitivity reaction? *British Journal of Dermatology*, **122** (2), 217–224.

94 Gomez Torrijos, E., Borja, J., Galindo, P.A. *et al.* (1997) Allergic contact dermatitis from mitomycin C. *Allergy*, **52** (6), 687.

95 McCune, J.S. & Holmberg, L.A. (2009) Busulfan in hematopoietic stem cell transplant setting. *Expert Opinion on Drug Metabolism and Toxicology*, **5** (8), 957–969.

96 Ljungman, P., Hassan, M., Békássy, A.N., Ringdén, O. & Oberg, G. (1995) Busulfan concentration in relation to permanent alopecia in recipients of bone marrow transplants. *Bone Marrow Transplantation*, **15** (6), 869–871.

97 Feingold, M.L. & Koss, L.G. (1969) Effects of long-term administration of busulfan. Report of a patient with generalized nuclear abnormalities, carcinoma of vulva, and pulmonary fibrosis. *Archives of Internal Medicine*, **124** (1), 66–71.

98 Haddow, A. & Timmis, G.M. (1953) Myleran in chronic myeloid leukaemia; chemical constitution and biological action. *Lancet*, **264** (6753), 207–208.

99 Haut, A. *et al.* (1961) Busulfan in the treatment of chronic myelocytic leukemia. The effect of long term intermittent therapy. *Blood*, **17**, 1–19.

100 Harrold, B.P. (1966) Syndrome resembling Addison's disease following prolonged treatment with busulphan. *British Medical Journal*, **1** (5485), 463–464.

101 Hymes, S.R., Simonton, S.C., Farmer, E.R., Beschorner, W.B., Tutschka, P.J. & Santos, G.W. (1985) Cutaneous busulfan effect in patients receiving bone-marrow transplantation. *Journal of Cutaneous Pathology*, **12** (2), 125–129.

102 Burns, W.A., McFarland, W. & Matthews, M.J. (1971) Toxic manifestations of busulfan therapy. *Medical Annals of the District of Columbia*, **40** (9), 567–572.

103 Kyle, R.A. & Dameshek, W. (1964) Porphyria cutanea tarda associated with chronic granulocytic leukemia treated with busulfan (Myleran). *Blood*, **23**, 776–785.

104 Kamil, N., Kamil, S., Ahmed, S.P., Ashraf, R., Khurram, M. & Ali, M.O. (2010) Toxic effects of multiple anticancer drugs on skin. *Pakistan Journal of Pharmaceutical Sciences*, **23** (1), 7–14.

105 Adrian, R.M., Hood, A.F. & Skarin, A.T. (1980) Mucocutaneous reactions to antineoplastic agents. *CA: A Cancer Journal for Clinicians*, **30** (3), 143–157.

106 Zackheim, H.S. (2003) Topical carmustine (BCNU) in the treatment of mycosis fungoides. *Dermatologic Therapy*, **16** (4), 299–302.

107 Zackheim, H.S., Epstein, E.H. Jr. & Crain, W.R. (1990) Topical carmustine (BCNU) for cutaneous T cell lymphoma: a 15-year experience in 143 patients. *Journal of the American Academy of Dermatology*, **22** (5 Pt 1), 802–810.

108 Zackheim, H.S., Epstein, E.H. Jr., McNutt, N.S., Grekin, D.A. & Crain, W.R. (1983) Topical carmustine (BCNU) for mycosis fungoides and related disorders: a 10-year experience. *Journal of the American Academy of Dermatology*, **9** (3), 363–374.

109 Frost, P. & DeVita, V.T. (1966) Pigmentation due to a new antitumor agent. Effects of topical application of BCNU [1,3-bis(2-chloroethyl)-1-nitrosourea]. *Archives of Dermatology*, **94** (3), 265–268.

110 Syrigou, E., Makrilia, N., Koti, I., Saif, M.W. & Syrigos, K.N. (2009) Hypersensitivity reactions to antineoplastic agents: an overview. *Anti-Cancer Drugs*, **20** (1), 1–6.

111 Pagani, M. (2010) The complex clinical picture of presumably allergic side effects to cytostatic drugs: symptoms, pathomechanism,

reexposure, and desensitization. *Medical Clinics of North America*, **94** (4), 835–852, xiii.

112 Lee, C., Gianos, M. & Klaustermeyer, W.B. (2009) Diagnosis and management of hypersensitivity reactions related to common cancer chemotherapy agents. *Annals of Allergy, Asthma and Immunology*, **102** (3), 179–187; quiz 187–189, 222.

113 Coyle, T., Bushunow, P., Winfield, J., Wright, J. & Graziano, S. (1992) Hypersensitivity reactions to procarbazine with mechlorethamine, vincristine, and procarbazine chemotherapy in the treatment of glioma. *Cancer*, **69** (10), 2532–2540.

114 Lehmann, D.F., Hurteau, T.E., Newman, N. & Coyle, T.E. (1997) Anticonvulsant usage is associated with an increased risk of procarbazine hypersensitivity reactions in patients with brain tumors. *Clinical Pharmacology and Therapeutics*, **62** (2), 225–229.

115 Giguere, J.K., Douglas, D.M., Lupton, G.P., Baker, J.R. & Weiss, R.B. (1988) Procarbazine hypersensitivity manifested as a fixed drug eruption. *Medical and Pediatric Oncology*, **16** (6), 378–380.

116 Serrone, L., Zeuli, M., Sega, F.M. & Cognetti, F. (2000) Dacarbazine-based chemotherapy for metastatic melanoma: thirty-year experience overview. *Journal of Experimental and Clinical Cancer Research*, **19** (1), 21–34.

117 Levy, A., Guitera, P., Kerob, D. *et al.* (2006) Hypersensitivity to dacarbazine in patients with metastatic malignant melanoma. *Annales de Dermatologie et de Venereologie*, **133** (2), 157–160.

118 Shepherd, G.M. (2003) Hypersensitivity reactions to chemotherapeutic drugs. *Clinical Reviews in Allergy and Immunology*, **24** (3), 253–262.

119 Beck, T.M., Hart, N.E. & Smith, C.E. (1980) Photosensitivity reaction following DTIC administration: report of two cases. *Cancer Treatment Reports*, **64** (4–5), 725–726.

120 Yung, C.W., Winston, E.M. & Lorincz, A.L. (1981) Dacarbazine-induced photosensitivity reaction. *Journal of the American Academy of Dermatology*, **4** (5), 541–543.

121 Treudler, R., Georgieva, J., Geilen, C.C. & Orfanos, C.E. (2004) Dacarbazine but not temozolomide induces phototoxic dermatitis in patients with malignant melanoma. *Journal of the American Academy of Dermatology*, **50** (5), 783–785.

122 Kennedy, R.D. & McAleer, J.J. (2001) Radiation recall dermatitis in a patient treated with dacarbazine. *Clinical Oncology (Royal College of Radiologists (Great Britain))*, **13** (6), 470–472.

123 Johnson, T.M., Rapini, R.P. & Duvic, M. (1987) Inflammation of actinic keratoses from systemic chemotherapy. *Journal of the American Academy of Dermatology*, **17** (2 Pt 1), 192–197.

124 Boyd, A.S. & Neldner, K.H. (1991) Hydroxyurea therapy. *Journal of the American Academy of Dermatology*, **25** (3), 518–524.

125 Salmon-Ehr, V., Leborgne, G., Vilque, J.P., Potron, G. & Bernard, P. (2000) Secondary cutaneous effects of hydroxyurea: prospective study of 26 patients from a dermatologic consultation. *Revue de Medecine Interne*, **21** (1), 30–34.

126 Layton, A.M., Sheehan-Dare, R.A., Goodfield, M.J. & Cotterill, J.A. (1989) Hydroxyurea in the management of therapy resistant psoriasis. *British Journal of Dermatology*, **121** (5), 647–653.

127 Kennedy, B.J., Smith, L.R. & Goltz, R.W. (1975) Skin changes secondary to hydroxyurea therapy. *Archives of Dermatology*, **111** (2), 183–187.

128 Kumar, B., Saraswat, A. & Kaur, I. (2002) Mucocutaneous adverse effects of hydroxyurea: a prospective study of 30 psoriasis patients. *Clinical and Experimental Dermatology*, **27** (1), 8–13.

129 Hernandez-Martin, A., Ros-Forteza, S. & de Unamuno, P. (1999) Longitudinal, transverse, and diffuse nail hyperpigmentation induced by hydroxyurea. *Journal of the American Academy of Dermatology*, **41** (2 Pt 2), 333–334.

130 Dahl, M.G. & Comaish, J.S. (1972) Long-term effects of hydroxyurea in psoriases. *British Medical Journal*, **4** (5840), 585–587.

131 Moschella, S.L. & Greenwald, M.A. (1973) Psoriasis with hydroxyurea. An 18-month study of 60 patients. *Archives of Dermatology*, **107** (3), 363–368.

132 Hendrix, J.D. Jr. & Greer, K.E. (1992) Cutaneous hyperpigmentation caused by systemic drugs. *International Journal of Dermatology*, **31** (7), 458–466.

133 Sigal, M., Crickx, B., Blanchet, P., Perron, J., Simony, J. & Belaïch, S. (1984) Cutaneous lesions induced by long-term use of hydroxyurea. *Annales de Dermatologie et de Venereologie*, **111** (10), 895–900.

134 Kelsey, P.R. (1992) Multiple longitudinal pigmented nail bands during hydroxyurea therapy. *Clinical and Laboratory Haematology*, **14** (4), 337–338.

135 Vomvouras, S., Pakula, A.S. & Shaw, J.M. (1991) Multiple pigmented nail bands during hydroxyurea therapy: an uncommon finding. *Journal of the American Academy of Dermatology*, **24** (6 Pt 1), 1016–1017.

136 Pirard, C., Michaux, J.L. & Bourlond, A. (1994) Longitudinal melanonychia and hydroxyurea. *Annales de Dermatologie et de Venereologie*, **121** (2), 106–109.

137 Delmas-Marsalet, B., Beaulieu, P., Teillet-Thiebaud, F., Jary, L. & Teillet, F. (1995) Longitudinal melanonychia induced by hydroxyurea: four case reports and review of the literature. *Nouvelle Revue Francaise d'Hematologie*, **37** (3), 205–210.

138 Kwong, Y.L. (1996) Hydroxyurea-induced nail pigmentation. *Journal of the American Academy of Dermatology*, **35** (2 Pt 1), 275–276.

139 Cakir, B., Sucak, G. & Haznedar, R. (1997) Longitudinal pigmented nail bands during hydroxyurea therapy. *International Journal of Dermatology*, **36** (3), 236–237.

140 Gropper, C.A., Don, P.C. & Sadjadi, M.M. (1993) Nail and skin hyperpigmentation associated with hydroxyurea therapy for polycythemia vera. *International Journal of Dermatology*, **32** (10), 731–733.

141 Varma, S. & Lanigan, S.W. (1999) Dermatomyositis-like eruption and leg ulceration caused by hydroxyurea in a patient with psoriasis. *Clinical and Experimental Dermatology*, **24** (3), 164–166.

142 Antonioli, E., Guglielmelli, P., Pieri, L. *et al.* (2012) Hydroxyurea-related toxicity in 3,411 patients with Ph'-negative MPN. *Americal Journal of Hematology*, **87**(5), 552–554.

143 Best, P.J., Daoud, M.S., Pittelkow, M.R. & Petitt, R.M. (1998) Hydroxyurea-induced leg ulceration in 14 patients. *Annals of Internal Medicine*, **128** (1), 29–32.

144 Haniffa, M.A. & Speight, E.L. (2006) Painful leg ulcers and a rash in a patient with polycythaemia rubra vera. Diagnosis: hydroxyurea-induced leg ulceration and dermatomyositis-like skin changes. *Clinical and Experimental Dermatology*, **31** (5), 733–734.

145 Daoud, M.S., Gibson, L.E. & Pittelkow, M.R. (1997) Hydroxyurea dermopathy: a unique lichenoid eruption complicating long-term therapy with hydroxyurea. *Journal of the American Academy of Dermatology*, **36** (2 Pt 1), 178–182.

146 Vassallo, C., Passamonti, F., Merante, S. *et al.* (2001) Muco-cutaneous changes during long-term therapy with hydroxyurea in chronic

myeloid leukaemia. *Clinical and Experimental Dermatology*, **26** (2), 141–148.

147 Eming, S.A., Peters, T., Hartmann, K., Scharffetter-Kochanek, K. & Mahrle, G. (2001) Lichenoid chronic graft-versus-host disease-like acrodermatitis induced by hydroxyurea. *Journal of the American Academy of Dermatology*, **45** (2), 321–323.

148 Senet, P., Aractingi, S., Porneuf, M., Perrin, P. & Duterque, M. (1995) Hydroxyurea-induced dermatomyositis-like eruption. *British Journal of Dermatology*, **133** (3), 455–459.

149 Callot-Mellot, C., Bodemer, C., Chosidow, O. *et al.* (1996) Cutaneous carcinoma during long-term hydroxyurea therapy: a report of 5 cases. *Archives of Dermatology*, **132** (11), 1395–1397.

150 Esteve, E., Georgescu, V., Heitzmann, P. & Martin, L. (2001) Multiple skin and mouth squamous cell carcinomas related to long-term treatment with hydroxyurea. *Annales de Dermatologie et de Venereologie*, **128** (8–9), 919–921.

151 De Benedittis, M., Petruzzi, M., Giardina, C., Lo Muzio, L., Favia, G. & Serpico, R. (2004) Oral squamous cell carcinoma during long-term treatment with hydroxyurea. *Clinical and Experimental Dermatology*, **29** (6), 605–607.

152 Sanchez-Palacios, C. & Guitart, J. (2004) Hydroxyurea-associated squamous dysplasia. *Journal of the American Academy of Dermatology*, **51** (2), 293–300.

153 Zaccaria, E., Cozzani, E. & Parodi, A. (2006) Secondary cutaneous effects of hydroxyurea: possible pathogenetic mechanisms. *Journal of Dermatological Treatment*, **17** (3), 176–178.

154 http://www.drugs.com/ppa/temozolomide.html (accessed 24 July 2013).

15 Antimetabolite Reactions

Emily Y. Chu and Heidi H. Kong

Dermatology Branch, National Cancer Institute, National Institutes of Health, Bethesda, MD, USA

Introduction

Antimetabolites are cytostatic agents that inhibit the use of natural chemicals in normal cellular biosynthetic reactions. These agents are often structurally similar to their endogenous target metabolites. Antimetabolites interfere with DNA and RNA synthesis, and as a result block cell division and tumor growth. They may be classified into one of three groups:
1. Folate antagonists (methotrexate, pemetrexed);
2. Pyrimidine analogs (capecitabine, fluorouracil, cytarabine, gemcitabine); and
3. Purine analogs (mercaptopurine, thioguanine, fludarabine, cladribine) (Figure 15.1; Tables 15.1 and Table 15.2).

Methotrexate

Methotrexate is commonly utilized as a component of regimens targeting both solid and hematologic malignancies. Methotrexate is a competitive inhibitor of the enzyme dihydrofolate reductase, which is essential for the synthesis of purine and thymidylate nucleotides required for assembling molecules of DNA and RNA. In addition, methotrexate partially inhibits the enzyme thymidylate synthetase, thereby blocking cell division. Methotrexate has been associated with a number of mucocutaneous adverse events (AEs), including hand-foot syndrome (HFS), skin ulceration, photo-recall reactions, photosensitivity, mucositis/stomatitis, reversible alopecia, and nail dystrophy.

Methotrexate is a relatively infrequent cause of chemotherapy-induced HFS. Administration of high-dose methotrexate for treatment of different types of malignancies has been shown to lead to tender inflamed palmo-plantar lesions in both adults and children [1–7], especially over pressure points [2]. In many of the reported cases, bullous reactions were observed [1,2,5,7]. HFS has been reported to arise after 24–72 hours of treatment, and up to 15 days after completion of therapy [1–4]. Histologic features include subepidermal bullae, keratinocyte necrosis, and perivascular lymphocytic inflammation [1,2]. HFS has been shown to respond to systemic steroid treatment and local wound care [7].

A well-documented AE of methotrexate treatment is cutaneous ulceration, most commonly occurring in plaques of psoriasis, but it can also occur in unaffected skin [8,9]. Several risk factors have been associated with the development of cutaneous toxicity, including initiation of therapy, dose escalation, co-administration with nonsteroidal anti-inflammatory drugs (NSAIDs), infection, and older age. Monitoring of methotrexate levels may therefore be helpful in determining the risk of developing cutaneous ulceration [10].

Photo-recall is a cutaneous AE in which areas of skin previously exposed to ultraviolet radiation develop significant erythema, mimicking the previously experienced photodermatitis [11]. The diagnosis is often made clinically, but characteristic features on biopsy include the presence of necrotic keratinocytes and superficial mild perivascular inflammation [11,12].

Oral mucositis commonly occurs, and empirical clinical experiences suggest that folic acid supplementation, dose splitting, and intravenous or intramuscular injection rather than oral therapy can ameliorate this AE [13,14].

Pemetrexed

Pemetrexed is a novel folate antagonist, which is indicated for use in combination with cisplatin for the treatment of mesothelioma and nonsmall cell lung cancer. It is a competitive inhibitor of

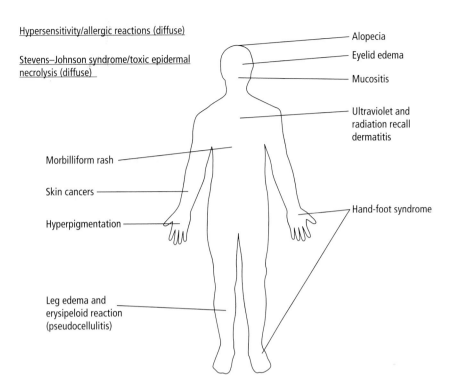

Figure 15.1 Location of antimetabolite-induced dermatologic toxicities.

Table 15.1 Classification of antimetabolites.

Folate antagonist	Methotrexate
	Pemetrexed
Pyrimidine analog	Capecitabine (prodrug of fluorouracil)
	Cytarabine
	Gemcitabine
Purine analog	Mercaptopurine
	Thioguanine
	Fludarabine
	Cladribine

reduced folate, inhibiting the activity of three enzymes involved in purine and pyrimidine synthesis: dihydrofolate reductase, thymidylate synthase, and glycinamide ribonucleotide formyl-transferase [15].

Rash has been frequently attributed to pemetrexed, with the rate of grade 3 or 4 skin toxicity ranging between 1% and 31% [16–18]. The occurrence of morbilliform drug eruptions has been suggested [19]. One case of acute generalized exanthematous pustulosis [20], and one case of Lyell syndrome (toxic epidermolytic necrosis) have been linked to pemetrexed [21].

Radiation recall dermatitis appears to be the most frequently reported cutaneous AE of pemetrexed [22–25]. The severity of reactions observed range from mild blanchable erythema to severe soft tissue necrosis within previous fields of irradiation [24,26], and topical and systemic steroids have anecdotally been reported to be effective [22,24].

Eyelid edema has been documented as a rare AE, with two published cases and a third cited in the Investigator's Brochure (April 2005) [19,25]. A patient developed edema of the eyelids only 8 days after initial treatment with pemetrexed. The edema responded to a course of dexamethasone, but reappeared with subsequent cycles. Similarly, leg edema occurred 10 days after initial administration, which recurred with additional cycles. The mechanism underlying this phenomenon is unknown.

Capecitabine

Capecitabine is a pro-drug of 5-fluorouracil that inhibits DNA synthesis in tumor cells, and is approved for treatment of metastatic breast and colon cancer. HFS/acral erythema (Figure 15.2) is the most commonly cited cutaneous AE, which may be a marker of antitumor efficacy [27]. A notable AE is the loss of fingerprints secondary to HFS, resulting in difficulty passing through airport customs [28]. Of 34 patients treated with capecitabine, 15 developed HFS [29], three with grade 3 and four with grade 2 reactions were able to continue therapy with dose reductions, dose discontinuation was required in one patient. In a case series of 10 patients, topical henna resulted in resolution of erythema within 1 week in eight patients (including three patients with grade 3 reactions), and partial response in the remaining two patients [30]. Celecoxib prevents HFS.

Cutaneous hyperpigmentation has been observed, including repigmentation within areas of pre-existing vitiligo (Figure 15.3) [31–33]. Longitudinal melanonychia has also been observed with

Table 15.2 Incidence of dermatologic adverse events to antimetabolites.

Drug name	Information source	Dermatologic adverse events			Nail changes	Hair modifications	Mucous membranes
		Cutaneous and subcutaneous toxicities					
Methotrexate	Package insert [114]	Rash: All: up to 10%		Photosensitivity All: ~3–10%		Alopecia: All: ~3–10%	Mucositis/stomatitis All: ~3–10%
Pemetrexed (Alimta)	Clarke et al. [16]	Rash /desquamation All: 100% Grade 3 or 4: 31%				Alopecia: 100% Grade 3 or 4: 0%	Mucositis/stomatitis All: 100% Grade 3 or 4: 5%
	Hanna et al. [17]	Rash All: 14% Grade 3 or 4: 1%				Alopecia: All: 6.4% Grade 3 or 4: 0%	Stomatitis All: 14.7% Grade 3 or 4: 1%
	Martin et al. [18]	Rash All: 59% Grade 3 or 4: 10%				Alopecia All: 21% Grade 3 or 4: 0%	Mucositis All: 37% Grade 3 or 4: 5%
Capecitabine (Xeloda)	Package insert [35]	Hand-foot syndrome All: 54% Grade 3 or 4: 17%	Dermatitis All: 27% Grade 3 or 4: 1%	Skin discoloration All: 7% Grade 3 or 4: <1%	Onycho-dystrophy All: 7%	Alopecia: All: 6% Grade 3 or 4: 0%	Stomatitis All: 25% Grade 3 or 4: 2%
Cytarabine	Cetkovska et al. [36]	Rash (including morbilliform eruptions, hand-foot syndrome, and other) All: ~50%					
	Lit [115]					Alopecia: All: 1–10%	Oral ulcerations All: >10%
							Perianal ulcerations All: >10%
Gemcitabine	Package insert [116]	Rash: All: up to 30% Grade 3 or 4: <1%		Pruritus: All: up to 13%		Alopecia: All: 15% Grade 3 or 4: <1%	Stomatitis: All: 10% Grade 3 or 4: <1%
	Chen et al. [58]	Edema: All: up to 20% Grade 3–4: <3%					
	Jeter et al. [72]	Photo-recall: All: up to 74%					
Mercaptopurine	Andersen et al. [82]	Rash: All: <1%					
	Cox et al. [77]	Hand-foot syndrome: All: up to 10%					
Thioguanine	Zackheim et al. [91]	Rash: All: <3%		Multiple skin cancers: All: <3%			Mucositis: All: <1%
	Zimm et al. [92]	Photosensitivity: All: <25%					
Fludarabine	Package insert [95]	Rash: All: up to 15%	Transfusion-associated graft-vs-host disease: All: <1%	Worsening of skin cancers: All: <1%			Mucositis: All: up to 9%
Cladribine	Package insert [104]	Rash: All: 27%	Injection site reactions: All: 19%	Pruritus: All: 6%			

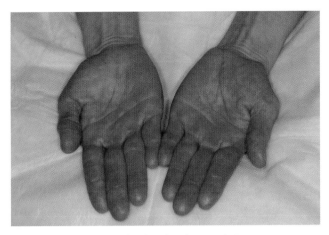

Figure 15.2 Capecitabine-induced acral erythema grade 1.

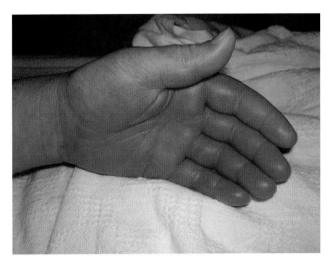

Figure 15.4 Cytarabine-induced acral erythema grade 2.

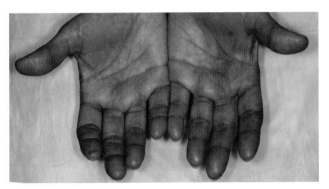

Figure 15.3 Hyperpigmentation to capecitabine grade 1.

Two cases of toxic epidermal necrolysis were reported in pediatric patients treated with intermediate [47] and high-dose [48] cytarabine. The reaction developed after the second and fifth days of treatment with both cases resulting in fatality.

Gemcitabine

Gemcitabine is a pyrimidine analog indicated for the treatment of ovarian, breast, nonsmall cell lung, and pancreatic cancers. The most common skin toxicities are rash (30%), edema (13–20%), pruritus (13%), alopecia (15%) [49,50], and photo-recall (<74%). Less frequently, HFS/acral erythema, an erysipeloid rash confined to edematous skin, localized skin sclerosis, linear immunoglobulin A (IgA) bullous dermatosis (Figure 15.5) [51], mucositis [52], pseudolymphoma [53], and anal pruritus occur [54]. Patients may rarely (<1%) experience more serious cutaneous toxicities including distal necrosis [55,56] and Stevens–Johnson syndrome/ toxic epidermal necrolysis (SJS/TEN) [57].

A transient fine pruritic maculopapular eruption over the trunk and extremities is reported in 30% of patients, developing [58] within 3–4 days of initiation. The eruption can be controlled with systemic antihistamines and corticosteroids despite continuation of therapy [58,59]. Cutaneous eruptions on rare occasions may be severe, requiring discontinuation of treatment. Histology of skin lesions may rarely suggest pseudolymphoma, but clinical history is important in ruling out this diagnosis [53].

Edema affects up to 20% of patients, with less than 3% experiencing severe edema [60]. It is generally not associated with cardiac, hepatic, or renal failure; however, rare cases (<1%) of fatal pulmonary edema have been reported [61]. In cases of generalized edema with dyspnea, discontinuation of gemcitabine with possible lung biopsy may be indicated [61]. Patients may develop bullae in addition to the peripheral edema [62]. High-dose systemic steroids may decrease and prevent severe generalized edema with subsequent infusions [61,63].

capecitabine therapy [34], as well as mucositis/stomatitis (25%), reversible alopecia (6%), and onychodystrophy (7%) [35].

Cytarabine

Cytarabine is used for acute and chronic types of leukemias and lymphoma. In a study of 172 patients, over 50% developed skin AEs, most commonly morbilliform eruptions and HFS (Figure 15.4) [36]. These events are dose dependent, and resolved with cessation of therapy. Other AEs include neutrophilic eccrine hidradenitis, toxic epidermal necrolysis, mucositis/stomatitis, reversible alopecia, and nail dystrophy [37]. HFS may recur upon rechallenge [38–41], with a more severe bullous reaction [37]. Treatment strategies based on anecdotal data include emollients, limb elevation, cold compresses, and systemic corticosteroids [42].

Neutrophilic eccrine hidradenitis [43–45] is classified as a neutrophilic dermatosis, presenting with erythematous asymptomatic plaques on the face, arms, and legs. Histologically, a neutrophilic infiltrate is present within and surrounding eccrine coils, with vacuolar degeneration and necrosis of the secretory epithelium, and involvement of apocrine glands [46].

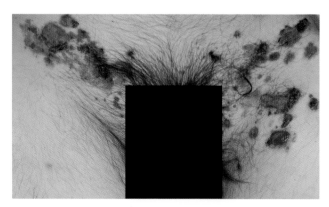

Figure 15.5 Gemcitabine-induced blistering rash grade 2.

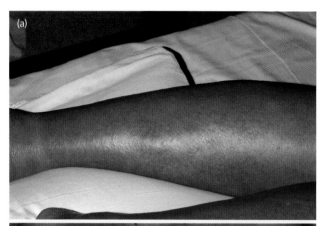

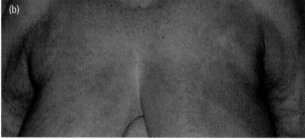

Figure 15.6 (a & b)Gemcitabine-induced rash grade 2.

An erysipeloid erythema largely confined to areas of edema can occur infrequently [64–67], within approximately 1–2 days of initiation and fades over a period of 2 weeks. It can be associated with warmth and tenderness, often raising concern for cellulitis (Figure 15.6). The reaction is time and dose limited and is reproducible upon reintroduction of gemcitabine [65]. Skin biopsies demonstrate nonspecific findings with moderate superficial perivascular lymphocytic infiltrate [64]. Management typically incorporates dose interruptions or steroids, and compression garments. Subsequent skin sclerosis and hyperpigmentation in areas affected by the erysipeloid eruption has been reported [64,66].

Radiation/photo-recall can occur [67–74], and is characterized by localized erythema, pain, swelling, scaling, blistering, or ulceration confined to the field of prior radiation. The dermatitis presents within hours to days of therapy, but radiation may have occurred days to years prior to treatment. Radiation recall may also affect mucosae and the central nervous system [72]. Primary treatment of recall reactions includes corticosteroids and interruption of therapy. Rechallenge with gemcitabine does not always result in recurrence.

HFS develops a few days after treatment and is characteristically localized to the palms and soles, followed by desquamation [75]. Management is primarily symptomatic, and can include keratolytics such as salicylic acid or urea-based creams and/or high-potency topical corticosteroids.

Drug-induced linear IgA has been described, with vesicular lesions developing within a few days of receiving gemcitabine. Diagnosis is based on immunofluorescence studies demonstrating linear IgA deposits along the basal membrane, and management includes drug interruption. Topical or short courses of systemic corticosteroids may speed resolution of skin lesions.

Pruritus ani has also been rarely associated during gemcitabine infusion [54], with resolution after discontinuation of the infusion. Symptoms recur with rechallenge; however, pretreatment with systemic or topical corticosteroids and pramoxine can prevent this recurrence [54].

Rare cases of painful distal necrosis of fingers and penis have been described in association with gemcitabine [55,56], with elevated antinuclear antibodies. Systemic corticosteroids may be helpful for treatment [55]. SJS/TEN has been reported in a patient treated with gemcitabine and radiation therapy [57]. Involvement of dermatology colleagues in the evaluation of this kind of toxicity is important. Discontinuation of the suspected drug is crucial to the management of SJS/TEN. Intensive skin management similar to that employed in burn units should be instituted.

Mercaptopurine

Mercaptopurine (6-MP) is a thiopurine antimetabolite indicated for the treatment of acute lymphocytic leukemia. Azathioprine is the prodrug of 6-MP. Dermatologic AEs include HFS/acral erythema (1–10%), alopecia (1%), eruptive nevi, hypersensitivity (<1%), possible neoplasms (<1%), and occasional mucositis.

HFS usually occurs within 2–4 weeks of initiating therapy, and biopsy shows parakeratosis, superficial perivascular lymphohistiocytic infiltrate, and rare apoptotic keratotinocytes [76,77].

Eruptive melanocytic nevi have been reported during the course of treatment with mercaptopurine or its prodrug, azathioprine [78–80]. The pathophysiology is uncertain; routine skin examinations are helpful in monitoring for concerning changes.

Hypersensitivity reactions occasionally occur, within 4 weeks of beginning therapy, but less commonly may occur within a few hours of treatment [81,82]. Symptoms include fever, chills, conjunctivitis, arthralgias, shortness of breath, nausea, vomiting, weakness, and occasionally shock [82]. Dermatologic examination may demonstrate acral violaceous papules [82], leg nodules [83], or vesiculopustules and plaques (with azathioprine) [81,83,84]. Laboratory findings include elevated liver transaminases, leukocytosis, and proteinuria. Histology from skin biopsies may rarely show acute lobular panniculitis with vasculitis and granulomatous inflammation [82]. Mercaptopurine should be promptly discontinued in patients with hypersensitivity reactions. Additionally, corticosteroids or anthihistamines may be considered [82,85]. Physical and laboratory findings resolve within 1–2 weeks.

Some studies have described a potential risk of secondary malignancies [86,87], including skin cancers and melanoma [88]. UVA photosensitivity has been cited as a partial explanation of the development of skin cancers in this population [89,90]. Patients treated with mercaptopurine who develop new, changing, or nonhealing skin lesions should be evaluated for possible skin cancers.

Thioguanine

Thioguanine (6-thioguanine) is a thiopurine analog used in the treatment of leukemia. Cutaneous toxicities are infrequent, and include drug eruptions, alopecia, and photosensitivity [91,92]. There have also been rare cases of multiple nonmelanoma skin cancers [93].

Thioguanine-associated drug rashes are characterized as maculopapular eruptions occurring within 2 months of initiating treatment [91]. Management includes dose modification and topical or oral steroids.

With intraperitoneal thioguanine, photosensitivity developed in six of 25 patients, likely as a result of UVA exposure synergizing with the accumulation of 6-thioguanine into DNA [90,92]. Increased sensitivity to sun is generally managed with avoidance of sun exposure as well as symptomatic treatment of affected skin.

Multiple skin cancers can develop in patients treated with thioguanine, including basal and squamous cell carcinomas [91]. Selective UVA photosensitivity has been suggested to partly explain the development of skin cancers [90]. Nonmelanoma skin cancers can be managed with surgical excision and/or destructive methods. Routine skin cancer surveillance is important to manage these tumors before there is continued local destruction of surrounding tissues or potential risk of metastasis.

Fludarabine

Fludarabine is a fluorinated purine antimetabolite approved for treatment of B-cell chronic lymphocytic leukemia. Dermatologic toxicities observed in patients receiving fludarabine are infrequent: worsening of skin cancers (<1%), rare cases of transfusion-associated graft versus host disease (GVHD) [94], mucositis (9%) [95], and worsening of psoriasis.

A few cases of exacerbation of skin cancers have been reported [96–99], with accelerated growth and invasion, or even metastatic disease [97,99]. Given the potential risk of aggressive skin cancers, timely surgical management of skin cancers with close observation should strongly be considered in patients treated with fludarabine.

Transfusion-associated GVHD is a quite rare but fatal complication associated with fludarabine. Immunocompetent allogeneic lymphocytes in blood products can engraft, proliferate, and develop an immunologic reaction against an immunodeficient or immunocompromised host [94,100]. Patients can develop fever, cutaneous eruption, and elevated transaminases. Skin biopsies demonstrate findings consistent with GVHD. The reports of transfusion-associated GVHD in patients treated with fludarabine suggest that the immunoablative effects of fludarabine may place some patients at risk for transfusion-associated GVHD. However, irradiation of cellular blood products reduces this risk.

Worsening of psoriasis may be seen with fludarabine treatment [101]. One report of a patient describes the onset of plaque psoriasis during treatment [101], yet other patients experience significant resolution of psoriatic lesions [102,103].

Cladribine

Cladribine is a chlorinated purine nucleoside analog indicated for the treatment of hairy cell leukemia. Rash (27%), injection site reactions (19%), pruritus (6%), erythema (6%), and SJS/TEN have been observed [104].

Extensive pruritus can progress to a generalized eruption, which may be maculopapular [105], vesicular [106], or purpuric [107–109]. The cutaneous findings generally appear a mean of 2 weeks after initiation of weeklong continuous infusion [106] or after subsequent cycles [105,107]. Histology of skin biopsies can demonstrate perivascular lymphocytic infiltrate, degranulated eosinophils (flame figures) [105], epidermal spongiosis [107], or features of erythema multiforme [108]. Vasculitic skin lesions associated with systemic vasculitis has been reported in a patient treated with cladribine [110].

A cutaneous eruption associated with cladribine may be accompanied by eosinophilia. Although some eruptions self-resolve, more extensive cutaneous involvement or symptomatic rashes can be managed effectively with systemic corticosteroids [105,107,111]. TEN has rarely been reported in association with cladribine [106]. As TEN is often fatal, discontinuation of the implicated agent is critical. Other rare cutaneous findings associated with cladribine include nonspecific eruptions in conjunction with transfusion-associated GVHD [112] and skin necrosis at the site of infusion [113].

References

1 Feizy, V., Namazi, M.R., Barikbin, B. & Ehsani, A. (2003) Methotrexate-induced acral erythema with bullous reaction. *Dermatology Online Journal*, **9**, 14.

2 Hellier, I., Bessis, D., Sotto, A., Margueritte, G. & Guilhou, J.J. (1996) High-dose methotrexate-induced bullous variant of acral erythema. *Archives of Dermatology*, **132**, 590–591.

3 Ikeda, H., Kawano, H., Kitaura, T., Kimura, A. & Kihira, K. (1999) Acral erythema associated with high-dose methotrexate infusion. *Annals of Pharmacotherapy*, **33**, 646.

4 Millot, F., Auriol, F., Brecheteau, P. & Guilhot, F. (1999) Acral erythema in children receiving high-dose methotrexate. *Pediatric Dermatology*, **16**, 398–400.

5 Morrell, D.S., Challgren, E., Eapen, M. & Esterly, N.B. (2002) Bullous acral erythema secondary to high-dose methotrexate. *Journal of Pediatric Hematology*, **24**, 240.

6 Postovsky, S. & Ben Arush, M.W. (2005) Acral erythema caused by high-dose methotrexate therapy in patients with osteogenic sarcoma. *Pediatric Hematology and Oncology*, **22**, 167–173.

7 Werchniak, A.E., Chaffee, S. & Dinulos, J.G. (2005) Methotrexate-induced bullous acral erythema in a child. *Journal of the American Academy of Dermatology*, **52**, S93–S95.

8 Kazlow, D.W., Federgrun, D., Kurtin, S. & Lebwohl, M.G. (2003) Cutaneous ulceration caused by methotrexate. *Journal of the American Academy of Dermatology*, **49**, S197–S198.

9 Pearce, H.P. & Wilson, B.B. (1996) Erosion of psoriatic plaques: an early sign of methotrexate toxicity. *Journal of the American Academy of Dermatology*, **35**, 835–838.

10 Del Pozo, J., Martinez, W., Garcia-Silva, J., Almagro, M., Pena-Penabad, C. & Fonseca, E. (2001) Cutaneous ulceration as a sign of methotrexate toxicity. *European Journal of Dermatology*, **11**, 450–452.

11 Goldfeder, K.L., Levin, J.M., Katz, K.A., Clarke, L.E., Loren, A.W. & James, W.D. (2007) Ultraviolet recall reaction after total body irradiation, etoposide, and methotrexate therapy. *Journal of the American Academy of Dermatology*, **56**, 494–499.

12 Andersen, K.E. & Lindskov, R. (1984) Recall of UVB-induced erythema in breast cancer patient receiving multiple drug chemotherapy. *Photo-Dermatology*, **1**, 129–132.

13 Kalb, R.E., Strober, B., Weinstein, G. & Lebwohl, M. (2009) Methotrexate and psoriasis: 2009 National Psoriasis Foundation Consensus Conference. *Journal of the American Academy of Dermatology*, **60**, 824–837.

14 Roenigk, H.H. Jr., Auerbach, R., Maibach, H., Weinstein, G. & Lebwohl, M. (1998) Methotrexate in psoriasis: consensus conference. *Journal of the American Academy of Dermatology*, **38**, 478–485.

15 Fuld, A.D., Dragnev, K.H. & Rigas, J.R. (2010) Pemetrexed in advanced non-small-cell lung cancer. *Expert Opinion on Pharmacotherapy*, **11**, 1387–1402.

16 Clarke, S.J., Abratt, R., Goedhals, L., Boyer, M.J., Millward, M.J. & Ackland, S.P. (2002) Phase II trial of pemetrexed disodium (ALIMTA, LY231514) in chemotherapy-naive patients with advanced non-small-cell lung cancer. *Annals of Oncology*, **13**, 737–741.

17 Hanna, N., Shepherd, F.A., Fossella, F.V. et al. (2004) Randomized phase III trial of pemetrexed versus docetaxel in patients with non-small-cell lung cancer previously treated with chemotherapy. *Journal of Clinical Oncology*, **22**, 1589–1597.

18 Martin, M., Spielmann, M., Namer, M. et al. (2003) Phase II study of pemetrexed in breast cancer patients pretreated with anthracyclines. *Annals of Oncology*, **14**, 1246–1252.

19 Guhl, G., Diaz-Ley, B., Sanchez-Perez, J., Jimenez, U. & Garcia-Diez, A. (2010) Pemetrexed-induced edema of the eyelid. *Lung Cancer (Amsterdam, Netherlands)*, **69**, 249–250.

20 Bracke, A., Van Marck, E. & Lambert, J. (2009) Acute generalized exanthematous pustulosis after pemetrexed, and recurrence after re-introduction. *Clinical and Experimental Dermatology*, **34**, 337–339.

21 Tummino, C., Barlesi, F., Tchouhadjian, C. et al. (2007) Severe cutaneous toxicity after Pemetrexed as second line treatment for a refractory non small cell lung cancer [in French]. *Revue Des Maladies Respiratoires*, **24**, 635–638.

22 Barlesi, F., Tummino, C., Tasei, A.M. & Astoul, P. (2006) Unsuccessful rechallenge with pemetrexed after a previous radiation recall dermatitis. *Lung Cancer (Amsterdam, Netherlands)*, **54**, 423–425.

23 Hureaux, J., Le Guen, Y., Tuchais, C., Savary, L. & Urban, T. (2005) Radiation recall dermatitis with pemetrexed. *Lung Cancer (Amsterdam, Netherlands)*, **50**, 255–258.

24 Khanfir, K. & Anchisi, S. (2008) Pemetrexed-associated radiation recall dermatitis. *Acta Oncologica (Stockholm, Sweden)*, **47**, 1607–1608.

25 Kurata, T., Tamura, K., Okamoto, I., Satoh, T., Nakagawa, K. & Fukuoka, M. (2006) Pemetrexed-induced edema of the eyelid. *Lung Cancer (Amsterdam, Netherlands)*, **54**, 241–242.

26 Spirig, C., Omlin, A., D'Addario, G. et al. (2009) Radiation recall dermatitis with soft tissue necrosis following pemetrexed therapy: a case report. *Journal of Medical Case Reports*, **3**, 93.

27 Chua, D., Wei, W.I., Sham, J.S. & Au, G.K. (2008) Capecitabine monotherapy for recurrent and metastatic nasopharyngeal cancer. *Japanese Journal of Clinical Oncology*, **38**, 244–249.

28 Wong, M., Choo, S.P. & Tan, E.H. (2009) Travel warning with capecitabine. *Annals of Oncology*, **20**, 1281.

29 Mackean, M., Planting, A., Twelves, C. et al. (1998) Phase I and pharmacologic study of intermittent twice-daily oral therapy with capecitabine in patients with advanced and/or metastatic cancer. *Journal of Clinical Oncology*, **16**, 2977–2985.

30 Yucel, I. & Guzin, G. (2008) Topical henna for capecitabine induced hand-foot syndrome. *Investigational New Drugs*, **26**, 189–192.

31 Schmid-Wendtner, M.H., Wendtner, C.M., Volkenandt, M. & Heinemann, V. (2001) Clinical picture: leopard-like vitiligo with capecitabine. *Lancet*, **358**, 1575.

32 Tavares-Bello, R. (2007) Capecitabine-induced hand-foot syndrome and cutaneous hyperpigmentation in an elderly vitiligo patient. *Journal of the European Academy of Dermatology and Venereology*, **21**, 1434–1435.

33 Villalon, G., Martin, J.M., Pinazo, M.I., Calduch, L., Alonso, V. & Jorda, E. (2009) Focal acral hyperpigmentation in a patient undergoing chemotherapy with capecitabine. *American Journal of Clinical Dermatology*, **10**, 261–263.

34 Paravar, T. & Hymes, S.R. (2009) Longitudinal melanonychia induced by capecitabine. *Dermatology Online Journal*, **15**, 11.

35 Package insert (2009) Xeloda (capecitabine). Genentech, Inc..

36 Cetkovska, P., Pizinger, K. & Cetkovsky, P. (2002) High-dose cytosine arabinoside-induced cutaneous reactions. *Journal of the European Academy of Dermatology and Venereology*, **16**, 481–485.

37 Crawford, J.H., Eikelboom, J.W. & McQuillan, A. (2002) Recurrent palmar-plantar erythrodysaesthesia following high-dose cytarabine treatment for acute lymphoblastic leukemia. *European Journal of Haematology*, **69**, 315–317.

38 Burgdorf, W.H., Gilmore, W.A. & Ganick, R.G. (1982) Peculiar acral erythema secondary to high-dose chemotherapy for acute myelogenous leukemia. *Annals of Internal Medicine*, **97**, 61–62.

39 Lokich, J.J. & Moore, C. (1984) Chemotherapy-associated palmar-plantar erythrodysesthesia syndrome. *Annals of Internal Medicine*, **101**, 798–799.

40 Peters, W.G. & Willemze, R. (1985) Palmar-plantar skin changes and cytarabine. *Annals of Internal Medicine*, **103**, 805.

41 Shall, L., Lucas, G.S., Whittaker, J.A. & Holt, P.J. (1988) Painful red hands: a side-effect of leukaemia therapy. *British Journal of Dermatology*, **119**, 249–253.

42 Nagore, E., Insa, A. & Sanmartin, O. (2000) Antineoplastic therapy-induced palmar plantar erythrodysesthesia ('hand-foot') syndrome. Incidence, recognition and management. *American Journal of Clinical Dermatology*, **1**, 225–234.

43 Harrist, T.J., Fine, J.D., Berman, R.S., Murphy, G.F. & Mihm, M.C. Jr. (1982) Neutrophilic eccrine hidradenitis. A distinctive type of neutrophilic dermatosis associated with myelogenous leukemia and chemotherapy. *Archives of Dermatology*, **118**, 263–266.

44 Keane, F.M., Munn, S.E., Buckley, D.A., Hopster, D., Mufti, G.J. & du Vivier, A.W. (2001) Neutrophilic eccrine hidradenitis in two neutropaenic patients. *Clinical and Experimental Dermatology*, **26**, 162–165.

45 Srivastava, M., Scharf, S., Meehan, S.A. & Polsky, D. (2007) Neutrophilic eccrine hidradenitis masquerading as facial cellulitis. *Journal of the American Academy of Dermatology*, **56**, 693–696.

46 Brehler, R., Reimann, S., Bonsmann, G. & Metze, D. (1997) Neutrophilic hidradenitis induced by chemotherapy involves eccrine and apocrine glands. *American Journal of Dermatopathology*, **19**, 73–78.

47 Figueiredo, M.S., Yamamoto, M. & Kerbauy, J. (1998) Toxic epidermal necrolysis after the use of intermediate dose of cytosine arabinoside. *Revista da Associacao Medica Brasileira*, **44**, 53–55.

48 Ozkan, A., Apak, H., Celkan, T., Yuksel, L. & Yildiz, I. (2001) Toxic epidermal necrolysis after the use of high-dose cytosine arabinoside. *Pediatric Dermatology*, **18**, 38–40.

49 Scheithauer, W., Schull, B., Ulrich-Pur, H. *et al.* (2003) Biweekly high-dose gemcitabine alone or in combination with capecitabine in patients with metastatic pancreatic adenocarcinoma: a randomized phase II trial. *Annals of Oncology*, **14**, 97–104.

50 Tonato, M., Mosconi, A.M. & Martin, C. (1995) Safety profile of gemcitabine. *Anti-Cancer Drugs*, **6** (Suppl. 6), 27–32.

51 del Pozo, J., Martinez, W., Yebra-Pimentel, M.T., Almagro, M., Pena-Penabad, C. & Fonseca, E. (2001) Linear immunoglobulin A bullous dermatosis induced by gemcitabine. *Annals of Pharmacotherapy*, **35**, 891–893.

52 Duvic, M., Talpur, R., Wen, S., Kurzrock, R., David, C.L. & Apisarnthanarax, N. (2006) Phase II evaluation of gemcitabine monotherapy for cutaneous T-cell lymphoma. *Clinical Lymphoma and Myeloma*, **7**, 51–58.

53 Marucci, G., Sgarbanti, E., Maestri, A., Calandri, C. & Collina, G. (2001) Gemcitabine-associated CD8+ CD30+ pseudolymphoma. *British Journal of Dermatology*, **145**, 650–652.

54 Hejna, M., Valencak, J. & Raderer, M. (1999) Anal pruritus after cancer chemotherapy with gemcitabine. *New England Journal of Medicine*, **340**, 655–656.

55 Banach, M.J. & Williams, G.A. (2000) Purtscher retinopathy and necrotizing vasculitis with gemcitabine therapy. *Archives of Ophthalmology*, **118**, 726–727.

56 Venat-Bouvet, L., Ly, K., Szelag, J.C. *et al.* (2003) Thrombotic microangiopathy and digital necrosis: two unrecognized toxicities of gemcitabine. *Anti-Cancer Drugs*, **14**, 829–832.

57 Sommers, K.R., Kong, K.M., Bui, D.T., Fruehauf, J.P. & Holcombe, R.F. (2003) Stevens-Johnson syndrome/toxic epidermal necrolysis in a patient receiving concurrent radiation and gemcitabine. *Anti-Cancer Drugs*, **14**, 659–662.

58 Chen, Y.M., Liu, J.M., Tsai, C.M., Whang-Peng, J. & Perng, R.P. (1996) Maculopapular rashes secondary to gemcitabine injection for non-small-cell lung cancer. *Journal of Clinical Oncology*, **14**, 1743–1744.

59 Kanai, M., Matsumoto, S., Nishimura, T. *et al.* (2010) Premedication with 20 mg dexamethasone effectively prevents relapse of extensive skin rash associated with gemcitabine monotherapy. *Annals of Oncology*, **21**, 189–190.

60 Azzoli, C.G., Miller, V.A., Ng, K.K. *et al.* (2003) Gemcitabine-induced peripheral edema: report on 15 cases and review of the literature. *American Journal of Clinical Oncology*, **26**, 247–251.

61 Pavlakis, N., Bell, D.R., Millward, M.J. & Levi, J.A. (1997) Fatal pulmonary toxicity resulting from treatment with gemcitabine. *Cancer*, **80**, 286–291.

62 Imen, A., Amal, K., Ines, Z., Sameh el, F., Fethi el, M. & Habib, G. (2006) Bullous dermatosis associated with gemcitabine therapy for non-small-cell lung carcinoma. *Respiratory Medicine*, **100**, 1463–1465.

63 Geffen, D.B. & Horowitz, J. (2000) Gemcitabine-induced severe extremity edema with muscle contractures and subsequent prevention with prednisone. *Israel Medical Association Journal*, **2**, 552–553.

64 Bessis, D., Guillot, B., Legouffe, E. & Guilhou, J.J. (2004) Gemcitabine-associated scleroderma-like changes of the lower extremities. *Journal of the American Academy of Dermatology*, **51**, S73–S76.

65 Brandes, A., Reichmann, U., Plasswilm, L. & Bamberg, M. (2000) Time- and dose-limiting erysipeloid rash confined to areas of lymphedema following treatment with gemcitabine–a report of three cases. *Anti-Cancer Drugs*, **11**, 15–17.

66 Chu, C.Y., Yang, C.H. & Chiu, H.C. (2001) Gemcitabine-induced acute lipodermatosclerosis-like reaction. *Acta Dermato-Venereologica*, **81**, 426–428.

67 Tan, D.H., Bunce, P.E., Liles, W.C. & Gold, W.L. (2007) Gemcitabine-related "pseudocellulitis": report of 2 cases and review of the literature. *Clinical Infectious Diseases*, **45**, e72–e76.

68 Burstein, H.J. (2000) Side effects of chemotherapy. Case 1. Radiation recall dermatitis from gemcitabine. *Journal of Clinical Oncology*, **18**, 693–694.

69 Schwartz, B.M., Khuntia, D., Kennedy, A.W. & Markman, M. (2003) Gemcitabine-induced radiation recall dermatitis following whole pelvic radiation therapy. *Gynecologic Oncology*, **91**, 421–422.

70 Fogarty, G., Ball, D. & Rischin, D. (2001) Radiation recall reaction following gemcitabine. *Lung Cancer (Amsterdam, Netherlands)*, **33**, 299–302.

71 Badger, J., Kang, S., Uzieblo, A. & Srinivas, S. (2005) Double diagnosis in cancer patients and cutaneous reaction related to gemcitabine: CASE 3. Photo therapy recall with gemcitabine following ultraviolet B treatment. *Journal of Clinical Oncology*, **23**, 7224–7225.

72 Jeter, M.D., Janne, P.A., Brooks, S. *et al.* (2002) Gemcitabine-induced radiation recall. *International Journal of Radiation Oncology, Biology, Physics*, **53**, 394–400.

73 Marisavljevic, D., Ristic, B. & Hajder, J. (2005) Gemcitabine-induced radiation recall dermatitis in a patient with resistant Hodgkin lymphoma. *American Journal of Hematology*, **80**, 91.

74 Zustovich, F., Pavei, P. & Cartei, G. (2006) Erysipeloid skin toxicity induced by gemcitabine. *Journal of the European Academy of Dermatology and Venereology*, **20**, 757–758.

75 Dalbagni, G., Russo, P., Sheinfeld, J. *et al.* (2002) Phase I trial of intravesical gemcitabine in bacillus Calmette-Guerin-refractory transitional-cell carcinoma of the bladder. *Journal of Clinical Oncology*, **20**, 3193–3198.

76 Wanat, K.A., Bandow, G.D. & Klekotka, P.A. (2008) Palmar-plantar erythrodysesthesia caused by mercaptopurine and mesalamine. *Archives of Dermatology*, **144**, 1079–1081.

77 Cox, G.J. & Robertson, D.B. (1986) Toxic erythema of palms and soles associated with high-dose mercaptopurine chemotherapy. *Archives of Dermatology*, **122**, 1413–1414.

78 Bovenschen, H.J., Tjioe, M., Vermaat, H. *et al.* (2006) Induction of eruptive benign melanocytic naevi by immune suppressive agents, including biologicals. *British Journal of Dermatology*, **154**, 880–884.

79 Happle, R. & Koopman, R.J. (1990) Acral nevi following chemotherapy. *Der Hautarzt; Zeitschrift für Dermatologie, Venerologie, und Verwandte Gebiete*, **41**, 331–332.

80 Kakrida, M., Orengo, I. & Markus, R. (2005) Sudden onset of Multiple nevi after administration of 6-mercaptopurine in an adult with Crohn's disease: a case report. *International Journal of Dermatology*, **44**, 334–336.

81 Garey, K.W., Streetman, D.S. & Rainish, M.C. (1998) Azathioprine hypersensitivity reaction in a patient with ulcerative colitis. *Annals of Pharmacotherapy*, **32**, 425–428.

82 Andersen, J.M. & Tiede, J.J. (1997) Serum sickness associated with 6-mercaptopurine in a patient with Crohn's disease. *Pharmacotherapy*, **17**, 173–176.

83 de Fonclare, A.L., Khosrotehrani, K., Aractingi, S., Duriez, P., Cosnes, J. & Beaugerie, L. (2007) Erythema nodosum-like eruption as a manifestation of azathioprine hypersensitivity in patients with inflammatory bowel disease. *Archives of Dermatology*, **143**, 744–748.

84 Jeurissen, M.E., Boerbooms, A.M., van de Putte, L.B. & Kruijsen, M.W. (1990) Azathioprine induced fever, chills, rash, and hepatotoxicity in rheumatoid arthritis. *Annals of the Rheumatic Diseases*, **49**, 25–27.

85 Glazier, K.D., Palance, A.L., Griffel, L.H. & Das, K.M. (2005) The ten-year single-center experience with 6-mercaptopurine in the treatment of inflammatory bowel disease. *Journal of Clinical Gastroenterology*, **39**, 21–26.

86 Disanti, W., Rajapakse, R.O., Korelitz, B.I., Panagopoulos, G. & Bratcher, J. (2006) Incidence of neoplasms in patients who develop sustained leukopenia during or after treatment with 6-mercaptopurine for inflammatory bowel disease. *Clinical Gastroenterology and Hepatology*, **4**, 1025–1029.

87 Schmiegelow, K., Al-Modhwahi, I., Andersen, M.K. *et al.* (2009) Methotrexate/6-mercaptopurine maintenance therapy influences the risk of a second malignant neoplasm after childhood acute lymphoblastic leukemia: results from the NOPHO ALL-92 study. *Blood*, **113**, 6077–6084.

88 Bouhnik, Y., Lemann, M., Mary, J.Y. *et al.* (1996) Long-term follow-up of patients with Crohn's disease treated with azathioprine or 6-mercaptopurine. *Lancet*, **347**, 215–219.

89 Guenova, E., Lichte, V., Hoetzenecker, W. *et al.* (2009) Nodular malignant melanoma and multiple cutaneous neoplasms under immunosuppression with azathioprine. *Melanoma Research*, **19**, 271–273.

90 O'Donovan, P., Perrett, C.M., Zhang, X. *et al.* (2005) Azathioprine and UVA light generate mutagenic oxidative DNA damage. *Science*, **309**, 1871–1874.

91 Zackheim, H.S., Glogau, R.G., Fisher, D.A. & Maibach, H.I. (1994) 6-Thioguanine treatment of psoriasis: experience in 81 patients. *Journal of the American Academy of Dermatology*, **30**, 452–458.

92 Zimm, S., Cleary, S.M., Horton, C.N. & Howell, S.B. (1988) Phase I/ pharmacokinetic study of thioguanine administered as a 48-hour continuous intraperitoneal infusion. *Journal of Clinical Oncology*, **6**, 696–700.

93 Zackheim, H.S. & Maibach, H.I. (1988) Treatment of psoriasis with 6-thioguanine. *Australasian Journal of Dermatology*, **29**, 163–167.

94 Leitman, S.F., Tisdale, J.F., Bolan, C.D. *et al.* (2003) Transfusion-associated GVHD after fludarabine therapy in a patient with systemic lupus erythematosus. *Transfusion*, **43**, 1667–1671.

95 Package insert (2007) Fludarabine injection. Bayer Healthcare Pharmaceuticals, Inc.

96 Davidovitz, Y., Ballin, A. & Meytes, D. (1997) Flare-up of squamous cell carcinoma of the skin following fludarabine therapy for chronic lymphocytic leukemia. *Acta Haematologica*, **98**, 44–46.

97 Rashid, K., Ng, R., Mastan, A., Sager, D. & Hirschman, R. (2005) Accelerated growth of skin carcinoma following fludarabine therapy for chronic lymphocytic leukemia. *Leukemia and Lymphoma*, **46**, 1051–1055.

98 Herr, D., Borelli, S., Kempf, W. & Trojan, A. (2005) Fludarabine: risk factor for aggressive behaviour of squamous cell carcinoma of the skin? *Annals of Oncology*, **16**, 515–516.

99 Larsen, C.R., Hansen, P.B. & Clausen, N.T. (2002) Aggressive growth of epithelial carcinomas following treatment with nucleoside analogues. *American Journal of Hematology*, **70**, 48–50.

100 Anderson, K.C. & Weinstein, H.J. (1990) Transfusion-associated graft-versus-host disease. *New England Journal of Medicine*, **323**, 315–321.

101 Jordan, J., Mey, U., Bieber, T. & Wilsmann-Theis, D. (2008) Paradoxical exacerbation of psoriasis during therapy with fludarabine. *European Journal of Dermatology*, **18**, 365–366.

102 Karadogan, I., Akca, S. & Undar, L. (1999) Resolution of psoriatic skin lesions with fludarabine. *American Journal of Medicine*, **107**, 300–301.

103 Smith, O.P., Hoffbrand, A.V. & Buckley, C. (1994) Fludarabine and psoriasis. *New England Journal of Medicine*, **330**, 1540–1541.

104 Package insert (2002) Cladribine injection. Ortho Biotech Products.

105 Rossini, M.S., de Souza, E.M., Cintra, M.L., Pagnano, K.B., Chiari, A.C. & Lorand-Metze, I. (2004) Cutaneous adverse reaction to 2-chlorodeoxyadenosine with histological flame figures in patients with chronic lymphocytic leukaemia. *Journal of the European Academy of Dermatology and Venereology*, **18**, 538–542.

106 Meunier, P., Castaigne, S., Bastie, J.N., Chosidow, O. & Aractingi, S. (1996) Cutaneous reactions after treatment with 2-chlorodeoxyadenosine. *Acta Dermato-Venereologica*, **76**, 385–386.

107 Robak, T., Sysa-Jedrzejowska, A., Robak, E., Dabkowski, J. & Blasinska-Morawiec, M. (1997) 2-chlorodeoxyadenosine (cladribine) induced allergic cutaneous reactions with eosinophilia in a patient with B-cell chronic lymphocytic leukemia. *Journal of Medicine*, **28**, 199–209.

108 Grey, M.R., Flanagan, N.G. & Kelsey, P.R. (2000) Severe skin rash in two consecutive patients treated with 2-chlorodeoxyadenosine for hairy cell leukaemia at a single institution. *Clinical and Laboratory Haematology*, **22**, 111–113.

109 Hendrick, A. (2001) Purpuric rash following treatment with 2-chlorodeoxyadenosine. *Clinical and Laboratory Haematology*, **23**, 67–68.

110 Tousi, B., D'Silva, R. & Papish, S. (2002) Systemic vasculitis complicating hairy cell leukaemia treatment with cladribine. *Clinical and Laboratory Haematology*, **24**, 259–260.

111 Rutella, S., Sica, S., Rumi, C. *et al.* (1996) Hypereosinophilia during 2-chlorodeoxyadenosine treatment for hairy cell leukaemia. *British Journal of Haematology*, **92**, 426–428.

112 Zulian, G.B., Roux, E., Tiercy, J.M. *et al.* (1995) Transfusion-associated graft-versus-host disease in a patient treated with Cladribine (2-chlorodeoxyadenosine): demonstration of exogenous DNA in various tissue extracts by PCR analysis. *British Journal of Haematology*, **89**, 83–89.

113 Zevin, S., Hershko, C. & Rosenmann, E. (1996) Halogenoderma of the forearm caused by 2-chlorodeoxyadenosine treatment. *American Journal of Hematology*, **53**, 209–210.

114 Package insert (2005) Methotrexate injection. Bedford Laboratories.

115 Litt, J.Z. (2008) *Litt's Drug Eruption Reference Manual*, 14th ed., Informa Healthcare, London.

116 Package insert (1996) Gemcitabine injection. Eli Lilly and Co.

16 Topoisomerase-Interacting Agents

Tomas Skacel[1,2], Roger von Moos[3] and Reinhard Dummer[4]

[1]Charles University, Prague, Czech Republic
[2]Amgen, Switzerland
[3]Cantonal Hospital Graubünden Chur, Switzerland
[4]Department of Dermatology, University Hospital Zurich, Zurich, Switzerland

Introduction

Topoisomerase inhibitors are agents designed to interfere with the action of the topoisomerase enzymes (topoisomerase I and II), which are enzymes that control the changes in the DNA structure, by catalyzing the breaking and rejoining of the phosphodiester backbone of DNA strands during the normal cell cycle. Topoisomerase I inhibitors bind to one strand of DNA, in contrast to type II inhibitors, which bind to both DNA strands. It is thought that topoisomerase inhibitors block the ligation step of the cell cycle, generating single and double-stranded breaks that disintegrate the genome. Introduction of these breaks subsequently leads to apoptosis and cell death. Topoisomerase inhibitors are divided according to which type of enzyme they inhibit. Topoisomerase I inhibitors include irinotecan, topotecan, and camptothecin, and all target type IA topoisomerases. Topoisomerase II inhibitors are tenipozid, etoposide, and most of the intercalating agents, anthracyclines (doxorubicin, pegylated liposomal doxorubicin (PLD), epirubicin, idarubicin) and derivates of anthracenedione (mitoxantrone). Topoisomerase inhibitors are considered important components for cancer chemotherapy treatments. Quinolones, which also inhibits topoisomerase, are used as antibacterial agents (Table 16.1) [1,2].

Topoisomerase I inhibitors

Irinotecan and topotecan

Irinotecan and topotecan are derivatives of camptothecin. Camptothecins interact specifically with the enzyme topoisomerase I which relieves torsional strain in the DNA by inducing reversible single-strand breaks. Current research suggests that the cytotoxicity of irinotecan is due to double-strand DNA damage produced during DNA synthesis when replication enzymes interact with the ternary complex formed by topoisomerase I, DNA, and either irinotecan or SN-38. Human cells cannot efficiently repair these double-strand breaks.

Irinotecan is indicated as a component of first-line therapy in combination with 5-fluorouracil and leucovorin for patients with metastatic carcinoma of the colon or rectum which has progressed following initial fluorouracil-based therapy. Topotecan is approved for treatment of metastatic carcinoma of the ovary after failure of initial or subsequent chemotherapy, small cell lung cancer sensitive disease after failure of first-line chemotherapy, and recurrent or persistent stage IV carcinoma of the cervix that is not amenable to curative treatment with surgery and/or radiation therapy. Topotecan is associated with the following dermatologic adverse events: alopecia up to 49% and rash in 16% of patients. Occasionally, pruritus and severe dermatitis is reported in patients treated with topotecan. Irinotecan is associated with alopecia in up to 60% of patients, excessive sweating in 16%, rash in 13%, and hand-foot syndrome (HFS) appears in 5% of patients. Mucositis and diarrhea are more common with irinotecan therapy than topotecan (88% and 29%, versus 32% and 18%, respectively).

Topoisomerase II inhibitors

Anthracyclines: Doxorubicin, liposomal doxorubicin, epirubicin and idarubicin

Anthracyclines are commonly used to treat hematologic malignancies such as leukemias, Hodgkin lymphoma, multiple myeloma, as well as solid tumors of the bladder, breast, stomach, lung, ovaries, thyroid, soft tissue sarcoma, and other locations. The most commonly used anthracyclines are epirubicin and doxorubicin. Examples of the most frequently administered

Dermatologic Principles and Practice in Oncology: Conditions of the Skin, Hair, and Nails in Cancer Patients, First Edition. Edited by Mario E. Lacouture.
© 2014 John Wiley & Sons, Inc. Published 2014 by John Wiley & Sons, Inc.

doxorubicin and epirubicin-containing regimens are EC/AC (epirubicin/Adriamycin® and cyclophosphamide), FEC/FAC (fluorouracil and EC/AC), AT (Adriamycin® and paclitaxel/docetaxel), TAC (docetaxel and AC) in breast cancer; ABVD (Adriamycin®, bleomycin, vinblastine, dacarbazine) in Hodgkin lymphoma and CHOP (cyclophosphamide, Adriamycin®, vincristine, prednisone) in non-Hodgkin lymphoma. PLD is used for metastatic breast cancer as well as for the treatment of ovarian cancer in combination with carboplatin or where the disease has progressed or reoccurred after platinum-based chemotherapy. Liposomes are microscopic phospholipid spheres that result in a distinct efficacy and toxicity profile for doxorubicin in animal models and early trials in humans, but their short half-life

hindered their ability to deliver agents effectively. A new type of liposome with segments of polyethylene glycol on the surface impedes uptake by the reticuloendothelial system and consequently heightens time in plasma, thereby conferring a longer half-life on pegylated liposomes. In various models, greater quantitites of doxorubicin was delivered to tumors when encapsulated in pegylated liposomes than unencapsulated drug. This alteration in delivery will also result in a distinct dermatologic adverse event profile, so that PLD will result in alopecia, HFS, and rash. Another indication of this agent is in the treatment of AIDS-related Kaposi sarcoma and tumor stage mycosis fungoides [3–6].

The most common dermatologic adverse events (AEs) associated with anthracyclines are alopecia, skin rash (intertrigo-like eruption, follicular pronounced scaly erythema; Figure 16.1), HFS (palmar and plantar erythema; Figure 16.2), nail changes (onycholysis, hyperpigmentation on the nail beds and Beau line), and ultraviolet (UV) and radiation recall. PLD of the anthracyclines has been associated with lower frequency of alopecia, but higher incidence of HFS.

Etoposide and teniposide
Etoposide and teniposide are semisynthetic derivatives of podophyllotoxin acting in the late S or early G_2 phase of the cell cycle, thus preventing cells from entering mitosis. The pharmacokinetic characteristics of both molecules are different. Teniposide is more extensively bound to plasma proteins and its cellular uptake is greater. Teniposide also has a lower systemic clearance, a longer half-life, and is excreted in the urine as a parent drug to a lesser extent than etoposide. Both drugs cause

Table 16.1 Classification of topoisomerase inhibitors.

Topoisomerase I inhibitors	
Camptothecin derivatives	Irinotecan and topotecan

Topoisomerase II inhibitors	
Anthracyclines	Doxorubicin, liposomal doxorubicin, daunorubicin, epirubicin, idarubicin
Actinomycin	Actinomycin D
Podophyllotoxin derivatives	Etoposide, teniposide
Anthracenedione	Mitoxantrone

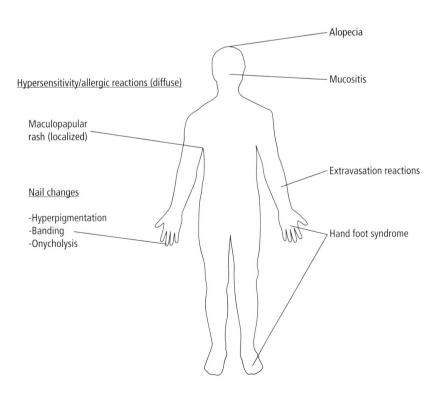

Figure 16.1 Location of topoisomerase-inhibitor induced dermatologic adverse events.

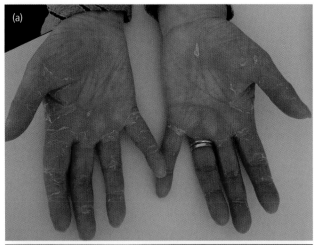

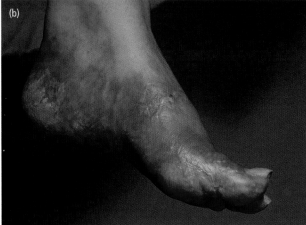

Figure 16.2 Hand-foot syndrome, palmar skin reaction (b). Hand-foot syndrome, plantar skin reaction.

dose-dependent single and double-stranded breaks in DNA and DNA protein cross-links. The mechanism of action is related to the inhibition of type II topoisomerase activity because teniposide does not intercalate into DNA or bind strongly to DNA. The cytotoxic effects of teniposide are related to the relative number of double-stranded DNA breaks produced in cells, which reflect the stabilization of a topoisomerase II-DNA intermediate.

Teniposide has a broad spectrum of antitumor activity against hematologic malignancies and various solid tumors. Notably, teniposide is active in certain subtypes of leukemias with acquired resistance to cisplatin, doxorubicin, amsacrine, daunorubicin, mitoxantrone, or vincristine. Teniposide is indicated for the treatment of refractory childhood acute lymphoblastic leukemia (ALL). It is also used in the treatment of refractory adult ALL and non-Hodgkin lymphoma. Etoposide has a broad therapeutic spectrum in oncology. It is used in some subtypes of leukemias, non-Hodgkin lymphoma, and many solid tumors, mainly testicular cancer, lung, ovarian cancer, and soft tissues sarcomas. The most common dermatologic AE occurring with etoposide is alopecia in 8–66%. Flushing, the episodic occurrence of diffuse

burning erythema on the face, upper part of the back and chest has been reported in connection with the administration of both cytostatics etoposide and teniposide. The etiology is unknown, but it is presumed to be due to cutaneous vasomotor instability. Specific treatment is not required unless it is moderate to severe. Other rare dermatologic AEs include various severe AEs in the spectrum of erythema multiforme, Stevens–Johnson syndrome and the life-threatening toxic epidermal necrolysis (TEN), also known as Lyell syndrome. Other mild dermatologic AEs such as hyperpigmentation and radiation recall dermatitis have also been reported. Mucositis and diarrhea appear in up to 6% and 13% of patients, respectively. Teniposide is associated with lower incidence of alopecia and rash (less than 10% and 3%, respectively) than etoposide, but has a higher incidence of mucositis and diarrhea (up to 76% and 33%, respectively).

Mitoxantrone

Mitoxantrone is a synthetic antineoplastic anthracenedione. It is indicated for advanced hormone-refractory prostate cancer and the initial therapy of acute nonlymphocytic leukemia (ANLL) in adults. Mitoxantrone is also indicated for reducing neurologic disability and/or the frequency of clinical relapses in patients with secondary (chronic) progressive, progressive relapsing, or worsening relapsing-remitting multiple sclerosis. The most common dermatologic AEs are alopecia (33–61%) and nail bed changes (11%). Type I allergic reactions have also been observed with mitoxantrone therapy. Hypersensitivity including urticaria and angioedema have also been reported. Treatment with antihistamines, systemic steroids or even adrenaline is indicated, depending on the severity of the allergic reaction. Mucositis and diarrhea were reported in 25% and 19%, respectively (Table 16.2).

Alopecia

Alopecia is a common AE of many cytotoxics, including the topoisomerase inhibitors. The anthracylines and etoposide are associated with the highest incidence of alopecia amongst topoisomerase inhibitors. Cells in hair follicles are altered in the S or G2 phase. The anagen phase of hair growth is interrupted which leads to hair loss. Two-thirds of patients lose their hair after treatment with etoposide or epirubicin and almost 90% of patients will experience alopecia after doxorubicin-based chemotherapy. Liposomal delivery of the anthracyclines has been associated with less alopecia.

Several treatment modalities have been evaluated to prevent alopecia: hypothermia, tourniquet pressure, and ImuVert. Hypothermia, through vasoconstriction, has demonstrated some benefit through the limitation of the amount of cytostatic agents in the scalp tissue. The scalp area needs to be cooled to minimum of 24°C for 5 minutes before and 20 minutes after administering chemotherapy. Tourniquet pressure is applied to the scalp in the form of a headband. Increased scalp pressure ranging 30–50 mmHg

Table 16.2 Pegylated liposomal doxorubicin (PLD) and hand-foot syndrome: dose and adverse event correlations.

Study/population	N	PLD regimen	Mean dose intensity of	Response rate (%)	Median progression	Incidence of PPE (% of patients)		
			PLD (mg/m²/wk)		(months)	All grades	Grade 3	Grade 4
Gordon et al. [31], platinum-resistant OC	239	50 mg/m² q 4 weeks	11.6	19.7	PFS: 7.2	49	22	1
Lorusso et al. [34], heavily pretreated OC	37	35 mg/m² q 3 weeks	10.8	13.5	mRD: 5.7	22	3	0
Campos et al. [35], recurrent OC, 40% platinum-paclitaxel-resistant disease (retrospective analysis)	72	40 mg/m² q 4 weeks (in 93% of patients)	10.0	26.7	TTDP: 5.3	21	8	0
Markman et al. [36], platinum-paclitaxel-refractory OC	49	40 mg/m² q 4 weeks	10.0	9	NR	18	0	0
Sehouli et al. [33], recurrent OC	64	20 mg/m² q 2 weeks	10.0	15.9	PFS: 4.3	48	5	0
Coleman et al. [32], metastatic BrCa	116	60 mg/m²/6 weeks (Arm A) 50 mg/m²/ 4 weeks (Arm B)	9.8 (Arm A) 11.9 (Arm B)	29 (Arm A) 31 (Arm B)	NR	33 (Arm A) 58 (Arm B)	2 (Arm A) 16 (Arm B)	
Al-Batran et al. [20], pretreated metastatic BrCa	46	40 vs 50 mg/m²	10.0	NR	NR	4.2%	0	0
Salzberg et al. [38], metastatic BrCa	58	40 mg/m² q 4 weeks	9.63	16	PFS: 3.5	52	14	3
Huober et al. [37], metastatic BrCa	125	40 mg/m² q 4 weeks	10.0	43	PFS: 7.2	30	6	1
Keller et al. [29], taxane refractory BrCa	301	50 mg/m² q 4 weeks	12.2	10	PFS: 2.9	37	18	1
O'Brien et al. [30]	509	50 mg/m² q 4 weeks	12.1	33	PFS: 6.9	48	17	0

BrCa, breast cancer; NR, no response; OC, ovarian cancer; PFS; Progression Free Survival ; PPE; Palmar–plantar erythrodysestehsia (PPE), ; mRD; mediam response duration; TTDP; time to disease progression.

above systolic blood pressure leads to a temporary decrease of blood flow and a limited exposure of hair proliferating cells to the topoisomerase inhibitors. Neither hypothermia nor the tourniquet method has been widely used in patients with malignancies having a high probability of metastasis of the scalp, such as lymphoproliferative disorders or breast carcinoma. ImuVert is an immunomodulator inducing production of interleukin-1, which protects the hair follicles. It may be administered via topical, subcutaneous, or intraperitoneal routes [7–9].

Hand-foot syndrome

HFS is also known as palmoplantar dysesthesia syndrome (PPDE), acral erythema, palmar-plantar erythrodysesthesia (PPE) or Burgdorf syndrome, which is characterized by painful, sharply demarcated, erythematous lesions of the palms, fingers, and soles of the feet, which might progress to a debilitating bullae and desquamation. Eythema and swelling most commonly appear on the thenar and hypothenar eminencies, as well as the lateral aspect of the fingers and the pads of the distal phalanges. The hands are affected more often than the feet and may be the only area involved. Less frequently, other areas of the skin may be involved, particularly those exposed to friction, occlusion, or frequent contact pressure, such as the axilla, groin, waist, inner side of knees, posterior side of elbows, anterior folding lines of wrists, sacral area, and bra line [10,11]. Neurologically, strength, reflexes and position senses are preserved despite potential functional limitations due to pain and swelling. The onset of symptoms has been reported within days of initiated chemotherapy, but the appearance of HFS can be delayed by up to 2–10 months. HFS symptoms are normally not reported before 2–3 courses of treatment. The natural course of HFS is self-limited upon dose reduction, delay of dosing or discontinuation and often resolves within 1–5 weeks after interrupting treatment.

HFS is most commonly associated with the administration of a wide range of cytostatics [12], but also it has been reported as a paraneoplastic phenomenon [13,14], following total body irradiation or after bone marrow transplantation. HFS might be an indicator of impending graft versus host disease (GVHD) [15,16]. Also, it is believed that HFS induced by one agent can be recalled following treatment with other chemotherapeutic agents. The most common chemotherapeutics associated with HFS are doxorubicin, mainly being PLD [17–20], flouropyrimidines especially capecitabine and fluorouracil administered in a continuous infusion and cytarabine. The pathogenesis of HFS is unclear. The causative agents most probably do not share the same pathogenesis: no common features of the different agents have been identified. Research in patients treated with PLD has suggested a likely mechanism of action for this agent. The drug is transported by sweat to the skin surface and penetrates into the stratum corneum, which might serve as a reservoir, allowing PLD penetration into deeper layers of skin. After penetration, free radicals are formed and damage epidermal cells, leading to HFS [21,22]. The palmar and plantar areas present a high density of eccrine sweat glands. The histologic findings are nonspecific and include vacuolar degeneration of the basal cell layer, mild spongiosis, keratinocyte necrosis, papillary dermal edema, lymphohistiocytic infiltrates, and partial separation of the epidermis from the dermis [5,23]. Perivascular infiltrates containing lymphocytes and eosinophils are present in the dermis.

Currently, there is no specific diagnostic test for HFS. The differential diagnosis includes TEN, erythromelalgia, erythema multiforme, Stevens–Johnson syndrome, vasculitis, and GVHD occurring in patients with ongoing bone marrow transplants.

The primary objective in the management of HFS is to prevent and/or reduce the severity of symptoms. In routine clinical practice numerous approaches are used: educating the patient, adjusting the topoisomerase inhibitors, regional cooling [24], administering corticosteroids (8 mg dexamthasone twice daily (bid) on days 1–5, 4 mg bid on day 6, 4 mg on day 7), and administering celecoxib [25–28].

PLD is approved in a dose of 50 mg/m^2 every 4 weeks as monotherapy in metastatic breast cancer [29,30] as well as in platinum-refractory ovarian cancer [31]. In clinical practice, oncologists were surprised by the high incidence of HFS (Table 16.2). Reducing PLD dose intensity is a standard approach used to reduce the risk of or to ameliorate HFS and has been used in patients with several tumor types including breast cancer and ovarian cancer [20,32–36]. Collectively studies demonstrate that PLD administered at a dose intensity of 10 mg/m^2/week, regardless of the dosing interval, is well tolerated and effective (Table 16.2) At this dose intensity most HFS is mild to moderate and potentially disabling HFS does not occur. This is supported by prospective community-based trials in Germany and Switzerland, where 40 mg/m^2 every 4 weeks and 20 mg/m^2 every 2 weeks are the most used regimens [37,38]. Only dose intensity modification for the prevention of HFS in patients treated with PLD has been evaluated in randomized clinical trials [32].

Hyperpigmentation

Hyperpigmentation is a common adverse reaction to cancer chemotherapy. This AE is frequently seen after treatment with alkylating agents, but it has also been reported after treatment with the topoisomerase inhibitors doxorubicin, epirubicin, and idarubicin. It may occur in various anatomic locations and its patterns may be related to various mechanisms of action. The anthracyclines have been implicated in hyperpigmented transverse bands of the nails as well as in mucocutaneous hyperpigmentation. Histologic findings showed increased melanin granules within all layers of the epidermis [39,40]. Nails and mucocutaneus changes occur within a few weeks after initiation of chemotherapy and gradually disappear over a period of months after therapy has been withdrawn. Management is limited to prevention of sun exposure and encouragement of rapid keratinocyte turnover leading to more rapid loss of melanin pigment, and decreased melanin synthesis. Topical retinoids, hydroquinones, and corticosteriods are the most beneficial treatment options.

Intertrigo

Intertrigo is an erythematous well-defined patch, localized to areas of skin-on-skin friction. Typical locations are the axilla, unframammary, and inguinal areas. The skin is usually warm, moist, tender, and pruritic or painful. Due to an impaired barrier, superinfection is very common. Candidal infections have been commonly reported; typical findings include the macroscopical presence of satellite pustules peripheral to the edge of the erythematous patches. Treatment with PLD is associated with up to 8% of intertrigo as an AE [41]. Differential diagnosis includes contact dermatitis, inverse psoriasis, erythrasma, and Hailey–Hailey disease. Intertriginous erythema requires treatment with cream paste including low potency topical corticosteroids and antibacterials and/or antifungals. It is essential to keep the affected areas clean and dry. In the case of candidal intertrigo the addition of topical azole (fluconazole, econazole) is recommended.

Nail changes

Various nails changes can be associated with topoisomerase inhibitors. The most common are pigmented transverse bands or diffuse nail hyperpigmentation. Other nail changes include nail discoloration (leukonychia), detachment of the nail from the nail bed (onycholysis), or transverse depressions of the nail plate, known as Beau lines. Extensive cytostatic treatment (more than six cycles) may predispose patients to mycotic superinfection (onychomycosis). Topoisomerase inhibitors and observed nail changes are listed in Appendix 16.1.

The management of nail changes has not been standardized. Dose reductions and delays of cytotoxic treatment are rarely considered, as risk: benefit ratio favors administration of systemic therapy to control cancer. Prevention of bacterial and/or mycotic infection as well as pain management is sometimes required. The nails will regrow normally after cessation of therapy. Differential diagnosis includes onychomycosis.

Extravasation of topoisomerase inhibitors

Extravasation at the infusion site has been reported in 0.1–6.5% of patients, which may result in erythema, swelling, pain, burning, and/or blue discoloration of the skin (see Chapter 28). Extravasation can result in tissue necrosis resulting in the need for debridement and skin grafting. Phlebitis has also been reported at the site of the infusion. A number of topoisomerase inhibitors can directly cause tissue necrosis as a result of drug extravasation: doxorubicin, idarubicin, and etoposide [42]. The most efficient preventive measure is educating the healthcare professionals about extravasation and the use of implanted central catheters. If extravasation with an anthracycline occurs, dexrazoxane (Savene®, Totect®) can be used. This substance inhibits DNA topoisomerase II the target of anthracycline chemotherapy. It binds topoisomerase II in a different step in the catalytic cycle than anthracyclines. This locks the enzyme in a form that is no longer affected by anthracycline.

Stevens–Johnson syndrome

Stevens–Johnson syndrome (SJS) is a limited form of toxic epidermal necrolysis (TEN) which is a life-threatening condition characterized by blister formations and erosions on mucous membranes and less than 30% of the body surface area. Involvement of more than 10% of the body surface area is considered an overlap between Stevens–Johnson syndrome and TEN. Although some cases are idiopathic, the majority of cases are caused by drugs (analgesics, antiepileptics, antibiotics), including topoisomerase inhibitors (etoposide) and possibly associated with coexisting viral infections. A careful allergologic work-up 4–6 weeks after the event is recommended [43].

Mucositis

Mucositis is a frequent complication of topoisomerase inhibitors that can impact on any part of the gastrointestinal tract (see Chapter 9). Mucositis affects many patients with hematologic malignancies and also a large number of patients with solid tumors. It is particularly associated with cytostatics that affect DNA synthesis, and is more often seen with the bolus dose rather than continuous infusion. Combinations with anthracyclines are often associated with mucositis, which usually occurs 3–7 days after administration [41]. It is characterized by painful erosions and aphthae in the mouth; however, the mucosal damage can occur anywhere along the gastrointestinal tract and may be manifested by diarrhea.

Radiation recall

Radiation recall dermatitis is an inflammatory skin reaction that occurs in previously irradiated body areas following chemotherapy administration (see Chapter 26). The mechanism of action is unknown. One hypothesis suggests that radiation induces heritable mutations within the surviving cells. The surviving cells spawn defective stem cells that are unable to tolerate the second insult of cytostatic therapy. The specific dose of radiation together with the dose of the chemotherapeutic agent may have a role in the pathogenesis. The histologic finding of radiation recall is characterized by apoptotic keratinocytes and vascular dilatation with atypical fibroblasts in the dermis. Radiation recall may appear with a latency period of months to years. Etoposide and doxorubicin are among the responsible topoisomerase agents. Doxorubicin is a radiosensitizer and radiation recall has been reported in up to 43% of patients. There are no established treatments for radiation recall. Anecdotal evidence suggests that cutaneous inflammation may be reduced by topical corticosteroids.

References

1 Mitscher, L.A. (2005) Bacterial topoisomerase inhibitors: quinolone and pyridone antibacterial agents. *Chemical Reviews*, **105** (2), 559–592.

2 Fisher, L.M. & Pan, X.S. (2008) Methods to assay inhibitors of DNA gyrase and topoisomerase IV activities. *Methods in Molecular Medicine*, **142**, 11–23.

3 English, J.C. 3rd, Toney, R. & Patterson, J.W. (2003) Intertriginous epidermal dysmaturation from pegylated liposomal doxorubicin. *Journal of Cutaneous Pathology*, **30**, 591–595.

4 Skelton, H., Linstrum, J. & Smith, K. (2002) Host-vs.-altered-host eruptions in patients on liposomal doxorubicin. *Journal of Cutaneous Pathology*, **29**, 148–153.

5 Lotem, M., Hubert, A., Lyass, O. et al. (2000) Skin toxic effects of polyethylene glycol-coated liposomal doxorubicin. *Archives of Dermatology*, **136**, 1475–1480.

6 Kim, R.J., Peterson, G., Kulp, B., Zanotti, K.M. & Markman, M. (2005) Skin toxicity associated with pegylated liposomal doxorubicin (40 mg^2) in the treatment of gynecologic cancers. *Gynecologic Oncology*, **97**, 374–378.

7 Hussein, A.M., Jimenez, J.J., McCall, C.A. & Yunis, A.A. (1990) Protection from chemotherapy-induced alopecia in a rat model. *Science*, **249**, 1564–1566.

8 Hussein, A.M. (1993) Chemotherapy-induced alopecia: new developments. *Southern Medical Journal*, **86**, 489–496, 505–506.

9 Hussein, A.M. (1995) Protection against cytosine arabinoside-induced alopecia by minoxidil in a rat animal model. *International Journal of Dermatology*, **34**, 470–473.

10 Abeloff, M.D., Armitage, J.O., Niederhuber, J.E., Kastan, M.B. & McKenna, W.G. (2004) *Clinical Oncology*, 3nd ed., Churchill Livingstone, Philadelphia, PA.

11 Baack, B.R. & Burgdorf, W.H. (1991) Chemotherapy-induced acral erythema. *Journal of the American Academy of Dermatology*, **24** (3), 457–461.

12 Kampmann, K.K., Graves, T. & Rogers, S.D. (1989) Acral erythema secondary to high-dose cytosine arabinoside with pain worsened by cyclosporine infusions. *Cancer*, **63** (12), 2482–2485.

13 Noble, J.P., Boisnic, S., Branchet-Gumila, M.C. & Poisson, M. (2002) Palmar erythema: cutanous marker of neoplasms. *Dermatology (Basel, Switzerland)*, **204**, 209–213.

14 Nielsen, M. (1985) Painful palmar-plantar erythema in myeloproliferative disease. *Archives of Dermatology*, **121**, 1240.

15 Crider, M.K., Jansen, J., Norins, A.L. & McHale, M.S. (1986) Chemotherapy-induced acral erythema in patients receiving bone marrow transplantation. *Archives of Dermatology*, **122** (9), 1023–1027.

16 Troussard, X., Dompmartin, A. & Dechaufour, F. (1993) Acral erythema and acute GVHD. *Bone Marrow Transplantation*, **11** (6), 501.

17 Lyass, O., Uziely, B., Ben-Yosef, R. *et al.* (2000) Correlation of toxicity with pharmacokinetics of pegylated liposomal doxorubicin (Doxil) in metastatic breast carcinoma. *Cancer*, **89** (5), 1037–1047.

18 Bhasin, S. Sunita, Gupta, D.K., Kataria, S.P., Saluja, S. & Sharma, M. (2005) Chemotherapy-induced palmer planter erythrodysesthesia. *Journal of the Association of Physicians of India*, **53**, 155–156.

19 Hui, Y.F. & Cortes, J.E. (2000) Palmar-plantar erythrodysesthesia syndrome associated with liposomal daunorubicin. *Pharmacotherapy*, **20** (10), 1221–1223.

20 Al-Batran, S.E., Meerpohl, H.G., von Minckwitz, G. *et al.* (2006) Reduced incidence of severe palmar-plantar erythrodysesthesia and mucositis in a prospective multicenter phase II trial with pegylated liposomal doxorubicin at 40 mg/m every 4 weeks in previously treated patients with metastatic breast cancer. *Oncology*, **70** (2), 141–146.

21 Lademann, J., Martschick, A., Jacobi, U. *et al.* (2005) Investigation of doxorubicin on the skin: a spectroscopic study to understand the pathogenesis of PPE. *Journal of Clinical Oncology*, **23** (Supplement), 5093.

22 von Moos, R., Thuerlimann, B.J., Aapro, M. *et al.* (2008) Pegylated liposomal doxorubicin-associated hand-foot syndrome: recommendations of an international panel of experts. *European Journal of Cancer*, **44** (6), 781–790.

23 Levine, L.E., Medenica, M.M., Lorincz, A.L., Soltani, K., Raab, B. & Ma, A. (1985) Distinctive acral erythema occurring during therapy for severe myelogenous leukemia. *Archives of Dermatology*, **121** (1), 102–104.

24 Molpus, K.L., Anderson, L.B., Craig, C.L. & Puleo, J.G. (2004) The effect of regional cooling on toxicity associated with intravenous infusion of pegylated liposomal doxorubicin in recurrent ovarian carcinoma. *Gynecol Oncol*, **93** (2), 513–516. PubMed PMID: 15099971.

25 Zimmerman, G.C., Keeling, J.H., Lowry, M., Medina, J., Von Hoff, D.D. & Burris, H.A. (1994) Prevention of docetaxel-induced erythrodysesthesia with local hypothermia. *Journal of the National Cancer Institute*, **86** (7), 557–558.

26 Drake, R.D., Lin, W.M., King, M., Farrar, D., Miller, D.S. & Coleman, R.L. (2004) Oral dexamethasone attenuates Doxil-induced palmar-plantar erythrodysesthesias in patients with recurrent gynecologic malignancies. *Gynecologic Oncology*, **94** (2), 320–324.

27 Vukelja, S.J., Baker, W.J., Burris, H.A. 3rd, Keeling, J.H. & Von Hoff, D. (1993) Pyridoxine therapy for palmar-plantar erythrodysesthesia associated with taxotere. *Journal of the National Cancer Institute*, **85** (17), 1432–1433.

28 Lin, E., Morris, J.S. & Ayers, G.D. (2002) Effect of celecoxib on capecitabine-induced hand-foot syndrome and antitumor activity. *Oncology (Williston Park, NY)*, **16** (12 Suppl. 14), 31–37.

29 Keller, A.M., Mennel, R.G., Georgoulias, V.A. *et al.* (2004) Randomized phase III trial of pegylated liposomal doxorubicin versus vinorelbine or mitomycin C plus vinblastine in women with taxane-refractory advanced breast cancer. *Journal of Clinical Oncology*, **22**, 3893–3901.

30 O'Brien, M.E., Wigler, N., Inbar, M. *et al.* (2004) Reduced cardiotoxicity and comparable efficacy in a phase III trial of pegylated liposomal doxorubicin HCl (CAELYX/Doxil) versus conventional doxorubicin for first-line treatment of metastatic breast cancer. *Annals of Oncology*, **15**, 440–449.

31 Gordon, A.N., Fleagle, J.T., Guthrie, D., Parkin, D.E., Gore, M.E. & Lacave, A.J. (2001) Recurrent epithelial ovarian carcinoma: a randomized phase III study of pegylated liposomal doxorubicin versus topotecan. *Journal of Clinical Oncology*, **19**, 3312–3322.

32 Coleman, R.E., Biganzoli, L., Canney, P. *et al.* (2006) A randomised phase II study of two different schedules of pegylated liposomal doxorubicin in metastatic breast cancer (EORTC-10993). *European Journal of Cancer*, **42**, 882–887.

33 Sehouli, J., Oskay-Ozcelik, G., Kuhne, J. *et al.* (2006) Biweekly pegylated liposomal doxorubicin in patients with relapsed ovarian cancer: results of a multicenter phase-II trial. *Annals of Oncology*, **17**, 957–961.

34 Lorusso, D., Naldini, A., Testa, A., D'Agostino, G., Scambia, G. & Ferrandina, G. (2004) Phase II study of pegylated liposomal doxorubicin in heavily pretreated epithelial ovarian cancer patients. May a new treatment schedule improve toxicity profile? *Oncology*, **67**, 243–249.

35 Campos, S.M., Penson, R.T., MacNeill, K.M. *et al.* (1999) A retrospective analysis of the clinical utility of doxil in recurrent ovarian cancer (ROC). *Proceedings of the American Society of Clinical Oncology*, **18**, 371a.

36 Markman, M., Kennedy, A., Webster, K., Peterson, G., Kulp, B. & Belinson, J. (2000) Phase 2 trial of liposomal doxorubicin (40 mg/m²) in platinum/paclitaxel-refractory ovarian and fallopian tube cancers and primary carcinoma of the peritoneum. *Gynecologic Oncology*, **78**, 369–372.

37 Huober, J., Fett, W., Nusch, A. *et al.* (2010) A multicentric observational trial of pegylated liposomal doxorubicin for metastatic breast cancer. *BMC Cancer*, **10**, 2.

38 Salzberg, M., Thurlimann, B., Hasler, U. *et al.* (2007) Pegylated liposomal doxorubicin (caelyx) in metastatic breast cancer: a community-based observation study. *Oncology*, **72**, 147–151.

39 Kroumpouzos, G., Travers, R. & Allan, A. (2002) Generalized hyperpigmentation with daunorubicin chemotherapy. *Journal of the American Academy of Dermatology*, **46** (2 Suppl.), 1–3.

40 Krutchik, A.N. & Buzdar, A.U. (1979) Pigmentation of the tongue and mucous membranes with cancer chemotherapy. *Southern Medical Journal*, **72**, 1615–1616.

41 Lotem, M., Hubert, A., Lyass, O. *et al.* (2000) Skin toxic effects of polyethylene glycolcoated liposomal doxorubicin. *Archives of Dermatology*, **136**, 1475–1480.

42 Ener, R.A., Meglathery, S.B. & Styler, M. (2004) Extravasation of systemic hemato-oncological therapies. *Annals of Oncology*, **15**, 858–862.

43 Wyatt, J.A., Leonard, G.D. & Sachs, D.L. (2006) Cutaneous reactions to chemotherapy and their management. *American Journal of Clinical Dermatology*, **7** (1), 45–63.

44 Product information (2009) Camptosar® irinotecan hydrochloride solution for intravenous injection. Pfizer, New York, NY.

45 Product information (2007) Campto® irinotecan hydrochloride concentrate for solution for infusion. Pfizer AG, Zürich, Switzerland.

46 Product information (2010) Hycamtin® IV injection, topotecan hydrochloride IV injection. GlaxoSmithKline, Research Triangle Park, NC.

47 Product information (2007) Hycamtin® oral capsules, topotecan oral capsules. GlaxoSmithKline, Research Triangle Park, NC.

48 Product information (2009) Hycamtin® IV injection, topotecan hydrochloride IV injection. GlaxoSmithKline AG, Münchenbuchsee, Switzerland.

49 van Warmerdam, L.J.C., ten Bokkel Huinink, W.W., Rodenhuis, S. *et al.* (1995) Phase I clinical and pharmacokinetic study of topotecan administered by a 24-hour continuous infusion. *Journal of Clinical Oncology*, **13**, 1768–1776.

50 Hochster, H., Liebes, L., Speyer, J. *et al.* (1994) Phase I trial of low-dose continuous topotecan infusion in patients with cancer: an active and well-tolerated regimen. *Journal of Clinical Oncology*, **12**, 553–559.

51 Product information (2008) Doxorubicin Ebewe® Doxorubicin hydrochloride solution for IV injection. Sandoz Pharmaceuticals AG, Steinhausen, Switzerland.

52 Carter, S.K. & Blum, R.H. (1974) New chemotherapeutic agents: bleomycin and adriamycin. *CA: A Cancer Journal for Clinicians*, **24**, 322–331.

53 Alagaratnam, T.T., Choi, T.K. & Ong, G.B. (1982) Doxorubicin and hyperpigmentation. *Australian and New Zealand Journal of Surgery*, **52**, 531.

54 Runne, U., Mitrenga, D. & Pfeiff, B. (1980) Braunes nagelbett, onycholyse und hautveraenderungen durch adriamycin und bleomycin. *Zeitschrift fur Hautkrankheiten*, **55**, 1590–1593.

55 Product information (2007) Doxil® IV injection, doxorubicin HCL liposome IV injection. Ortho Biotech Products,LP, Raritan, NJ.

56 Product information (2008) Caelyx® IV injection, doxorubicin HCL liposome IV injection. Janssen-Cilag AG, Baar, Switzerland.

57 Skelton, H., Linstrum, J. & Smith, K. (2002) Host-vs-altered-host eruptions in patients on liposomal doxorubicin. *Journal of Cutaneous Pathology*, **29**, 148–153.

58 Product information (2009) Zavedos® idarubicin hydrochloride solution for intravenous injection and intravenous powder for solution. Pfizer AG, Zürich, Switzerland.

59 Weiss, R.B., Sarosy, G., Clagett-Carr, K., Russo, M. & Leyland-Jones, B. (1986) Anthracycline analogs: the past, present, and future (review). *Cancer Chemotherapy and Pharmacology*, **18**, 185–197.

60 Hurteloup, P. & Ganzina, F. (1986) Clinical studies with new anthracyclines: epirubicin, idarubicin, esorubicin (review). *Drugs Under Experimental and Clinical Research*, **12**, 233–246.

61 Bonfante, V., Ferrari, L., Villani, F. & Bonadonna, G. (1983) Phase I study of 4-demethoxydaunorubicin. *Investigational New Drugs*, **1**, 161–168.

62 Lopez, M., Contegiacomo, A., Vici, P. *et al.* (1989) A prospective randomized trial of doxorubicin versus idarubicin in the treatment of advanced breast cancer. *Cancer*, **64**, 2431–2436.

63 Lopez, M., Di Lauro, L., Papaldo, P., Lazzaro, B., Ganzina, F. & Di Pietro, N. (1986) Phase II trial with oral idarubicin in advanced breast cancer. *Investigational New Drugs*, **4**, 39–42.

64 Ganzina, F., Pacciarini, M.A. & Di Pietro, N. (1986) Idarubicin (4-demethoxydaunorubicin). A preliminary overview of preclinical and clinical studies. *Investigational New Drugs*, **4**, 85–105.

65 Stuart, N.S.A., Cullen, M.H., Priestman, T.J., Blackledge, G.R. & Tyrrell, C.J. (1988) A phase II study or oral idarubicin (4-demethoxydaunorubicin) in advanced breast cancer. *Cancer Chemotherapy and Pharmacology*, **21**, 351–354.

66 Product information (1997) Idamycin®, idarubicin. Adria Laboratories, Columbus, OH.

67 Product information (2006) Cerubidine® Daunorubicin intravenous powder for solution. Sanofi-Aventis SA, Meyrin, Switzerland.

68 Product information (1999) Cerubidine®, daunorubicin. Ben Venue Laboratories, Bedford, OH, USA.

69 Kelly, T.M., Fishman, L.M. & Lessner, H.E. (1984) Hyperpigmentation with daunorubicin therapy. *Archives of Dermatology*, **120**, 262–263.

70 Dragon, L.H. & Braine, H.G. (1979) Necrosis of the hand after daunorubicin infusion distal to an arteriovenous fistula. *Annals of Internal Medicine*, **91**, 58–59.

71 Wong, K.Y. & Lampkin, B.C. (1983) Anthracycline toxicity. *American Journal of Pediatric Hematology*, **5**, 93–97.

72 Product information (2003) Ellence(R), epirubicin hydrochloride. Pharmacia & Upjohn Company, Kalamazoo, MI.

73 Cersosimo, R.J. & Hong, W.K. (1986) Epirubicin: a review of the pharmacology, clinical activity, and adverse effects of an adriamycin analogue. *Journal of Clinical Oncology*, **4**, 425–439.

74 Product information (2006) Epirubicin Ebewe® Doxorubicin hydrochloride solution for IV injection. Sandoz Pharmaceuticals AG, Steinhausen, Switzerland.

75 Product information (2004) Cosmegen®, dactinomycin. Merck & Co., Whitehouse Station, NJ.

76 Product information (2009) Cosmegen®, dactinomycin. Lundbeck Pharmaceuticals Ireland Ltd., Dublin, Ireland.

77 Gilman, A.G., Rall, T.W., Nies, A.S. *et al.* (eds) (1990) *The Pharmacological Basis of Therapeutics*, 8th ed., Pergamon Press, New York, NY.

78 Product information (2008) Novantron® mitoxantrone hydrochloride solution for IV injection. MEDA Pharma GmbH, Wangen-Brüttisellen, Switzerland.

79 Dharmasena, F., Chu, A.C., Goldman, J.M. & Galton, D.A. (1985) Mitoxantrone induced asteatosis. *Lancet*, **2**, 101.

80 Anderson, K.C. & Cohen, G.I. (1982) Garnich MB: phase II trial of mitoxantrone. *Cancer Treatment Reports*, **66**, 1929–1931.

81 Anderson, K.C., Garnick, M.B., Meshad, M.W. *et al.* (1983) Phase I trial of mitozantrone by 24 hours continuous infusions. *Cancer Treatment Reports*, **67**, 435–438.

82 Taylor, W.B., Cantwell, B.M.J., Roberts, J.T. & Harris, A.L. (1986) Allergic reactions to mitoxantrone (letter). *Lancet*, **1**, 1439.

83 Bedikian, A.Y., Stroehlein, J., Korinek, J., Karlin, D., Valdivieso, M. & Bodey, G.P. (1983) Phase II evaluation of dihydroxyanthracenedione (DHAD, NSC 301739) in patients with metastatic colorectal cancer. *American Journal of Clinical Oncology*, **6**, 45–48.

84 Smith, I.E. (1983) Mitoxantrone (novantrone): a review of experimental and early clinical studies. *Cancer Treatment Reviews*, **10**, 103–115.

85 Arlin, Z.A., Friedland, M.L. & Atamer, M.A. (1984) Selective alopecia with mitoxantrone. *New England Journal of Medicine*, **310**, 1464.

86 Estey, E.H., Keating, M.J., McCredie, K.B., Bodey, G.P. & Freireich, E.J. (1983) Phase II trial of mitoxantrone in refractory acute leukemia. *Cancer Treatment Reports*, **67**, 389–390.

87 Product information (2000) VePesid®, etoposide. Bristol Laboratories, Princeton, NJ.

88 Product information (2010) Vepesid® etoposide. Bristol-Myers Squibb SA, Baar, Switzerland.

89 Perry, M.C., Moertel, C.G., Schutt, A.J., Reitemeier, R.J. & Hahn, R.G. (1976) Phase II studies of dianhydrogalactitol and VP-16-213 in colorectal cancer. *Cancer Treatment Reports*, **60**, 1247–1250.

90 Nissen, N.I., Hansen, H.H., Pedersen, H., Stroyer, I., Dombernowsky, P. & Hessellund, M. (1975) Clinical trial of the oral form of a new podophyllotoxin derivative, VP-16-213 (NSC-141540), in patients with advanced neoplastic disease. *Cancer Chemotherapy Reports. Part 1*, **59**, 1027–1029.

91 Jungi, W.F., Senn, H.J., Beckman, C., Flury, R., Frei, P. & Holdener, E. (1975) Therapeutic experiences using the new podophyllotoxin derivative VP 16213 in human malignant tumors. *Schweizerische Medizinische Wochenschrift*, **105**, 1365–1369.

92 Schey, S.A., Cooper, J. & Summerhayes, M. (1992) The "handfoot syndrome" occurring with chronic administration of etoposide (letter). *European Journal of Haematology*, **48**, 118–119.

93 Williams, B.J., Roth, D.J. & Callen, J.P. (1993) Ultraviolet recall associated with etoposide and cyclophosphamide therapy. *Clinical and Experimental Dermatology*, **18**, 452–453.

94 Obermair, A. & Vavra, N. (1995) Letters to the editor (letter). *Gynecologic Oncology*, **57**, 436.

95 Jameson, C.H. & Solanki, D.L. (1983) Stevens-Johnson syndrome associated with etoposide therapy. *Cancer Treatment Reports*, **67**, 1050–1051.

96 Product information (2010) Etopophos® IV injection, etoposide phosphate IV injection. Baxter Healthcare Corporation, Deerfield, IL.

97 Product information (2006) Etopophos® etoposide phosphate IV injection. Bristol-Myers Squibb SA, Baar, Switzerland.

98 Product information. (2011) Vumon(R), teniposide. Bristol-Myers Squibb, Princeton, NJ.

Appendix 16.1 Dermatologic adverse event of topoisomerase inhibitors.

Drug name	Information source	Dermatologic adverse events — Cutaneous and subcutaneous	Nail	Hair	Mucous membranes
Irinotecan (CPT-11, Camptosar)	Prod Info [44]	Rash All: 13–14.3% Grade 3 or 4: 1–2%; Exfoliative dermatitis All: 0%; Sweating All: 16%		Alopecia All: 46.1–60%	Stomatitis All: 12%
Topotecan (Hycamtin)	Prod Info [45]	Skin reaction All: 0.1% to 1%		Alopecia All: 60%	Stomatitis All: 0.1–10%
	Prod Info IV [46]	Rash incl. pruritus, rash erythematous, urticaria, dermatitis, bullous eruption and maculopapular rash) All: 16%		Alopecia All: 49%	Stomatitis All: 18% Grade 3: 1% Grade 4: <1%
	Prod Info oral [47]			Alopecia All: 10–20% Grade 3 or 4: 0–0.1%	
	Prod Info IV [48]	Exanthema All: 1–10%		Alopecia All: 16–31%	Stomatitis All: 17%
	van Warmerdam et al. [49]			Alopecia All: 80%	
	Hochster et al. [50]			Alopecia All: 5%	
Doxorubicin (Adriamycin)	Prod Info [51]	Hyperpigmentation All: 0.01–0.1%; Photosensitivity, radiation recall syndrome All: 0.01–0.1%; Urticaria All: 0.01–0.1%; Exanthema, pruritus, acral erythema All: <0.01%	Hyperpigmentation All: 0.01–0.1%	Alopecia All: 90–100%	Stomatitis and esophagitis reported
	Carter & Blum [52]			Alopecia All: 100%	Stomatitis All: 80%
	Alagaratnam et al. [53] Runne et al. [54]		Oncholysis reported		

(Continued)

Drug name	Information source	Dermatologic adverse events			
		Cutaneous and subcutaneous	Nail	Hair	Mucous membranes
Pegylated doxorubicin (Doxil, Caelyx)	Prod Info [55]	Rash (Ovarian cancer) All: 28.5% Grade 3 or 4: 4.2% (Multiple myeloma) All: 22% (AIDS-related Kaposi sarcoma) All: 1–5% Hand-foot syndrome (Ovarian cancer) All: 50.6% Grade 3 or 4: 23.8% (Multiple myeloma) All: 19% (AIDS-related Kaposi sarcoma) All: 3.4%		Alopecia (AIDS-related Kaposi sarcoma) All: 8.9%	Stomatitis (Ovarian cancer) All: 41.4% Grade 3 or 4: 8.3% (Multiple myeloma) All: 20% Grade 3: 2% Grade 4: 0% (AIDS-related Kaposi's sarcoma) All: 6.8%
	Prod Info [56]	Rash All: 17.3% Grade 3 and 4: 2.4% Hand-foot syndrome All: 37.7% Grade 3: 19% Grade 4: <1% Dry skin, abnormal pigmentation, skin discoloration, pruritus, erythema, skin desquamation, dermatitis, exfoliative dermatitis, maculopapular rash All: 1–10% Sweating, acne, urticaria, ecchymosis, exanthema All: 0.1–1%	Nail changes All: 1–10%	Alopecia All: 13.4% Grade 3 and 4: 0.6%	Stomatitis All: 28.1% Grade 3 and 4: 5.5% Mucositis All: 1–10% Gingivitis All: 0.1–1% Mucomembranous disease All: 14.5% Grade 3 and 4: 3.1%
	Skelton et al. [57]	Cutaneous eruptions/skin lesion reported			
Idarubicin (Idamycin)	Prod Info [58]	Rash All: 25% Grade 3 and 4: 0% Local skin reaction All: 15% Grade 3 and 4: 0.5% Pruritus, Radiation recall syndrome All: 1–10% Urticaria, Hyperpigmentation All: 0.1–1% Acral erythema: 0.01–0.1%	Hyperpigmentation All: 0.1–1%	Alopecia All: 70% Grade 3 and 4: 35%	Mucositis All: 58% Grade 3 and 4: 12% Stomatitis All: >10%
	Weiss et al. [59] Hurteloup & Ganzina et al. [60] Bonfante et al. [61] Lopez et al. [62,63] Ganzina et al. [64]			Alopecia All: 25–30%	

Reference	Rash	Photosensitivity	Hyperpigmentation	Alopecia	Mucositis/Stomatitis
Hurteloup & Ganzina et al. [60] Bonfante et al. [61] Ganzina et al. [64]					Stomatitis All: 11%
Stuart et al. [65]	Rash reported				
Prod Info [66]	Urticaria and bullous erythrodermatous rash of the palms and soles reported				
Daunorubicin (Daunomycin) Prod Info [67]	Erythema, exanthema, urticaria, hyperpigmentation All: 0.01–0.1%			Alopecia All: 100%	Stomatitis All: 15%
Prod Info [68]				Alopecia All: most patients	Mucositis reported
Kelly et al. [69]	Hyperpigmentation reported				
Dragon & Braine [70]	Digital necrosis reported				
Wong & Lampkin [71]					Mucositis reported
Epirubicin (Ellence, Pharmorubicin, Epirubicin Ebewe) Prod Info [72] Cersosimo & Hong [73]	Rash reported	Photosensitivity, radiation recall syndrome, urticaria reported	Hyperpigmentation, nail changes reported	Alopecia All: 25–100% (average 70%)	Mucositis, mainly stomatitis All: 1% to 60%
Prod Info [74]	Rash, skin changes, urticaria All: >10%	Photosensitivity, radiation recall syndrome All: 1–10%	Hyperpigmentation All: 0.1–1%	Alopecia All: most patients Grade 2 to 4: 20%	Mucositis (stomatitis and esophagitis) All: 1–10% Mucosal ulceration, hyperpigmentation of the oral mucosa All: 0.1–1%

(Continued)

Drug name	Information source	Dermatologic adverse events				Mucous membranes
		Cutaneous and subcutaneous		Nail	Hair	
Actinomycin D (Dactinomycin)	Prod Info [75]	Skin eruptions, acne, erythema, hyperpigmentation of previously irradiated skin reported	Radiation recall syndrome reported		Alopecia of previously irradiated skin reported	Severe oropharyngeal mucositis with concurrent radiation therapy, ulcerative stomatitis, esophagitis, enteritis reported
		Epidermiolysis, erythema (with regional limb perfusion) reported				
	Prod Info [76]	Acne, exanthema, epidermiolysis, hyperpigmentation of previously irradiated skin reported			Alopecia reported	Stomatitis ulcerosa, cheilitis, esophagitis, proctitis reported
	Gilman et al. [77]					Stomatitis, cheilitis, glossitis, proctitis All: 1–10%
						Severe oropharyngeal mucositis with concurrent radiation therapy, oral ulcerations reported
Mitoxantrone (Novantrone)	Prod Info [78]	Rash All: 1–10%		Tissue necrosis reported	Alopecia All: 61%	Mucositis All: 10%
		Ecchymosis All 11%	Blue skin discoloration All: 0.1–1%	Nail changes reported		Stomatitis All: 19%
	Dharmasena et al. [79]	Severe pruritus and skin desquamation caused by progressive dry skin (asteatosis) in 4 of 18 patients				
	Anderson et al. [80,81]	Mild phlebitis and a blue discoloration of the veins reported				
	Taylor et al. [82] Bedikian et al. [83] Anderson & Cohen [80]	Erythematous maculopapular eruptions reported				

Drug	Reference	Dermatologic/skin reactions	Flushing	Allergic / nail changes	Alopecia	Mucositis / Stomatitis
	Smith [84]				Severe alopecia All: 0.4% Mild alopecia All: 11%	Mucositis All: 4%
	Arlin et al. [85]				Selective loss of white hair reported	
Etoposide (Vepesid)	Estey et al. [86] Bedikian et al. [83]					Mucositis All: 26–54%
	Prod Info [87]	Rash, urticaria and/or pruritus reported				Stomatitis, mucositis All: 1–6%
	Prod Info [88]	Stevens–Johnson syndrome, toxic epidermal necrolysis, skin pigmentation, pruritus, urticaria, rash All: 0.01–0.1%			Alopecia All: 66%	Stomatitis, mucositis All: 1–10%
	Prod Info [87] Perry et al. [89] Nissen et al. [90] Jungi et al. [91]				Alopecia All: 8–93%	
	Schey et al. [92]	Hand-foot syndrome reported				
	Williams et al. [93]	Ultraviolet recall reported				
	Schey et al. [92] Obermair & Vavra [94]			Oncholysis of the finger and toe nails reported		
	Jameson & Solanki [95]	Stevens–Johnson syndrome, toxic epidermal necrolysis reported				
Etoposide phosphate (Etophos)	Prod Info [96]	Rash All: 3%	Flushing All: 2%	Allergic reactions (including rash, urticaria and/or pruritus) reported	Alopecia All: 33–44%	Mucositis All: 11%
	Prod Info [97]	Stevens–Johnson syndrome, toxic epidermal necrolysis, skin pigmentation, pruritus, urticaria, rash All: 0.01–0.1%			Alopecia All: 33–44%	Mucositis All: 11% Stomatitis All: 1–10%
Teniposide (Vumon, VM-26)	Prod Info [98]					Mucositis All: up to 76%

17 Epidermal Growth Factor Receptor Inhibitor Reactions

Yevgeniy Balagula and Mario E. Lacouture

Dermatology Service, Memorial Sloan-Kettering Cancer Center, New York, NY, USA

Introduction

Epidermal growth factor receptor inhibitors (EGFRIs) such as gefitinib, erlotinib, afatinib, lapatinib, cetuximab, and panitumumab are widely employed for the treatment of solid malignancies. While their use has significantly reduced the incidence of systemic toxicities such as myelosuppression, they are associated with dermatologic adverse events (AEs) affecting the skin and its adnexae. This chapter reviews the spectrum of dermatologic AEs associated with EGFRIs, their clinical presentation, underlying mechanisms, potential risk factors, and available management strategies.

Epidermal growth factor receptor inhibitors

In skin, epidermal growth factor receptor (EGFR) [1] is found in proliferating keratinocytes in the basal and suprabasal layers of the epidermis, outer layers of the hair follicle, pilosebaceous and eccrine sweat glands [2,3]. The EGFR pathway has a critical role in regulating keratinocyte proliferation, differentiation, migration, and survival [4,5]. Multiple agents targeting the EGFR have been developed and can be classified into two categories based on the domain of the receptor they target (Table 17.1) [4]. Monoclonal antibodies (e.g., cetuximab and panitumumab) have a high affinity for the extracellular domain of the receptor and their binding results in receptor internalization and degradation, with subsequent inhibition of activity. In contrast, erlotinib and afatinib are small molecule inhibitors that target the intracellular tyrosine kinase portion of the receptor by competing with adenosine triphosphate (ATP). Lapatinib is a low molecular weight inhibitor with dual activity against EGFR and ErbB2 (Her2/neu) [6]. All of these agents lead to a set of dermatologic AEs that are considered as class-based effects (Figure 17.1).

Dermatologic adverse events of EGFRIs

Papulopustular (acneiform) rash
Clinical presentation
Cetuximab, panitumumab, erlotinib, and afatinib are all associated with a papulopustular (acneiform) rash, which is the most clinically significant AE (Table 17.2) [7]. The rash is characterized by erythematous papules and/or pustules affecting the seborrheic-rich areas, and is indistinguishable from agent to agent (Figure 17.2; Table 17.2) [7]. Thus, it most commonly manifests on the scalp and face, particularly involving the cheeks, nose, nasolabial folds, chin, perioral regions, and the forehead [8,9]. While the upper trunk is frequently affected, the rash can less commonly involve the lower trunk, buttocks, and the extremities [10]. The palmoplantar surfaces are always spared [8,9,11]. The onset of signs and symptoms is variable, although the rash most commonly manifests within the first 2–4 weeks of therapy [12]. Dysesthesias, accompanied by erythema and edema may precede the manifestation of the rash. Upon further progression, purulent material and debris accumulate in a form of crusts overlying the lesions, which do not necessarily indicate an underlying infection. After reaching its peak intensity at approximately 4 weeks, spontaneous partial improvement may occur, even despite continued EGFRI therapy [11,13,14]. Following the resolution of acute lesions, persistent erythema, hyperpigmentation, and multiple telangiectasias may remain [15]. In most people, there are no permanent sequelae, but the erythema and hyperpigmentation can persist for months or years [16].

Dermatologic Principles and Practice in Oncology: Conditions of the Skin, Hair, and Nails in Cancer Patients, First Edition. Edited by Mario E. Lacouture.
© 2014 John Wiley & Sons, Inc. Published 2014 by John Wiley & Sons, Inc.

Of note, the rash associated with lapatinib appears to have different clinical behavior and presentation compared to with other EGFRI-induced eruptions. With predilection for truncal involvement, it infrequently affects the face and generally is less severe [17].

In addition to affecting cosmetically sensitive areas, the papulopustular rash may be associated with physical symptoms of pain, pruritus, burning, and irritation in approximately 62% of patients [18,19]. The rash has been shown to have a negative impact on patients' quality of life (QoL), as measured by a dermatology-specific questionnaire, Skindex-16. The Skindex-16 is a patient-reported outcome tool that grades three domains represented by 16 symptoms, with a total score ranging from 0

(no impact on QoL) to 100 (greatest impact on QoL). While symptoms (median score 45.8) and functioning (median score 23.3) domains are clearly impacted by the rash, the greatest impact was found on the emotional domain (median score 57.1) [20]. With increasing rash severity, there was a significantly diminished QoL among all three domains. The papulopustular rash tends to be mild (grade 1) to moderate (grade 2) in severity (Table 17.2) [14,21]. However, higher grades of the rash (grade 3 or higher) affecting the minority of patients may result in dose modification or cessation of therapy [22], with 76% and 32% of oncology practitioners interrupting or discontinuing EGFRIs because of rash [23]. These unplanned treatment modifications can potentially compromise clinical outcome.

Histopathologic findings and underlying pathophysiology

The most frequently altered structure appears to be the hair follicle [24]. In general, two predominant histopathologic patterns can be observed: superficial perifolliculitis, with an inflammatory infiltrate surrounding ectatic and hyperkeratotic follicular infundibula, and neutrophilic suppurative folliculitis [25]. There is thinning of the stratum corneum, which loses its normal basket-weave-like configuration [25]. Changes in the pilosebaceous glands are noted, characterized by their small size, poorly differentiated sebocytes and keratinocytes, and inflammatory cell infiltrate [24]. Epidermal atrophy, dyskeratosis, and dysmaturation can be seen to a variable degree [26]. Interestingly, evidence of dysregulated differentiation of keratinocytes in the epidermal

Table 17.1 Classification of epidermal growth factor receptor inhibitors.

Small molecule inhibitors	
Erlotinib	Reversible
Gefitinib	Reversible
Afatinib	Irreversible
Lapatinib (dual EGFR-Her 2)	Reversible
Monoclonal antibodies	
Cetuximab	Chimeric
Panitumumab	Fully humanized
Pertuzumab (dimerization)	Humanized

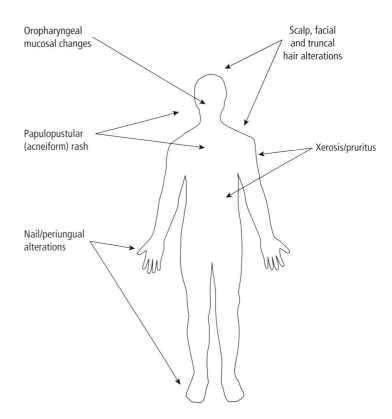

Figure 17.1 Anatomic location of epidermal growth factor receptor inhibitor inhibitor-induced dermatologic adverse events.

Table 17.2 Incidence of dermatologic adverse events to epidermal growth factor receptor inhibitors.

Drug name (Trade)	Information Source	Dermatologic adverse events		Nail/periungual	Hair	Mucous membranes
		Cutaneous and subcutaneous				
Cetuximab (Erbitux)	[8,65,66]	Rash All grades: 90%; Grade 3–4: 10% Xerosis All: –; Grade 3–4: 4%	Pruritus All grades: 10%; Grade 3–4: 1%	All grades: 16%; Grade 3–4: <1%	Alopecia All grades: 5%; Trichomegaly 12%	All grades: 11%; Grades 3–4: <1%
Panitumumab (Vectibix)	[67]	Rash All grades: 57%; Grade 3–4: 7% Xerosis All:10%; Grade 3–4: 0%	Pruritus All grades: 57%; Grade 3–4: 2%	All grades: 25%; Grade 3–4: 2%	Trichomegaly 6%	All grades: 6%; Grades 3–4: <1%
Erlotinib (Tarceva)	[8,22,68,69]	Rash All grades: 75%; Grade 3–4: 9% Xerosis All:12%; Grade 3–4: 0%	Pruritus All grades: 13%; Grade 3–4: <1%	All grades: 14%; Grade 3–4: <1%	Alopecia All grades: 6%; Trichomegaly 11%	All grades: 19%; Grades 3–4: <1%
Lapatinib (Tykerb)	[70,71]	Rash All grades: 47%; Grade 3–4: 3% Xerosis All:13% ; Grade 3–4: <1%	Pruritus All grades: 12%; Grade 3–4: <1%	All grades: 11%; Grade 3–4: <1%	Alopecia All grades: 13%;	All grades: 44%; Grades 3–4: 0%
Gefitinib (Iressa)	[72,73]	Rash All grades: 47%; Grade 3–4: 2% Xerosis All:11% ; Grade 3–4: 0%	Pruritus All grades: 8%; Grade 3–4: <1%	All grades: 3%; Grade 3–4: <1%	–	All grades: 1%; Grades 3–4: –

layer is also evident in skin unaffected by the rash. Biopsy of normal-appearing skin in patients treated with EGFRIs reveals compact orthokeratosis with loss of basket weave appearance, dyskeratosis, disruption of hair follicle architecture, reflecting abnormal process of terminal corneocyte differentiation [24].

It is currently hypothesized that the primary event underlying the development of the rash is direct inhibition of the EGFR, which results in increased and premature keratinocyte differentiation, increased cellular attachment with diminished cell migration and reduced keratinocyte proliferation [27]. In addition, there is a marked inflammatory response, with T lymphocytes, monocytes, and neutrophils [27], induced by keratinocyte release of cytokines and chemokines, including CCL2 and CCL5 [27]. Alternatively, alteration of follicular epithelium and pilosebaceous unit, with keratinocyte apoptosis may serve as a trigger of the inflammatory response [24]. Recent histopathologic investigations demonstrated higher pAKT (signal transduction marker), diminished p27 (negative growth regulator) and K16 (hyperproliferation marker) expression, reduced epidermal atrophy, and follicular neutrophilic infiltrate in skin of patients treated with lapatinib compared with cetuximab,

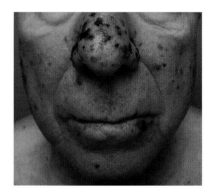

Figure 17.2 Papulopustular eruption secondary to epidermal growth factor receptor inhibitors that may affect up to 90% of treated patients.

erlotinib, and panitumumab [26]. These findings correlate with the reduced severity of clinically observed rash to lapatinib [26].

In contrast to acne, no comedonal lesions (blackheads) or cysts are seen and the distribution of EGFRI-induced rash extends outside the areas usually affected by acne. Whereas sebaceous gland hyperplasia is seen in acne vulgaris, hypoplasia and glandular distortion is noted in EGFRI-affected skin [24]. Similarly, typical antiacne interventions, such as topical retinoic acids and benzoyl peroxide, are not effective in ameliorating papulopustular rash and cause significant irritation [7].

Management

There are two management approaches to patients treated with EGFRIs. Treatment may be instituted in a prophylactic manner in an attempt to prevent or diminish anticipated dermatologic toxicities. Alternatively, reactive therapy may be employed following their manifestations. Regardless, all patients should be counseled and educated about the spectrum of toxicities expected to occur throughout therapy prior to initiation of EGFRIs. In addition, specific lifestyle modifications that may ameliorate dermatologic adverse events should be recommended (Table 17.3).

In recent years most efforts have concentrated on pre-emptive strategies for a papulopustular rash. Multiple randomized controlled trials (RCTs) have been conducted thus far with variable results (Table 17.4) [28–32]. Based on these outcomes, prophylactic therapy with a skin treatment regimen consisting of 100 mg doxycycline bid, sunscreen, moisturizer, and hydrocortisone 1%, or 100 mg/day minocycline is recommended. Pending further evidence, the authors recommend offering prophylactic therapy to all patients who are starting therapy with EGFRIs.

Smoking during therapy with erlotinib is associated with a lower incidence of rash, attributed to induction of CYP4503A4 and subsequent enhanced clearance of the drug [33,34]. In patients with nonsmall lung cancer treated with erlotinib, older age (≥70 years) was associated with a more severe rash (≥ grade 3; 16% vs. 6% of younger patients, respectively) [35]. This is in contrast to mCRC patients treated with cetuximab, among which younger age (≤70 years) was associated with a higher rate of grade 3 rash (6% vs. 1% in older patients) [36]. Male gender in this population was also associated with an increased rate of grade 3 papulopustular rash (7% vs. 3%) and the risk was additive, with 8% of younger males who experienced grade 3 rash [36]. Skin color, as measured by the Fitzpatrick skin phototype (SPT) system (ranges from I, pale skin, burns easily upon sun exposure, through VI, black skin, does not burn upon sun exposure), may also correlate with rash severity, with 0% of SPT V–VI and 5% of SPT III–IV patients presenting with a lower incidence of ≥ grade 3 rash when compared with patients with SPT I–II (63%) [37]. This may be explained by the critical role of EGFR in mediating keratinocyte proliferation and survival following the exposure to UVR [38]. Clinically, the rash frequently affects photoexposed regions such as the face, V-shaped area of the chest, and the upper back. Nevertheless, the prophylactic use of a sunscreen with a sun protection factor of 60 failed to either prevent or attenuate EGFRI-induced papulopustular rash in a recently conducted placebo-controlled RCT [32].

As an alternative, therapy may be initiated following the rash manifestation. However, the use of various agents has been based on anecdotal evidence and expert recommendations. Reactive treatment is guided by the severity of the eruption, using the National Cancer Institute's Common Terminology Criteria for Adverse Events version 4.0 (NCI CTCAE v.4). While this latest version has allowed more accurate assessments than its predecessors, its application in routine clinical care is limited [39,40]. To compensate for deficiencies of CTCAE, a new classification scale was recently designed by a Multinational Association for Supportive Care in Cancer (MASCC) skin toxicity group to address dermatologic toxicities specific to EGFRIs [41]. Taking into consideration the severity of the rash at presentation, the treatment with a combination of topical and/or oral corticosteroids and antibiotics is recommended (Figure 17.3). These recommendations are based on several management guidelines proposed in recent years, stemming from expert opinions of clinicians and limited clinical data [7,15,16,42]. Dose modification or treatment interruption according to package insert may be necessary in cases of high grade rash. Benzoyl peroxide, topical retinoic acid, and pimecrolimus, utilized in treatment of acne vulgaris and dermatitis, should be avoided [7,12,28,42].

The pre-emptive and reactive use of semisynthetic tetracycline antibiotics is partially based on their anti-inflammatory properties stemming from inhibition of matrix metalloproteinases [16]. Microorganisms are not thought to be the primary culprit in the pathophysiology of the rash, but 38% of patients were shown to have secondary infections, including bacterial (29%), with *Staphylococcus aureus* being the most common pathogen (22.6%),

Table 17.3 Life-style modifications to diminish dermatologic toxicities of epidermal growth factor receptors inhibitors.

Papulopustular rash	Xerosis/pruritus	Nail/periungual toxicities
Broad-spectrum (UVA/UVB) sunscreen with SPF ≥30	Minimize the frequency and duration of hot showers	Avoid wearing tight-fitting shoes
Physical blockers (zinc oxide, titanium dioxide)		
Limit excessive sun exposure	Use lukewarm water to shower and wash dishes	Keep nails short
Use thick, alcohol-free emollients	Eliminate the use of alcohol containing products	Avoid exposure to harsh, irritative chemicals
Avoid over-the-counter antiacne medications	Emollients to moisturize dry skin twice a day	Moisturize periungual areas
	Avoid antibacterial soaps	Minimize frequent water immersion/dish washing

Table 17.4 Results of randomized controlled trials in prophylactic therapy for epidermal growth factor receptor inhibitors (EGFRI) associated papulopustular rash.

EGFRI	Intervention	Schedule	Study results
Cetuximab	Oral minocycline 100 mg versus placebo along with topical tazarotene 0.05% cream applied to one side of the face	Minocycline 100 mg/day at dinnertime Tazarotene 0.05% twice daily, at morning and bedtime. Both agents started on the same day with cetuximab	• Significant reduction of total facial lesion counts at weeks 1–4 • Lower proportion of patients reporting severe pruritus at week 4 in minocycline versus placebo (20% vs. 50%; $p = 0.05$) • No observed clinical benefit of topical tazarotene • High incidence of irritation due to tazarotene
Panitumumab	Oral doxycycline 100 mg, skin moisturizer, sunscreen (UVA/UVB, PABA free, SPF >15), topical 1% hydrocortisone cream versus reactive treatment as per investigator	Oral doxycycline 100 mg twice a day, skin moisturizer applied in the morning, sunscreen before going outdoors, 1% hydrocortisone cream at bedtime All agents started 1 day prior to the first dose of panitumumab and continued weeks 1–6	• Greater than 50% reduction in incidence of specific ≥grade 2 skin toxicities in a pre-emptive arm • Reduction in all-grade acneiform rash in a pre-emptive vs. reactive arm (77% vs. 85%) • Reduction of all-grade paronychia in a pre-emptive vs. reactive arm (17% vs. 36%) • Improved dermatologic QoL in a pre-emptive arm
EGFRIs (gefitinib, cetuximab, erlotinib, or an investigational agent within the same class)	Oral tetracycline 500 mg versus placebo	Oral tetracycline 500 mg twice a day for 4 weeks started within 7 days of trial enrollment	• No significant difference in incidence of the rash between tetracycline and placebo treated patients (70% vs. 76%; $p = 0.61$) • Reduction of rash severity by week 4 Grade 2 was seen in 17% in tetracycline arm vs. 55% in placebo arm; $p = 0.04$ • Significant reduction of pruritus, burning, stinging, and irritation at 4 weeks
EGFRIs (gefitinib, cetuximab, erlotinib, or an investigational agent within the same class)	Oral tetracycline 500 mg versus placebo	Oral tetracycline 500 mg twice a day for 4 weeks	• No significant difference in incidence of the rash between tetracycline and placebo treated patients during the first 4 weeks (82% vs. 75%), which was grade ≥2 in 52% vs 44%; $p = 0.62$ • No difference in dermatologic QoL (e.g., skin burning, pain, irritation)
EGFRIs (erlotinib, cetuximab or other agents within this class)	Sunscreen with SPF of 60 (7.5% titanium dioxide and 7.5% zinc oxide) versus a placebo	Sunscreen with SPF 60 applied twice a day for 4 weeks started within 3 days of randomization	• No significant difference in incidence of rash in sunscreen arm versus placebo during the 4 weeks (78% vs. 80%; $p = 1.00$) • No significant difference in rash severity or dermatologic QoL

and methicillin-resistant *S. aureus* in 5.4% of patients. While less common, infections with Gram-negative organisms, including *Pseudomonas aeruginosa* and *Klebsiella* were observed, and 23.5% of patients had polymicrobial infections. The most common areas of involvement were limited to seborrheic rich areas, typically affected by the papulopustular rash. Infections with a dermatophyte or virus were found in 5.9% and 2.7% of patients, respectively [43]. These findings support the importance of remaining vigilant for signs and symptoms of secondary superinfection and prompt initiation of appropriate antimicrobial therapy.

Xerosis and pruritus

Direct receptor inhibition in the epidermis results in aberrant terminal differentiation with loss of basket weave appearance, compact orthokeratosis, and reduced granular layer. These changes are not limited to skin directly affected by the papulopustular rash [24], providing an explanation why xerosis

typically involves larger surface areas. Additionally, it takes approximately 14 days for keratinocytes to migrate to stratum corneum after the terminal division. This latency period explains why xerosis typically manifests after 4–6 weeks of EGFRI therapy, in contrast to a more rapid onset of the papulopustular rash [8]. Up to 100% of patients treated with EGFRIs for more than 6 months may be affected by xerosis, which is diffuse and is characterized by dry, scaly, and pruritic skin [44]. Uncontrolled xerosis can progress to painful fissuring of skin, which most often involves distal tufts of fingers and toes, heels, periungual skin, and dorsal surface of the interphalangeal joints (Figure 17.4) [8,9].

Patients should be counseled prior to initiation of EGFRI therapy to modify their lifestyles with the goal of minimizing xerosis. Long hot showers should be avoided and the use of tepid water when bathing and washing dishes should be encouraged. Similarly, the use of any skin care products that would promote skin dryness, such as alcohol-containing moisturizers, antibacterial

Papulopustular Rash

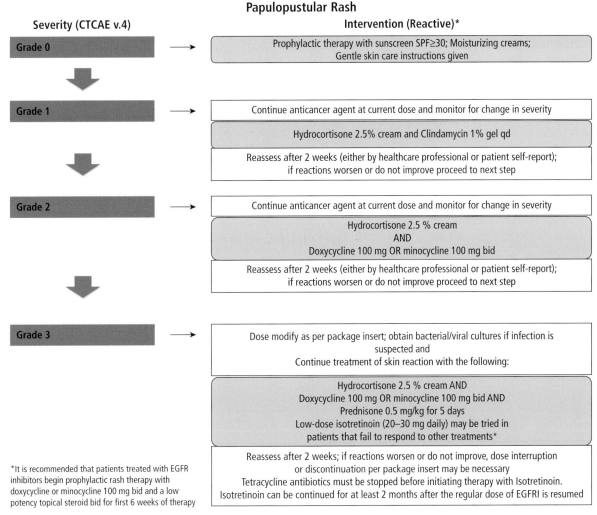

Severity (CTCAE v.4)	Intervention (Reactive)*
Grade 0	Prophylactic therapy with sunscreen SPF≥30; Moisturizing creams; Gentle skin care instructions given
Grade 1	Continue anticancer agent at current dose and monitor for change in severity
	Hydrocortisone 2.5% cream and Clindamycin 1% gel qd
	Reassess after 2 weeks (either by healthcare professional or patient self-report); if reactions worsen or do not improve proceed to next step
Grade 2	Continue anticancer agent at current dose and monitor for change in severity
	Hydrocortisone 2.5 % cream AND Doxycycline 100 mg OR minocycline 100 mg bid
	Reassess after 2 weeks (either by healthcare professional or patient self-report); if reactions worsen or do not improve proceed to next step
Grade 3	Dose modify as per package insert; obtain bacterial/viral cultures if infection is suspected and Continue treatment of skin reaction with the following:
	Hydrocortisone 2.5 % cream AND Doxycycline 100 mg OR minocycline 100 mg bid AND Prednisone 0.5 mg/kg for 5 days Low-dose isotretinoin (20–30 mg daily) may be tried in patients that fail to respond to other treatments*
	Reassess after 2 weeks; if reactions worsen or do not improve, dose interruption or discontinuation per package insert may be necessary Tetracycline antibiotics must be stopped before initiating therapy with Isotretinoin. Isotretinoin can be continued for at least 2 months after the regular dose of EGFRI is resumed

*It is recommended that patients treated with EGFR inhibitors begin prophylactic rash therapy with doxycycline or minocycline 100 mg bid and a low potency topical steroid bid for first 6 weeks of therapy

Figure 17.3 Treatment algorithm for epidermal growth factor receptor inhibitor-associated papulopustular (acneiform) rash.

soaps, and over-the-counter antiacne creams should be minimized. Management options for xerosis include topical and systemic approaches (Figure 17.5). In general, topical therapy should rely on the use of creams or ointments such as zinc oxide (40%), petroleum jelly, Eucerin, and Cetaphil [42]. Zinc oxide (20–30%), or cyanoacrylate glue (Super Glue) can be utilized to manage symptomatic fissures [10,42]. Xerotic dermatitis, characterized by erythematous, inflamed, and ichthyotic skin can be treated with a short course of topical corticosteroids to minimize pruritus and scratching.

EGFRI-associated pruritus may be significant, interfering with patients' sleep and daily activities. Cooling emollients or creams prior to their application to skin may provide partial and temporary symptomatic relief. Sarna Ultra cream, containing antipruritic ingredient pramoxine 1% and menthol (0.5%), may be effective in ameliorating symptoms [42]. For more pronounced pruritus, therapy may be enhanced with topical corticosteroids. Sedating first-generation oral antihistamines such as diphenhydramine and hydroxizine may be administered

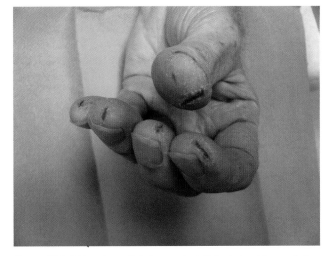

Figure 17.4 Epidermal growth factor receptor inhibitor-induced fissures that are associated with significant pain and may interfere with activities of daily living.

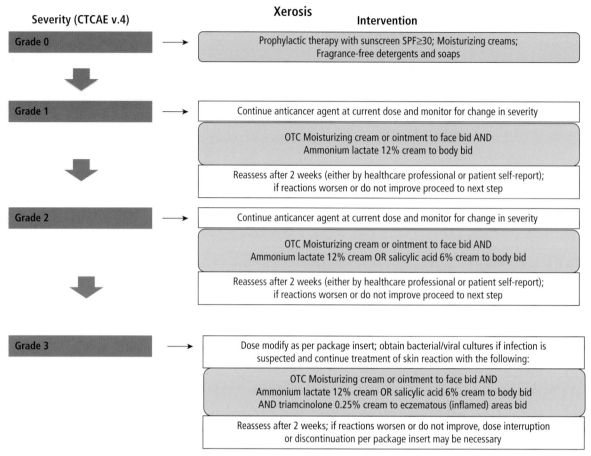

Figure 17.5 Treatment algorithm for epidermal growth factor receptor inhibitor-associated xerosis.

at bedtime to diminish pruritus at night. In cases of severe and intractable pruritus, GABA agonists (e.g., gabapentin, pregabalin) or aprepitant may be an alternative in patients in whom symptomatic relief has not been attained with other strategies (for additional information see Chapter 12) [42].

The disruption of a normally protective epidermal barrier is further compounded by pruritus-induced scratching that compromises intact skin and may predispose patients to skin and soft tissue infections, emphasizing the need for monitoring for signs and symptoms of secondary superinfection. In case of infection, treatment with an appropriate antimicrobial coverage should be instituted after obtaining cultures.

Hyperpigmentation

In contrast to other classes of targeted agents such as multikinase inhibitors sunitinib and sorafenib, which can induce pigmentary abnormalities by their direct interaction with cell surface receptors, hyperpigmentation due to EGFRIs appears to be post-inflammatory in nature, although spontaneous hyperpigmentation arising *de novo* has been reported. It is a late adverse event, typically manifesting after 1–2 months of therapy [42]. There is a tendency for its development in African-American patients and it can be exacerbated by UVR exposure, highlighting the

importance of counseling patients for sun avoidance and sunscreen use prior to therapy. Gradual resolution over weeks to months can usually be expected following discontinuation of therapy but the use of hydroquinone, azelaic acid, or laser treatments may facilitate improvement [42].

Telangiectasias

Telangiectasias tend to manifest later in the course of therapy, predominately distributed in the areas affected by the rash [42,45]. Formation of the network of dilated vessels may be attributed to growth of endothelial cells towards the regions of necrotic keratinocytes, and may explain the predilection of telangiectasias to arise in the vicinity of the papulopustular rash [27]. Discontinuation of EGFRIs is typically followed by measured resolution but cosmetic improvement can be accomplished with the use of a pulsed-dye laser, which targets hemoglobin [42].

Mucosal toxicities

While the use of EGFRIs has reduced the incidence and severity of mucosal changes compared to conventional cytotoxic chemotherapy, mucosal surfaces are not entirely spared. The manifestation of mucosal involvement differs from the characteristic mucositis associated with chemotherapy and its pathogenesis has not been precisely defined. Thus far, multiple terms such as mucositis, stomatitis, and aphthous ulcerations have been used to categorize this toxicity (for additional information see Chapter 9) [9,13,21,46]. Conjunctivitis due to either direct irritation by elongated and thickened eyelashes (trichomegaly) or xerophthalmia, meibomitis, and squamous blepharitis can be observed [47]. Minimally symptomatic aphthous ulcerations measuring 2–3 mm in size have been observed in oral and genital mucosa [8,9], and ulceration of the nasal mucosa, which may be secondary to bacterial overgrowth, has also been reported [48]. Xerosis of the vaginal mucosa in association with dysuria can also occur [49]. Manifestation may also be limited to a burning sensation without clinically overt lesions [13,21].

Corticosteroid (dexamethasone)-containing mouthwash can be used to manage symptomatic patients [50]. Additionally, localized application of 0.1% triamcinolone acetonide in an emollient dental paste (Orabase) may be of benefit for discrete aphthous ulcerations. For nasal ulcerations or erosions, intranasal mupirocin can be utilized based on the premise that dryness with *S. aureus* colonization has a role. Xerosis involving genital mucosa can be ameliorated with the use of lubricating agents [50].

Hair alterations

Considering the localization of EGFR to the outer root sheath of the hair follicle, it is not unexpected that this class of agents has been associated with a wide spectrum of hair alterations. Depending on the anatomic site, paradoxical changes can be observed, including hair loss, slowed and accelerated growth rate. The onset of alopecia occurs late, typically manifesting after several months of EGFRI therapy [27]. One pattern is nonscarring inflammatory alopecia that is patchy in distribution and tends to involve the crown of the scalp (Figure 17.6) [51]. Predominance

of neutrophils or plasma cells with multinucleated giant cells can be seen, reflecting an acute and a more chronic process, respectively [51]. It is important to note that scarring alopecia can develop following significant scalp inflammation and pustular lesions, highlighting the importance of aggressive approach to treatment in order to prevent permanent hair loss [42]. There is a paradoxical increased growth of thick and dark hair on the face and extremities [8,45,52]. Trichomegaly, characterized by elongated and rigid eyelashes (Figure 17.7), can result in significant corneal injury if growth is directed toward the eye (trichiasis) [53]. Hair alterations manifesting 2–3 months of therapy have been reported to affect 18% and 15% of patients treated with cetuximab and erlotinib, respectively [8]. Higher incidence is observed with prolonged exposure. In one series 87.5%, 62.5%, and 56% of patients maintained on EGFRIs for longer than 6 months demonstrated hair abnormalities, trichomegaly, and hypertrichosis, respectively, highlighting the subacute and/or chronic nature of EGFRI-related toxicities [44].

Laser epilation, waxing, threading, plucking, or topical application of eflornithine cream may be used to manage increased hair growth [50]. Trimming of long eyelashes should generally be avoided and patients with trichiasis and ocular involvement should be referred to an ophthalmologist for epilation therapy to diminish the risk of corneal ulceration [54].

Nail and periungual involvement

Therapy with EGFRIs can affect the nail plate and periungual tissues. The overall nail growth rate is diminished and there is increased fragility (brittle nails) [45]. Paronychia is the main manifestation of periungual tissue involvement, which affects 10–15% and 24% of patients undergoing therapy with cetuximab and gefitinib and panitumumab, respectively, and up to 56% of patients on EGFRI therapy for more than 6 months [10,44,55]. Similar to hair modifications, paronychia develops after several months of therapy, with the onset ranging from 20 days to 6

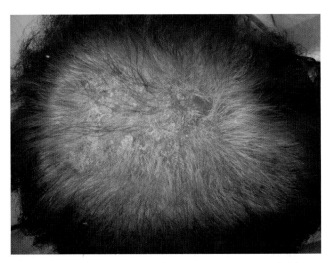

Figure 17.6 Reversible nonscarring inflammatory alopecia associated with epidermal growth factor receptor inhibitors.

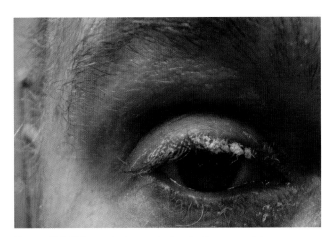

Figure 17.7 Trichomegaly that may lead to significant corneal damage, including erosions and ulcerations.

months [56]. Characteristic erythema and swelling of the lateral nail fold may affect any finger or toe but has a predilection for great toe and thumbs (Figure 17.8) [8,9]. In some cases, pyogenic granuloma-like changes with friable granulation tissue develop, which can bleed with minor physical trauma [9,45]. Persistence of symptoms for several months may be observed despite interruption of treatment, therefore management is suggested over dose modifications or interruptions [14]. Similar to papulopustular rash, secondary superinfection with Gram-negative bacteria such as *Klebsiella pneumoniae* and *Pseudomonas aeruginosa* and Gram-positive organisms such as *S. aureus*, including methicillin-resistant strains, may complicate clinical presentation [43,57]. Candidal species are less commonly the culprit [57].

EGFRI-induced changes in stratum corneum and thinning of the epidermis result in increased skin fragility and may promote penetration of nail plate fragments into adjacent tissue and elicit characteristic clinical manifestations [27]. Therapeutic approaches are based on the severity of presentation and may include a combination of topical and oral agents (Figure 17.9). One should

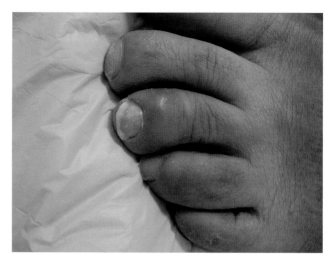

Figure 17.8 Paronychia due to epidermal growth factor receptor inhibitors that can be associated with significant pain and interfere with activities of daily living.

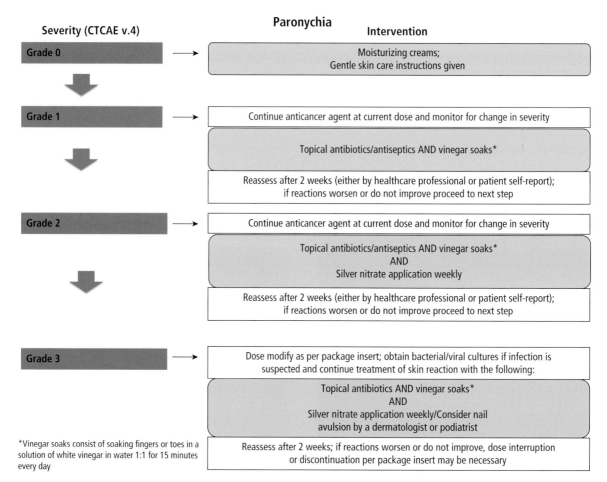

Figure 17.9 Treatment algorithms for paronychia.

remain vigilant for signs and symptoms of a superinfection, which should be cultured and treated with appropriate antimicrobial therapy. Electrodessication, cryosurgery, and nail plate avulsion may be utilized in more severe cases [56]. Patients with brittle nails may be treated with biotin 2.5 mg a day and a topical nail strengthener [58].

Interaction of EGFRIs with conventional cytotoxic chemotherapy and radiotherapy

Multiple currently used treatment protocols combine EGFRIs with cytotoxic chemotherapy agents and/or radiation therapy. While combination therapy may potentiate their therapeutic efficacy, the risk of dermatologic toxicities may be modified. Addition of EGFRIs to radiotherapy has been shown to increase the risk of high grade (grade 3–4) radiation dermatitis, mucositis, and rash (RR = 2.39, 95% CI 1.8–3.2; $p < 0.001$; RR = 1.8, 95% CI 1.5–2; $p < 0.001$; and RR = 3.1, 95% CI 2.1–4.6; $p < 0.001$, respectively) [59]. Enhanced toxicity was particularly pronounced when panitumumab was combined with radiation therapy and docetaxel/cisplatin 75%; 95% CI 37.7–93.7%) and erlotinib with radiation and cisplatin (56%; 95% CI 36.6–73.7%) in contrast to radiotherapy alone (13.1%; 95% CI 6.5–24.8%) [59]. Inhibition of EGFR renders keratinocytes more prone to injury associated with radiotherapy, stemming from impaired repair mechanisms and increased keratinocyte apoptosis [59]. Paradoxical sparing of skin from the papulopustular rash in regions previously treated (>3 months) with radiation has also been documented [60], attributed to radiation-induced marked reduction in EGFR expressing hair follicles and sebaceous glands [61].

A recent meta-analysis demonstrated increased incidence and risk of high grade papulopustular rash when cetuximab is combined with cytotoxic chemotherapy as compared to cetuximab monotherapy (10.3% vs 6.5%, respectively, RR = 1.6, 95% CI 1.2–2.0%, $p < 0.0001$) [62]. In contrast, a significantly lower incidence of all-grade rash was seen in patients treated with erlotinib in combination with chemotherapy (RR = 0.84; 95% CI 0.77–0.93; $p = 0.001$), while no significant difference was observed for high grade rash to combination therapy (RR = 1.02; 95% CI 0.74–1.42; $p = 0.89$) [63]. Future investigations are needed to elucidate potential reasons for these observations.

Conclusions

Dermatologic AEs of EGFRIs have emerged as a "class-effect" of this type of targeted agents. Although rarely life-threatening, they may affect patients' QoL, add a financial burden to the overall costs [64], and result in dose modifications and treatment interruptions, which may limit patients' exposure to potentially life-prolonging therapy. Future emphasis should be placed on developing evidence-based management guidelines, for which a multidisciplinary approach would be critical.

References

1 Yarden, Y. & Sliwkowski, M.X. (2001) Untangling the ErbB signalling network. *Nature Reviews. Molecular Cell Biology*, **2**, 127–137.

2 Nanney, L.B., Stoscheck, C.M., King, L.E. Jr., Underwood, R.A. & Holbrook, K.A. (1990) Immunolocalization of epidermal growth factor receptors in normal developing human skin. *Journal of Investigative Dermatology*, **94**, 742–748.

3 Nanney, L.B., Magid, M., Stoscheck, C.M. & King, L.E. Jr. (1984) Comparison of epidermal growth factor binding and receptor distribution in normal human epidermis and epidermal appendages. *Journal of Investigative Dermatology*, **83**, 385–393.

4 Mendelsohn, J. & Baselga, J. (2003) Status of epidermal growth factor receptor antagonists in the biology and treatment of cancer. *Journal of Clinical Oncology*, **21**, 2787–2799.

5 Jost, M., Kari, C. & Rodeck, U. (2000) The EGF receptor: an essential regulator of multiple epidermal functions. *European Journal of Dermatology*, **10**, 505–510.

6 Mendelsohn, J. & Baselga, J. (2006) Epidermal growth factor receptor targeting in cancer. *Seminars in Oncology*, **33**, 369–385.

7 Perez-Soler, R., Delord, J.P., Halpern, A. *et al.* (2005) HER1/EGFR inhibitor-associated rash: future directions for management and investigation outcomes from the HER1/EGFR inhibitor rash management forum. *The Oncologist*, **10**, 345–356.

8 Roe, E., Garcia Muret, M.P., Marcuello, E., Capdevila, J., Pallares, C. & Alomar, A. (2006) Description and management of cutaneous side effects during cetuximab or erlotinib treatments: a prospective study of 30 patients. *Journal of the American Academy of Dermatology*, **55**, 429–437.

9 Busam, K.J., Capodieci, P., Motzer, R., Kiehn, T., Phelan, D. & Halpern, A.C. (2001) Cutaneous side-effects in cancer patients treated with the antiepidermal growth factor receptor antibody C225. *British Journal of Dermatology*, **144**, 1169–1176.

10 Hu, J.C., Sadeghi, P., Pinter-Brown, L.C., Yashar, S. & Chiu, M.W. (2007) Cutaneous side effects of epidermal growth factor receptor inhibitors: clinical presentation, pathogenesis, and management. *Journal of the American Academy of Dermatology*, **56**, 317–326.

11 Jacot, W., Bessis, D., Jorda, E. *et al.* (2004) Acneiform eruption induced by epidermal growth factor receptor inhibitors in patients with solid tumours. *British Journal of Dermatology*, **151**, 238–241.

12 Scope, A., Lieb, J.A., Dusza, S.W. *et al.* (2009) A prospective randomized trial of topical pimecrolimus for cetuximab-associated acnelike eruption. *Journal of the American Academy of Dermatology*, **61**, 614–620.

13 Hidalgo, M., Siu, L.L., Nemunaitis, J. *et al.* (2001) Phase I and pharmacologic study of OSI-774, an epidermal growth factor receptor tyrosine kinase inhibitor, in patients with advanced solid malignancies. *Journal of Clinical Oncology*, **19**, 3267–3279.

14 Saltz, L.B., Meropol, N.J., Loehrer, P.J. Sr., Needle, M.N., Kopit, J. & Mayer, R.J. (2004) Phase II trial of cetuximab in patients with refractory colorectal cancer that expresses the epidermal growth factor receptor. *Journal of Clinical Oncology*, **22**, 1201–1208.

15 Lynch, T.J. Jr., Kim, E.S., Eaby, B., Garey, J., West, D.P. & Lacouture, M.E. (2007) Epidermal growth factor receptor inhibitor-associated cutaneous toxicities: an evolving paradigm in clinical management. *The Oncologist*, **12**, 610–621.

16 Melosky, B., Burkes, R., Rayson, D., Alcindor, T., Shear, N. & Lacouture, M. (2009) Management of skin rash during EGFR-targeted monoclonal antibody treatment for gastrointestinal malignancies: Canadian recommendations. *Current Oncology*, **16**, 16–26.

17 Lacouture, M.E., Laabs, S.M., Koehler, M. *et al.* (2009) Analysis of dermatologic events in patients with cancer treated with lapatinib. *Breast Cancer Research and Treatment*, **114**, 485–493.

18 Li, T. & Perez-Soler, R. (2009) Skin toxicities associated with epidermal growth factor receptor inhibitors. *Targeted Oncology*, **4**, 107–119.

19 Wagner, L.I. & Lacouture, M.E. (2007) Dermatologic toxicities associated with EGFR inhibitors: the clinical psychologist's perspective. Impact on health-related quality of life and implications for clinical management of psychological sequelae. *Oncology (Williston Park, NY)*, **21**, 34–36.

20 Joshi, S.S., Ortiz, S., Witherspoon, J.N. *et al.* (2010) Effects of epidermal growth factor receptor inhibitor-induced dermatologic toxicities on quality of life. *Cancer*, **116**, 3916–3923.

21 Cunningham, D., Humblet, Y., Siena, S. *et al.* (2004) Cetuximab monotherapy and cetuximab plus irinotecan in irinotecan-refractory metastatic colorectal cancer. *New England Journal of Medicine*, **351**, 337–345.

22 Shepherd, F.A., Rodrigues Pereira, J., Ciuleanu, T. *et al.* (2005) Erlotinib in previously treated non-small-cell lung cancer. *New England Journal of Medicine*, **353**, 123–132.

23 Boone, S.L., Rademaker, A., Liu, D., Pfeiffer, C., Mauro, D.J. & Lacouture, M.E. (2007) Impact and management of skin toxicity associated with anti-epidermal growth factor receptor therapy: survey results. *Oncology*, **72**, 152–159.

24 Guttman-Yassky, E., Mita, A., De Jonge, M. *et al.* (2010) Characterisation of the cutaneous pathology in non-small cell lung cancer (NSCLC) patients treated with the EGFR tyrosine kinase inhibitor erlotinib. *European Journal of Cancer*, **46**, 2010–2019.

25 Agero, A.L., Dusza, S.W., Benvenuto-Andrade, C., Busam, K.J., Myskowski, P. & Halpern, A.C. (2006) Dermatologic side effects associated with the epidermal growth factor receptor inhibitors. *Journal of the American Academy of Dermatology*, **55**, 657–670.

26 Nardone, B., Nicholson, K., Newman, M. *et al.* (2010) Histopathologic and immunohistochemical characterization of rash to human epidermal growth factor receptor 1 (HER1) and HER1/2 inhibitors in cancer patients. *Clinical Cancer Research*, **16**, 4452–4460.

27 Lacouture, M.E. (2006) Mechanisms of cutaneous toxicities to EGFR inhibitors. *Nature Reviews: Cancer*, **6**, 803–812.

28 Scope, A., Agero, A.L., Dusza, S.W. *et al.* (2007) Randomized double-blind trial of prophylactic oral minocycline and topical tazarotene for cetuximab-associated acne-like eruption. *Journal of Clinical Oncology*, **25**, 5390–5396.

29 Jatoi, A., Rowland, K., Sloan, J.A. *et al.* (2008) Tetracycline to prevent epidermal growth factor receptor inhibitor-induced skin rashes: results of a placebo-controlled trial from the North Central Cancer Treatment Group (N03CB). *Cancer*, **113**, 847–853.

30 Jatoi, A., Dakhil, S.R., Sloan, J.A. *et al.* (2011) Prophylactic tetracycline does not diminish the severity of epidermal growth factor receptor (EGFR) inhibitor-induced rash: results from the North Central Cancer Treatment Group (Supplementary N03CB). *Supportive Care in Cancer*, **19**, 1601–1607.

31 Lacouture, M.E., Mitchell, E.P., Piperdi, B. *et al.* (2010) Skin toxicity evaluation protocol with panitumumab (STEPP), a phase II, open-label, randomized trial evaluating the impact of a pre-emptive skin treatment regimen on skin toxicities and quality of life in patients with metastatic colorectal cancer. *Journal of Clinical Oncology*, **28**, 1351–1357.

32 Jatoi, A., Thrower, A., Sloan, J.A. *et al.* (2010) Does sunscreen prevent epidermal growth factor receptor (EGFR) inhibitor-induced rash? Results of a placebo-controlled trial from the North Central Cancer Treatment Group (N05C4). *The Oncologist*, **15**, 1016–1022.

33 Hughes, A.N., O'Brien, M.E., Petty, W.J. *et al.* (2009) Overcoming CYP1A1/1A2 mediated induction of metabolism by escalating erlotinib dose in current smokers. *Journal of Clinical Oncology*, **27**, 1220–1226.

34 Hamilton, M., Wolf, J.L., Rusk, J. *et al.* (2006) Effects of smoking on the pharmacokinetics of erlotinib. *Clinical Cancer Research*, **12**, 2166–2171.

35 Wheatley-Price, P., Ding, K., Seymour, L., Clark, G.M. & Shepherd, F.A. (2008) Erlotinib for advanced non-small-cell lung cancer in the elderly: an analysis of the National Cancer Institute of Canada Clinical Trials Group Study BR.21. *Journal of Clinical Oncology*, **26**, 2350–2357.

36 Jatoi, A., Green, E.M., Rowland, K.M. Jr., Sargent, D.J. & Alberts, S.R. (2009) Clinical predictors of severe cetuximab-induced rash: observations from 933 patients enrolled in north central cancer treatment group study N0147. *Oncology*, **77**, 120–123.

37 Lai, S.E., Minnelly, L., O'Keeffe, P. *et al.* (2007) Influence of skin color in the development of erlotinib-induced rash: a report from the SERIES clinic. *ASCO Annual Meeting Proceedings Part I*, **25** (18 Suppl), 9127.

38 Peus, D., Vasa, R.A., Meves, A., Beyerle, A. & Pittelkow, M.R. (2000) UVB-induced epidermal growth factor receptor phosphorylation is critical for downstream signaling and keratinocyte survival. *Photochemistry and Photobiology*, **72**, 135–140.

39 Edgerly, M. & Fojo, T. (2008) Is there room for improvement in adverse event reporting in the era of targeted therapies? *Journal of the National Cancer Institute*, **100**, 240–242.

40 Trotti, A., Colevas, A.D., Setser, A. & Basch, E. (2007) Patient-reported outcomes and the evolution of adverse event reporting in oncology. *Journal of Clinical Oncology*, **25**, 5121–5127.

41 Lacouture, M.E., Maitland, M.L., Segaert, S. *et al.* (2010) A proposed EGFR inhibitor dermatologic adverse event-specific grading scale from the MASCC skin toxicity study group. *Supportive Care in Cancer*, **18**, 509–522.

42 Burtness, B., Anadkat, M., Basti, S. *et al.* (2009) NCCN Task Force Report: management of dermatologic and other toxicities associated with EGFR inhibition in patients with cancer. *Journal of the National Comprehensive Cancer Network*, **7** (Suppl. 1), S5–S21; quiz S22–S24.

43 Eilers, R.E. Jr., Gandhi, M., Patel, J.D. *et al.* (2010) Dermatologic infections in cancer patients treated with epidermal growth factor receptor inhibitor therapy. *Journal of the National Cancer Institute*, **102**, 47–53.

44 Osio, A., Mateus, C., Soria, J.C. *et al.* (2009) Cutaneous side-effects in patients on long-term treatment with epidermal growth factor receptor inhibitors. *British Journal of Dermatology*, **161**, 515–521.

45 Segaert, S. & Van Cutsem, E. (2005) Clinical signs, pathophysiology and management of skin toxicity during therapy with epidermal growth factor receptor inhibitors. *Annals of Oncology*, **16**, 1425–1433.

46 Rowinsky, E.K., Schwartz, G.H., Gollob, J.A. *et al.* (2004) Safety, pharmacokinetics, and activity of ABX-EGF, a fully human anti-epidermal growth factor receptor monoclonal antibody in patients

with metastatic renal cell cancer. *Journal of Clinical Oncology*, **22**, 3003–3015.

47 Melichar, B. & Nemcova, I. (2007) Eye complications of cetuximab therapy. *European Journal of Cancer Care*, **16**, 439–443.

48 Lee, M.W., Seo, C.W., Kim, S.W. *et al.* (2004) Cutaneous side effects in non-small cell lung cancer patients treated with Iressa (ZD1839), an inhibitor of epidermal growth factor. *Acta Dermato-Venereologica*, **84**, 23–26.

49 Herbst, R.S., LoRusso, P.M., Purdom, M. & Ward, D. (2003) Dermatologic side effects associated with gefitinib therapy: clinical experience and management. *Clinical Lung Cancer*, **4**, 366–369.

50 Segaert, S., Chiritescu, G., Lemmens, L., Dumon, K., Van Cutsem, E. & Tejpar, S. (2009) Skin toxicities of targeted therapies. *European Journal of Cancer*, **45** (Suppl. 1), 295–308.

51 Graves, J.E., Jones, B.F., Lind, A.C. & Heffernan, M.P. (2006) Nonscarring inflammatory alopecia associated with the epidermal growth factor receptor inhibitor gefitinib. *Journal of the American Academy of Dermatology*, **55**, 349–353.

52 Van Doorn, R., Kirtschig, G., Scheffer, E., Stoof, T.J. & Giaccone, G. (2002) Follicular and epidermal alterations in patients treated with ZD1839 (Iressa), an inhibitor of the epidermal growth factor receptor. *British Journal of Dermatology*, **147**, 598–601.

53 Lane, K. & Goldstein, S.M. (2007) Erlotinib-associated trichomegaly. *Ophthalmic Plastic and Reconstructive Surgery*, **23**, 65–66.

54 Basti, S. (2007) Ocular toxicities of epidermal growth factor receptor inhibitors and their management. *Cancer Nursing*, **30**, S10–S16.

55 Giusti, R.M., Shastri, K.A., Cohen, M.H., Keegan, P. & Pazdur, R. (2007) FDA drug approval summary: panitumumab (Vectibix). *The Oncologist*, **12**, 577–583.

56 Fox, L.P. (2007) Nail toxicity associated with epidermal growth factor receptor inhibitor therapy. *Journal of the American Academy of Dermatology*, **56**, 460–465.

57 Eames, T., Grabein, B., Kroth, J. & Wollenberg, A. (2010) Microbiological analysis of epidermal growth factor receptor inhibitor therapy-associated paronychia. *Journal of the European Academy of Dermatology and Venereology*, **24**, 958–960.

58 Hochman, L.G., Scher, R.K. & Meyerson, M.S. (1993) Brittle nails: response to daily biotin supplementation. *Cutis: Cutaneous Medicine for the Practitioner*, **51**, 303–305.

59 Tejwani, A., Wu, S., Jia, Y., Agulnik, M., Millender, L. & Lacouture, M.E. (2009) Increased risk of high-grade dermatologic toxicities with radiation plus epidermal growth factor receptor inhibitor therapy. *Cancer*, **115**, 1286–1299.

60 Bossi, P., Liberatoscioli, C., Bergamini, C. *et al.* (2007) Previously irradiated areas spared from skin toxicity induced by cetuximab in six patients: implications for the administration of EGFR inhibitors in previously irradiated patients. *Annals of Oncology*, **18**, 601–602.

61 Lacouture, M.E., Hwang, C., Marymont, M.H. & Patel, J. (2007) Temporal dependence of the effect of radiation on erlotinib-induced skin rash. *Journal of Clinical Oncology*, **25**, 2140; author reply 2141.

62 Balagula, Y., Wu, S., Su, X., Dusza, S.W. & Lacouture, M.E. (2010) The effect of cytotoxic chemotherapy on the risk of high-grade acneiform rash with cetuximab in cancer patients: a meta-analysis. *Journal of Clinical Oncology*, **28**, 15 (suppl; abstr 9072).

63 Jia, Y., Lacouture, M.E., Su, X. & Wu, S. (2009) Risk of skin rash associated with erlotinib in cancer patients: a meta-analysis. *Journal of Supportive Oncology*, **7**, 211–217.

64 Abraham, T., Rademaker, A., Ortiz, S. *et al.* (2008) Economic impact associated with the management of dermatologic adverse drug reactions (dADRs) induced by EGFR inhibitors (EGFRIs) in lung cancer. *Journal of Clinical Oncology*, **26**, (suppl.) abstract 19094.

65 Food and Drug Administration website (2004) Erbitux package insert Imclone Systems Incorporated and Bristol-Myers Squibb Company, Branchburg and Princeton, NJ. Available from: http://www.accessdata.fda.gov/drugsatfda_docs//label/2004/125084lbl.pdf (accessed 7 April 2013).

66 Motzer, R.J., Amato, R., Todd, M. *et al.* (2003) Phase II trial of antiepidermal growth factor receptor antibody C225 in patients with advanced renal cell carcinoma. *Investigational New Drugs*, **21**, 99–101.

67 U.S. Food and Drug Administration website (2009) Vectibix package insert. Amgen ITO, CA. Available from: http://www.accessdata.fda.gov/drugsatfda_docs/label/2009/125147s080lbl.pdf (accessed 7 April 2013).

68 Lilenbaum, R., Axelrod, R., Thomas, S. *et al.* (2008) Randomized phase II trial of erlotinib or standard chemotherapy in patients with advanced non-small-cell lung cancer and a performance status of 2. *Journal of Clinical Oncology*, **26**, 863–869.

69 Tarceva package insert. Available from: www.tarceva.com (accessed 7 April 2013).

70 Tykerb (lapatinib) package insert. Available from: http://www.fda.gov/Safety/MedWatch/SafetyInformation/ucm200945.htm (accessed 7 April 2013).

71 Toi, M., Iwata, H., Fujiwara, Y. *et al.* (2009) Lapatinib monotherapy in patients with relapsed, advanced, or metastatic breast cancer: efficacy, safety, and biomarker results from Japanese patients phase II studies. *British Journal of Cancer*, **101**, 1676–1682.

72 Thatcher, N., Chang, A., Parikh, P. *et al.* (2005) Gefitinib plus best supportive care in previously treated patients with refractory advanced non-small-cell lung cancer: results from a randomised, placebo-controlled, multicentre study (Iressa Survival Evaluation in Lung Cancer). *Lancet*, **366**, 1527–1537.

73 Gefitinib package insert. Available from: http://www.cancer.gov/cancertopics/druginfo/fda-gefitinib (accessed 7 April 2013).

18 Small Molecule Multikinase Inhibitors

Caroline Robert[1], Vincent Sibaud[2] and Christine Mateus[1]

[1]Dermatology Department, Cancer Institute Gustave Roussy, Villejuif, France
[2]Oncodermatology Department and Clinical Research Unit, Claudius Regaud Institute, Cancer Comprehensive Center, Toulouse, France

Introduction

With increasing knowledge of mechanisms involved in cancer, new drugs with innovative mechanisms of action have been developed. Targeted therapies rely on the concept of specifically inhibiting biologic events implicated in oncogenic processes. These oncogenic pathways mediate their effects via a cascade of enzymatic reactions, mostly tyrosine phosphorylations that sequentially activate involved proteins. In cancer cells, receptors or intracellular kinases are often activated in an abnormal and uncontrolled fashion [1]. This activation can result from somatic modifications: mutational events, gene amplifications or mutations, or gene product overexpression.

There are two possible strategies for inhibiting a protein kinase. Using small molecules designed to inhibit enzymatic activity; the suffix -ib is usually used to name these molecules. The other strategy uses monoclonal antibodies (mAb, suffix -ab) that bind to ligands or receptors to prevent their interaction and the subsequent pathway activation.

Targeted agents can also aim at inhibiting the tumor neovascularization, as for antiangiogenic agents targeting vascular endothelial growth factor receptors (VEGFRs) [2]. Contrary to what could have been expected, the effects of targeted therapies are not limited to the cancer cells and are unfortunately associated with many adverse events (AEs). Dermatologic AEs are among the most frequently observed [3], and can impact patients' quality of life.

In this chapter, we review the dermatologic AEs of antiangiogenic agents (sorafenib, sunitinib, and pazopanib), of kit, platelet-derived growth factor receptor (PDGFR), and bcr-abl inhibitors (imatinib, dasatinib, and nilotinib), and of mammalian target of rapamycin (mTOR) inhibitors (everolimus and temsirolimus) (Figure 18.1).

Kit, PDGFR and bcr-abl inhibitors: imatinib, nilotinib, dasatinib

Drugs, indications, and mechanisms of action

Imatinib (Gleevec®), nilotinib (Tasigna®), and dasatinib (Sprycel®) inhibit c-kit, PDGFR, and the bcr-abl fusion protein (Philadelphia chromosome; Ph+), characteristic for chronic myeloid leukemia (CML). The c-kit receptor CD117 is activated by mutation in the majority of gastrointestinal stromal tumors (GIST), the bcr-abl protein is the product of the translocation between chromosomes 9 and 22 found in CML. PDGFRα is involved in hypereosinophilic syndrome and TEL-PDGFRβ in chronic myelomonocytic leukemia (CMmoL).

Therefore these drugs are indicated in the treatment of GIST, CML, some hypereosinophilic syndromes, and CMmoL. Nilotinib and dasatinib can be used in imatinib-refractory Ph+ CML and acute lymphoblastic leukemia (ALL) (Table 18.1).

Imatinib

Imatinib (Gleevec®) is relatively well tolerated and induces mainly hematologic and digestive disorders: nausea, vomiting, abdominal pain, and diarrhea. Dermatologic AEs are common but rarely severe, with a prevalence ranging 9.5–69% [2,3–9].

Edema predominating on the face, more visible on the periorbital areas in the morning and inferior parts of the body in the evening, is one of the most common AEs. It is reported in 63–84% of cases and appears on average 6 weeks after therapy [5,10]. Epiphora, or visual obstruction due to intense eyelid edema, ptosis, blepharoconjonctivits, or retinal edema, can occur. Edema can also be more diffuse with substantial weight gain and even pleural and/or peritoneal effusions or cerebral edema [11]. The pathophysiology is unclear and is thought to be caused by

Dermatologic Principles and Practice in Oncology: Conditions of the Skin, Hair, and Nails in Cancer Patients, First Edition. Edited by Mario E. Lacouture.
© 2014 John Wiley & Sons, Inc. Published 2014 by John Wiley & Sons, Inc.

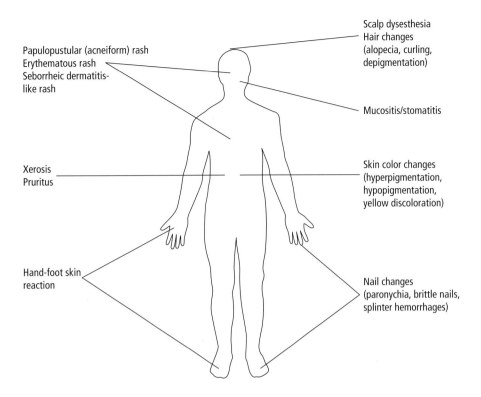

Figure 18.1 Anatomic location of dermatologic adverse events induced by small molecule multikinase inhibitors.

Table 18.1 Kit and platelet-derived growth factor receptor (PDGFR) inhibitors: drugs and indications.

INN	Trade name	Indications
Imatinib	Gleevec	**Ph⁺ CML**, if bone marrow transplantation is not considered as first-line therapy, or after failure of interferon alpha treatment, or in accelerated phase or in blast crisis
		Relapsed or refractory **Ph⁺ ALL**
		Myelodysplastic/myeloproliferative syndromes associated with PDGFR gene rearrangements
		Hypereosinophilic syndrome at an advanced stage and/or **chronic eosinophilic leukemia** associated with a FIP1L1-PDGFR-alpha rearrangement
		Kit (CD 117)-positive unresectable and/or metastatic malignant **gastrointestinal stromal tumors**
		Unresectable and/or relapsing and/or metastatic **dermatofibrosarcoma protuberans**
Dasatinib	Sprycel	**Ph⁺ CML** in the chronic and accelerated phase, in the event of resistance or intolerance to prior therapy with imatinib
Nilotinib	Tasigna	**Ph⁺ CML** in the chronic, accelerated, or blast phase, in the event of resistance or intolerance to prior therapy with imatinib
		Ph⁺ CML and ALL in the lymphoid blast phase, in the event of resistance or intolerance to prior therapy

ALL, acute lymphoblastic leukemia; CML, chronic myeloid leukemia;HCC, hepatocellular carcinoma; GIST, gastrointestinal stromal tumor; Ph+, Philadelphia+; RCC, renal cell cancer.

modification of interstitial fluid homeostasis linked to PDGFR inhibition [3].

Maculopapular eruptions (rash) involving the trunk and limbs, sometimes associated with pruritus, occur in up to 50% of patients, appearing on average 9 weeks after treatment initiation [5,10]. It is usually mild–moderate, self-limiting, and easily manageable with antihistamines and/or topical steroids [9].

Histopathology demonstrates nonspecific perivascular mononuclear cell infiltrates [5,10].

More severe eruptions (grades 3 and 4), erythrodermas [5], Stevens–Johnson syndrome [12–17], acute generalized exanthematous pustulosis [18,19], and a case of drug reaction with eosinophilia and systemic symptoms (DRESS) [20] have been reported.

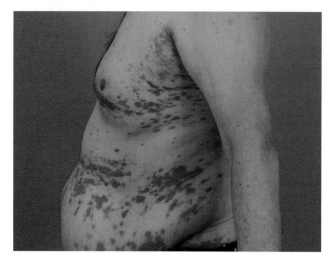

Figure 18.2 Imatinib-induced lichenoid rash.

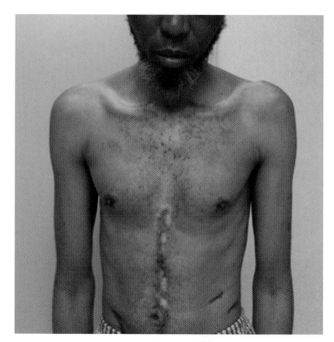

Figure 18.3 Imatinib-induced hypopigmentation.

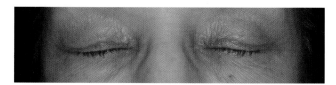

Figure 18.4 Periorbital edema induced by dasatinib.

Exacerbations of psoriasis or psoriasiform eruptions with diffuse erythemato-squamous rashes [5,21], and nonfollicular pustular eruptions similar to pustular psoriasis have been observed, developing within a period of 1–7 months after treatment initiation [21]. Erythematous plaques surrounded by desquamative collarette resembling pytiriasis rosea, with histology showing spongiosis, associated with a lymphocytic superficial perivascular infiltrate were described [22,23]. Several cases of palmoplantar hyperkeratoses and nail dystrophies have also been reported [24].

Lichenoid eruptions (Figure 18.2), sometimes associated with mucosal erosive or lichenoid intrabuccal, may appear [25–31], presenting as red–purple papules localized symmetrically on the trunk and limbs. Lichenoid infiltrates around the basal membrane and apoptotic keratinocytes are seen on the pathologic skin histopathology.

Localized or diffuse pigmentary AEs are frequently reported. Homogeneous depigmentation, particularly in patients with black (Figure 18.3) or tanned skin (phototype 5–6) has been reported in 16–40% of patients [5,32,33]. Diffuse skin and hair depigmentation associated with disappearance of lentigines has been described [34]. Conversely, hyperpigmentation and repigmentation of the skin and hair have also been reported [5,35,36]. These pigmentary changes are reversible upon treatment discontinuation and might be caused by the inhibition of c-kit, which is involved in melanogenesis via the transcription factor MITF [37,38]. Hair depigmentation is more commonly seen with the kit/PDGF/VEGFR inhibitor sunitinib [3,33]. Moreover, urticaria, neutrophilic dermatosis, vascular purpura [39], pseudolymphoma [40], and photosensitive eruptions have been reported [5,41]. Eruptions and edema seem to be dose-dependent [5,7]. This suggests pharmacologic and not immunologic mechanisms in the development of these AEs [4].

Nilotinib and dasatinib

Nilotinib-associated rash is reported in 17–35% of patients, pruritus in 13–24%, alopecia in 10%, and xerosis in 13–17%. The majority of the cases are grade 1–2, and a dose-dependent effect is also demonstrated [42,43]. Edema can also be present, albeit less frequently than with imatinib. Rare cases of pigmentary disorders and Sweet syndrome have also been reported.

The most frequent dermatologic AEs with dasatinib are localized or diffuse maculopapular rashes (13–27%), often with pruritus (11%) [22]. Mucositis and stomatitis develops in 16% of the patients [44,45]. Other manifestations like hyperhidrosis, xerosis, alopecia, photosensitivity, pigmentary disorders, and panniculitis have rarely been described [46,47].

Management

Moderate periorbital edema (Figure 18.4) does not require any specific treatment. In cases of diffuse and severe edema, a diuretic can be prescribed with attention to electrolyte monitoring.

The majority of eruptions can be managed with antihistamines and topical treatments (emollients and/or topical corticosteroids) and do not require treatment discontinuation. However, because most of the reported AEs are dose dependent, in the case of severe or persistent manifestations uncontrolled by symptomatic treatments, a dose reduction accompanied by a short-acting systemic corticosteroid may be attempted. In cases of severe and

Table 18.2 Antiangiogenic small molecule inhibitors, molecular targets, and indications.

INN	Trade name	Targets	Indications
Sorafenib	Nexavar	VEGFR-2,-3, KIT, PDGFR-α, -β, Flt3, RAF	RCC HCC
Sunitinib	Sutent	VEGFR-1-3, KIT, PDGFR-α, -β, Flt3,	RCC GIST[a]
Pazopanib	Votrient	VEGFR-1-3, PDGFR-α,-β, KIT	RCC

GIST, gastrointestinal stromal tumor; HCC, hepatocellular carcinoma; RCC, renal cell cancer.
[a]After disease progression on or intolerance to imatinib.

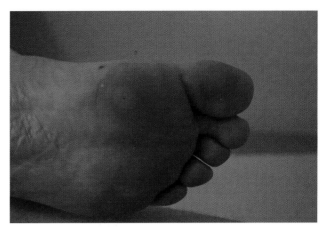

Figure 18.5 Hand-foot skin reaction to sorafenib/sunitinib.

potentially life-threatening dermatologic AEs, the agent should be discontinued and not reintroduced.

Antiangiogenic agents: sorafenib, sunitinib axitinib, regorafenib, and pazopanib

Tumor neoangiogenesis is a one of the key processes of tumor progression and key players include VEGF/VEGFR [48], αvβ3 and αvβ5 integrins, FGF-2, angiopoietins 1 and 2 [49].

Antiangiogenic agents can target the ligand VEGF or its receptors (VEGFR). The inhibition of VEGFR can be achieved by the use of a monoclonal antibody that binds VEGF and prevents it from binding to its receptors or by using small molecules that inhibit the kinase activity of the intracellular portion of the VEGFR. For the small molecules, the inhibition spectrum is not limited to VEGFR, as they are multikinase inhibitors (Table 18.2). They are indicated in the treatment of renal cell cancer, hepatocellular carcinoma, and GIST (Table 18.2).

Like most of the so-called targeted agents, antiangiogenic small molecule inhibitors have various AEs. High blood pressure (with all three compounds), glomerulopathy, and hypothyroidism with sunitinib are some examples. However, mucocutaneous manifestations are usually the most prominent AEs and frequently impact patients' quality of life, often threatening adherence [3,50,51].

Cutaneous AEs that are common to sorafenib, sunitinib and pazopanib are as follow.

Hand-foot skin reaction
Hand-foot skin reaction (HFSR) is the major dermatologic AE of antiangiogenic multikinase inhibitors. It usually appears during the first 5 weeks and affects 10–63% of patients treated with sorafenib, with 2–36% being grade 3 in severity [52–58]; 10–28% with sunitinib (4–12% grade 3) [59–62], and 11% with pazopanib (2% grade 3) [63–65].

The clinical appearance of antiangiogenic HFSR differs from the hand-foot syndrome (HFS) with cytotoxic chemotherapies like capecitabine, 5-fluorouracil (FU), pegylated doxorubicin, or cytarabine [66–68]. First, the lesions are predominantly located on pressure (Figure 18.5) or friction areas (metatarsal heads, heels, sides of the feet, metacarpophalangeal joints). Second, they rapidly become hyperkeratotic, whereas in classic chemotherapy-associated HFSR, hyperkeratosis is usually seen later in the course of the disease, and the lesions remain inflammatory, erythematous, and possibly desquamative for several weeks or months before hyperkeratosis. However, inflammation is also frequent in antiangiogenic HFSR with erythema, desquamation, and even bullous lesions, with an erythematous ring surrounding the lesions [3,50,69]. The HFSR is classically bilateral and symmetrical [70]. Areas of pre-existing hyperkeratotic lesions seem to confer a predisposition for painful sole involvement [70,71]. Lesions can be very painful, interfering with the everyday activities, such as walking or holding objects. Prodromes with tingling, numbness, and pin and needles feelings of the hands and feet are frequently reported as well as a painful sensation induced by contact with hot objects [69].

The pathophysiology of HFSR is still unclear. It is not observed with imatinib, which blocks PDGFR, or with the VEGF ligand blocker bevacizumab, suggesting that it is directly linked to the inhibition of one at least of the VEGFRs targeted by the three compounds. The description of lesions with the same clinical appearance elsewhere than on the feet and hands, on chronically microtraumatized contact areas (e.g., the elbows, amputation stump, or old scars) suggests that HFSR could be the equivalent of a Koebner phenomenon [72–74].

The main pathologic abnormalities observed are keratinocyte necrosis and/or horizontal vacuolar degeneration, with or without acanthosis, spongiosis, exocytosis, dilatation of the dermal vessels with a perivascular lymphocytic infiltrate, and sometimes eccrine squamous syringometaplasia [70,74,75]. Sequential pathologic modifications were found during the course of the treatment with changes in the stratum spinosum–stratum granulosum during the first month and then in the stratum corneum with hyperkeratosis and focal parakeratosis after the first month [75].

Management

The impact of HFSR on quality of life has been clearly demonstrated, using generic dermatologic scales [74] or scales that have been more specifically developed for this syndrome. This effect is clearly dose dependent and may improve with dose reductions or treatment interruptions. Management has only been evaluated by one controlled study and is heavily based on prescribers' experience and advised by experts' consensus [76]. The following management is recommended.

Preventing measures

The patients must be clearly informed that a HFSR might occur, and ideally, they should have hands and feet examined prior to treatment initiation. A podiatric examination and preventive treatments of pre-existing hyperkeratotic areas by mechanical or chemical keratolytic measures (topical 10–50% urea, 3–6% salicylic acid creams) may reduce the incidence of all-grade HFSR and delay its onset. Emollients can be used to prevent dryness and cracking. Prescription of orthopedic soles or inserts may also be helpful in patients with unbalanced sole pressure areas.

Patients should be advised to wear comfortable and flexible shoes and to avoid rubbing and trauma.

Treatment

Treatment is based on symptomatic measures and dose adjustment, because no treatments have been evaluated in controlled settings.

Therapeutic measures are proposed according to the three HFSR severity grades (NCI CTCAE v.4)

Grade 1: Supportive measures using moisturizing creams, keratolytic agents such as 10–40% urea and/or 1–10% salicylic acid creams or ointments on the palms and soles. Cushioning of the affected regions with gel or foam-based shock absorber soles and soft shoes are recommended. Antiangiogenic multikinase inhibitor treatment is maintained at the same dosage.

Grade 2: The same symptomatic measures as for grade 1 should be promptly initiated; potent topical corticosteroids (clobetasol) can be prescribed on inflammatory lesions for a few weeks. Analgesic treatment should be considered if needed. A dose reduction of 50% should be considered until the HFSR returns to grade 0 or 1 in the event of a second episode of grade 2 HFSR, or when it becomes intolerable. If toxicity resolves to grade 0–1, re-escalation to the initial dose should be carried out. Decisions whether to re-escalate dose after the second or third occurrence of grade 2 HFSR should be based on clinical judgment and patient preference. If toxicity does not resolve to grade 0–1 despite dose reduction, treatment should be interrupted for a minimum of 7 days and until toxicity has resolved to grade 0–1. When resuming treatment after dose interruption, treatment should

begin at reduced dose. If toxicity is maintained at grade 0–1 at reduced dose for a minimum of 7 days, the initial (registered) dose is recommended.

Grade 3: Symptomatic measures as described for grade 2 HFSR as well as antiseptic treatment of blisters and erosions. Treatment should be interrupted for a minimum of 7 days and until toxicity is grade 0–1. When resuming treatment after dose interruption, treatment should begin at reduced dose. If toxicity is maintained at grade 0–1 at reduced dose for a minimum of 7 days, initial dose should be given again. On the second occurrence of grade 3 HFSR, decision whether to re-escalate dose should be based on clinical judgment and patient preference. The same principle applies for the decision whether to discontinue therapy after the third occurrence of grade 3 HFSR.

No systemic therapy has demonstrated any beneficial effect for HFSR; oral pyridoxine or systemic steroids have not been found to be effective, but pain control may be necessary.

Subungual splinter hemorrhages

Ranging between 3–70%, these occur with the compounds sorafenib, sunitinib, pazopanib but their frequency is often underestimated because of absent symptoms. They appear as painless longitudinal black lines, predominantly beneath the distal part of the nail plate, during the first weeks of therapy. They can be clinically identical to those observed in certain systemic diseases such as rheumatoid arthritis, systemic lupus, or endocarditis, but they are not associated with distant embolic or thrombotic processes, unlike these conditions. Inhibition of the VEGFR coupled with local microtraumas could explain the symptom. They disappear progressively after treatment and do not require any intervention [69,71,77].

Erythematous rashes

Various erythematous rashes are observed with sorafenib, sunitinib, and pazopanib, usually appearing within the first weeks. They are not well characterized, and occur in 13–24% of patients with sunitinib [78,79], 10–60% with sorafenib [69,78,80], and 6–8% with pazopanib [63–65]. They can predominate on the face, especially with sorafenib (Figure 18.6) [69]. The most frequently reported histologic aspect is a superficial perivascular lymphocytic infiltrate. They can disappear spontaneously despite continued treatment but therapy interruption may be necessary in some cases. A case of erythema multiforme has been published [81] and signs of severity such as mucosal involvement, epidermal detachment and general signs (fever, elevated hepatic enzymes), which can be associated with severe manifestations, toxic epidermal necrolysis, or a DRESS syndrome should always be evaluated.

Hair modifications

Largely underreported in the literature, hair modifications are almost always associated with these drugs. It may only be a minor texture change, with hair usually becoming dryer and curlier. Alopecia occurs in 21–44% of patients on sorafenib [69,80,82]

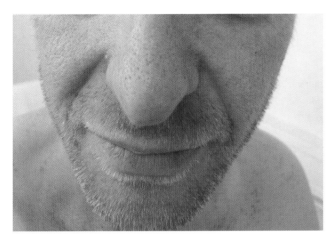

Figure 18.6 Sorafenib-induced rash.

but less frequently with sunitinib (5–21%) and pazopanib (8–10%) [63–65]. It is usually moderate and develops gradually after several weeks or months, and can be associated with alopecia in other regions (trunk, arms, pubis).

It is not unusual to see hair growing back even though patients are still on therapy with sorafenib. New growing hair is then usually curlier than before treatment (authors' personal observations). These changes have not been shown to be associated with thyroid or iron study abnormalities in uncontrolled assessments.

Reversible hair depigmentation is observed with sunitinib (7–14%) [78,83,84] and pazopanib (27–44%) [63,64]. It can affect all body hair areas: head, beard, eyelashes, and eyebrows. With sunitinib, which is given 4 weeks on and 2 weeks off, characteristic discoloration can occur with successive depigmented bands related to periods of treatment and normally pigmented bands associated with periods off treatment. This phenomenon is reversible upon discontinuation of treatment after 2–3 weeks [84,85]. The underlying mechanism of the depigmentation is likely an inhibition of the c-kit pathway; however, other factors may have a role because other kit inhibitors such as imatinib, dasatinib, or nilotinib do not induce such systematic hair depigmentation.

Xerosis
The skin becomes dryer with these agents [3,69] but symptomatic emollient treatments are usually effective.

Genital involvement
Genital rash with erythematous, desquamative psoriasiform or lichenoid lesions can be observed in the genital areas of both genders, with an unknown incidence [51,86]. Lesions can involve the vulvar or scrotal areas, and extend to the inguinal region, and occasionally result in phimosis. Histolopathology reveals a psoriasiform or lichenoid pattern. Such genital rashes have been observed with sorafenib, sunitinib, and pazopanib (C. Robert,

personal observations) [86]. Treatment with topical steroids can be considered after ruling out a bacterial or fungal infection. A temporary dose modification is sometimes necessary, resulting in a rapid improvement of the symptoms.

Mucositis
Stomatitis and cheilitis have been reported in 19–35% of sunitinib treated patients, and 19–26% with sorafenib [62,69,78,87]. Lesions usually occur during the first weeks of treatment, can be painful and impair alimentation. They are dose dependent and may require dose modifications [78]. Patients frequently present with functional disorders without apparent lesions, which rapidly improve during the 2-week treatment-free interval with sunitinib.

AEs specifically related to sunitinib
Skin discoloration
A yellow appearance of the skin is seen with sunitinib. It is rapidly reversible and decreases during the 2 weeks off treatment. It is probably caused by the bright yellow color of the drug itself [3].

Facial edema
A mild to moderate facial edema occurs in 4.5–24% of patients treated with sunitinib [88]. Hypothyroidism, which is a frequent complication of sunitinib, can exacerbate this edema.

AEs related specifically to sorafenib
Eruptive nevi
Several cases of eruptive nevi have been published with sorafenib therapy [82,89]. Nevi present as homogeneous macules of few millimeters on the face, trunk, or limbs, including the palmoplantar areas. Pathologically, the lesions present as junctional nevi. Because of the prosenescence effect of BRAF protein in wild-type BRAF cells [90,91], it can be hypothesized that the nevi eruption could be linked to an "anti-senescence effect" with the appearance and the development of subclinical pre-existing nevi.

Early facial erythematous rash
A face and scalp rash is frequently seen during the first days or weeks of treatment with sorafenib. It involves the centrofacial area and scalp, resembling seborrhoeic dermatitis. It is commonly associated with scalp dysesthesia or pain. This AE is not systematically reported although it is quite frequent in the authors' experience, and usually disappears after a few weeks.

Squamous cell proliferations: keratoacanthomas and squamous cell carcinomas
Keratoacanthomas (KA) and squamous cell carcinomas (SCC) have been reported during sorafenib therapy [92–95]. These lesions can be multiple and occur several weeks to months after initiating treatment, with an estimated incidence of less than 10%. Beside the contexts of uncommon genetic diseases like Ferguson Smith or Muir–Torre syndromes, KA is a rare lesion preferentially occurring on sun-exposed areas and presenting

as a fast-growing dome-shaped nodule with a central keratotic crust. It does not give rise to metastases and can occasionally spontaneously regress. Pathologically, it is almost undistinguishable from a well-differentiated SCC, with an exoendophytic proliferation and a crateriform zone of well-differentiated squamous epithelium surrounding a central keratotic plug. The existence of KA is still controversial because for some authors this entity should be assimilated to a well-differentiated form of SCC [96–98]. In contrast to KA, SCC is a malignancy that does not regress spontaneously and can metastasize. It is a frequent skin tumor, mostly related to sun exposure or to precancerous lesions like actinic keratoses. However, SCC with sorafenib do not appear as the typical and frequently reported cutaneous SCC. They exhibit clinical and pathologic aspects similar to KA, and are usually described pathologically as KA-like SCC with nests of atypical cells invading the dermis, as well as a crateriform pattern with bulging borders reminiscent of KA, and are not always located on sun-exposed areas [92]. Until now, no metastases from KA or SCC induced by sorafenib has been reported and they have behaved as low aggressiveness tumors.

It could be deduced that this AE is caused by RAF inhibition. Indeed, no KA or SCC has been reported with drugs targeting molecules inhibited by sorafenib other than RAF proteins (i.e., PDGFR, FLT3, or VEGFR), like sunitinib (VEGFR, KIT, PDGFR, FLT3), or imatinib (kit, PDGFR) for example. This reasoning proved to be correct because similar tumors are now described with the use of two new agents that specifically target RAF proteins, particularly mutant BRAF: BRAF^{V600E} [99–101]. The BRAF pathway is activated in more than 65% of melanomas resulting from a BRAF^{V600E} mutation in 40–50% of cases, and NRAS mutation in 15–20% of cases [102].

The mechanism for the development of skin tumors with sorafenib and RAF inhibitors is likely a paradoxical RAF-MEK-ERK pathway activation via BRAF wild-type cells, especially if they carry a mutant RAS protein [103–106].

It is recommended that patients' skin should be carefully monitored, and that KA/SCC should be completely resected; simple shaving with partial resection should not be performed.

In addition to KA and SCC, more or less inflammatory follicular cystic lesions are frequently observed with sorafenib: keratosis pilaris [80], microcysts, dystrophic follicular cystic lesions, perforating folliculitis [69,80,92]. Association of these lesions with KA/SCC in the same patients suggests that they represent various aspects of a spectrum of lesions ranging from benign cystic lesions to borderline (KA) and malignant skin tumors (SCC) [92].

mTOR inhibitors: everolimus and temsirolimus

Drugs and mechanisms of action

These drugs inhibit the serine or threonine kinase mTOR after binding to the intracellular protein FKBP-12 inducing downstream dephosphorylation of the mTOR molecular targets(i.e., 4E-BP1 and S6K1), and ultimately inhibition of the PI3K-AKT-mTOR signaling pathway. This particular signaling pathway has a critical role in tumor cell biology, especially in regulating cell growth, survival, proliferation, apoptosis, and angiogenesis [107–109].

Two compounds are approved against metastatic renal cell cancer: temsirolimus (Torisel®), and everolimus (Afinitor®). They are associated with various AEs: hematologic (e.g., anemia, neutropenia, lymphopenia, thrombocytopenia), metabolic (e.g., hypertriglyceridemia, hypercholesterolemia, hyperglycemia, hypocalcemia), asthenia, diarrhea, nausea, and interstitial pneumonia, but mucocutaneous AEs are the most frequent.

Skin manifestations

Rashes and papulopustular eruptions

Rash develops in 25–61% of patients on everolimus and 43–76% on temsirolimus. Usually mild to moderate (0–6% grade 3–4), it appears during the first weeks of treatment. Patients rarely require dose modifications or treatment interruption. However, rashes are described as maculopapular, papulopustular (Figure 18.7), or acneiform eruptions in 30–40% of the patients. A nonspecific neutrophilic dermoepidermal infiltrate has been found pathologically. Therapeutic management is currently, and by analogy, based on that proposed for anti-EGFR inhibitors. Pruritus is a common symptom that could be treated with topical or oral corticosteroids and antihistamines.

The incidence of true maculopapular rashes is not known; they seem much less frequent than papulopustular ones. Pathologic examination of a rash of this kind occurring with temsirolimus revealed an eosinophilic infiltrate with epidermal spongiosis [110].

Stomatitis – oral ulcerations

Mucositis resembling aphthous ulcers are very common: in up to 40% with everolimus and 70% with temsirolimus [111–118]. These AEs are dose dependent and can result in a dose reduction or treatment interruption, especially in the case of painful oral ulcers that impact patients' food intake.

A sensation of a dry mouth has also been reported in 5–11% of patients treated with everolimus and a dysgeusia has been

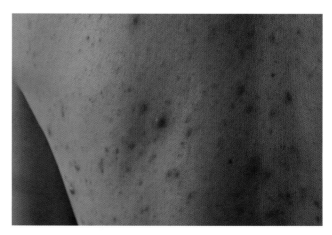

Figure 18.7 Everolimus-induced rash.

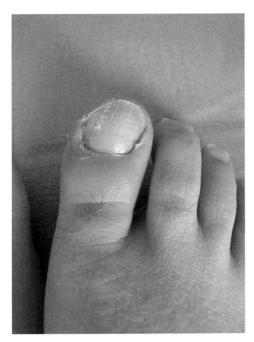

Figure 18.8 Nail plate modification and perionyxis with mTOR inhibitor.

observed with both compounds [112,113,115–117]. Management of these AEs relies on symptomatic measures: topical or systemic analgesics, topical corticosteroids (clobetasol ointment applied four times a day to lesions), and dose modifications.

Paronychia – pyogenic granulomas

Nail involvement, sometimes described as nail dystrophy or thinning of the nail plate, has been reported in 5–46% of the cases.

Paronychia and/or pyogenic granulomas localized on the lateral nail folds (Figure 18.8) are similar to those with EGFR inhibitors, and the incidence is unknown. Management relies on symptomatic measures depending on severity, including topical antibiotics, antiseptics (povidone-iodine ointments), cryotherapy, silver nitrate chemical cauterization, and partial nail avulsion.

Xerosis and pruritus

Xerosis and pruritus are common (20% and 30%, respectively) and are sometimes associated. Edema is also reported in up to 35% of patients [88,114,119].

Conclusions

Targeted anticancer small molecule kinase inhibitors induce various and unique skin manifestations that can significantly impact patients' quality of life and adherence to therapy. Close interactions between prescribers and dermatologists is highly recommended for these patients in order to inform them of the risk before the treatments are initiated, to describe and report new

AEs, and to introduce preventive and treatment measures to alleviate the manifestations. Furthermore, study of these AEs represents a considerable source of information concerning the mechanisms governing skin homeostasis.

References

1 Krause, D.S. & Van Etten, R.A. (2005) Tyrosine kinases as targets for cancer therapy. *New England Journal of Medicine*, **353** (2), 172–187.

2 Ellis, L.M. & Hicklin, D.J. (2008) VEGF-targeted therapy: mechanisms of anti-tumour activity. *Nature Reviews: Cancer*, **8** (8), 579–591.

3 Robert, C., Soria, J.C., Spatz, A. *et al.* (2005) Cutaneous side-effects of kinase inhibitors and blocking antibodies. *Lancet Oncology*, **6** (7), 491–500.

4 Breccia, M., Carmosino, I., Russo, E., Morano, S.G., Latagliata, R. & Alimena, G. (2005) Early and tardive skin adverse events in chronic myeloid leukaemia patients treated with imatinib. *European Journal of Haematology*, **74** (2), 121–123.

5 Valeyrie, L., Bastuji-Garin, S., Revuz, J. *et al.* (2003) Adverse cutaneous reactions to imatinib (STI571) in Philadelphia chromosome-positive leukemias: a prospective study of 54 patients. *Journal of the American Academy of Dermatology*, **48** (2), 201–206.

6 Basso, F.G., Boer, C.C., Correa, M.E. *et al.* (2009) Skin and oral lesions associated to imatinib mesylate therapy. *Supportive Care in Cancer*, **17** (4), 465–468.

7 Brouard, M. & Saurat, J.H. (2001) Cutaneous reactions to STI571. *New England Journal of Medicine*, **345** (8), 618–619.

8 Kantarjian, H., Sawyers, C., Hochhaus, A. *et al.* (2002) Hematologic and cytogenetic responses to imatinib mesylate in chronic myelogenous leukemia. *New England Journal of Medicine*, **346** (9), 645–652.

9 Deininger, M.W., O'Brien, S.G., Ford, J.M. & Druker, B.J. (2003) Practical management of patients with chronic myeloid leukemia receiving imatinib. *Journal of Clinical Oncology*, **21** (8), 1637–1647.

10 Scheinfeld, N. (2006) Imatinib mesylate and dermatology part 2: a review of the cutaneous side effects of imatinib mesylate. *Journal of Drugs in Dermatology*, **5** (3), 228–231.

11 Hensley, M.L. & Ford, J.M. (2003) Imatinib treatment: specific issues related to safety, fertility, and pregnancy. *Seminars in Hematology*, **40** (2 Suppl. 2), 21–25.

12 Hsiao, L.T., Chung, H.M., Lin, J.T. *et al.* (2002) Stevens–Johnson syndrome after treatment with STI571: a case report. *British Journal of Haematology*, **117** (3), 620–622.

13 Severino, G., Chillotti, C., De Lisa, R., Del Zompo, M. & Ardau, R. (2005) Adverse reactions during imatinib and lansoprazole treatment in gastrointestinal stromal tumors. *Annals of Pharmacotherapy*, **39** (1), 162–164.

14 Vidal, D., Puig, L., Sureda, A. & Alomar, A. (2002) Sti571-induced Stevens–Johnson syndrome. *British Journal of Haematology*, **119** (1), 274–275.

15 Pavithran, K. & Thomas, M. (2005) Imatinib induced Stevens–Johnson syndrome: lack of recurrence following re-challenge with a lower dose. *Indian Journal of Dermatology, Venereology and Leprology*, **71** (4), 288–289.

16 Sanchez-Gonzalez, B., Pascual-Ramirez, J.C., Fernandez-Abellan, P., Belinchon-Romero, I., Rivas, C. & Vegara-Aguilera, G. (2003) Severe

skin reaction to imatinib in a case of Philadelphia-positive acute lymphoblastic leukemia. *Blood*, **101** (6), 2446.

17 Mahapatra, M., Mishra, P. & Kumar, R. (2007) Imatinib-induced Stevens–Johnson syndrome: recurrence after re-challenge with a lower dose. *Annals of Hematology*, **86** (7), 537–538.

18 Brouard, M.C., Prins, C., Mach-Pascual, S. & Saurat, J.H. (2001) Acute generalized exanthematous pustulosis associated with STI571 in a patient with chronic myeloid leukemia. *Dermatology (Basel, Switzerland)*, **203** (1), 57–59.

19 Schwarz, M., Kreuzer, K.A., Baskaynak, G., Dorken, B. & le Coutre, P. (2002) Imatinib-induced acute generalized exanthematous pustulosis (AGEP) in two patients with chronic myeloid leukemia. *European Journal of Haematology*, **69** (4), 254–256.

20 Le Nouail, P., Viseux, V., Chaby, G., Billet, A., Denoeux, J.P. & Lok, C. (2006) Drug reaction with eosinophilia and systemic symptoms (DRESS) following imatinib therapy. *Annales de Dermatologie et de Venereologie*, **133** (8–9 Pt 1), 686–688.

21 Woo, S.M., Huh, C.H., Park, K.C. & Youn, S.W. (2007) Exacerbation of psoriasis in a chronic myelogenous leukemia patient treated with imatinib. *Journal of Dermatology*, **34** (10), 724–726.

22 Brazzelli, V., Prestinari, F., Roveda, E. *et al.* (2005) Pityriasis rosea-like eruption during treatment with imatinib mesylate: description of 3 cases. *Journal of the American Academy of Dermatology*, **53** (5 Suppl. 1), S240–S243.

23 Konstantopoulos, K., Papadogianni, A., Dimopoulou, M., Kourelis, C. & Meletis, J. (2002) Pityriasis rosea associated with imatinib (STI571, Gleevec). *Dermatology (Basel, Switzerland)*, **205** (2), 172–173.

24 Deguchi, N., Kawamura, T., Shimizu, A. *et al.* (2006) Imatinib mesylate causes palmoplantar hyperkeratosis and nail dystrophy in three patients with chronic myeloid leukaemia. *British Journal of Dermatology*, **154** (6), 1216–1218.

25 Kuraishi, N., Nagai, Y., Hasegawa, M. & Ishikawa, O. (2010) Lichenoid drug eruption with palmoplantar hyperkeratosis due to imatinib mesylate: a case report and a review of the literature. *Acta Dermato-Venereologica*, **90** (1), 73–76.

26 Gomez Fernandez, C., Sendagorta Cudos, E., Casado Verrier, B., Feito Rodriguez, M., Suarez Aguado, J. & Vidaurrazaga Diaz de Arcaya, C. (2010) Oral lichenoid eruption associated with imatinib treatment. *European Journal of Dermatology*, **20** (1), 127–128.

27 Kawakami, T., Kawanabe, T. & Soma, Y. (2009) Cutaneous lichenoid eruption caused by imatinib mesylate in a Japanese patient with chronic myeloid leukaemia. *Acta Dermato-Venereologica*, **89** (3), 325–326.

28 Sendagorta, E., Herranz, P., Feito, M. *et al.* (2009) Lichenoid drug eruption related to imatinib: report of a new case and review of the literature. *Clinical and Experimental Dermatology*, **34** (7), e315–e316.

29 Dalmau, J., Peramiquel, L., Puig, L., Fernandez-Figueras, M.T., Roe, E. & Alomar, A. (2006) Imatinib-associated lichenoid eruption: acitretin treatment allows maintained antineoplastic effect. *British Journal of Dermatology*, **154** (6), 1213–1216.

30 Prabhash, K. & Doval, D.C. (2005) Lichenoid eruption due to imatinib. *Indian Journal of Dermatology, Venereology and Leprology*, **71** (4), 287–288.

31 Ena, P., Chiarolini, F., Siddi, G.M. & Cossu, A. (2004) Oral lichenoid eruption secondary to imatinib (Glivec). *Journal of Dermatological Treatment*, **15** (4), 253–255.

32 Arora, B., Kumar, L., Sharma, A., Wadhwa, J. & Kochupillai, V. (2004) Pigmentary changes in chronic myeloid leukemia patients treated with imatinib mesylate. *Annals of Oncology*, **15** (2), 358–359.

33 Tsao, A.S., Kantarjian, H., Cortes, J., O'Brien, S. & Talpaz, M. (2003) Imatinib mesylate causes hypopigmentation in the skin. *Cancer*, **98** (11), 2483–2487.

34 Campbell, T., Felsten, L. & Moore, J. (2009) Disappearance of lentigines in a patient receiving imatinib treatment for familial gastrointestinal stromal tumor syndrome. *Archives of Dermatology*, **145** (11), 1313–1316.

35 Etienne, G., Cony-Makhoul, P. & Mahon, F.X. (2002) Imatinib mesylate and gray hair. *New England Journal of Medicine*, **347** (6), 446.

36 McPherson, T., Sherman, V. & Turner, R. (2009) Imatinib-associated hyperpigmentation, a side effect that should be recognized. *Journal of the European Academy of Dermatology and Venereology*, **23** (1), 82–83.

37 Dippel, E., Haas, N., Grabbe, J., Schadendorf, D., Hamann, K. & Czarnetzki, B.M. (1995) Expression of the c-kit receptor in hypomelanosis: a comparative study between piebaldism, naevus depigmentosus and vitiligo. *British Journal of Dermatology*, **132** (2), 182–189.

38 Cario-Andre, M., Ardilouze, L., Pain, C., Gauthier, Y., Mahon, F.X. & Taieb, A. (2006) Imatinib mesilate inhibits melanogenesis in vitro. *British Journal of Dermatology*, **155** (2), 493–494.

39 Hamm, M., Touraud, J.P., Mannone, L., Klisnick, J., Ponnelle, T. & Lambert, D. (2003) Imatinib-induced purpuric vasculitis. *Annales de Dermatologie et de Venereologie*, **130** (8–9 Pt 1), 765–767.

40 Clark, S.H., Duvic, M. & Prieto, V.G. (2003) Mycosis fungoides-like reaction in a patient treated with Gleevec. *Journal of Cutaneous Pathology*, **30** (4), 279–281.

41 Rousselot, P., Larghero, J., Raffoux, E. *et al.* (2003) Photosensitization in chronic myelogenous leukaemia patients treated with imatinib mesylate. *British Journal of Haematology*, **120** (6), 1091–1092.

42 Kantarjian, H., Giles, F., Wunderle, L. *et al.* (2006) Nilotinib in imatinib-resistant CML and Philadelphia chromosome-positive ALL. *New England Journal of Medicine*, **354** (24), 2542–2551.

43 Kantarjian, H.M., Giles, F., Gattermann, N. *et al.* (2007) Nilotinib (formerly AMN107), a highly selective BCR-ABL tyrosine kinase inhibitor, is effective in patients with Philadelphia chromosome-positive chronic myelogenous leukemia in chronic phase following imatinib resistance and intolerance. *Blood*, **110** (10), 3540–3546.

44 Talpaz, M., Shah, N.P., Kantarjian, H. *et al.* (2006) Dasatinib in imatinib-resistant Philadelphia chromosome-positive leukemias. *New England Journal of Medicine*, **354** (24), 2531–2541.

45 Hochhaus, A., Kantarjian, H.M., Baccarani, M. *et al.* (2007) Dasatinib induces notable hematologic and cytogenetic responses in chronic-phase chronic myeloid leukemia after failure of imatinib therapy. *Blood*, **109** (6), 2303–2309.

46 Heidary, N., Naik, H. & Burgin, S. (2008) Chemotherapeutic agents and the skin: an update. *Journal of the American Academy of Dermatology*, **58** (4), 545–570.

47 Assouline, S., Laneuville, P. & Gambacorti-Passerini, C. (2006) Panniculitis during dasatinib therapy for imatinib-resistant chronic myelogenous leukemia. *New England Journal of Medicine*, **354** (24), 2623–2624.

48 Ferrara, N., Gerber, H.P. & LeCouter, J. (2003) The biology of VEGF and its receptors. *Nature Medicine*, **9** (6), 669–676.

49 Bjornsti, M.A. & Houghton, P.J. (2004) The TOR pathway: a target for cancer therapy. *Nature Reviews: Cancer*, **4** (5), 335–348.

50 Robert, C. (2007) Cutaneous side effects of antiangiogenic agents. *Bulletin Du Cancer*, **94 Spec No**, S260–S264.

51 Robert, C., Mateus, C., Spatz, A., Wechsler, J. & Escudier, B. (2009) Dermatologic symptoms associated with the multikinase inhibitor sorafenib. *Journal of the American Academy of Dermatology*, **60** (2), 299–305.

52 Abou-Alfa, G.K., Schwartz, L., Ricci, S. *et al.* (2006) Phase II study of sorafenib in patients with advanced hepatocellular carcinoma. *Journal of Clinical Oncology*, **24** (26), 4293–4300.

53 Blumenschein, G.R. Jr., Gatzemeier, U., Fossella, F. *et al.* (2009) Phase II, multicenter, uncontrolled trial of single-agent sorafenib in patients with relapsed or refractory, advanced non-small-cell lung cancer. *Journal of Clinical Oncology*, **27** (26), 4274–4280.

54 Cheng, A.L., Kang, Y.K., Chen, Z. *et al.* (2009) Efficacy and safety of sorafenib in patients in the Asia-Pacific region with advanced hepatocellular carcinoma: a phase III randomised, double-blind, placebo-controlled trial. *Lancet Oncology*, **10** (1), 25–34.

55 Escudier, B., Eisen, T., Stadler, W.M. *et al.* (2009) Sorafenib for treatment of renal cell carcinoma: final efficacy and safety results of the phase III treatment approaches in renal cancer global evaluation trial. *Journal of Clinical Oncology*, **27** (20), 3312–3318.

56 Llovet, J.M., Di Bisceglie, A.M., Bruix, J., *et al.* (2008) Design and endpoints of clinical trials in hepatocellular carcinoma. *Journal of the National Cancer Institute*, **100** (10), 698–711.

57 Ratain, M.J., Eisen, T., Stadler, W.M. *et al.* (2006) Phase II placebo-controlled randomized discontinuation trial of sorafenib in patients with metastatic renal cell carcinoma. *Journal of Clinical Oncology*, **24** (16), 2505–2512.

58 Ryan, C.W., Goldman, B.H., Lara, P.N. Jr. *et al.* (2007) Sorafenib with interferon alfa-2b as first-line treatment of advanced renal carcinoma: a phase II study of the Southwest Oncology Group. *Journal of Clinical Oncology*, **25** (22), 3296–3301.

59 Demetri, G.D., van Oosterom, A.T., Garrett, C.R. *et al.* (2006) Efficacy and safety of sunitinib in patients with advanced gastrointestinal stromal tumour after failure of imatinib: a randomised controlled trial. *Lancet*, **368** (9544), 1329–1338.

60 Gore, M.E., Szczylik, C., Porta, C. *et al.* (2009) Safety and efficacy of sunitinib for metastatic renal-cell carcinoma: an expanded-access trial. *Lancet Oncology*, **10** (8), 757–763.

61 Motzer, R.J., Hutson, T.E., Tomczak, P. *et al.* (2007) Sunitinib versus interferon alfa in metastatic renal-cell carcinoma. *New England Journal of Medicine*, **356** (2), 115–124.

62 Motzer, R.J., Rini, B.I., Bukowski, R.M. *et al.* (2006) Sunitinib in patients with metastatic renal cell carcinoma. *Journal of the American Medical Association*, **295** (21), 2516–2524.

63 Hurwitz, H.I., Dowlati, A., Saini, S. *et al.* (2009) Phase I trial of pazopanib in patients with advanced cancer. *Clinical Cancer Research*, **15** (12), 4220–4227.

64 Sternberg, C.N., Davis, I.D., Mardiak, J. *et al.* (2010) Pazopanib in locally advanced or metastatic renal cell carcinoma: results of a randomized phase III trial. *Journal of Clinical Oncology*, **28** (6), 1061–1068.

65 Hutson, T.E., Davis, I.D., Machiels, J.P. *et al.* (2010) Efficacy and safety of pazopanib in patients with metastatic renal cell carcinoma. *Journal of Clinical Oncology*, **28** (3), 475–480.

66 Susser, W.S., Whitaker-Worth, D.L. & Grant-Kels, J.M. (1999) Mucocutaneous reactions to chemotherapy. *Journal of the American Academy of Dermatology*, **40** (3), 367–398; quiz 399–400.

67 von Moos, R., Thuerlimann, B.J., Aapro, M. *et al.* (2008) Pegylated liposomal doxorubicin-associated hand-foot syndrome: recommendations of an international panel of experts. *European Journal of Cancer*, **44** (6), 781–790.

68 Webster-Gandy, J.D., How, C. & Harrold, K. (2007) Palmar-plantar erythrodysesthesia (PPE): a literature review with commentary on experience in a cancer centre. *European Journal of Oncology Nursing*, **11** (3), 238–246.

69 Autier, J., Escudier, B., Wechsler, J., Spatz, A. & Robert, C. (2008) Prospective study of the cutaneous adverse effects of sorafenib, a novel multikinase inhibitor. *Archives of Dermatology*, **144** (7), 886–892.

70 Lipworth, A.D., Robert, C. & Zhu, A.X. (2009) Hand-foot syndrome (hand-foot skin reaction, palmar-plantar erythrodysesthesia): focus on sorafenib and sunitinib. *Oncology*, **77** (5), 257–271.

71 Autier, J., Mateus, C., Wechsler, J., Spatz, A. & Robert, C. (2008) Cutaneous side effects of sorafenib and sunitinib. *Annales de Dermatologie et de Venereologie*, **135** (2), 148–153; quiz 147, 154.

72 Sibaud, V., Delord, J.P. & Chevreau, C. (2009) Sorafenib-induced hand-foot skin reaction: a Koebner phenomenon? *Targeted Oncology*, **4** (4), 307–310.

73 Boone, S.L., Jameson, G., Von Hoff, D. & Lacouture, M.E. (2009) Blackberry-induced hand-foot skin reaction to sunitinib. *Investigational New Drugs*, **27** (4), 389–390.

74 Lacouture, M.E., Reilly, L.M., Gerami, P. & Guitart, J. (2008) Hand foot skin reaction in cancer patients treated with the multikinase inhibitors sorafenib and sunitinib. *Annals of Oncology*, **19** (11), 1955–1961.

75 Yang, C.H., Lin, W.C., Chuang, C.K. *et al.* (2008) Hand-foot skin reaction in patients treated with sorafenib: a clinicopathological study of cutaneous manifestations due to multitargeted kinase inhibitor therapy. *British Journal of Dermatology*, **158** (3), 592–596.

76 Lacouture, M.E., Wu, S., Robert, C. *et al.* (2008) Evolving strategies for the management of hand-foot skin reaction associated with the multitargeted kinase inhibitors sorafenib and sunitinib. *The Oncologist*, **13** (9), 1001–1011.

77 Robert, C., Faivre, S., Raymond, E., Armand, J.P. & Escudier, B. (2005) Subungual splinter hemorrhages: a clinical window to inhibition of vascular endothelial growth factor receptors? *Annals of Internal Medicine*, **143** (4), 313–314.

78 Lee, W.J., Lee, J.L., Chang, S.E. *et al.* (2009) Cutaneous adverse effects in patients treated with the multitargeted kinase inhibitors sorafenib and sunitinib. *British Journal of Dermatology*, **161** (5), 1045–1051.

79 Motzer, R.J., Hutson, T.E., Tomczak, P. *et al.* (2009) Overall survival and updated results for sunitinib compared with interferon alfa in patients with metastatic renal cell carcinoma. *Journal of Clinical Oncology*, **27** (22), 3584–3590.

80 Kong, H.H. & Turner, M.L. (2009) Array of cutaneous adverse effects associated with sorafenib. *Journal of the American Academy of Dermatology*, **61** (2), 360–361.

81 MacGregor, J.L., Silvers, D.N., Grossman, M.E. & Sherman, W.H. (2007) Sorafenib-induced erythema multiforme. *Journal of the American Academy of Dermatology*, **56** (3), 527–528.

82 Kong, H.H., Sibaud, V., Chanco Turner, M.L., Fojo, T., Hornyak, T.J. & Chevreau, C. (2008) Sorafenib-induced eruptive melanocytic lesions. *Archives of Dermatology*, **144** (6), 820–822.

83 Rosenbaum, S.E., Wu, S., Newman, M.A., West, D.P., Kuzel, T. & Lacouture, M.E. (2008) Dermatological reactions to the multitargeted tyrosine kinase inhibitor sunitinib. *Supportive Care in Cancer*, **16** (6), 557–566.

84 Robert, C., Spatz, A., Faivre, S., Armand, J.P. & Raymond, E. (2003) Tyrosine kinase inhibition and grey hair. *Lancet*, **361** (9362), 1056.

85 Hartmann, J.T. & Kanz, L. (2008) Sunitinib and periodic hair depigmentation due to temporary c-KIT inhibition. *Archives of Dermatology*, **144** (11), 1525–1526.

86 Billemont, B., Barete, S. & Rixe, O. (2008) Scrotal cutaneous side effects of sunitinib. *New England Journal of Medicine*, **359** (9), 975–976; discussion 976.

87 Suwattee, P., Chow, S., Berg, B.C. & Warshaw, E.M. (2008) Sunitinib: a cause of bullous palmoplantar erythrodysesthesia, periungual erythema, and mucositis. *Archives of Dermatology*, **144** (1), 123–125.

88 Guevremont, C., Alasker, A. & Karakiewicz, P.I. (2009) Management of sorafenib, sunitinib, and temsirolimus toxicity in metastatic renal cell carcinoma. *Current Opinion in Supportive and Palliative Care*, **3** (3), 170–179.

89 Bennani-Lahlou, M., Mateus, C., Escudier, B. *et al.* (2008) Eruptive nevi associated with sorafenib treatment. *Annales de Dermatologie et de Venereologie*, **135** (10), 672–674.

90 Dhomen, N., Reis-Filho, J.S., da Rocha Dias, S. *et al.* (2009) Oncogenic Braf induces melanocyte senescence and melanoma in mice. *Cancer Cell*, **15** (4), 294–303.

91 Wajapeyee, N., Serra, R.W., Zhu, X., Mahalingam, M. & Green, M.R. (2008) Oncogenic BRAF induces senescence and apoptosis through pathways mediated by the secreted protein IGFBP7. *Cell*, **132** (3), 363–374.

92 Arnault, J.P., Wechsler, J., Escudier, B. *et al.* (2009) Keratoacanthomas and squamous cell carcinomas in patients receiving sorafenib. *Journal of Clinical Oncology*, **27** (23), e59–e61.

93 Dubauskas, Z., Kunishige, J., Prieto, V.G., Jonasch, E., Hwu, P. & Tannir, N.M. (2009) Cutaneous squamous cell carcinoma and inflammation of actinic keratoses associated with sorafenib. *Clinical Genitourinary Cancer*, **7** (1), 20–23.

94 Kong, H.H., Cowen, E.W., Azad, N.S., Dahut, W., Gutierrez, M. & Turner, M.L. (2007) Keratoacanthomas associated with sorafenib therapy. *Journal of the American Academy of Dermatology*, **56** (1), 171–172.

95 Kwon, E.J., Kish, L.S. & Jaworsky, C. (2009) The histologic spectrum of epithelial neoplasms induced by sorafenib. *Journal of the American Academy of Dermatology*, **61** (3), 522–527.

96 Clausen, O.P., Aass, H.C., Beigi, M. *et al.* (2006) Are keratoacanthomas variants of squamous cell carcinomas? A comparison of chromosomal aberrations by comparative genomic hybridization. *Journal of Investigative Dermatology*, **126** (10), 2308–2315.

97 Cribier, B., Asch, P. & Grosshans, E. (1999) Differentiating squamous cell carcinoma from keratoacanthoma using histopathological criteria. Is it possible? A study of 296 cases. *Dermatology (Basel, Switzerland)*, **199** (3), 208–212.

98 Hodak, E., Jones, R.E. & Ackerman, A.B. (1993) Solitary keratoacanthoma is a squamous-cell carcinoma: three examples with metastases. *American Journal of Dermatopathology*, **15** (4), 332–342; discussion 343–352.

99 Flaherty, K., Puzanov, I., Sosman, J. *et al.* (2009) Phase I study of PLX4032: proof of concept for V600E BRAF mutation as a therapeutic target in human cancer. *Journal of Clinical Oncology*, **27**, 9000.

100 Kefford, R., Arkenau, H.T., Brown, M.P. *et al.* (2010) Selective inhibition of oncogenic BRAF V600E/K/D by GSK2118436: evidence of clinical activity in subjects with metastatic melanoma. *Pigment Cell and Melanoma Research*, **23** (suppl; abstr 912).

101 Robinson, M.J. & Cobb, M.H. (1997) Mitogen-activated protein kinase pathways. *Current Opinion in Cell Biology*, **9** (2), 180–186.

102 Dhomen, N. & Marais, R. (2009) BRAF signaling and targeted therapies in melanoma. *Hematology/Oncology Clinics of North America*, **23** (3), 529–545, ix.

103 Heidorn, S., Milagre, C., Whittaker, S. *et al.* (2010) Kinase-dead BRAF and oncogenic RAS cooperate to drive tumor progression through CRAF. *Cell*, **140**, 209–221.

104 Joseph, E.W., Pratilas, C.A., Poulikakos, P.I. *et al.* (2010) The RAF inhibitor PLX4032 inhibits ERK signaling and tumor cell proliferation in a V600E BRAF-selective manner. *Proceedings of the National Academy of Sciences of the United States of America*, **107** (33), 14903–14908.

105 Mateus, C. & Robert, C. (2009) New drugs in oncology and skin toxicity. *La Revue de Medecine Interne*, **30** (5), 401–410.

106 Poulikakos, P., Zhang, C., Bollag, G., Shokat, K. & Rosen, N. (2010) RAF inhibitors transactivate RAF dimers and ERK signalling in cells with wild-type BRAF. *Nature*, **464**, 427–431.

107 Bjelogrlic, S.K., Srdic, T. & Radulovic, S. (2006) Mammalian target of rapamycin is a promising target for novel therapeutic strategy against cancer. *Journal of the Balkan Union of Oncology*, **11** (3), 267–276.

108 Sehgal, S.N. (1998) Rapamune (RAPA, rapamycin, sirolimus): mechanism of action immunosuppressive effect results from blockade of signal transduction and inhibition of cell cycle progression. *Clinical Biochemistry*, **31** (5), 335–340.

109 Nguyen, A., Hoang, V., Laquer, V. & Kelly, K.M. (2009) Angiogenesis in cutaneous disease: part I. *Journal of the American Academy of Dermatology*, **61** (6), 921–942, quiz 943–944.

110 Gandhi, M., Kuzel, T. & Lacouture, M. (2009) Eosinophilic rash secondary to temsirolimus. *Clinical Genitourinary Cancer*, **7** (2), E34–E36.

111 Amato, R.J., Jac, J., Giessinger, S., Saxena, S. & Willis, J.P. (2009) A phase 2 study with a daily regimen of the oral mTOR inhibitor RAD001 (everolimus) in patients with metastatic clear cell renal cell cancer. *Cancer*, **115** (11), 2438–2446.

112 Atkins, M.B., Hidalgo, M., Stadler, W.M. *et al.* (2004) Randomized phase II study of multiple dose levels of CCI-779, a novel mammalian target of rapamycin kinase inhibitor, in patients with advanced refractory renal cell carcinoma. *Journal of Clinical Oncology*, **22** (5), 909–918.

113 Atkins, M.B., Yasothan, U. & Kirkpatrick, P. (2009) Everolimus. *Nature Reviews Drug Discovery*, **8** (7), 535–536.

114 Ellard, S.L., Clemons, M., Gelmon, K.A. *et al.* (2009) Randomized phase II study comparing two schedules of everolimus in patients with recurrent/metastatic breast cancer: NCIC Clinical Trials Group IND.163. *Journal of Clinical Oncology*, **27** (27), 4536–4541.

115 Motzer, R.J., Escudier, B., Oudard, S. *et al.* (2008) Efficacy of everolimus in advanced renal cell carcinoma: a double-blind, randomised, placebo-controlled phase III trial. *Lancet*, **372** (9637), 449–456.

116 O'Donnell, A., Faivre, S., Burris, H.A. 3rd *et al.* (2008) Phase I pharmacokinetic and pharmacodynamic study of the oral mammalian target of rapamycin inhibitor everolimus in patients

with advanced solid tumors. *Journal of Clinical Oncology*, **26** (10), 1588–1595.

117 Tabernero, J., Rojo, F., Calvo, E. *et al.* (2008) Dose- and schedule-dependent inhibition of the mammalian target of rapamycin pathway with everolimus: a phase I tumor pharmacodynamic study in patients with advanced solid tumors. *Journal of Clinical Oncology*, **26** (10), 1603–1610.

118 Punt, C.J., Boni, J., Bruntsch, U., Peters, M. & Thielert, C. (2003) Phase I and pharmacokinetic study of CCI-779, a novel cytostatic cell-cycle inhibitor, in combination with 5-fluorouracil and leucovorin in patients with advanced solid tumors. *Annals of Oncology*, **14** (6), 931–937.

119 Raymond, E., Alexandre, J., Faivre, S. *et al.* (2004) Safety and pharmacokinetics of escalated doses of weekly intravenous infusion of CCI-779, a novel mTOR inhibitor, in patients with cancer. *Journal of Clinical Oncology*, **22** (12), 2336–2347.

19 Antimicrotubule Agents

Claus Garbe

Center for Dermatooncology, University Hospital, Tuebingen, Germany

Introduction

Microtubules are the target of a number of natural product-derived anticancer drugs. Microtubules are highly dynamic assemblies of the protein tubulin. They readily polymerize and depolymerize in cells, and they undergo two interesting kinds of dynamics, dynamic instability and treadmilling, both crucial to mitosis. Microtubule dynamics are highly regulated during the cell cycle by endogenous regulators. In addition, many antitumor drugs and natural compounds alter the polymerization dynamics of microtubules, blocking mitosis, and inducing cell death by apoptosis. These drugs include several that inhibit microtubule polymerization, namely, the vinca alkaloids and estramustine (Table 19.1). Conversely, paclitaxel and docetaxel stimulate microtubule polymerization and stabilize microtubules. Importantly, considerable evidence indicates that, at lower concentrations, these drugs have a common mechanism of action; they suppress the dynamics of microtubules without appreciably changing the mass of microtubules in the cell [1].

Taxanes

The taxanes are diterpenes produced by the plants of the genus Taxus (yews). Taxanes include paclitaxel (Taxol®) and docetaxel (Taxotere®). Paclitaxel was originally derived from the Pacific yew tree. The principal mechanism of the taxane class of drugs is the disruption of microtubule function by stabilizing guanosine diphosphate (GDP)-bound tubulin in the microtubule.

Paclitaxel initially received approval in 1992 for ovarian cancer; since then approvals include advanced breast cancer and non-small cell lung cancer (NSCLC). Paclitaxel is also widely used off-label for various other tumors. Docetaxel was first approved

in 1996 for metastatic breast cancer, and then for breast cancer, NSCLC, prostate cancer, gastric adenocarcinoma, and head and neck squamous cell carcinoma (SCC).

As taxanes are hydrophobic, they require solvents to enable parenteral administration, mainly Cremophor EL® or polysorbate for docetaxel. Cremophor EL® is a nonionic solubilizer and emulsifier obtained by causing ethylene oxide to react with castor oil in a molar ratio of 35:1. The main component is glycerol-polyethylene glycol ricinoleate, which, together with fatty acid esters of polyethylene glycol, represents the hydrophobic portion. The smaller, hydrophilic part consists of polyethylene glycols and ethoxylated glycerol. Cremophor EL has been widely used as the vehicle for a number of hydrophobic pharmacologic agents, including propofol, diazepam, and cyclosporine. Notably, the concentration of Cremophor EL in the therapeutic dose of parenteral paclitaxel is relatively high compared with other agents. In contrast, docetaxel is solubilized in another polyoxyethylated surfactant, polysorbate 80 (Tween 80®), for clinical use.

These solvents contribute to the main toxicities, especially hypersensitivity reactions (HSR), peripheral neuropathy, and myelosuppression. Cremophor EL can also leach plasticizers from polyvinyl chloride tubing, which can result in severe anaphylactic reactions. To decrease HSR, corticosteroids and antihistamines are standard premedication with taxanes.

In early trials with paclitaxel, a high incidence of acute HSR characterized by respiratory distress, hypotension, angioedema, generalized urticaria, and rash were observed [2–6]. Prolongation of the infusion time has been proposed in order to decrease HSR. Despite premedications with corticosteroids and histamine antagonists, minor reactions (e.g., flushing and rash) still occur in approximately 40% of all patients, and nearly 3% of patients experience potentially life-threatening reactions [7,8]. Prolonging the infusion does not eliminate the risk of HSR. Docetaxel has been known to cause infusion-related reactions in the absence of

Dermatologic Principles and Practice in Oncology: Conditions of the Skin, Hair, and Nails in Cancer Patients, First Edition. Edited by Mario E. Lacouture.
© 2014 John Wiley & Sons, Inc. Published 2014 by John Wiley & Sons, Inc.

premedication; however, these reactions have occurred at a decreased frequency when compared with paclitaxel and can be effectively managed by premedication with corticosteroids and antihistamines [5].

Nanoparticle albumin-bound paclitaxel (nab-Paclitaxel, Abraxane®) is a solvent-free albumin-bound nanoparticle formulation that does not require solvents for parenteral administration. This eliminates the need for premedication with steroids or antihistamines. nab-Paclitaxel binds to gp60, the albumin receptor on endothelial cells, which activates caveolin-1 with formation of caveolae, then transporting the conjugate to the extracellular space, including the tumor interstitium, where SPARC (secreted protein, acidic and rich in cysteine) is selectively secreted by the tumors and binds to albumin conjugate with subsequent release of paclitaxel. Neither HSR nor cutaneous adverse events (AEs) were reported in phase II–III trials with nab-Paclitaxel [9–11].

Clinical features

HSR is the most severe AE, mainly with paclitaxel and less frequently with docetaxel. It occurs during the first infusion in more than 50% of affected patients and in others during the second infusion (Figure 19.1). Symptoms manifest during the first minutes of infusion, and Table 19.2 summarizes the characteristic symptoms. Evidence suggests that the solvents Cremophor EL and Tween 80® are the hypersensitivity culprits. Cremophor EL was shown to induce histamine release with HSR in dogs [4, 5]. The hypersensitivity reaction seems to be a dose-dependent intolerance reaction and not a type I allergic reaction, although it simulates many symptoms of the latter. HSR occurred in nearly one-third of treated patients before the introduction of premedication [8]. Since the early 1990s, when premedications where routinely used, the frequency of hypersensitivity reaction dropped to around 10% [2, 12].

In HSR, dyspnea with or without bronchospasm is observed most frequently (80%), followed by cutaneous reactions with erythematous flush and urticaria (75 %) and by changes of blood pressure (60%), mainly hypotension [2]. Close monitoring is required. The first 5 minutes of the infusion the patient should be under surveillance, and regular measurement of pulse and blood pressure are obligatory.

Alopecia of different degrees induced by taxanes is a common problem and has been observed in 20% of patients treated by paclitaxel monotherapy [13]. However, paclitaxel is frequently combined, reaching alopecia of more than 60% [14]. Thirty-five percent of patients developed alopecia under single-agent therapy with docetaxel [15], with nab-Paclitaxel alopecia reaches 77% [10].

Nail toxicity and onycholysis occurred in 5 of 21 patients who received six courses of weekly paclitaxel. It did not occur in

Table 19.1 Classification of antimicrotubule agents.

Taxanes	Paclitaxel, albumin-bound paclitaxel, docetaxel
Vinca alkaloids	Vincristine, vinblastine, vinorelbine
Estradiol derivative	Estramustine

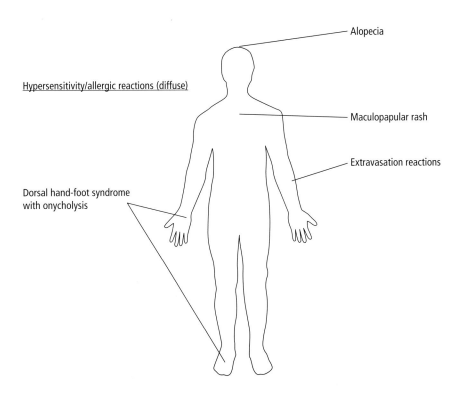

Figure 19.1 Anatomic location of dermatologic adverse events to antimicrotubule agents.

patients who received fewer cycles or those treated every 3 weeks. Prolonged weekly paclitaxel and other taxanes cause onycholysis in some patients, which may be precipitated by sunlight, so patients should protect their nails from sunlight [16, 17].

Nail toxicity is more frequent under docetaxel [18], reported in 88.5% of patients, with grade 3 toxicity in 11% [19]. Symptoms include subungual and splinter hemorrhages and hyperkeratosis, paronychia, loosening or separation of the nail from the nail bed, hyperpigmentation, and Beau–Rail lines, which indicate cessation of nail growth. For many patients, nail changes are associated with psychologic distress, considerable pain, and ambulatory and functional impairment in 32% [19–21] which can lead to discontinuation of treatment [19, 21, 22]. The severity of nail changes depends on the number of treatment cycles (appearing after the second cycle) and cumulative dose [19, 21].

A distinct type of hand-foot syndrome (HFS) has been reported with multidrug chemotherapy protocols that include paclitaxel and docetaxel, with a frequency of 10% and 5%, respectively (Figure 19.2 [23, 24]. Taxane-induced HFS develops with cumulative doses and more frequently with weekly schedule than those every 3 weeks. It is a class-based effect, as weekly paclitaxel and docetaxel resulted in 4 of 20 patients developing HFS. Clinically, the HFS to taxanes is distinct from that of anthracyclines, antimetabolites, or multikinase inhibitors (Table 19.3). In taxane-induced HFS, eryhtematous or violaceous plaques, which may blister, develop on the dorsum of the hands, especially over the thenar and hypothenar eminences, and over the Achilles tendon and malleoli. Consequently, Childress and Lokich [25] have suggested that HFS associated with taxanes be called PATEO or "periarticular thenar erythema and onycholysis." Histopathology shows hyperkeratosis, acanthosis, and focal areas of hydropic

degeneration of the basal cell layer and a dense neutrophilic dermal infiltrate with nuclear dust [26]. Prevention of taxane-induced HFS and onycholysis is possible with the use of frozen glove and sock therapy, which is lower in controlled studies in the frozen gloved hand than the control hand (p = 0.0001). Onycholysis in the frozen gloved hand was grade 1–2 in 11% and 51% in the control hand. Moreover, skin toxicity was grade 1–2 in 27%in the frozen gloved hand and 59% in the control hand.

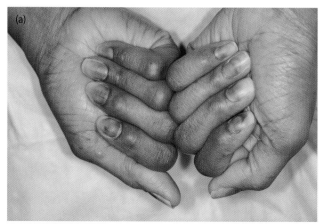

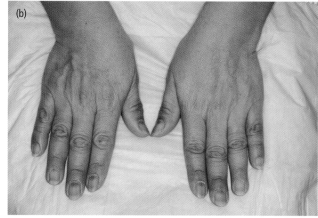

Figure 19.2 (a) Hand-foot syndrome with subungual hemorrhages due to taxanes. (b) Taxane induced onycholysis as part of PATEO (periarticular thenar erythema with onycholysis). (Photos courtesy of Mario Lacouture.)

Table 19.2 Symptoms of the hypersensitivity reaction due to paclitaxel and docetaxel.

Dyspnea	Chest tigthness	Back pain
Tachycardia	Urticaria	Erythematous flush
Hypertension	Hypotension	Extreme anxiety

Table 19.3 Characteristics of hand-foot syndrome to taxanes, anthracyclines/antimetabolites, and multikinase inhibitors.

Drug class	Taxanes	Anthracyclines/antimetabolites	Multikinase inhibitors
Drug names	Docetaxel, paclitaxel	Doxorubicin, liposomal doxorubicin, capecitabine, 5-fluorouracil	Sorafenib, sunitinib, pazopanib
Schedule specific	No	Yes	No
Location in hands	Dorsal: 1st and 5th fingers	Ventral: diffuse palmar	Ventral: digit tips, over joints, thenar and hypothenar
Location in feet	Dorsal: Achilles tendon, malleoli	Ventral: diffuse soles	Ventral: heels, forefoot
Onycholysis	Yes	No	No

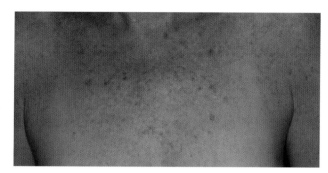

Figure 19.3 Maculopapular-induced rash to taxanes. (Photos courtesy of Mario Lacouture.)

Maculopapular rashes have been reported with paclitaxel monotherapy in 13% of patients [13] and their frequency increases to more than 20% with combination regimens (Figure 19.3) [14]. Variants include bullous fixed drug eruption [27], erythema multiforme [28, 29], and acute generalized exanthematous pustulosis [30].

Scleroderma-like cutaneous lesions induced by paclitaxel and by docetaxel have been reported, with biopsy showing dermal fibrosis [31–33], suggesting that these are a unique cutaneous adverse event caused by taxanes [31].

Cutaneous lupus erythematosus induced by paclitaxel has been reported twice [34] Similarly, four patients on docetaxel developed subacute cutaneous lupus erythematosus (SCLE)-like photodistributed eruptions. Histopathology showed an atrophying interface dermatitis with mucin deposition. Immunofluorescence revealed granular epidermal keratinocyte deposition of IgG and C5, consistent with SCLE [35].

Cutaneous photosensitivity induced by paclitaxel in combination with trastuzumab has been reported. The eruption appeared on the dorsal aspect of the patient's hands, forearms, legs, and face consisting of erythema, edema, and vesicles, and was associated with distal onycholysis. Aberrations in various parameters of the metabolism of porphyrins were observed in urine and erythrocytes. Sun avoidance and withdrawal of paclitaxel was followed by resolution of the rash and a return to the normal pattern of porphyrins biosynthesis [36]. Paclitaxel-associated photosensitive conditions have only been reported in nine patients: onycholysis in five, erythema multiforme and onycholysis in two, photo-recall phenomenon in one. The skin lesions developed on sun-exposed areas, usually after the patient had received several weekly doses of paclitaxel, and resolved following drug discontinuation [29]. However, the anecdotal benefit of topical or oral corticosteroids has been demonstrated in settings where interruption or discontinuation of a taxane was not a therapeutic option.

Radiation recall dermatitis has been reported under treatments with paclitaxel and docetaxel [37]. Two patients after having finished irradiation of the brain and receiving docetaxel, developed a severe erythema of the irradiated skin and large areas of moist erosions with crust (CTCAE grade 4) [38].

Extravasation of paclitaxel and docetaxel causes cutaneous toxicity of WHO grade 2–3 with slow spontaneous resolution in about 2 months [39, 40]. In some patients, a delayed vesicant reaction to paclitaxel extravasation resulting in severe necrosis was reported [41].

Treatment of choice and prognosis

The hypersensitivity reaction to paclitaxel or docetaxel can be avoided in about 20% of patients by standard premedication, which usually consists of 20 mg dexamethasone, 300 mg cimetidine, and 50 mg diphenhydramine. Premedication recommendations and treatment of HSR are as follow.

Premedication:
• 20 mg dexamethasone orally 12 and 6 hours before paclitaxel or docetaxel and 20 mg IV just before treatment;
• 50 mg diphenhydramine orally and IV in same schedule as dexamethasone;
• 300 mg cimetidine orally just before treatment;
• Slowly withdraw the patient (if possible) from any beta-blocker medication that could potentiate a reaction or make it harder to treat.

Treatment set-up:
• IV access must be established, preferentially as a venous port;
• Blood pressure monitoring must be available;
• The nurse should remain in the room for at least 5 minutes after the start of each infusion, as most hypersensitivity reactions begin in the early minutes of the infusion.

Treatment of reactions:
• Discontinue taxol;
• Administer epinephrine 0.35–0.5 mL IV every 15–20 minutes until the reaction subsides or a total of six doses are given;
• If hypotension is present that does not respond to epinephrine, administer IV fluids;
• If wheezing is present that is not responsive to epinephrine, administer 0.35 mL nebulized albuterol solution;
• Administer 50 mg diphenhydramine IV;
• Although corticosteroids have no effect on the initial reaction, they have been shown to block "late" allergic reactions to a variety of substances. Thus, 125 mg methylprednisolone IV (or its equivalent) may be administered to prevent recurrent or ongoing allergy manifestations [2].

Despite premedication, 10% of patients treated with paclitaxel will still develop a HSR. Despite these interventions, many patients with taxane-responsive cancers still present with HSR and would benefit from the reintroduction of therapy. Feldweg et al. [42] described a 6- to 7-hour standard desensitization protocol for the management of patients with severe HSRs to taxanes. The protocol was safe for 17 patients, who received a total of 77 planned courses of taxane chemotherapy.

The standard 12-step desensitization protocol combined gradual increases in the rate of infusion and concentration of the taxane, administering the total dose over 5.8 hours. The target dose is calculated based on the patient's body surface area. Three different infusion solutions – A, B, and C – with different

Table 19.4 Standard three-solution, 12-step desensitization protocol for a total paclitaxel dose of 300 mg [42].

Total dose	300 mg	Solution concentration (mg/mL)	Dose in each solution (mg)
Solution A	250 mL	0.012	3.0*
Solution B	250 mL	0.120	30.0*
Solution C	250 mL	1.200	300.0*

Step	Solution	Rate (mL/hour)	Time (min)	Administered dose (mg)	Cumulative dose (mg)
1	A	2	15	0.006	0.006
2	A	5	15	0.015	0.021
3	A	10	15	0.030	0.051
4	A	20	15	0.060	0.111
5	B	5	15	0.150	0.261
6	B	10	15	0.300	0.561
7	B	20	15	0.600	1.161
8	B	40	15	1.200	2.361
9	C	10	15	3.000	5.361
10	C	20	15	6.000	11.361
11	C	40	15	12.000	23.361
12	C	75	184.4	276.639	300.000

*The sum of the doses in solutions A, B, and C equals 333 mg. Total dose infused is 300 mg.
Total time = 5.8 hours. Total dose = 300 mg.

concentrations of paclitaxel are used. The rate of the infusion is adjusted every 15 minutes, with each step delivering approximately twice the dose of the previous step [42]. The standard 12-step protocol, with an infusion of 300 mg paclitaxel as an example, is shown in Table 19.4.

Alopecia can be reduced to half in the majority of patients treated with paclitaxel or docetaxel by scalp cooling [43–50]. Hair conservation could be obtained when scalp temperature is reduced to a level ≤25°C, 15 minutes before, during, and 15 minutes after the infusion [47].

Zimmermann et al. [51] described their experience in preventing HFS in a patient treated with docetaxel by cooling with iced water. Dexamethasone may prevent HFS [52], and it is routinely given as a premedication.

Surgical implantation of central venous ports for the application of chemotherapy is probably one of the most effective measures in order to prevent extravasation at peripheral venous accesses [53]. In case of signs of extravasation, the infusion should immediately be stopped. Local injections of saline solution are effective in diluting the vesicants [54]. The injection of hyaluronidase (250 IU diluted in 6 mL normal saline) subcutaneously into and around a taxane extravasation site causes the local symptoms of the extravasation to subside [55]. Additionally, topical cooling has been recommended in the management of extravasation of vesicants. In conclusion, the

application of hyaluronidase is probably the most effective treatment modality in taxane extravasations [56, 57].

Vinca alkaloids

The naturally occurring compounds of the vinca alkaloid family, vinblastine and vincristine, were isolated from the leaves of the periwinkle plant Catharanthus roseus. The clinical efficacies in combination therapies has led to the development of novel semisynthetic analogs: vinorelbine, vindesine, and vinflunine.

Tubulins and microtubules are the main targets of the vinca alkaloids, which deeply polymerize microtubules and destroy mitotic spindles at high concentrations. At low but clinical relevant concentrations vinblastine does not deeply polymerize spindle microtubules, yet it powerfully blocks mitoses.

Clinical features
With vindesine and vinorelbine as single agents alopecia was observed in 52% and 32% of patients, respectively. Mostly, alopecia is moderate and total alopecia is rarely observed [58].

Localized cutaneous reactions, most often consisting of erythematous macules over the injected vein, have been reported with vinca alkaloids [59]. Local reactions have been seen in 5% of patients with vindesine and 16% with vinorelbine [58].

Rashes are rare with vinca alkaloids, with few reports. Typically, patients develop a papulo-erythematous eruption on the whole body 4–7 days after administration, with rapid improvement after the therapy completion [60].

Vinca alkaloids are included in the group of agents with the highest destructive power for skin necrosis. Cytotoxic drugs cause pain, erythema, discoloration of the overlying epidermis, and tissue necrosis when they leak outside a vein; however, leaving such material in the subcutaneous space implicates the risk of the material being incorporated into cell nuclei and gradually destroying the tissue, thus causing late ulceration [61].

Treatment of choice and prognosis
The extravasated fluid is evacuated best by aspiration through the original needle. Then 250 IU hyaluronidase diluted in 6 mL normal saline should be administered through the indwelling needle if still in place, otherwise by six subcutaneous injections with a 25-gauge needle around the extravasation area. Corticosteroids or cold packs should not be applied.

Estramustine phosphate sodium

Estramustine is an orally available disodium salt, monohydrate, of estramustine phosphate, a synthetic molecule that combines estradiol and nornitrogen mustard through a carbamate link. Estramustine and its major metabolite estramustine bind to microtubule-associated proteins and tubulin, thereby inhibiting microtubule dynamics and leading to anaphase arrest; this agent also exhibits antiandrogenic effects.

Estramustine is mainly used to treat androgen-independent prostate cancer. The toxicities of treatment have not been greater than predicted when used in combination [62, 63].

The main dermatologic AEs of estramustine are edema, thrombosis, and breast tenderness. Other side effects include alopecia and fatigue. Dermatologic AEs including easy bruising (3%), pruritus (2%), and xerosis (2%) [62]. Treatment modalities remain symptomatic, and in most cases treatments with moisturizers are successful.

References

1 Jordan, M.A. (2002) Mechanism of action of antitumor drugs that interact with microtubules and tubulin. *Current Medicinal Chemistry: Anti-cancer Agents*, **2**, 1–17.

2 Weiss, R.B., Donehower, R.C., Wiernik, P.H. *et al.* (1990) Hypersensitivity reactions from taxol. *Journal of Clinical Oncology*, **8**, 1263–1268.

3 Wiernik, P.H., Schwartz, E.L., Strauman, J.J., Dutcher, J.P., Lipton, R.B. & Paietta, E. (1987) Phase I clinical and pharmacokinetic study of taxol. *Cancer Research*, **47**, 2486–2493.

4 Lorenz, W., Reimann, H.J., Schmal, A. *et al.* (1977) Histamine release in dogs by Cremophor E1 and its derivatives: oxethylated oleic acid is the most effective constituent. *Agents and Actions*, **7**, 63–67.

5 Bernstein, B.J. (2000) Docetaxel as an alternative to paclitaxel after acute hypersensitivity reactions. *Annals of Pharmacotherapy*, **34**, 1332–1335.

6 Michaud, L.B. (1997) Methods for preventing reactions secondary to Cremophor EL. *Annals of Pharmacotherapy*, **31**, 1402–1404.

7 ten Tije, A.J., Verweij, J., Loos, W.J. & Sparreboom, A. (2003) Pharmacological effects of formulation vehicles : implications for cancer chemotherapy. *Clinical Pharmacokinetics*, **42**, 665–685.

8 Rowinsky, E.K., Eisenhauer, E.A., Chaudhry, V., Arbuck, S.G. & Donehower, R.C. (1993) Clinical toxicities encountered with paclitaxel (Taxol). *Seminars in Oncology*, **20**, 1–15.

9 Gradishar, W.J., Tjulandin, S., Davidson, N. *et al.* (2005) Phase III trial of nanoparticle albumin-bound paclitaxel compared with polyethylated castor oil-based paclitaxel in women with breast cancer. *Journal of Clinical Oncology*, **23**, 7794–7803.

10 Green, M.R., Manikhas, G.M., Orlov, S. *et al.* (2006) Abraxane, a novel Cremophor-free, albumin-bound particle form of paclitaxel for the treatment of advanced non-small-cell lung cancer. *Annals of Oncology*, **17**, 1263–1268.

11 Roy, V., LaPlant, B.R., Gross, G.G., Bane, C.L. & Palmieri, F.M. (2009) Phase II trial of weekly nab (nanoparticle albumin-bound)-paclitaxel (nab-paclitaxel) (Abraxane) in combination with gemcitabine in patients with metastatic breast cancer (N0531). *Annals of Oncology*, **20**, 449–453.

12 Markman, M., Kennedy, A., Webster, K., Kulp, B., Peterson, G. & Belinson, J. (2000) Paclitaxel-associated hypersensitivity reactions: experience of the gynecologic oncology program of the Cleveland Clinic Cancer Center. *Journal of Clinical Oncology*, **18**, 102–105.

13 Grau, J.J., Caballero, M., Verger, E., Monzo, M. & Blanch, J.L. (2009) Weekly paclitaxel for platin-resistant stage IV head and neck cancer patients. *Acta Oto-Laryngologica*, **129**, 1294–1299.

14 Mok, T.S., Wu, Y.L., Thongprasert, S. *et al.* (2009) Gefitinib or carboplatin-paclitaxel in pulmonary adenocarcinoma. *New England Journal of Medicine*, **361**, 947–957.

15 Krzakowski, M., Ramlau, R., Jassem, J. *et al.* (2010) Phase III trial comparing vinflunine with docetaxel in second-line advanced non-small-cell lung cancer previously treated with platinum-containing chemotherapy. *Journal of Clinical Oncology*, **28**, 2167–2173.

16 Hussain, S., Anderson, D.N., Salvatti, M.E., Adamson, B., McManus, M. & Braverman, A.S. (2000) Onycholysis as a complication of systemic chemotherapy: report of five cases associated with prolonged weekly paclitaxel therapy and review of the literature. *Cancer*, **88**, 2367–2371.

17 Flory, S.M., Solimando, D.A., Jr., Webster, G.F., Dunton, C.J., Neufeld, J.M. & Haffey, M.B. (1999) Onycholysis associated with weekly administration of paclitaxel. *Annals of Pharmacotherapy*, **33**, 584–586.

18 Baker, J., Ajani, J., Scotte, F. *et al.* (2009) Docetaxel-related side effects and their management. *European Journal of Oncology Nursing*, **13**, 49–59.

19 Hong, J., Park, S.H., Choi, S.J. *et al.* (2007) Nail toxicity after treatment with docetaxel: a prospective analysis in patients with advanced non-small cell lung cancer. *Japanese Journal of Clinical Oncology*, **37**, 424–428.

20 Scotte, F., Tourani, J.M., Banu, E. *et al.* (2005) Multicenter study of a frozen glove to prevent docetaxel-induced onycholysis and cutaneous toxicity of the hand. *Journal of Clinical Oncology*, **23**, 4424–4429.

21 Winther, D., Saunte, D.M., Knap, M., Haahr, V. & Jensen, A.B. (2007) Nail changes due to docetaxel–a neglected side effect and nuisance for the patient. *Supportive Care in Cancer*, **15**, 1191–1197.

22 Poikonen, P., Sjostrom, J., Klaar, S. *et al.* (2004) Skin toxicity as a risk factor for major infections in breast cancer patients treated with docetaxel. *Acta Oncologica (Stockholm, Sweden)*, **43**, 190–195.

23 Bafaloukos, D., Papadimitriou, C., Linardou, H. *et al.* (2004) Combination of pegylated liposomal doxorubicin (PLD) and paclitaxel in patients with advanced soft tissue sarcoma: a phase II study of the Hellenic Cooperative Oncology Group. *British Journal of Cancer*, **91**, 1639–1644.

24 Bafaloukos, D., Linardou, H., Aravantinos, G. *et al.* (2010) A randomized phase II study of carboplatin plus pegylated liposomal doxorubicin versus carboplatin plus paclitaxel in platinum sensitive ovarian cancer patients: a Hellenic Cooperative Oncology Group study. *BMC Medicine*, **8**, 3.

25 Childress, J. & Lokich, J. (2003) Cutaneous hand and foot toxicity associated with cancer chemotherapy. *Am J Clin Oncol*, **26**, 435–436.

26 Cruz, A., Temu, T., Hines-Telang, G. & Kroumpouzos, G. (2011) Paclitaxel-induced neutrophilic adverse reaction and acral erythema. *Acta Dermato-Venereologica*, **91**, 86–87.

27 Baykal, C., Erkek, E., Tutar, E., Yuce, K. & Ayhan, A. (2000) Cutaneous fixed drug eruption to paclitaxel; a case report. *European Journal of Gynaecological Oncology*, **21**, 190–191.

28 Hiraki, A., Aoe, K., Murakami, T., Maeda, T., Eda, R. & Takeyama, H. (2004) Stevens-Johnson syndrome induced by paclitaxel in a patient with squamous cell carcinoma of the lung: a case report. *Anticancer Research*, **24**, 1135–1137.

29 Cohen, P.R. (2009) Photodistributed erythema multiforme: paclitaxel-related, photosensitive conditions in patients with cancer. *Journal of Drugs in Dermatology*, **8**, 61–64.

30 Weinberg, J.M., Egan, C.L., Tangoren, I.A., Li, L.J., Laughinghouse, K.A. & Guzzo, C.A. (1997) Generalized pustular dermatosis following paclitaxel therapy. *International Journal of Dermatology*, **36**, 559–560.

31 Kupfer, I., Balguerie, X., Courville, P., Chinet, P. & Joly, P. (2003) Scleroderma-like cutaneous lesions induced by paclitaxel: a case study. *Journal of the American Academy of Dermatology*, **48**, 279–281.

32 Konishi, Y., Sato, H., Sato, N., Fujimoto, T., Fukuda, J. & Tanaka, T. (2010) Scleroderma-like cutaneous lesions induced by paclitaxel and carboplatin for ovarian carcinoma, not a single course of carboplatin, but re-induced and worsened by previously administered paclitaxel. *Journal of Obstetrics and Gynaecology Research*, **36**, 693–696.

33 Kawakami, T., Tsutsumi, Y. & Soma, Y. (2009) Limited cutaneous systemic sclerosis induced by paclitaxel in a patient with breast cancer. *Archives of Dermatology*, **145**, 97–98.

34 Adachi, A. & Horikawa, T. (2007) Paclitaxel-induced cutaneous lupus erythematosus in patients with serum anti-SSA/Ro antibody. *Journal of Dermatology*, **34**, 473–476.

35 Chen, M., Crowson, A.N., Woofter, M., Luca, M.B. & Magro, C.M. (2004) Docetaxel (taxotere) induced subacute cutaneous lupus erythematosus: report of 4 cases. *Journal of Rheumatology*, **31**, 818–820.

36 Cohen, A.D., Mermershtain, W., Geffen, D.B. *et al.* (2005) Cutaneous photosensitivity induced by paclitaxel and trastuzumab therapy associated with aberrations in the biosynthesis of porphyrins. *Journal of Dermatological Treatment*, **16**, 19–21.

37 Magne, N., Benezery, K., Otto, J., Namer, M. & Lagrange, J.L. (2002) Radiation recall dermatitis after docetaxel and external beam radiotherapy. Report of two cases and review of the literature. *Cancer Radiotherapie: Journal de la Societe Francaise de Radiotherapie Oncologique*, **6**, 281–284.

38 Giesel, B.U., Kutz, G.G. & Thiel, H.J. (2001) Recall dermatitis caused by re-exposure to docetaxel following irradiation of the brain. Case report and review of the literature. *Strahlentherapie Und Onkologie*, **177**, 487–493.

39 Stanford, B.L. & Hardwicke, F. (2003) A review of clinical experience with paclitaxel extravasations. *Supportive Care in Cancer*, **11**, 270–277.

40 Ho, C.H., Yang, C.H. & Chu, C.Y. (2003) Vesicant-type reaction due to docetaxel extravasation. *Acta Dermato-Venereologica*, **83**, 467–468.

41 Herrington, J.D. & Figueroa, J.A. (1997) Severe necrosis due to paclitaxel extravasation. *Pharmacotherapy*, **17**, 163–165.

42 Feldweg, A.M., Lee, C.W., Matulonis, U.A. & Castells, M. (2005) Rapid desensitization for hypersensitivity reactions to paclitaxel and docetaxel: a new standard protocol used in 77 successful treatments. *Gynecologic Oncology*, **96**, 824–829.

43 Auvinen, P.K., Mahonen, U.A., Soininen, K.M. *et al.* (2010) The effectiveness of a scalp cooling cap in preventing chemotherapy-induced alopecia. *Tumori*, **96**, 271–275.

44 Ridderheim, M., Bjurberg, M. & Gustavsson, A. (2003) Scalp hypothermia to prevent chemotherapy-induced alopecia is effective and safe: a pilot study of a new digitized scalp-cooling system used in 74 patients. *Supportive Care in Cancer*, **11**, 371–377.

45 Grevelman, E.G. & Breed, W.P. (2005) Prevention of chemotherapy-induced hair loss by scalp cooling. *Annals of Oncology*, **16**, 352–358.

46 Lemenager, M., Genouville, C., Bessa, E.H. & Bonneterre, J. (1995) Docetaxel-induced alopecia can be prevented. *Lancet*, **346**, 371–372.

47 Lemenager, M., Lecomte, S., Bonneterre, M.E., Bessa, E., Dauba, J. & Bonneterre, J. (1997) Effectiveness of cold cap in the prevention of docetaxel-induced alopecia. *European Journal of Cancer*, **33**, 297–300.

48 Bulow, J., Friberg, L., Gaardsting, O. & Hansen, M. (1985) Frontal subcutaneous blood flow, and epi- and subcutaneous temperatures during scalp cooling in normal man. *Scandinavian Journal of Clinical and Laboratory Investigation*, **45**, 505–508.

49 Gregory, R.P., Cooke, T., Middleton, J., Buchanan, R.B. & Williams, C.J. (1982) Prevention of doxorubicin-induced alopedia by scalp hypothermia: relation to degree of cooling. *British Medical Journal (Clinical Research Ed.)*, **284**, 1674.

50 Satterwhite, B. & Zimm, S. (1984) The use of scalp hypothermia in the prevention of doxorubicin-induced hair loss. *Cancer*, **54**, 34–37.

51 Zimmerman, G.C., Keeling, J.H., Lowry, M., Medina, J., Von Hoff, D.D. & Burris, H.A. (1994) Prevention of docetaxel-induced erythrodysesthesia with local hypothermia. *Journal of the National Cancer Institute*, **86**, 557–558.

52 Drake, R.D., Lin, W.M., King, M., Farrar, D., Miller, D.S. & Coleman, R.L. (2004) Oral dexamethasone attenuates Doxil-induced palmar-plantar erythrodysesthesias in patients with recurrent gynecologic malignancies. *Gynecologic Oncology*, **94**, 320–324.

53 Biffi, R., Pozzi, S., Agazzi, A. *et al.* (2004) Use of totally implantable central venous access ports for high-dose chemotherapy and peripheral blood stem cell transplantation: results of a monocentre series of 376 patients. *Annals of Oncology*, **15**, 296–300.

54 Scuderi, N. & Onesti, M.G. (1994) Antitumor agents: extravasation, management, and surgical treatment. *Annals of Plastic Surgery*, **32**, 39–44.

55 Bertelli, G., Dini, D., Forno, G.B. *et al.* (1994) Hyaluronidase as an antidote to extravasation of Vinca alkaloids: clinical results. *Journal of Cancer Research and Clinical Oncology*, **120**, 505–506.

56 Zhu, Q.C., Li, A.M., Luo, R.C., Liang, W.J., Dai, M. & Chen, X.H. (2007) Efficacy of chitosan and hyaluronidase on skin damage caused by docetaxel extravasation in rats. *Ai Zheng*, **26**, 346–350.

57 Ascherman, J.A., Knowles, S.L. & Attkiss, K. (2000) Docetaxel (taxotere) extravasation: a report of five cases with treatment recommendations. *Annals of Plastic Surgery*, **45**, 438–441.

58 Furuse, K., Fukuoka, M., Kuba, M. *et al.* (1996) Randomized study of vinorelbine (VRB) versus vindesine (VDS) in previously untreated stage IIIB or IV non-small-cell lung cancer (NSCLC). The Japan Vinorelbine Lung Cancer Cooperative Study Group. *Annals of Oncology*, **7**, 815–820.

59 Arias, D., Requena, L., Hasson, A. *et al.* (1991) Localized epidermal necrolysis (erythema multiforme-like reaction) following intravenous injection of vinblastine. *Journal of Cutaneous Pathology*, **18**, 344–346.

60 Nakashima, H., Fujimoto, M. & Tamaki, K. (2005) Cutaneous reaction induced by vincristine. *British Journal of Dermatology*, **153**, 225–226.

61 Morenod, V., Dauden, E., Abajo, P., Bartolome, B., Fraga, J. & Garcia-Diez, A. (2002) Skin necrosis from extravasation of vinorelbine. *Journal of the European Academy of Dermatology and Venereology*, **16**, 488–490.

62 Hudes, G. (1997) Estramustine-based chemotherapy. *Seminars in Urologic Oncology*, **15**, 13–19.

63 Kreis, W. & Budman, D. (1999) Daily oral estramustine and intermittent intravenous docetaxel (Taxotere) as chemotherapeutic treatment for metastatic, hormone-refractory prostate cancer. *Seminars in Oncology*, **26**, 34–38.

20 Histone Deacetylase Inhibitors, Proteasome Inhibitors, Demethylating Agents, Arsenicals, and Retinoids

Najla Al-Dawsari[1], Shannon C. Trotter[2] and Francine Foss[3]

[1]Dhahran Health Center, Saudi Aramco Medical Service Organization, Saudi Arabia
[2]Division of Dermatology, Ohio State University, Columbus, OH, USA
[3]Yale University School of Medicine, New Haven, CT, USA

The clinical presentation of dermatologic adverse events (AEs) to histone deacetylase (HDAC) inhibitors, proteasome inhibitors, demethylating agents, arsenicals, and retinoids is varied (Figure 20.1).

Histone deacetylase inhibitors

Vorinostat

Vorinostat is an oral histone deacetylase inhibitor that is Food and Drug Administration (FDA) approved for the management of cutaneous T-cell lymphoma (CTCL) in patients with progressive, persistent, or recurrent disease during or after treatment with two systemic therapies. Vorinostat acts by causing accumulation of acetylated histones, induction of apoptosis, and cell cycle arrest in cancer cells including Sézary cells [1].

Clinical features and pathogenesis

Cutaneous AEs in patients receiving vorinostat include alopecia and leukonychia. During phase IIB trials of vorinostat 17.6% of patients developed alopecia. The type of alopecia was not described but may have been consistent with anagen effluvium secondary to the antiapoptotic effect of vorinostat [2,3]. Rare case reports of scarring alopecia with chemotherapy have been reported [4].

Apparent leukonychia was described in three patients 6–9 months after receiving vorinostat [5]. Apparent leukonychia refers to a whitish opacity of the nails that fades with pressure and is caused by nail bed insults [6]. In the case of vorinostat, the apparent leukonychia could be related to the repression of endothelial nitric oxide causing compromise of the endothelial cell function seen in HDAC inhibitors [5].

Treatment and prognosis

Chemotherapy-induced alopecia is usually reversible within 3–6 months of discontinuing chemotherapy [3]. A randomized double-blind controlled trial using topical minoxidil 2% twice a day during and 4 months after discontinuing chemotherapy showed a statistically significant shortening of duration of baldness compared with placebo in patients with chemotherapy-induced alopecia [7]. The leukonychia required no treatment and disappeared within 3–10 months after discontinuing vorinostat [5].

Romidepsin

Romidepsin is an intravenous histone deacetylase inhibitor that has recently proven to be effective in patients with CTCL. Romidepsin is FDA approved for patients with CTCL who have received at least one systemic medication [8].

Clinical features and pathogenesis

Cutaneous AEs are rare with romidepsin and include increased incidence of oral candidiasis [9]. Dermatitis medicamentosa (drug rash) developed in one patient during a multicenter study. The rash was mild and did not require discontinuing romidepsin. The was no mention of clinical course and treatment [9]. Drug rashes are variable and range between 2–3% of hospitalized patients. Most of drug rashes are generalized morbilliform drug exanthems and, less commonly, urticaria and pruritus [10,11]. Severe drug rashes are rare and include Stevens–Johnson syndrome (SJS), toxic epidermal necrolysis (TEN), hypersensitivity syndrome, anticoagulant-induced skin necrosis, and vasculitis along with serum sickness and angioedema [12]. The most common pathogenesis of drug reactions is a non-immediate induced allergic reaction caused by activation of T cells leading

Dermatologic Principles and Practice in Oncology: Conditions of the Skin, Hair, and Nails in Cancer Patients, First Edition. Edited by Mario E. Lacouture.

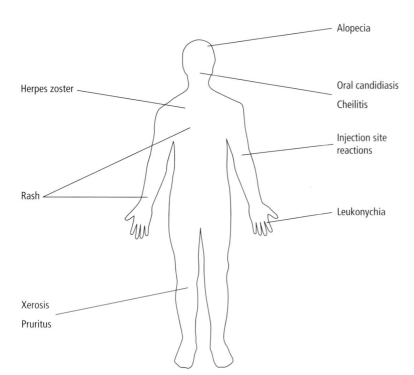

Alopecia

Herpes zoster

Oral candidiasis

Cheilitis

Injection site reactions

Rash

Leukonychia

Xerosis

Pruritus

Figure 20.1 Location of histone deacetylase and proteasome inhibitor, arsenical, and retinoid-induced dermatologic adverse events.

to the production of multiple cytokines including interferon-γ, tumor necrosis factor-α (TNF-α), interleukin 2 (IL-2), and the cytotoxic markers perforin and granzyme [13].

Treatment

Treatment for mild oral candidiasis includes clotrimazole troches (10 mg 5 times daily), nystatin suspension of 100 000 IU/mL (4–6 mL 4 times daily), or 1–2 nystatin pastilles (200 000 IU each, 4 times daily). The treatment should be continued for 7–14 days (evidence level II). Moderate to severe cases are treated with oral fluconazole (100–200 mg/day) for 7–14 days. In patients not responding to fluconazole, itraconazole solution (200 mg/day) or posaconazole suspension (400 mg twice daily for 3 days, then 400 mg/day for up to 28 days) are recommended (evidence level II). Voriconazole and amphotericin B are used for severe refractory disease [14].

Prophylactic prechemotherapy oral care with management of pulpoperiapical and periodontal disease along with continuous maintenance of good oral hygiene are important factors in preventing oral disease during chemotherapy [15].

Drug rashes secondary to chemotherapy are approached like any other drug reaction. Mild rashes resolve upon discontinuation of the offending drug. Topical and systemic steroids are used as needed. Serious rashes (SJS/TEN) require supportive care with emphasis on nutrition, fluid replacement, and prevention of secondary bacterial skin infections through aseptic care. Patients should be handled in a similar way to burns patients. Direct communication between the oncologist and the dermatologist is important in making decisions regarding discontinuing or replacing the treatment [12,16].

Proteasome inhibitors

Bortezomib

Bortezomib (Velcade®) is approved for the management of patients with relapsed multiple myeloma post transplantation and as a second-line treatment for patients with multiple myeloma who are not suitable for transplantation [17]. Bortezomib is also approved for the management of patients with mantle cell lymphoma who have received at least one prior therapy [18].

Botrezomib is a proteasome inhibitor that inhibits the degradation of NF-κB, which activates multiple pathways in the myeloma and mantle cell signaling. It also increases apoptosis of plasma cells and mantle cells and inhibits IL-6, insulin-like growth factor (IGF-1), vascular endothelial growth factor (VEGF), and TNF-α. These cytokines are important in the development of myeloma cells in the bone marrow. Bortezomib also inhibits angiogenesis in both multiple myeloma and mantle cell lymphoma [17,18].

Clinical features and pathogenesis

An observational analysis of three prospective clinical trials in 47 patients treated with bortezomib showed dermatologic AEs in 13% of patients (Figure 20.2). Three patients developed erythematous nodules on various locations (Figure 20.1). One patient developed nodules on trunk alone. Another patient had nodules on trunk and limbs while a third patient presented with nodules on trunk, neck, and face. Two patients developed papules and plaques and one patient developed a morbilliform exanthem and ulcerations on the trunk. The mean time of onset was 30–65

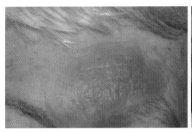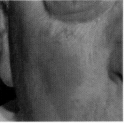

Figure 20.2 Bortezomib-induced rash to the forehead and the cheek. (Photo courtesy of Dr. Mario E. Lacouture.)

days. In patients developing nodules, papules, and plaques, histopathology showed interface dermatitis with variable degrees of perivascular and periadnexal inflammation, spongiosis, and apoptotsis of keratinocytes. The morbilliform exanthem showed lymphocytic perivascular inflammation with few neutrophils [19].

A study examining three phase II studies of patients with non-Hodgkin lymphoma identified 26 patients with an erythematous maculopapular rash during treatments. Most of the rashes developed after at least two or three treatment cycles. Fewer patients developed the rash after the first cycle of treatment. The rash usually resolved 5–7 days following the last dose of the cycle and was not dose dependent. Some patients experienced mild pruritus but in general the rash was asymptomatic. Biopsies of six patients showed non-necrotizing small vessel cutaneous vasculitis. There was no associated systemic vasculitis. Patients who developed the rash had better response rate to treatment with bortezomib. Patients rechallenged with bortezomib developed the same rash. However, none of the patients developed systemic adverse reactions [20]. Bortezomib-associated cutaneous vasculitis maybe attributed to the overproduction of proinflammatory cytokines compensating for the loss of the proteasome activity [21].

Sweet syndrome, an acute neutrophilic dermatosis characterized by tender erythematous nodules and plaques associated with fever and leukocytosis, was reported following administration of bortezomib in at least six cases [22,23]. Patients developed Sweet syndrome at variable times after starting each cycle. Histopathology of the cases of Sweet syndrome showed typical neutrophilic-rich infiltrate at the upper dermis. Leukocytoclastic vasculitis was not observed. One case had histiocytes predominant infiltrate. Another case had a significant number of CD30+ lymphocytes. The pathogenesis behind the development of Sweet syndrome is poorly understood [23–26].

Treatment and prognosis

The eruptions presenting as papules, nodules, or plaques along with the morbilliform eruption resolved within 1 week after treatment with low dose prednisone with or without antihistamines [19]. Patients who developed small vessel vasculitis had mild pruritus which responded to topical steroids [20,21].

The administration of IV methylprednisolone helped speed the resolution of Sweet syndrome. However, upon restarting

bortezomib for the next cycle, some patients experienced a severe flare of Sweet syndrome. Most patients tolerated Sweet syndrome if bortezomib was administered along with systemic steroids [23–25]. For a summary see Table 20.1 [18–24].

Demethylating agents

5-Azacitidine and decitabine

Demethylating agents are compounds that inhibit DNA methylation abnormalities commonly seen in hematopoietic neoplasms leading to cell cycle arrest and apoptosis [27]. 5-Azacitidine (Vidaza®) and decitabine (Dacogen®) are approved demethylating agents for the management of myelodysplastic syndrome. Both drugs are occasionally used alone or in combination with other chemotherapies for management of acute and chronic leukemias [28,29].

Clinical features and pathogenesis

The administration of 5-azacitidine is commonly associated with injection site reactions. In about half of patients treated, injection site reactions presented as erythematous plaques during the first 5 days of therapy. Biopsies of involved areas did not show any inflammation which makes the pathogenesis most likely related to direct chemical irritation caused by the treatment [30].

No reports of cutaneous AEs with decitabine were reported except for one case of neutrophilic eccrine hidradenitis that started 2 weeks after the first course of decatibine [31]. The pathogeneses maybe related to direct toxic effect of chemotherapy on sweat glands [32].

Treatment and prognosis

Cutaneous lesions secondary to 5-azacitidine injections resolved spontaneously 1 week after stopping the injections [30]. Spontaneous resolution of neutrophilic eccrine hidradenitis usually occurs in 1–2 weeks. Systemic and topical steroids and dapsone may be helpful; however, the efficacy has been proven only in case reports [31,33,34].

Arsenicals

Arsenic trioxide

Arsenic trioxide (Trisenox®) is an organic intravenous arsenical compound approved for the management of nonresponsive or relapsed acute promyelocytic leukemia (APL) not responding to all-*trans* retinoic acid (ATRA). Arsenic trioxide is also proven to be effective in multiple myeloma, myelodysplastic syndrome, and solid tumors such as colon and renal cancer. It induces terminal differentiation of leukemia cells, apoptosis, and accumulation of reactive oxygen radicals. It also inhibits NF-κB that promotes cells' survival [35].

Table 20.1 Dermatologic adverse events of bortezomib.

Cutaneous side effects	Clinical appearance	Histopathology	Time of onset	Duration of rash	Treatment	Effects of rechallenge	Mechanism of rash
Nonspecific dermatitis	Papules, nodules or plaques	Interface dermatitis with variable degrees of perivascular and periadnexal inflammation + spongiosis and apoptotsis of keratinocytes	30–65 days	One week after stopping offending drug	Oral steroids +/– antihistamines Evidence level V	No reports	Unknown
	Morbiliform exanthum	Lymphocytic perivascular inflammation with few neutrophils					
	Erythematous maculopapular rash	Non-necrotizing small vessels vasculitis	Majority after 2–3 Treatment cycles	5–7 days after last dose in the cycle	Topical steroids Evidence level V	Rash reappeared with no worsening	Overproduction of proinflammatory cytokines compensating for the loss of the proteasome activity
Sweet syndrome	Tender erythematous nodules and plaques + Fever and leukocytosis	Nuetrophilic rich infiltrate in the upper dermis	Variable	Variable IV steroids helped speed the resolution	IV methylprednisolone Level V evidence	Worsening of the rash (IV steroids + bortezomib patients had milder tolerated rash)	Unknown

Clinical features and pathogenesis

Cutaneous AEs secondary to arsenic trioxide were infrequent during phase I trials [36]. In phase II trials by Litzow et al. [37], 43% of APL patients developed a nonspecific dermatitis, which was considered mild/moderate in nature. There was no observed increase in skin cancer. During the past several years, an increased incidence of recurrent herpes zoster was noticed in patients receiving arsenic trioxide for APL, multiple myeloma, and colon cancer [38,39,73].

Herpes zoster infection is an acute reactivation of latent varicella zoster virus in the affected dermatome. Infection is usually reactivated by stress, trauma, or immunosuppression, sometimes with no apparent cause. The disease presents with multiple grouped vesicles on an erythematous base following a dermatome. Before the rash appears, patients complain of pruritus, tingling, or pain. Multiple dermatomes are rarely affected [40]. Patients on arsenic trioxide developing herpes zoster had normal leukocyte count and differential. Most patients presented within the first year of treatment. No cases of disseminated herpes or zoster were reported. Patients had zoster

did not develop other opportunistic infections. As patients with multiple myeloma have intact cell-mediated immunity and patients with APL had normal counts in the cases presented, arsenic trioxide was most likely responsible for the recurrence [38,39]. The mechanism of zoster reactivation is not clear, but could be explained by the studies showing arsenic inhibition of antigen presenting cells, particularly the TA3 subtype [41].

Treatment and prognosis

Patients who developed herpes zoster secondary to arsenic trioxide did not experience complicated localized infections and responded well to antiviral drugs. Current antiviral recommendations for noncomplicated herpes zoster infection with normal renal function are acyclovir (800 mg every 4 hours) for 7–10 days; famciclovir (500 mg every 8 hours) for 7 days; and valacyclovir (1000 mg every 8 hours) for 7 days (level I evidence) [42,43]. Treatment in the first 72 hours is recommended [15]. The herpes zoster vaccine given to patients above 60 years old helped reduce the incidence of post herpetic neuralgia along with duration and severity of attacks [44]. However, the vaccine is contraindicated in patients undergoing hematopoietic stem cell transplant and patients with cellular immunodeficiency [45].

Retinoids

Bexarotene, all-*trans* retinoic acid or tretinoin, and alitretinoin

Retinoids are an important class of drugs used to treat cancer. The clinical results of retinoids can be explained by their effect on gene transcription within cells. Consequently, many of their cutaneous reactions are a class effect. However, some of the retinoids also have unique adverse cutaneous findings associated with their use.

Bexarotene

Bexarotene is a selective retinoid X receptor (RXR) agonist that blocks cell cycle progression. It stimulates apoptosis and differentiation. It inhibits angiogenesis and metastasis and prevents multidrug resistance [46]. Oral bexarotene (Targretin® capsules) is a synthetic retinoid that is approved for the treatment of the skin manifestations of cutaneous T-cell lymphoma in patients who have already tried at least one systemic therapy [47]. Topical bexarotene (Targretin® gel) is approved for the treatment of patients with stage IA and IB cutaneous T-cell lymphoma that is persistent or refractory to other therapies or for patients not tolerating other therapies [48].

All-*trans* retinoic acid

ATRA, also known as tretinoin, is a systemic retinoid that is effective in the treatment of APL. Tretinoin capsules (Vesanoid®) are indicated for the induction of remission in patients with APL, French-American-British (FAB) classification M3 (including the M3 variant), characterized by the presence of the t(15;17) translocation and/or the presence of the *PML/RAR*α gene, who are refractory to or who have relapsed from anthracycline chemotherapy, or from whom anthracycline-based chemotherapy is contraindicated. Tretinoin capsules are to be used for the induction of remission only [49].

Alitretinoin

Alitretinoin, also known as 9-*cis* retinoic acid, is a first generation retinoid and a unique panagonist, capable of binding to all six known retinoid receptors (RAR-α, -β, -γ, and RXR-α, -β, -γ) [50]. It comes as an oral and topical form. In the United States, alitretinoin is approved as a topical preparation (Panretin® gel, Ligand Pharmaceuticals). Topical alitretinoin is indicated for the treatment of cutaneous AIDS-related Kaposi sarcoma. Alitretinoin is not indicated when systemic therapy against Kaposi sarcoma is required [51]. The oral form of alitretinoin (Toctino®, Basilea, Switzerland) is used in the United Kingdom to treat refractory chronic hand dermatitis [52]. There have been clinical trials in the United States investigating systemic alitretinoin's role as an

antineoplastic agent, but it does not currently have FDA approval [53–55].

Clinical features and pathogenesis
Class effects

As a class of drugs, the retinoids demonstrate various degrees of dermatitis or skin irritation, including xerosis or dry skin, pruritus, and cheilitis. Nonetheless, some of the retinoid drugs also exhibit other skin reactions.

Bexarotene

Adverse cutaneous events related to oral bexarotene include transient exfoliative dermatitis at the initiation of treatment which characteristically responds well to emollients. Patients may also experience pruritus. However, it is difficult to discern if the pruritus is a result of bexarotene or related to the CTCL itself, or a combination thereof. The pruritus may be related to xerosis secondary to the reduction transglutamase synthesis caused by bexarotene [56]. Topical bexarotene (Targretin® gel) is commonly associated with cutaneous, especially irritant reactions (for additional information see Chapter 29).

All-*trans* retinoic acid

Xerosis and cheilitis are common but mild AEs of ATRA [57]. Scrotal ulcers are rare but are a well-documented complication of ATRA. Adults and children as young as 10 years can develop ulcers. The clinical presentation of the ulcers can vary. Ulcerations associated with ATRA can be single or multiple, painless or painful. They typically develop 10–30 days after starting treatment. Some ulcers are associated with a preceding exfoliative dermatitis and have sharp borders surrounded by erythema. The base of the ulcer is purulent or sometimes have a black eschar. Some patients have fever accompanying the ulcers.

The pathogenesis is possibly related to overproduction of superoxide and the release cytokines stimulated by ATRA leading to tissue damage and ulceration [58–61]. Histopathology shows ulceration with a neutrophilic infiltrate and foci of necrosis. Bacterial, viral, and fungal cultures are negative.

Alitretinoin

Alitretinoin displays cutaneous AEs similar to the other retinoid drugs. The most common skin AEs include dermatitis or xerosis. These findings are attributed to alitretinoin's effect on gene expression which controls the process of cellular differentiation and proliferation in both normal and neoplastic cells [62,63].

Cutaneous AEs to alitretinoin can vary based on the preparation used. Clinical trials involving topical alitretinoin have focused on the treatment of Kaposi sarcoma. Application site dermatitis was a common finding, but self-limited in most cases [64–66].

Oral administration of alitretinoin results in more systemic or widespread cutaneous AEs. Dry skin was the most common skin reaction observed in cancer clinical trials with alitretinoin

[53–55]. Patients complained of dry cracking skin on the trunk and extremities of various degrees. Other cutaneous AEs included alopecia, exfoliative dermatitis, cheilitis (dry lips), and mucocutaneous infections such oral candidiasis and herpes simplex. Less commonly reported dermatologic AEs included dry mouth, hair disorders, and nail disorders. No specifics were provided on the types of hair and nail disorders observed.

Treatment and prognosis
Retinoid class effects
Cutaneous reactions associated with retinoids are typically a class effect. Xerosis or dry skin can be best managed through the generous application of emollients, such as ointments or creams containing urea, salicylic acid, or ammonium lactate. In addition, modification of bathing routine can be beneficial. Bathing should be done on a daily basis but for short time intervals and using lukewarm water followed by a generous application of emollients. For inflamed skin associated with xerosis, mid-potency topical corticosteroids may be necessary in conjunction with frequent moisturization to restore the skin barrier. Antihistamines may be beneficial for pruritus associated with dry skin or as an independent AE of alitretinoin or bexarotene. Although not demonstrated in the studies mentioned, several studies have shown retinoid AEs to be dose dependent. Decreasing the patient's dose or frequency of application may result in decreased cutaneous AEs. Moreover, a preventative approach when initiating systemic retinoid therapy benefits the patient, with the focus on preventing skin breakdown and potential infection. Patients should be advised to moisturize their skin, lips, nose, and eyes regularly during systemic retinoid therapy. In addition, they should be instructed on how to care for eroded areas that may occur due to excessive dryness. Appropriate therapies include topical antibiotics until the area has healed or the use of oral antibiotics if an infection is severe [14,67]. Overall prognosis for patients using alitretinoin, bexarotene, and ATRA is good. The cutaneous AEs are usually reversible [48,49,51,57].

Bexarotene
Decreasing frequency, brief discontinuation, and use of moisturizers helped alleviate the symptoms associated with topical bexarotene. Patients who developed leukocytoclastic vasculitis stopped the treatment with topical bexarotene [48].

All-trans retinoic acid
The treatment for scrotal ulcerations includes wound care, topical antibacterials to prevent secondary bacterial infections, and topical steroids as needed. Viral and bacterial cultures should be collected to exclude infections before the initiation of treatment. Rarely, patients with painful ulcers require systemic steroids.

Alitretinoin
Mucocutaneous infections like oral candidiasis can be treated with clotrimazole troches (10 mg 5 times daily), nystatin

suspension of 100 000 IU/mL (4–6 mL 4 times daily), or 1–2 nystatin pastilles (200 000 IU each, 4 times daily). The treatment duration should be for 7–14 days (evidence level II). Moderate to severe cases are treated with oral fluconazole (100–200 mg/day) for 7–14 days. In patients not responding to fluconazole, itraconazole solution (200 mg/day) or posaconazole suspension (400 mg twice daily for 3 days, then 400 mg/day for up to 28 days) are recommended (evidence level II). Voriconazole and amphotericin B are used for severe refractory disease [68].

The treatment of cutaneous herpetic infections is based on the type of cutaneous disease, initial versus recurrent episodes, and HIV or immunosuppression status. There are several antiviral drugs available to treat cutaneous herpes infections that vary based on dosing and cost. In a systematic review evaluating the herpes treatment in cancer patients, acyclovir was shown to be effective in preventing herpes labialis. There was no evidence that valacyclovir is more efficacious than acyclovir, or that higher doses of valacyclovir are more effective than lower doses. The recommended dosing schedule for initial and recurrent episodes of herpes labialis are listed in Table 20.2. Disseminated infections require intravenous antivirals such as acyclovir [69–71]. See Table 20.3 for a summary [14,50–72].

Table 20.2 Management of orolabial herpes and varicella-zoster virus infections.

Herpes simplex infection	Drug and dosage
Recurrent orolabial herpes	Penciclovir: 1% cream applied q 2 hours × 4 days
	Famciclovir: 1.5 g PO × 1 dose
	Valacyclovir: 2 g PO BID × 1 day
Immunocompromised setting mucocutaneous herpes	Recommend use until all mucocutaneous lesions are healed:
	Acyclovir: 400 mg PO TID or 200 mg PO 5×/day
	Famciclovir: 500 mg PO BID
	Valacyclovir: 1 g PO BID
Varicella-zoster virus infections	
Zoster	Acyclovir: 20 mg/kg (800 mg max) PO QID × 5 days
Adult immunocompromised	Acyclovir: 10 mg/kg (500 mg/m^2) IV Q8 hours × 7–10 days

Table 20.3 Dermatologic adverse events to retinoids.

Causative agent/agents	Adverse events (AEs)	Treatment
Oral bexarotene Oral alitretinoin Oral all-*trans* retinoic acid (ATRA)	Transient exfoliative dermatitis +/− chelitis (dry lips) +/− pruritus	Generous application of emollients Bathing for short time intervals using lukewarm water Mid-potency topical corticosteroids for inflamed skin Antihistamines for pruritus Decreasing drug dose or frequency
Topical bexarotene Topical alitretinoin	Redness, irritation at site of application	Decreasing frequency Topical emollients Topical corticosteroids Usually self-limited
Topical bexarotene	Rash at site of application	Decreasing frequency Topical emollients Topical corticosteroids Usually self-limited
Oral all-*trans* retinoic acid (ATRA)	Vesiculobullous rash Leukocytoclastic vasculitis Scrotal ulcers	No details discussed in studies Required discontinuation of medication Viral and bacterial cultures to exclude infections Wound care Topical antibacterials Topical steroids as needed Systemic steroids for painful ulcers

References

1 Duvic, M. & Vu, J. (2007) Update on the treatment of cutaneous T-cell lymphoma (CTCL): focus on vorinostat. *Biologics*, **1**, 377–392.

2 Olsen, E.A., Kim, Y.H., Kuzel, T.M. *et al.* (2007) Phase IIb multicenter trial of vorinostat in patients with persistent, progressive, or treatment refractory cutaneous T-cell lymphoma. *Journal of Clinical Oncology*, **25**, 3109–3115.

3 Botchkarev, V.A. (2003) Molecular mechanisms of chemotherapy-induced hair loss. *Journal of Investigative Dermatology*, **8**, 72–75.

4 Tallon, B., Blanchard, E. & Goldberg, L.J. (2010) Permanent chemotherapy-induced alopecia: case report and review of the literature. *Journal of the American Academy of Dermatology*, **63**, 333–336.

5 Bartell, H.L. & Olsen, E.A. (2009) Leukonychia related to vorinostat. *Archives of Dermatology*, **145**, 1338–1339.

6 Grossman, M. & Scher, R.K. (1990) Leukonychia. Review and classification. *International Journal of Dermatology*, **29**, 535–541.

7 Duvic, M., Lemak, N.A., Valero, V. *et al.* (1996) A randomized trial of minoxidil in chemotherapy-induced alopecia. *Journal of the American Academy of Dermatology*, **35**, 74–78.

8 Grant, C., Rahman, F., Piekarz, R. *et al.* (2010) Romidepsin: a new therapy for cutaneous T-cell lymphoma and a potential therapy for solid tumors. *Expert Review of Anticancer Therapy*, **10**, 997–1008.

9 Whittaker, S.J., Demierre, M.F., Kim, E.J. *et al.* (2010) Final results from a multicenter, international, pivotal study of romidepsin in refractory cutaneous T-cell lymphoma. *Journal of Clinical Oncology*, **28**, 4485–4491.

10 Arndt, K.A. & Jick, H. (1976) Rates of cutaneous reactions to drugs. *Journal of the American Medical Association*, **235**, 918–923.

11 Bigby, M. (2001) Rates of cutaneous reactions to drugs. *Archives of Dermatology*, **137**, 765–770.

12 Roujeau, J.-C. & Stern, R.S. (1994) Severe adverse cutaneous reactions to drugs. *New England Journal of Medicine*, **331**, 1272–1285.

13 Torres, M.J., Mayorga, C. & Blanca, M. (2009) Nonimmediate allergic reactions induced by drugs: pathogenesis and diagnostic tests. *Journal of Investigational Allergology and Clinical Immunology*, **19**, 80–90.

14 Pappas, P.G., Kauffman, C.A., Andes, D. *et al.* (2009) Clinical practice guidelines for the management of candidiasis: 2009 update by the Infectious Diseases Society of America. *Clinical Infectious Diseases*, **48**, 503–535.

15 Sonis, S. & Kunz, A. (1988) Impact of improved dental services on the frequency of oral complications of cancer therapy for patients with non-head-and-neck malignancies. *Oral Surgery, Oral Medicine, and Oral Pathology*, **65**, 19–22.

16 Kathleen, A. (2003) Remlinger cutaneous reactions to chemotherapy drugs: the art of consultation. *Archives of Dermatology*, **139**, 77–81.

17 Richardson, P.G., Mitsiades, C., Schlossman, R. *et al.* (2008) Bortezomib in the front-line treatment of multiple myeloma. *Expert Review of Anticancer Therapy*, **8**, 1053–1072.

18 Field-Smith, A., Morgan, G.J. & Davies, F.E. (2006) Bortezomib (Velcade™) in the Treatment of multiple myeloma. *Therapeutics and Clinical Risk Management*, **2**, 271–279.

19 Wu, K.L., Heule, F., Lam, K. & Sonneveld, P. (2006) Pleomorphic presentation of cutaneous lesions associated with the proteasome inhibitor bortezomib in patients with multiple myeloma. *Journal of the American Academy of Dermatology*, **55**, 897–900.

20 Gerecitano, J., Goy, A., Wright, J. *et al.* (2006) Drug-induced cutaneous vasculitis in patients with non- Hodgkin lymphoma treated with the novel proteasome inhibitor bortezomib: a possible surrogate marker of response. *British Journal of Haematology*, **134**, 391–39.

ef.: 8888.

21 Min, C.K., Lee, S., Kim, Y.J. *et al.* (2006) Cutaneous leucoclastic vasculitis (LV) following bortezomib therapy in a myeloma patient; association with pro-inflammatory cytokines. *European Journal of Haematology*, **76**, 265–268.

22 Cohen, P.R. & Kurzrock, R. (2003) Sweet's syndrome revisited: a review of disease concepts. *International Journal of Dermatology*, **42**, 761–778.

23 Van Regenmortel, N., Van de Voorde, K., De Raeve, H. *et al.* (2005) Bortezomib-induced Sweet's syndrome. *Haematologica*, **90**, 116–117.

24 Thomas, M., Cavelier Balloy, B., Andreoli, A., Briere, J. & Petit, A. (2009) Bortezomib-induced neutrophilic dermatosis with CD30+ lymphocytic infiltration. *Annales de Dermatologie et de Venereologie*, **136**, 438–442.

25 Thuillier, D., Lenglet, A., Chaby, G. *et al.* (2009) Bortezomib-induced eruption: sweet syndrome? Two case reports. *Annales de Dermatologie et de Venereologie*, **136**, 427–430.

26 Murase, J.E., Wu, J.J., Theate, I., Cole, G.W., Barr, R.J. & Dyson, S.W. (2009) Bortezomib-induced histiocytoid Sweet syndrome. *Journal of the American Academy of Dermatology*, **60**, 496–497.

27 Leone, G., Voso, M.T., Teofili, L. & Lübbert, M. (2003) Inhibitors of DNA methylation in the treatment of hematological malignancies and MDS. *Clinical Immunology (Orlando, Florida)*, **109**, 89–102.

28 Jones, P.A., Taylor, S.M. & Wilson, V.L. (1983) Inhibition of DNA methylation by 5-azacytidine. *Recent Results in Cancer Research. Fortschritte Der Krebsforschung. Progres Dans Les Recherches Sur Le Cancer*, **84**, 202–211.

29 Oki, Y., Aoki, E. & Issa, J.P. (2007) Decitabine: bedside to bench. *Critical Reviews in Oncology*, **61**, 140–152.

30 Goldsmith, S.M., Sherertz, E.F., Powell, B.L. & Hurd, D.D. (1991) Cutaneous reactions to azacitidine. *Archives of Dermatology*, **127**, 1847–1848.

31 Ng, E.S., Aw, D.C., Tan, K.B. *et al.* (2010) Neutrophilic eccrine hidradenitis associated with decitabine. *Leukemia Research*, **34**, 130–132.

32 Brehler, R., Reimann, S., Bonsmann, G. & Metze, D. (1997) Neutrophilic hidradenitis induced by chemotherapy involves eccrine and apocrine glands. *American Journal of Dermatopathology*, **73-78**.

33 Shear, N.H., Knowles, S.R., Shapiro, L. & Poldre, P. (1996) Dapsone in prevention of recurrent neutrophilic eccrine hidradenitis. *Journal of the American Academy of Dermatology*, **35**, 819–822.

34 Beutner, K.R., Packman, C.H. & Markowitch, W. (1986) Neutrophilic eccrine hidradenitis associated with Hodgkin's disease and chemotherapy. A case report. *Archives of Dermatology*, **122**, 809–811.

35 Emadi, A. & Gore, S.D. (2010) Arsenic trioxide: an old drug rediscovered. *Blood Reviews*, **24**, 191–199.

36 Fox, E., Razzouk, B.I., Widemann, B.C. *et al.* (2008) Phase 1 trial and pharmacokinetic study of arsenic trioxide in children and adolescents with refractory or relapsed acute leukemia, including acute promyelocytic leukemia or lymphoma. *Blood*, **111**, 566–573.

37 Litzow, M.R., Lee, S., Bennett, J.M. *et al.* (2006) A phase II trial of arsenic trioxide for relapsed and refractory acute lymphoblastic leukemia. *Haematologica*, **91**, 1105–1108.

38 Tanvetyanon, T. & Nand, S. (2004) Herpes zoster during treatment with arsenic trioxide. *Annals of Hematology*, **83**, 198–200.

39 Au, W.Y. & Kwong, Y.L. (2005) Frequent varicella zoster reactivation associated with therapeutic use of arsenic trioxide: portents of an old scourge. *Journal of the American Academy of Dermatology*, **53**, 890–892.

40 McCrary, M.L., Severson, J. & Tyring, S.K. (1999) Varicella zoster virus. *Journal of the American Academy of Dermatology*, **41**, 1–14.

41 Harrison, M.T. & McCoy, K.L. (2001) Immunosuppression by arsenic: a comparison of cathepsin L inhibition and apoptosis. *International Immunopharmacology*, **4**, 647–656.

42 Tyring, S.K., Beutner, K.R., Tucker, B.A., Anderson, W.C. & Crooks, R.J. (2000) Antiviral therapy for herpes zoster: randomized, controlled clinical trial of valacyclovir and famciclovir therapy in immunocompetent patients 50 years and older. *Archives of Family Medicine*, **9**, 863–869.

43 Wood, M.J., Kay, R., Dworkin, R.H., Soong, S.J. & Whitley, R.J. (1996) Oral acyclovir therapy accelerates pain resolution in patients with herpes zoster: a meta-analysis of placebo-control. *Clinical Infectious Diseases*, **22**, 341–347.

44 Oxman, M.N., Levin, M.J., Johnson, G.R. *et al.* (2005) A vaccine to prevent herpes zoster and postherpetic neuralgia in older adults. *New England Journal of Medicine*, **352**, 2271–2284.

45 Harpaz, R., Ortega-Sanchez, I.R. & Seward, J.F. (2008) Centers for disease control and prevention, prevention of herpes zoster: recommendations of the Advisory Committee on Immunization Practices (ACIP). *MMWR. Recommendations and Reports: Morbidity and Mortality Weekly Report. Recommendations and Reports*, **57**, 1–30.

46 Qu, L. & Tang, X. (2010) Bexarotene: a promising anticancer agent. *Cancer Chemotherapy and Pharmacology*, **65**, 201–205.

47 Wong, S.F. (2001) Oral bexarotene in the treatment of cutaneous T-cell lymphoma. *Annals of Pharmacotherapy*, **35**, 1056–1065.

48 Breneman, D., Duvic, M., Kuzel, T., Yocum, R., Truglia, J. & Stevens, V.J. (2002) Phase 1 and 2 trial of bexarotene gel for skin-directed treatment of patients with cutaneous T-cell lymphoma. *Archives of Dermatology*, **138**, 325–332.

49 Vesanoid package insert. Available from: http://news.cancerconnect.com/druginserts/Tretinoin.pdf (accessed 9 April 2013).

50 Lehmann, J.M., Jong, L., Fanjul, A. *et al.* (1944) Retinoids selective for retinoid X receptor response pathways. *Science*, **258**, 19466–1992.

51 FDA package insert Panretin gel 0.1%. Available from: http://www.accessdata.fda.gov/drugsatfda_docs/label/1999/20886lbl.pdf (accessed 9 April 2013).

52 Ruzicka, T., Larsen, F.G., Galewicz, D. *et al.* (2004) Oral alitretinoin (9-cis-retinoic acid) therapy for chronic hand dermatitis in patients refractory to standard therapy: results of a randomized, double-blind, placebo-controlled, multicenter trial. *Archives of Dermatology*, **140**, 1453–1459.

53 Soignet, S.L., Benedetti, F., Fleischauer, A. *et al.* (1998) Clinical study of 9-cis retinoic acid (LGD1057) in acute promyelocytic leukemia. *Leukemia*, **12**, 1518–1521.

54 Aboulafia, D.M., Norris, D., Henry, D. *et al.* (2003) 9-cis-retinoic acid capsules in the treatment of AIDS-related Kaposi sarcoma: results of a phase 2 multicenter clinical trial. *Archives of Dermatology*, **139**, 178–186.

55 Arrieta, O., González-De la Rosa, C.H., Aréchaga-Ocampo, E. *et al.* (2010) Randomized phase II trial of all-trans-retinoic acid with chemotherapy based on paclitaxel and cisplatin as first-line treatment in patients with advanced non-small-cell lung cancer. *Journal of Clinical Oncology*, **28**, 3463–3471.

56 Duvic, M., Hymes, K., Heald, P. *et al.* (2001) Bexarotene is effective and safe for treatment of refractory advanced-stage cutaneous T-cell

lymphoma: multinational phase II-III trial results. *Journal of Clinical Oncology*, **19**, 2456–2471.

57 Frankel, S.R., Eardley, A., Heller, G. *et al.* (1994) All-trans retinoic acid for acute promyelocytic leukemia: results of the New York Study. *Annals of Internal Medicine*, **120**, 278–286.

58 Mourad, Y.A., Jabr, F. & Salem, Z. (2005) Scrotal ulceration induced by all-trans retinoic acid in a patient with acute promyelocytic leukemia. *International Journal of Dermatology*, **44**, 68–69.

59 Lee, H.Y., Ang, A.L., Lim, L.C., Thirumoorthy, T. & Pang, S.M. (2010) All-trans retinoic acid-induced scrotal ulcer in a patient with acute promyelocytic leukaemia. *Clinical and Experimental Dermatology*, **35**, 91–92.

60 Shimizu, D., Nomura, K., Matsuyama, R. *et al.* (2005) Scrotal ulcers arising during treatment with all-trans retinoic acid for acute promyelocytic leukemia. *Internal Medicine (Tokyo, Japan)*, **44**, 480–483.

61 Simzar, S., Rotunda, A.M. & Craft, N. (2005) Scrotal ulceration as a consequence of all-trans-retinoic acid (ATRA) for the treatment of acute promyelocytic leukemia. *Journal of Drugs in Dermatology*, **4**, 231–232.

62 Sami, N. & Harper, J.C. (2007) Topical retinoids. In: S.E. Wolverton (ed), *Comprehensive Dermatologic Drug Therapy*, pp. 625–641. WB Saunders, Philadelphia.

63 Patton, T.J., Zirwas, M.J. & Wolverton, S.E. (2007) Systemic retinoids. In: S.E. Wolverton (ed), *Comprehensive Dermatologic Drug Therapy*, pp. 275–300. WB Saunders, Philadelphia.

64 Morganroth, G.S. (2002) Topical 0.1% alitretinoin gel for classic Kaposi sarcoma. *Archives of Dermatology*, **138**, 542–543.

65 Duvic, M., Friedman-Kien, A.E., Looney, D.J. *et al.* (2000) Topical treatment of cutaneous lesions of acquired immunodeficiency syndrome-related Kaposi sarcoma using alitretinoin gel: results of phase 1 and 2 trials. *Archives of Dermatology*, **136**, 1461–1469.

66 Shalita, A.R. (1987) Mucocutaneous and systemic toxicity of retinoids: monitoring and management. *Dermatologica*, **175**, 151–157.

67 Saurat, J.H. (1992) Side effects of systemic retinoids and their clinical management. *Journal of the American Academy of Dermatology*, **27**, 23–28.

68 Glenny, A.M., Fernandez Mauleffinch, L.M., Pavitt, S., Pavitt, S. & Walsh, T. (2009) Interventions for the prevention and treatment of herpes simplex virus in patients being treated for cancer. *Cochrane Database of Systematic Reviews*, 1, CD006706.

69 Huber, M.A. (2003) Herpes simplex type-1 virus infection. *Quintessence International (Berlin, Germany: 1985)*, **34**, 453–467.

70 Chakrabarty, A., Pang, K., Wu, J. *et al.* (2004) Emerging therapies for herpes viral infections (types 1–8). *Expert Opinion on Emerging Drugs*, **9**, 237–256.

71 Balfour, H.H., Jr., Bean, B., Laskin, O.L. *et al.* (1983) Acyclovir halts progression of herpes zoster in immunocompromised patients. *New England Journal of Medicine*, **308**, 1448–1453.

72 Brady, R. & Bernstein, D. (2004) Treatment of herpes simplex infections. *Antiviral Research*, **61**, 73–81.

73 Nouri, K., Ricotti, C.A., Jr., Bouzari, N., Chen, H., Ahn, E. & Bach, A. (2006) The incidence of recurrent herpes simplex and herpes zoster infection during treatment with arsenic trioxide. *Journal of Drugs in Dermatology*, **5**, 182–185.

21 Miscellaneous Reactions

Katharina C. Kaehler[1], Christine B. Boers-Doets[2], Mario E. Lacouture[3] and Axel Hauschild[1]

[1]Department of Dermatology, University Hospital Schleswig-Holstein Campus, Kiel, Germany
[2]Department of Clinical Oncology, Leiden University Medical Center, Leiden, The Netherlands
[3]Dermatology Service, Memorial Sloan-Kettering Cancer Center, New York, NY, USA

Introduction

This chapter focuses on various agents that are used against solid and hematopoietic tumors through distinct mechanisms of action. L-asparaginase catalyzes the conversion of L-asparagine to aspartic acid and ammonia, resulting in the depletion of asparagine, inhibition of protein synthesis, cell cycle arrest in the G1 phase, and apoptosis in susceptible leukemic cells. Bleomycin forms complexes with iron that reduce molecular oxygen to superoxide and hydroxyl radicals which cause single and double-stranded breaks in DNA. Thalidomide and lenalidomide inhibit tumor necrosis factor α (TNF-α) production and angiogenesis, they stimulate T cells, and reduce serum levels of the cytokines vascular endothelial growth factor (VEGF) and basic fibroblast growth factor (bFGF). Their dermatologic adverse event (AE) profile is as distinct as their mechanism of action, therefore the understanding of these untoward events is critical for their optimal use (Figure 21.1; Table 21.1).

L-Asparaginase

Asparaginase hydrolyzes L-asparagine to L-aspartic acid and ammonia in leukemic cells, resulting in the depletion of asparagine, inhibition of protein synthesis, cell cycle arrest in the G1 phase, and apoptosis in susceptible leukemic cells. Asparagine is critical to protein synthesis in leukemic cells; some cells cannot synthesize this amino acid *de novo* because of absent or deficient expression of the enzyme asparagine synthase. Its antileukemic effect is believed to result from the depletion of circulating asparagine, which is not essential for normal cells but for most malignant lymphoblastic cells. The sources of L-asparaginase used clinically are bacterial: an *Escherichia coli*, *Erwinia carotovora*,

or an *Erwinia chrysanthemi* derivative (crisantaspase (Erwinase)) [1]. It is also available in a polyethylene glycol form: PEG-asparaginase. The *E. carotovora*-derived form of asparaginase is typically reserved for cases of asparaginase hypersensitivity.

The enzyme L-asparaginase has been used in the treatment of lymphoblastic malignancies in children since 1970 [2]. Asparaginase (Elspar®) is a component of a multiagent regimen for the treatment of acute lymphoblastic leukemia (ALL) and is also used against some mast cell tumors [1].

Unlike other chemotherapies, it can be given as an intramuscular, subcutaneous, or intravenous injection without tissue irritation. The recommended dose of asparaginase is 6000 IU/m² intramuscularly or intravenously three times a week [3].

The AEs related to L-asparaginase include nausea, vomiting, myelotoxicity, hepatic failure, and hypersensitivity reactions [3]. Asparaginase has minimal bone marrow toxicity. Its main AEs are allergic reactions (including anaphylaxis), pancreatitis, diabetes, and coagulation abnormalities that may lead to intracranial thrombosis or hemorrhage [2].

Allergic reactions

The incidence of allergic reactions ranges 6–43%, with anaphylactic reactions occurring in <10% of patients [4]. The overall risk of a reaction per dose is 5–8% with an increase to 33% after the fourth dose [5]. The risk of serious allergic reactions is higher in patients with prior exposure to asparaginase or other *Escherichia coli*-derived L-asparaginases [4]. Third, a previous exposure to bleomycin [4], with hypersensitivity reactions in 24% of patients exposed months or years earlier. Other risk factors include doses higher than 6000 IU/m²/day and single-agent chemotherapy [4]. The clinical features are those typical of type I reactions: they occur within an hour of administration and present with pruritus, dyspnea, urticaria, and hypotension. Life-threatening anaphylaxis may ensue. Evans *et al.* reported that 44%

Dermatologic Principles and Practice in Oncology: Conditions of the Skin, Hair, and Nails in Cancer Patients, First Edition. Edited by Mario E. Lacouture.
© 2014 John Wiley & Sons, Inc. Published 2014 by John Wiley & Sons, Inc.

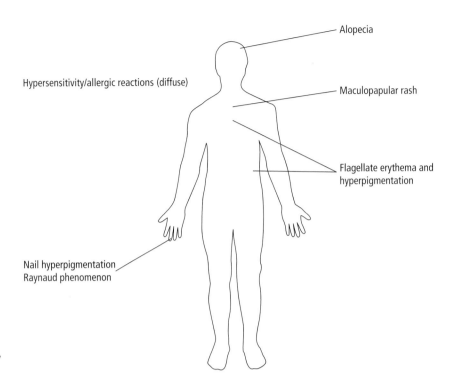

Hypersensitivity/allergic reactions (diffuse)

Alopecia

Maculopapular rash

Flagellate erythema and hyperpigmentation

Nail hyperpigmentation
Raynaud phenomenon

Figure 21.1 Location of miscellaneous agent-induced dermatologic adverse events (L-asparaginase, bleomycin, thalidomide, lenalidomide).

Table 21.1 Classification of miscellaneous agents.

Hydrolytic enzyme	L-asparaginase
Glycopeptide antibiotic	Bleomycin
Glutamic acid derivative	Thalidomide
Thalidomide derivative	Lenalidomide

of the patients with reactions had anaphylaxis. The pathogenetic mechanisms of hypersensitivity to L-asparaginase are not fully explained, but an immunoglobulin E (IgE) mediated hypersensitivity has been demonstrated with the Prausnitz–Küstner test in five patients. In eight patients with allergy, anaphylaxis could be explained by complement activation induced by the formation of immunocomplexes of L-asparaginase and specific IgM and IgG antibodies [4].

Toxic epidermal necrolysis (TEN) has been reported once in the literature, and twice to Medwatch, the United States' Food and Drug Administration's reporting system for AEs [6]. However, localized pain and edema at the injection site are very common [7].

Observation of patients for 1 hour after administration of asparaginase in a setting with resuscitation equipment and other agents necessary to treat anaphylaxis is recommended. Discontinue asparaginase in patients with serious allergic reactions.

Skin tests used to diagnose or prevent hypersensitivity reactions are of no value because they can give false-positive or false-negative results [4]. There are several possibilities in the treatment of patients who have developed hypersensitivity reactions and

need to continue therapy. Discontinuation of E. coli-derived L-asparaginase and substitution with Erwinia-derived L-asparaginase or PEG-asparaginase is advised [8,9]. However, cross-reactivity has been reported during the first dose of Erwinia-derived formulation, or the patient may produce specific antibodies to the drug, which could provoke anaphylaxis. Therefore, in cases of hypersensitivity to E. coli and Erwinia-derived L-asparaginase, the option is to use PEG-asparaginase, which is less immunogenic than the two other forms and is tolerated in more than 70% of cases of patients with allergies to the other two versions [4]. Unfortunately, the availability of Erwinia-derived L-asparaginase and PEG-asparaginase is limited, so premedication or desensitization protocols are necessary alternatives. Premedication with steroids and antihistamines as part of a desensitization protocol in 16 patients with previous allergic reactions to L-asparaginase allowed for completion of chemotherapy in approximately 70% [4].

Bleomycin

Bleomycin is a glycopeptide antibiotic produced by the bacterium *Streptomyces verticillus*. The forms used in oncology are primarily bleomycin A_2 and B_2. Bleomycin works by causing breaks in DNA. It has been used singly or in combination for the management of head and neck squamous cell carcinoma, external genitalia (penis and vulva) and cervix; Hodgkin lymphoma (as a component of the ABVD regimen); non-Hodgkin lymphoma; testis carcinoma, and as intrapleural therapy for malignant pleural effusion.

Bleomycin may be given by the intramuscular, intravenous, subcutaneous, or intrapleural routes.

AEs include pulmonary toxicities (10%), idiosyncratic reactions (1%), and integument and mucous membrane reactions (50%). Fever, chills and vomiting, anorexia and weight loss are frequently reported AEs. Pain at the tumor site, phlebitis, and other local reactions were reported infrequently. Malaise was also reported as part of postmarketing surveillance [10].

Dermatologic AEs usually develop in the second and third week of treatment, after a cumulative dose of 150–300 units, whereas pulmonary fibrosis occurs at doses >400 units [11]. This drug may inadvertently affect the skin, mucous membranes, hair and nails in 50% of the patients, producing many AEs including "flagellate" erythema (scratch dermatitis) (Figure 21.2), hyperpigmentation, Raynaud phenomenon, gangrene, fibrosis, neutrophilic eccrine hidradenitis (NEH), alopecia, edema, nail changes, and other miscellaneous reactions [12–18]. One case of fatal fulminant angioedema involving the skin and lungs has been reported [10]. Two cases of Steven–Johnsons syndrome (SJS) are reported in the literature and eight in Medwatch (Appendix 21.1).

Flagellate erythema

Flagellate erythema is a characteristic AE of bleomycin, which occurs in 8–66% of treated patients. Clinically, erythematoviolaceous linear streaks on the trunk and/or shoulders develop [16,19–36]. This AE is considered to be dose dependent, occurring at doses >100 IU, although it has also been reported after 14–15 IU [19,25–27,30]. The time between administration of bleomycin and onset of flagellate erythema varies from 12–24 hours [21,25,26,28] to 6 months [36]. The occurrence of flagellate dermatitis is not dependent on the route of administration, as it has been reported after intrapleural [20,21,28,34,36], intraperitoneal [31], and intracutaneous [19] injection.

Histologically, flagellate erythema is characterized by hyperkeratosis in the epidermis with focal parakeratosis, irregular acanthosis, spongiosis, exocytosis of lymphocytes, and an increase of melanin. Dermal edema, vasodilatation, and a perivascular lymphocytic infiltrate are also typical histologic features [20,26,27]. In some cases, pruritus as part of the flagellate erythema is reported. The pathogenesis of flagellate erythema is believed to be scratching-induced microtrauma, which causes drug extravasation from blood vessels. Even with a negative patch test, flagellate erythema may recur upon rechallenge [30]. There is also evidence for enhanced toxicity of bleomycin in combination with heat [37]. The pathogenesis of flagellate hyperpigmentation is still not completely clear, possible hypotheses include postinflammatory hyperpigmentation [21]; a negative influence on epidermal turnover with prolongation of contact between melanocytes and keratinocytes [20]; slower turnover of keratinocytes with blockage of melanocytes in the pigment synthesis phase [5]; or accumulation of bleomycin in skin may lead to a fixed drug eruption due to direct effects on keratinocytes [22]. Injections of bleomycin into normal human skin induced inflammatory reactions with persistent postinflammatory hyperpigmentation.

Raynaud phenomenon and gangrene

Reports of Raynaud phenomenon after treatment with combination chemotherapy involving bleomycin exist [38–44], and also after local intralesional application of bleomycin for recalcitrant warts [45–48]. Raynaud phenomenon is frequently observed in patients with Kaposi sarcoma and HIV treated with bleomycin, and a decreased amount of capillaries in the nail fold has been found in this patient population [49,50].

Vascular endothelial cell injury in small blood vessels is considered to be a possible cause for Raynaud phenomenon [51]. Further development of acral gangrene has been reported [39,40,52], while gangrene without prior onset of Raynaud phenomenon has been reported [52,53]. The incidence of Raynaud phenomenon is independent of the route of administration or dosage of bleomycin.

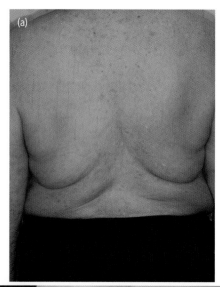

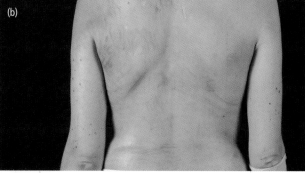

Figure 21.2 (a & b) Bleomycin-induced flagellate dermatitis and hyperpigmentation grade 2. (Picture courtesy of Dr. J Toonstra, University Medical Centre Utrecht, The Netherlands.)

Histologically, a leukocytoclastic vasculitis, leading to ischemic necrosis can be detected [53]. Bleomycin seems to enhance TNF-α synthesis, which induces a procoagulant effect in blood vessels by increasing tissue factor and tissue plasminogen-activator inhibitor production, and by decreasing endothelial thrombomodulin and protein C activation [54]. Thus, bleomycin-induced TNF-α may be an important pathogenic cornerstone in the development of Raynaud phenomenon.

Bleomycin-induced scleroderma
Systemic sclerodermatous changes have been reported, with [55–58] male patients predominantly affected, with cumulative dose of bleomycin varying between 51 and 780 IU.

In vitro, bleomycin upregulates mRNA expression of extracellular matrix proteins in human lung and dermal fibroblasts [59,60]. Newly synthesized collagen by bleomycin-treated fibroblasts is rapidly degraded [61], suggesting that increased collagen degradation may be responsible for the remodeling process. Also, bleomycin enhances mRNA expression for transforming growth factor β (TGF-β) and connective tissue growth factor in skin fibroblasts [60]. Both are fibrogenic cytokines and have an important role in the development of tissue fibrosis. Human lung fibroblasts enhance chemotactic activity for both neutrophils and monocytes in response to bleomycin, suggesting that fibroblasts modulate inflammatory cell recruitment [62]. In mice, repeated local injection of bleomycin resulted in dermal sclerosis mimicking human scleroderma, and consequently has been established as a mouse model for scleroderma [63,64].

Neutrophilic eccrine hidradenitis
NEH has been associated with the combination agents including bleomycin, cytarabine, doxorubicin, vincristine, cisplatin, and dacarbazine [65,66].

Fever and a nonspecific skin eruption – with erythema, pain, and edema of the skin – are common symptoms of NEH, appearing 1–2 weeks after drug administration. Lesions can appear on the extremities, trunk, and face, which can mimic cellulitis when severe. Generalized lesions resembling erythema multiforme have been reported [67]. Clinically, erythematous plaques and nodules appear, and histologically a neutrophilic infiltrate of eccrine glands (sweat glands) with cell degeneration. There are various possible mechanisms, including the direct toxic effects on sweat glands, as part of a neutrophilic dermatosis, or it may represent a paraneoplastic condition. Histology of bleomycin-injected human skin also showed necrosis of the eccrine epithelium associated with prominent neutrophilic infiltrates, in a condition resembling NEH [68]. In summary, eccrine (sweat) glands may be highly susceptible to the toxic effects of bleomycin.

Acute generalized exanthematous pustulosis
Acute generalized exanthematous pustulosis (AGEP) is a rare skin AE, characterized by an acute generalized erythema with a number of pustules and systemic symptoms such as a high fever, most frequently developing after drug administration, especially antibiotics. A case of AGEP in a patient treated with bleomycin, etoposide, and cisplatin has been reported [69], and was confirmed by patch testing. Additionally, an unusual report of a case of Stevens–Johnson syndrome (SJS) resembling AGEP, was induced by peplomycin, a bleomycin analog [70].

Alopecia
Bleomycin is one of the chemotherapeutic agents known to cause alopecia through inhibition of anagen and hair follicle apoptosis. The growth of isolated organ-cultured human anagen hair follicles is inhibited by TGF-β1 and follicles can be induced to enter a regression process that resembles the early stages of a catagen-like transformation [71,72]. As bleomycin induces TGF-β in several cell types, TGF-β may have an important role in bleomycin-induced alopecia.

Nail changes
Nail dystrophy and fingernail loss were reported following intralesional bleomycin injections for periungual warts [73,74]. Bleomycin has also the potential to induce nail pigmentation. The pigment is located in horizontal or vertical bands, which may be brown or blue, and generally grow out with the nail [16]. Converesely, it has been suggested that the pigmentation occurs in the nail bed [75]. Much drug-induced nail pigmentation is the result of increased melanin production by nail matrix melanocytes.

The majority of dermatologic AEs induced by bleomycin are manageable and require symptomatic treatment. As bleomycin is excreted renally, patients with an impaired renal function should be monitored carefully.

Thalidomide

Thalidomide is a synthetic derivative of glutamic acid (alpha-phthalimido-glutarimide) with teratogenic, immunomodulatory, anti-inflammatory and antiangiogenic properties. Thalidomide acts primarily by inhibiting both the production of TNF-α in stimulated peripheral monocytes and the activity of interleukin and interferon. This agent also inhibits polymorphonuclear chemotaxis and monocyte phagocytosis. In addition, thalidomide inhibits proangiogenic factors such as VEGF and bFGF, thereby inhibiting angiogenesis.

Thalidomide in combination with other agents, such as doxorubicin and dexamethasone, or melphalan and prednisone, is indicated for the treatment of multiple myeloma, and for the acute treatment of the cutaneous manifestations of erythema nodosum leprosum [76].

For multiple myeloma, thalidomide is administered in combination with dexamethasone in 28-day treatment cycles [76]. The most frequently reported AEs in multiple myeloma trials are constipation, sensory neuropathy, confusion, hypocalcemia, edema, dyspnea, thrombosis/embolism, and rash/desquamation (occurring in ≥20% of patients and with a frequency of ≥10% in patients treated with thalidomide/dexamethasone compared with dexamethasone alone). Also drowsiness, peripheral neuropathy, dizziness, and leukopenia are reported [76].

Cases of exfoliative [77] and erythrodermic reactions [78], allergic vasculitis and thrombocytopenic purpura [79], TEN [80], and psoriasis exacerbation [81] have been reported with the use of thalidomide. Acne, alopecia, dry skin, eczematous rash, exfoliative dermatitis, ichthyosis, perifollicular thickening, skin necrosis, seborrhea, sweating, urticaria, and vesiculobullous rash are seen [76]. In an open-label clinical trial of 87 patients with multiple myeloma, subjects were treated with thalidomide alone (50 patients) or thalidomide and dexamethasone (37 patients) [82]. Skin reactions (including maculopapular, morbilliform, seborrhoeic, or nonspecific dermatitis) occurred in 46% of patients taking thalidomide and in 43% of those taking thalidomide combined with dexamethasone. In this study, moderate rashes resulted in altered dosing and severe rashes led to permanent discontinuation of treatment. Three of the 16 patients who developed a rash in the thalidomide and dexamethasone arm developed severe skin reactions (one each of erythema multiforme, exfoliative erythroderma, and TEN) which required hospitalization and discontinuation of thalidomide. Patients with HIV are more likely to experience hypersensitivity reactions; three of eight male patients treated for severe aphthous oropharyngeal ulceration with thalidomide experiencing such reaction (fever, widespread erythematous macular rash, and tachycardia), requiring drug discontinuation [83].

In myeloma trials, rash and/or desquamation developed in 30.4% of the safety population (n = 204)with no grade 3–4 rash or desquamation reported. Dry skin appeared in 20.6%, of which 3.9% was grade 3 [76]. Rashes and/or fever occurred in 20 (36%) of the 56 patients; there was no apparent relationship between AE and the starting dosage of thalidomide. Overall, the mean time to the onset of the reaction was 7–13 days. The rashes were pruritic, maculopapular eruptions, or diffusely erythematous and occurred primarily on the trunk and proximal parts of the limbs. Seven (47%) of 15 patients with rashes also had fever and five had fever alone [84]. There was one report of SJS in the literature and 11 cases in Medwatch. Of TEN, two cases have been reported in the literature and 16 in Medwatch [6].

In case of maculopapular, morbilliform, or other dermatitis associated with pruritus, in the absence of systemic signs and symptoms, the rash should be managed symptomatically by application of moisturizers, oral antihistamines, plus oral or topical corticosteroids. If the rash is associated with signs and symptoms of a type I hypersensitivity reaction, is bullous, or if SJS or TEN is suspected, use of thalidomide should not be resumed [76]. Hall *et al.* [82] advises physicians to use caution and preferably not to prescribe thalidomide in combination with other drugs strongly associated with TEN. Furthermore, caution should be exercised when using the combination of thalidomide and dexamethasone for newly diagnosed multiple myeloma until this interaction is further elucidated.

Lenalidomide

Lenalidomide is a thalidomide analog with potential antineoplastic activity. Lenalidomide inhibits TNF-α production, stimulates T cells, reduces serum levels of the cytokines VEGF and bFGF, and inhibits angiogenesis. This agent also promotes G1 cell cycle arrest and apoptosis of malignant cells [85] and is a potent human teratogen [86].

Lenalidomide in combination with dexamethasone is indicated for the treatment of multiple myeloma [86] and for patients with transfusion-dependent anemia due to low or intermediate risk myelodysplastic syndromes (MDS) associated with a 5q deletion [87].

Lenalidomide/dexamethasone AEs include neutropenia (39.4%), fatigue (27.2%), asthenia (17.6%), constipation (23.5%), muscle cramp (20.1%), thrombocytopenia (18.4%), anaemia (17.0%), diarrhoea (14.2%), and rash (10.2%) [85].

Within multiple myeloma, a very common AE (≥1/10) is rash, which can be morbilliform (Figure 21.3), urticarial, dermatitic, or acneform. Common events (≥1 in 100 to <1 in 10) of lenalidomide are face edema, dry skin, pruritus, erythema, folliculitis, skin hyperpigmentation, exanthema, increased sweating, night sweats, and alopecia. Uncommon AEs (≥1 in 1000 to <1 in 100) are erythema nodosum, urticaria, angioedema, eczema, erythrosis, erythematous rash, pruritic rash, papular rash, hyperkeratosis, skin fissures, acne, dermatitis acneiform, lichen sclerosus,

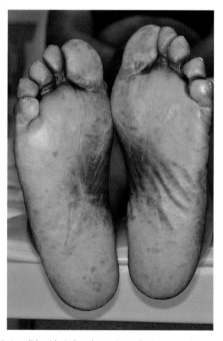

Figure 21.3 Lenalidomide-induced xerosis grade 1.

decubitus ulcer, pigmentation lip, prurigo, rosacea, photosensitivity reaction, seborrheic dermatitis, skin burning sensation, skin desquamation, and skin discoloration. Rare AEs (≥1 in 10 000 to <1 in 1000) are SJS, and TEN [86].

Within MDS, dermatologic AEs include pruritus (41.9%), rash (35.8%), dry skin (14.2%), contusion (8.1%), night sweats (8.1%), increased sweating (6.8%), ecchymosis (5.4%), erythema (5.4%), skin desquamation, erythema multiforme, and acute febrile neutrophilic dermatosis. Twelve reports of SJS and one report of TEN have also been reported and one biopsy-confirmed case of SJS [88].

Lenalidomide must be discontinued for rash associated with type I reaction signs and symptoms, for exfoliative or bullous rash, or if SJS or TEN is suspected, and should not be resumed. Patients with a history of serious rash associated with thalidomide treatment should not receive lenalidomide [86].

References

1 Bitish National Formulary. (2009) Other antineoplastic drugs. *British National Formulary (BNF 57)*, p. 476. BMJ Group and RPS Publishing, United Kingdom.

2 Duval, M., Suciu, S., Ferster, A. *et al.* (2002) Comparison of *Escherichia coli*-asparaginase with *Erwinia*-asparaginase in the treatment of childhood lymphoid malignancies: results of a randomized European Organisation for Research and Treatment of Cancer-Children's Leukemia Group phase 3 trial. *Blood*, **99**, 2734–2739.

3 Lundbeck Worldwide. (2010) Full prescribing information L-asparaginase. Available from: http://www.lundbeckinc.com/USA/products/hematology_oncology/elspar/usa_els_pi_april_10.pdf (accessed 9 April 2013).

4 Pagani, M. (2010) The complex clinical picture of presumably allergic side effects to cytostatic drugs: symptoms, pathomechanism, reexposure, and desensitization. *Medical Clinics of North America*, **94**, 835–852, xiii.

5 Guillet, G., Guillet, M.H., de Meaux, H. *et al.* (1986) Cutaneous pigmented stripes and bleomycin treatment. *Archives of Dermatology*, **122**, 381–382.

6 Sorrell, J., West, D.P., Bennett, C.L., Raisch, D.W. & Lacouture, M.E. (2009) Life-threatening dermatologic toxicities to cancer drug therapy: an assessment of the published peer-reviewed literature [abstract of ASCO Annual Meeting Proceedings]. *Journal of Clinical Oncology*, **27** (15 Suppl), e20592.

7 Dinndorf, P.A., Gootenberg, J., Cohen, M.H., Keegan, P. & Pazdur, R. (2007) FDA drug approval summary: pegaspargase (Oncaspar®) for the first-line treatment of children with Acute Lymphoblastic Leukemia (ALL). *The Oncologist*, **12** (8), 991–998.

8 Beard, M.E., Crowther, D., Galton, D.A. *et al.* (1970) L-asparaginase in treatment of acute leukaemia and lymphosarcoma. *British Medical Journal*, **1** (5690), 191–195.

9 Ohnuma, T., Holland, J.F. & Meyer, P. (1972) Erwinia carotovora asparaginase in patients with prior anaphylaxis to asparaginase from E. coli. *Cancer*, **30**, 376–381.

10 Teva Generics. (2007) Full prescribing information bleomycin. Available from: http://www.tevausa.com/assets/base/products/pi/Bleomycin_PI_7-2007.pdf (accessed 9 April 2013).

11 D'Cruz, D. (2000) Autoimmune diseases associated with drugs, chemicals and environmental factors. *Toxicology Letters*, **112–113**, 421–432.

12 Cohen, I.S., Mosher, M.B., O'Keefe, E.J., Klaus, S.N. & De Conti, R.C. (1973) Cutaneous toxicity of bleomycin in therapy. *Archives of Dermatology*, **107**, 553–555.

13 Dantzig, P.I. (1974) Immunosuppressive and cytotoxic drugs in dermatology. *Archives of Dermatology*, **110**, 393–406.

14 Werner, Y. & Törnberg, B. (1976) Cutaneous side effects of bleomycin therapy. *Acta Dermato-Venereologica*, **56**, 155–158.

15 Nixon, D.W., Pirozzi, D. & York, R.M. (1981) Dermatologic changes after systemic cancer therapy. *Cutis: Cutaneous Medicine for the Practitioner*, **27**, 181–194.

16 DeSpain, J.D. (1992) Dermatologic toxicity of chemotherapy. *Seminars in Oncology*, **19**, 501–507.

17 Remlinger, K.A. (2003) Cutaneous reactions to chemotherapy drugs: the art of consultation. *Archives of Dermatology*, **139**, 77–81.

18 Yagoda, A., Mukherji, B., Young, C. *et al.* (1972) Bleomycin, an antitumor antibiotic: clinical experience in 274 patients. *Annals of Internal Medicine*, **77**, 861–870.

19 Abess, A., Keel, D.M. & Graham, B.S. (2003) Flagellate hyperpigmentation following intralesional bleomycin treatment of verruca plantaris. *Archives of Dermatology*, **139**, 337–339.

20 Fernandez-Obregon, A.C., Hogan, K.P. & Bibro, M.K. (1985) Flagellate pigmentation from intrapleural bleomycin. A light microscopy and electron microscopy study. *Journal of the American Academy of Dermatology*, **13**, 464–468.

21 Polla, B.S., Merot, Y., Saurat, J.H. & Slosman, D. (1986) Flagellate pigmentation from bleomycin. *Journal of the American Academy of Dermatology*, **14**, 690.

22 Lindae, M.L., Hu, C.H. & Nickoloff, B.J. (1987) Pruritic erythematous linear plaques on the neck and back. *Archives of Dermatology*, **123**, 393–398.

23 Rademaker, M., Meyrick-Thomas, R.H. & Lowe, D.G. (1987) Linear streaking due to bleomycin. *Clinical and Experimental Dermatology*, **12**, 457–459.

24 Lazar, A.P. & Lazar, P. (1988) Streaky pigmentation in a patient with acquired immune deficiency syndrome (AIDS). *Cutis: Cutaneous Medicine for the Practitioner*, **42**, 397–398.

25 Vignini, M., Miori, L., Brusamoliono, E. & Pelfini, C. (1989) Linear streaking after bleomycin administration. *Clinical and Experimental Dermatology*, **14**, 261.

26 Cortina, P., Garrido, J.A., Tomas, J.F., Unamuno, P. & Armijo, M. (1990) 'Flagellate' erythema from bleomycin. With histopathological findings suggestive of inflammatory oncotaxis. *Dermatologica*, **180** (2), 106–109.

27 Miori, L., Vignini, M. & Rabbiosi, G. (1990) Flagellate dermatitis after bleomycin: a histological and immunohistochemical study. *American Journal of Dermatopathology*, **12**, 598–602.

28 Duhra, P., Ilchyshyn, A. & Das, R.N. (1991) Bleomycin-induced flagellate erythema. *Clinical and Experimental Dermatology*, **16**, 216–217.

29 Tsuji, T. & Sawabe, M. (1993) Hyperpigmentation in striae distensae after bleomycin treatment. *Journal of the American Academy of Dermatology*, **28**, 503–505.

30 Mowad, C.M., Nguyen, T.V., Elenitsas, R. & Leyden, J.J. (1994) Bleomycin-induced flagellate dermatitis: a clinical and histopathological review. *British Journal of Dermatology*, **131**, 700–702.

31 Zaki, I., Haslam, P. & Scerri, L. (1994) Flagellate erythema after intraperitoneal bleomycin. *Clinical and Experimental Dermatology*, **19**, 366–367.

32 Mullai, N., Khokha, N. & Shimoto, G. (1998) Bleomycin cutaneous toxicity. *Journal of Clinical Oncology*, **16**, 1625–1627.

33 Yamamoto, T., Yokozeki, H. & Nishioka, K. (1998) Dermal sclerosis in the lesional skin of 'flagellate' erythema (scratch dermatitis) induced by bleomycin. *Dermatology (Basel, Switzerland)*, **297**, 399–400.

34 Rubeiz, N.G., Salem, Z., Dibbs, R. & Kibbi, A.G. (1999) Bleomycin-induced urticarial flagellate drug hypersensitivity reaction. *International Journal of Dermatology*, **38** (2), 140–141.

35 Nigro, M.G. & Hsu, S. (2001) Bleomycin-induced flagellate pigmentation. *Cutis; Cutaneous Medicine for the Practitioner*, **68**, 285–286.

36 von Hilsheimer, G.E. & Norton, S.A. (2002) Delayed bleomycin-induced hyperpigmentation and pressure on the skin. *Journal of the American Academy of Dermatology*, **46** (4), 642–643.

37 Braun, J. & Hahn, G.M. (1975) Enhanced cell killing by bleomycin and 43 degrees hyperthermia and the inhibition of recovery from potentially lethal damage. *Cancer Research*, **35**, 2921–2927.

38 Total Health Care (2012) Total health-care Available at: http://www.total-health-care.com/raynauds-disease/raynaud-duration-after-bleomycin.html (accessed 9 April 2013).

39 Hladunewich, M., Sawka, C., Fam, A. & Franssen, E. (1997) Raynaud's phenomenon and digital gangrene as a consequence of treatment for Kaposi's sarcoma. *Journal of Rheumatology*, **24**, 2371–2375.

40 Reiser, M., Bruns, C., Hartmann, P., Salzberger, B., Diehl, V. & Fätkenheuer, G. (1998) Raynaud's phenomenon and acral necrosis after chemotherapy for AIDS-related Kaposi's sarcoma. *European Journal of Clinical Microbiology and Infectious Diseases*, **17**, 58–60.

41 Fertakos, R.J. & Mintzer, D.M. (1992) Digital gangrene following chemotherapy for AIDS-related Kaposi's sarcoma. *American Journal of Medicine*, **93**, 581–582.

42 Elomaa, I., Pajunen, M. & Virkkunen, P. (1984) Raynaud's phenomenon progressing to gangrene after vincristine and bleomycin therapy. *Acta Medica Scandinavica*, **216**, 323–326.

43 Vayssairat, M., Gaitz, J.P. & Bamberger, N. (1993) Digital gangrene, HIV infection and bleomycin treatment. *Journal of Rheumatology*, **20**, 921.

44 Snauwaert, J. & Degreef, H. (1984) Bleomycin-induced Raynaud's phenomenon and acral sclerosis. *Dermatologica*, **169**, 172–174.

45 Epstein, E. (1991) Intralesional bleomycin and Raynaud's phenomenon. *Journal of the American Academy of Dermatology*, **24**, 785–786.

46 Gregg, L.J. (1992) Intralesional bleomycin and Raynaud's phenomenon. *Journal of the American Academy of Dermatology*, **27**, 279–280.

47 de Pablo, P., Aguillar, A. & Gallego, M.A. (1992) Raynaud's phenomenon and intralesional bleomycin. *Acta Dermato-Venereologica*, **72**, 465.

48 Vanhooteghem, O., Richert, B. & de la Brassinne, M. (2001) Raynaud phenomenon after treatment of verruca vulgaris of the sole with intralesional injection of bleomycin. *Pediatric Dermatology*, **18**, 249–251.

49 Caumes, E., Guermonprez, G., Katlama, C. & Gentilini, M. (1992) AIDS-associated mucocutaneous Kaposi's sarcoma treated with bleomycin. *AIDS (London, England)*, **6**, 1483–1487.

50 Gill, P.S., Rarick, M., McCutchan, J.A. *et al.* (1991) Systemic treatment of AIDS related Kaposi's sarcoma: results of a randomized trial. *American Journal of Medicine*, **90**, 427–433.

51 Bellmunt, J., Navarro, M., Morales, S. *et al.* (1990) Capillary microscopy is a potentially useful method for detecting bleomycin vascular toxicity. *Cancer*, **65**, 303–309.

52 Surville-Barland, J., Caumes, E., Ankri, A., Francès, C., Katlama, C. & Chosidow, O. (1998) Bleomycin-induced digital gangrene. *European Journal of Dermatology*, **8**, 221.

53 Correia, O., Ribas, F., Azevedo, R., Rodrigues, H. & Delgado, L. (2000) Gangrene of the fingertips after bleomycin and methotrexate. *Cutis: Cutaneous Medicine for the Practitioner*, **66**, 271–274.

54 Wakefield, P.E., James, W.D., Samlaska, C.P. & Meltzer, M.S. (1991) Tumor necrosis factor. *Journal of the American Academy of Dermatology*, **24**, 675–685.

55 Finch, W.R., Rodnan, G.P., Buckingham, R.B., Prince, R.K. & Winkelstein, A. (1980) Bleomycin-induced scleroderma. *Journal of Rheumatology*, **7**, 651–659.

56 Kerr, L.D. & Spiera, H. (1992) Scleroderma in association with the use of bleomycin: a report of 3 cases. *Journal of Rheumatology*, **19**, 294–296.

57 Kim, K.-H., Yoon, T.-J., Oh, C.W., Ko, G.H. & Kim, T.H. (1996) A case of bleomycin-induced scleroderma. *Journal of Korean Medical Science*, **11**, 454–456.

58 Passiu, G., Cauli, A., Atzeni, F. *et al.* (1999) Bleomycin-induced scleroderma: report of a case with a chronic course rather than the typical acute/subacute self-limiting form. *Clinical Rheumatology*, **18**, 422–424.

59 Clark, J.C., Starcher, B.C. & Uitto, J. (1980) Bleomycin-induced synthesis of type I procollagen by human lung skin fibroblasts in culture. *Biochimica et Biophysica Acta*, **631**, 359–370.

60 Yamamoto, T., Eckes, B. & Krieg, T. (2000) Bleomycin increases steady-state levels of type I collagen, fibronectin and decorin gene expression in human skin fibroblasts. *Archives of Dermatological Research*, **292**, 556–561.

61 Sterling, K.M., Jr, DiPetrillo, T.A., Kotch, J.P. & Cutroneo, K.R. (1982) Bleomycin induced increase of collagen turnover in IMR-90 fibroblasts: an *in vitro* model of connective tissue restructuring during lung fibrosis. *Cancer Research*, **42**, 3502–3506.

62 Sato, E., Koyama, S. & Robbins, R.A. (2000) Bleomycin stimulates lung fibroblast and epithelial cell lines to release eosinophil chemotactic activity. *European Respiratory Journal*, **16**, 951–958.

63 Yamamoto, T., Takagawa, S., Katayama, I. *et al.* (1999) Animal model of sclerotic skin. I: local injections of bleomycin induce sclerotic skin mimicking scleroderma. *Journal of Investigative Dermatology*, **112**, 456–462.

64 Yamamoto, T. (2002) Animal model of sclerotic skin induced by bleomycin: a clue to the pathogenesis of and therapy for scleroderma? *Clinical Immunology (Orlando, Florida)*, **102**, 209–216.

65 Beutner, K.R., Packman, C.H. & Markowitch, W. (1986) Neutrophilic eccrine hidradenitis associated with Hodgkin's disease and chemotherapy: a case report. *Archives of Dermatology*, **122**, 809–811.

66 Scallan, P.J., Kettler, A.H., Levy, M.L. & Tschen, J.A. (1988) Neutrophilic eccrine hidradenitis: evidence implicating bleomycin as a causative agent. *Cancer*, **62**, 2532–2536.

67 Thorisdottir, K., Tomecki, K.J., Bergfeld, W.F. & Andresen, S.W. (1993) Neutrophilic eccrine hidradenitis. *Journal of the American Academy of Dermatology*, **28** (5 Pt 1), 775–777.

68 Templeton, S.F., Solomon, A.R. & Swerlick, R.A. (1994) Intradermal bleomycin injections into normal human skin: a histopathologic and immunopathologic study. *Archives of Dermatology*, **130**, 577–583.

69 Altaykan, A., Boztepe, G., Erkin, G., Ozkaya, O. & Ozden, E. (2004) Acute generalized exanthematous pustulosis induced by bleomycin and confirmed by patch testing. *Journal of Dermatological Treatment*, **15**, 231–234.

70 Umebayashi, Y., Enomoto, H. & Ogasawara, M. (2004) Drug eruption due to peplomycin: an unusual form of Stevens–Johnson syndrome with pustules. *Journal of Dermatology*, **31**, 802–805.

71 Philpott, M.P., Sanders, D., Westgate, G.E. & Kealey, T. (1994) Human hair growth in vitro: a model for the study of hair follicle biology. *Journal of Dermatological Science*, **7**, S55–S72.

72 Soma, T., Ogo, M., Suzuki, J., Takahashi, T. & Hibino, T. (1998) Analysis of apoptotic cell death in human hair follicles *in vivo* and *in vitro*. *Journal of Investigative Dermatology*, **111**, 948–954.

73 Gonzalez, U.F., Gil, C.M.C., Martinez, A.A., Rodriguez, G.P., de Paz, S.F. & García-Pérez, A. (1986) Cutaneous toxicity of intralesional bleomycin administration in the treatment of periungual warts. *Archives of Dermatology*, **122**, 974–975.

74 Willer, R.A.W. (1984) Nail dystrophy following intralesional injections of bleomycin for a periungual wart. *Archives of Dermatology*, **120**, 963–964.

75 Shetty, M.R. (1977) Case of pigmented banding of the nail caused by bleomycin. *Cancer Treatment Reports*, **61**, 501–502.

76 Thalidomid. (2010) Full prescribing information thalidomide. Available at: http://www.thalomid.com/thalomid_pi.aspx (accessed 9 April 2013)

77 Salafia, A. & Kharkar, R.D. (1988) Thalidomide and exfoliative dermatitis. *International Journal of Leprosy*, **56**, 625.

78 Bielsa, I., Teixido, J., Ribera, M. & Ferrandiz, C. (1994) Erythroderma due to thalidomide: report of two cases. *Dermatology (Basel, Switzerland)*, **189**, 179–181.

79 Koch, H.P. (1985) Thalidomide and congeners as anti-inflammatory agents. *Progress in Medicinal Chemistry*, **22**, 165–242.

80 Rajkumar, S.V., Gertz, M.A. & Witzig, T.E. (2000) Life-threatening toxic epidermal necrolysis with thalidomide therapy for myeloma. *New England Journal of Medicine*, **343**, 972–973.

81 Dobson, C.M. & Parslew, R.A. (2003) Exacerbation of psoriasis by thalidomide in Behçet's syndrome. *British Journal of Dermatology*, **149**, 432–433.

82 Hall, V.C., El-Azhary, R.A., Bouwhuis, S. & Rajkumar, S.V. (2003) Dermatologic side effects of thalidomide in patients with multiple myeloma. *Journal of the American Academy of Dermatology*, **48**, 548–552.

83 Williams, I., Weller, I.V., Malni, A., Anderson, J. & Waters, M.F. (1991) Thalidomide hypersensitivity in AIDS. *Lancet*, **337**, 436–437.

84 Haslett, P., Tramontana, J., Burroughs, M., Hempstead, M. & Kaplan, G. (1997) Adverse reactions to thalidomide in patients infected with human immunodeficiency virus. *Clinical Infectious Diseases*, **24**, 1223–1227.

85 National Cancer Institute. (2009) Cancer Drug Information lenalidomide. Available from: http://www.cancer.gov/cancertopics/druginfo/lenalidomide (accessed 9 April 2013).

86 Celgene. (2011) Summary of product characteristics lenalidomide. Available from: http://www.medicines.org.uk/emc/medicine/19841/SPC/Revlimid%C2%AE/ (accessed 9 April 2013).

87 Lenalidomide. Full prescribing information lenalidomide. Available from: http://www.revlimid.com/pdf/REVLIMID_PI.pdf (accessed 31 January 2011).

88 Drugs.com. Lenalidomide side effects. Available from: http://www.drugs.com/sfx/lenalidomide-side-effects.html (accessed 9 April 2013).

Appendix 21.1 Incidence of dermatologic adverse events to miscellaneous agents (L-asparaginase, bleomycin, thalidomide, lenalidomide).

Drug name (Trade)	Dermatologic adverse events				
	Cutaneous and subcutaneous	TEN/SJS	Nail	Hair	Mucous membranes
L-asparaginase (Asparaginase, Elspar)	Allergic skin reactions: All: 6–43% [4] Grade 3–4: with *E. coli*-asparaginase 2.5% [2], with *Erwinia*-asparaginase 2.6% [2]	TEN: 1 literature report [6] 2 Medwatch reports [6]	–	–	–
Bleomycin (Blenoxane)	Integument membranes 50% [10]: flagellate erythema [10] rash [10] striae [10] vesiculation [10], hyperpigmentation [10] tenderness of the skin [10], hyperkeratosis [10] pruritus [10] scleroderma [10] Raynaud phenomenon (rare) [38]	SJS: 2 literature reports [6] 8 Medwatch reports [6]	Nail changes [10]	Alopecia [10]	Mucous membranes 50% [10], stomatitis [10]

(Continued)

Drug name (Trade)	Dermatologic adverse events				
	Cutaneous and subcutaneous	**TEN/SJS**	**Nail**	**Hair**	**Mucous membranes**
Thalidomide (Thalomid)	Rash/desquamation: rash all: 64% [82] acne [76] eczematous rash [76] exfoliative dermatitis [76], ichthyosis [76] perifollicular thickening [76] skin necrosis [76] seborrhea [76] sweating [76] urticaria [76] vesiculobullous rash [76] rash grade 3–4: 3.9% [76] dry skin: all: 20.6% [76] dry skin: grade 3–4: 0% [76]	SJS: 1 literature report [6] 11 Medwatch reports [6] TEN: 2 literature reports [6] 16 Medwatch reports [6]	–	Alopecia [76]	–
Lenalidomide (Revlimid)	Within MM patients: All grades: rash: 21.2% [87] increased sweating: 9.9% [87] dry skin: 9.3% [87] pruritus: 7.6% [87] Within MDS patients: pruritus: 41.9% [87] rash: 35.8% (0.6 grade 3) [87] dry skin: 14.2% [87] contusion: 8.1% night sweats: 8.1% [87] increased sweating: 6.8% [87] ecchymosis: 5.4% [87] erythema: 5.4% [87]	SJS: 12 reports [88] TEN:1 report [88]	–	–	–

MDS, myelodysplastic syndromes; MM, multiple myeloma; SJS: Stevens–Johnson syndrome, TEN: toxic epidermal necrolysis [6].

22 Skin Toxicities due to Biotherapy

Kathryn T. Ciccolini[1], Katharina C. Kaehler[2], Mario E. Lacouture[1] and Axel Hauschild[2]

[1]Dermatology Service, Memorial Sloan-Kettering Cancer Center, New York, NY, USA
[2]University of Kiel, Kiel, Germany

Biotherapy has been used in medicinal practice since Edward Jenner's inoculation of cowpox to induce immunity in 1876 [1]. The acceptance of the immune surveillance theory of cancer development allowed for future use of this innovative new approach to cancer treatment [2,3]. Over the past few decades, biotherapy has been more clearly elucidated through novel research tools [2,4–6].

Biotherapy shifts the balance of the immune system to reject malignant cell growth by building an immune response that overcomes the immunosuppressive tumor microenvironment [7–9]. This shift allows immune cells to target and destroy malignant cells that would otherwise evade immunosurveillance [10] through mechanisms such as tumor escape, immunoediting, and tumor-induced immunosuppression [3]. The basic goals of anticancer biotherapy are to stimulate immunocompetence, create tumor-specific immunity, and induce tumor regression, when used with other cancer treatments [2].

Interferon α2b (IFN-α2b) and interleukin-2 (IL-2) are antitumor biotherapy cytokines that are approved for the treatment of certain cancers (Table 22.1) [2]. Cytokines regulate the immune response, hematopoiesis, inflammation, wound repair, and tissue development, and are profoundly involved in cellular growth and differentiation [4,11]. The first class of cytokines includes lymphokines and monokines. The second and third classes include growth factors and colony stimulating factors [11,12]. Dermatologic adverse events (AEs) with these agents have a characteristic presentation described in this chapter (Figure 22.1).

Interferon α

IFN-α are cytokines with antiviral, antiproliferative, antineoplastic, and immunomodulatory properties [11,13]. Endogenous IFN-α is produced and secreted by the majority of white blood cells [11].

They produce many systemic effects but, most importantly, they stimulate direct inhibition and toxicity to normal and malignant cells, and augment immune recognition [14,15]. Although IFN-α are generated mainly in response to viral or microbial infection, they contribute significantly to the immune response shift towards the rejection of cancer [14]. Recombinant forms of IFN-α are most frequently utilized in the clinical setting, whereas the natural form is uncommonly used in oncologic indications [14]. The mechanism of action of IFN-α has not been fully elucidated [16].

Interferon α2b

IFN-α2b is prepared using recombinant DNA technology in genetically modified *Escherichia coli* [17–19]. It is administered intramuscularly, intravenously, subcutaneously, or directly into the lesion (intralesional) [19,20]. Indications include AIDS-related Kaposi sarcoma, follicular lymphoma, hairy cell leukemia, and melanoma [19,21].

Dermatologic AEs to IFN-α

The main dermatologic AEs of IFN-α are alopecia [13,22–25], autoimmune cutaneous disorders, most commonly new onset psoriasis or exacerbation [13,22,24,26–39], rashes (Figure 22.2 and Figure 22.3) [13,22–24,33,34], and injection site reactions [13,22,23,28,35]. Cutaneous AEs to IFN-α have been reported in 5–12% of patients, and are usually mild to moderate in severity [13]. These dermatologic AEs usually resolve without pharmacologic management or dose modifications, and improve within 24–48 hours of cessation of therapy [13,23].

IFN-α alopecia has been reported in 8–38% of patients [36,37], as a result of cell growth inhibition and direct cytotoxic effects on the follicular cells [22,23]. Most patients describe mild loss of hair; however, excessive eyelash growth [24], hair discoloration [23,25], Pohl–Pinkus hair constriction [25], and telogen effluvium [25,28] have also been reported.

Dermatologic Principles and Practice in Oncology: Conditions of the Skin, Hair, and Nails in Cancer Patients, First Edition. Edited by Mario E. Lacouture.
© 2014 John Wiley & Sons, Inc. Published 2014 by John Wiley & Sons, Inc.

Autoimmunity and effective tumor immunity have been considered as two sides of the immune phenomenon, suggesting autoimmunity as a correlate of therapeutic benefit [15]. Patients on IFN-α therapy have been reported to experience autoimmune reactions such as exacerbation of psoriasis [13,24,27–29,31] in ≤5% of patients [37], new onset psoriasis [13,24,26,28, 29,31], anasarca [13], eosinophilic fasciitis [13], paraneoplastic pemphigus [13], systemic lupus erythematosus [13], and cutaneous vasculature changes [28,38]. Psoriasis is a chronic autoimmune disorder of the skin characterized by inflammation of the dermis and abnormal epidermal proliferation [39] which may be exacerbated or triggered by IFN-α therapy and may have an inverse relationship with psoriasis and disease progression [13,27,29]. Data suggest that IFN-α has a role in psoriasis pathophysiology [27]; psoriasis patients have increased levels of autoantibodies against IFN-α, increased IFN-α in sera, and IFN-α has been encountered in psoriatic lesions (Figure 22.4) [24,27,29].

The clinical presentation of rashes resulting from IFN-α has not been systematically described, but in ≤25% [37] the rashes are generalized [22], maculopapular [24], or unspecified [13]. Pruritus [13,22,23], xerosis [13], and urticaria [23,24] are frequently associated. Development of vesiculopapules [13] and unspecified skin lesions [40] have also been reported. The underlying mechanisms are not well understood but include the expression of adhesion molecules by dermal vascular endothelial cells, and cytokine overproduction causing increased vascular permeability [13].

Injection site reactions develop in ≤20% of patients [22,37] and are described as erythematous [22,28], indurated [22,28], hard [13], painful nodules [13,28], and edematous [13]. Ulceration [28], eczematous reactions [23], or tissue necrosis [13,28,36] are rarely reported. Frequent changes of injection sites have been found to be an adequate approach to prevent further, or worsening of site reactions [23]. A local enhancement of cutaneous immunity, cutaneous infarction related to capillary and venous thrombosis, hypercoagulation, and cytokine overproduction are believed to underlie these reactions [13].

Interleukins

Interleukins (IL) are cytokines that have pleiotropic effects on innate and cellular immunity. IL also have antineoplastic properties [41]. The name interleukin derives from the ability of cytokines to communicate between (inter) various white blood cells (leukins) [11,42].

Table 22.1 Classification of biotherapies.

Recombinant biologic response modifier Antitumor biotherapy Cytokine	Interferon-α2b (Intron A) [4,13]
Recombinant biologic response modifier Antitumor biotherapy Cytokine	Interleukin-2 (Aldesleukin) [4]

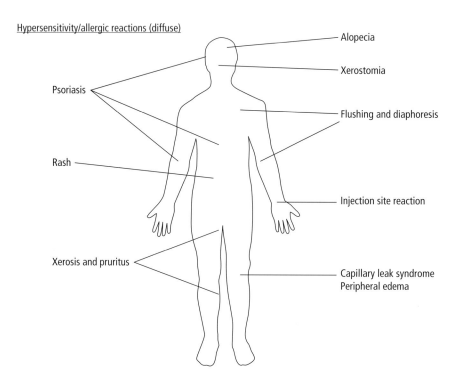

Hypersensitivity/allergic reactions (diffuse)

Alopecia

Xerostomia

Psoriasis

Flushing and diaphoresis

Rash

Injection site reaction

Xerosis and pruritus

Capillary leak syndrome
Peripheral edema

Figure 22.1 Anatomic location of dermatologic adverse events to interferon-α2b and interleukin-2.

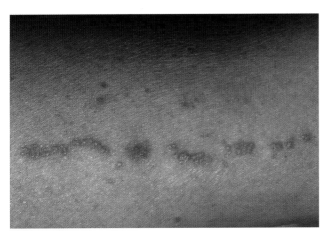

Figure 22.2 Lichen ruber-type reaction to interferon α.

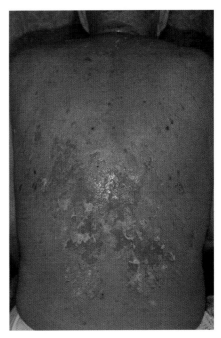

Figure 22.4 Exacerbation of Hailey–Hailey disease (benign familial pemphigus) by interferon α.

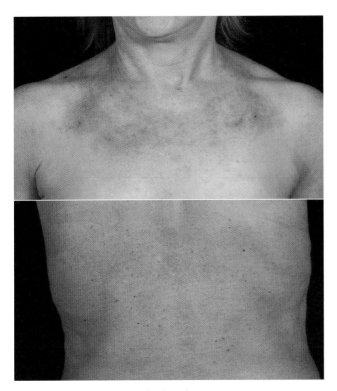

Figure 22.3 Interferon α-induced rash grade 1.

Interleukin 2

IL-2 is a secretory product of T cells that alters immunity by binding to specific immune cell receptors [43,44]. IL-2 stimulates T-cell proliferation, as well as lymphoid cell (B cells, lymphokine activate killer cells, natural killer) expansion. This leads to a secondary release of other cytokines including interferons, tumor necrosis factor (TNF), and IL-1, inducing cytolytic activity in a tumor antigen nonspecific and specific manner [11,12,43–53] The only preparation available for clinical use is aldesleukin (Proleukin); a recombinant version of IL-2 that is administered

intravenously or subcutaneously [54–56]. Approved indications include metastatic renal cell carcinoma and metastatic melanoma (as monotherapy, or in combination regimens) in adults [54,57,58].

Dermatologic AEs to IL-2

IL-2 treatment is associated with various AEs that virtually involve every organ system [44]; however, the main AE is capillary leak syndrome [14,51,53,59–63], leading to edema [48,51–53,59, 61,62,64–67] and erythematous macular rashes [44,46,48, 49–53,59,61–63,65,66,68–79], erythema nodosum [50], desquamation [44,48,49,53,59,62,63,65,69,73,80], xerosis [59,65], urticaria [73,77], burning [44,50,51,53,59,61,63], pruritus [44, 46,48–53,59,61–68,70,71,73,75,80,81], and dermatitis [44,46,49, 50,53,59,63,80]. Additional AEs include bullous eruptions [50,51,61,65,71,80,82], injection site reactions (Figure 22.5 and Figure 22.6) [48,51,79,83], iodinated radiographic contrast allergy [48,61], psoriasis exacerbation [44,48,49,53,59–61,63], and cutaneous bacterial infections [44,48,63]. The pathophysiology underlying these events is likely cutaneous inflammation [59]. Appearance of AE may occur on the first to third day [50,53, 59,61,65,69,71], reversing within approximately 24–48 hours of therapy cessation [46,48,49,51,53,67]. Most dermatologic AEs are dose dependent, but relatively mild, reversible, and do not require altered dosing [48,50,53,59,63,80].

Fluid shift from the vascular space to the interstitial tissue resulting from an increased vascular permeability is one of the major AEs with IL-2 [48,63,67]. This fluid redistribution manifests as peripheral edema, and can affect areas such as the face, neck,

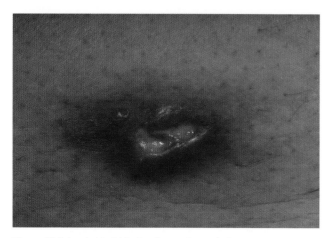

Figure 22.5 Interleukin-2 injection site reaction grade 1.

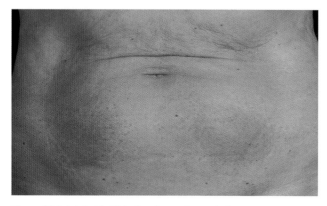

Figure 22.6 Interleukin-2 injection site reaction grade 2.

and bilateral lower extremities [48,80]. It is thought to result from IL-2 induced neutrophil activation and binding to endothelial cells, resulting in thromboxane release and consequent vasodilatation. Furthermore, heightened C -reactive protein synthesis and increased levels of complement proteins result in vasodilatation and increased vascular permeability [48]. When severe, it may limit dosing, as decreased systemic vascular resistance and increased capillary permeability leads to intravascular fluid loss in soft tissues [67].

Rashes occur in 20–100% of patients on IL-2 [49,69,70,74,75–78]. The intracellular communication of cytokines within skin, and increased expression of intercellular adhesion molecule 1 (ICAM-1) in keratinocytes likely results in the characteristic rash [49,50,59,71,83]. A macular erythema with burning and pruritus on the head and neck that begins 24–72 hours after IL-2 administration has been described. Although one study reported postinflammatory desquamation lasting 14–20 days [71], occasional generalization followed by desquamation occurs within 48–72 hours of cessation of therapy [46,49–51,53].

References

1 Waldmann, T.A. (2003) Immunotherapy: past, present and future. *Nature Medicine*, **9**, 269–277.
2 Shelton, B.K., Ziegfeld, C.R. & Olsen, M.M. (2004) *Sidney Kimmel Comprehensive Cancer Center at Johns Hopkins University. The Manual of Cancer Nursing*, 2nd ed., Lippincott Williams & Wilkins, Philadelphia.
3 Swann, J.B. & Smyth, M.J. (2007) Immune surveillance of tumors. *Journal of Clinical Investigation*, **117**, 1137–1146.
4 Oldham, R.K. & Dillman, R.O. (2009) *Principles of Cancer Biotherapy*, 5th ed., Springer, London, New York.
5 Sandstrom, S.K. (1996) Nursing management of patients receiving biological therapy. *Seminars in Oncology Nursing*, **12**, 152–162.
6 Finn, O.J. (2008) Molecular origins of cancer: cancer immunology. *New England Journal of Medicine*, **358**, 2704–2715.
7 Ribas, A., Butterfield, L.H., Glaspy, J.A. & Economou, J.S. (2003) Current developments in cancer vaccines and cellular immunotherapy. *Journal of Clinical Oncology*, **21**, 2415–2432.
8 Immunotherapy: Cancer and the Power of Your (Health after 50): The John Hopkins Medical Letter. (2011) 22, 4–5.
9 National Cancer Institute; US National Institutes of Health (2006) Biologic therapies for cancer: questions and answers. Available from: http://www.cancer.gov/cancertopics/factsheet/Therapy/biological (accessed 10 April 2013).
10 Hoos, A., Eggermont, A.M.M., Janetzki, S. et al. (2010) Improved endpoints for cancer immunotherapy trials. *Journal of the National Cancer Institute*, **102**, 1388–1397.
11 Corwin, E.J. (2000) Understanding cytokines. Part I: physiology and mechanism of action. *Biological Research for Nursing*, **2**, 30–40.
12 Newton, S., Jackowski, C. & Marrs, J. (2002) Biotherapy skin reaction. *Clinical Journal of Oncology Nursing*, **6**, 181–182.
13 Stafford-Fox, V. & Guindon, K.M. (2000) Cutaneous reactions associated with alpha interferon therapy. *Clinical Journal of Oncology Nursing*, **4**, 164–168.
14 DeVita, V.T., Theodore, S.L. & Rosenberg, A.S. (2008) *Cancer: Principles and Practice of Oncology*, 8th ed., Wolters Kluwer/Lippincott Williams & Wilkins, Philadelphia.
15 Ferrantini, M., Capone, I. & Belardelli, F. (2007) Interferon-α and cancer: mechanisms of action and new perspectives of clinical use. *Biochimie*, **89**, 884–893.
16 Lexicomp Online. Interferon-alfa stability: actions. Available from: http://online.lexi.com/crlsql/servlet/crlonline (accessed on 2 May 2011).
17 US Food and Drug Administration. Interferon alfa-2b: drug details original approval. Available from: http://www.accessdata.fda.gov/scripts/cder/drugsatfda/ (accessed 10 April 2013).
18 US Food and Drug Administration. Interferon alfa-2b: label and approval history. Available from: http://www.accessdata.fda.gov/scripts/cder/drugsatfda/ (accessed 10 April 2013).
19 Schering Corporation (2011) Intron-A product information: package insert. Available from: http://www.spfiles.com/piintrona.pdf (accessed 10 April 2013).
20 Thomson Reuters. Interferon alfa-2b mechanism of action and pharmacokinetics. Available from: http://www.micromedexsolutions.com/ (accessed 5 May 2013).

21 Thomson Reuters. Interferon alfa-2b clinical applications: Dosing and indications: FDA-labeled indications Available from: http://www.micromedexsolutions.com/ (accessed 5 May 2013).

22 Sleijfer, S., Bannink, M., Van Gool, A.R., Kruit, W.H.J. & Stoter, G. (2005) Side effects of interferon-α therapy. *Pharmacy World and Science*, **27**, 423–431.

23 Guillot, B., Blazquez, L., Bessis, D., Dereure, O. & Guilhou, J.J. (2004) A prospective study of cutaneous adverse events induced by low-dose alpha-interferon treatment for malignant melanoma. *Dermatology (Basel, Switzerland)*, **208**, 49–54.

24 Quesada, J.R., Talpaz, M. & Rios, A. (1986) Clinical toxicity of interferons in cancer patients: a review. *Journal of Clinical Oncology*, **4**, 234–243.

25 Tosti, A., Misciali, C., Bardazzi, F., Fanti, P.A. & Varotti, C. (1992) Telogen effluvium due to recombinant interferon alpha-2b. *Dermatology (Basel, Switzerland)*, **184**, 124–125.

26 Jucgla, A., Marcoval, J., Curco, N. & Servitje, O. (1991) Psoriasis with articular involvement induced by interferon alfa [6]. *Archives of Dermatology*, **127**, 910–911.

27 Quesada, J.R. & Gutterman, J.U. (1986) Psoriasis and alpha-interferon. *Lancet*, **1**, 1466–1468.

28 Chang, L.W., Liranzo, M. & Bergfeld, W.F. (1995) Cutaneous side effects associated with interferon-alpha therapy: a review. *Cutis: Cutaneous Medicine for the Practitioner*, **56**, 144.

29 Bergman, R., Ramon, M., Wildbaum, G. *et al.* (2009) Psoriasis patients generate increased serum levels of autoantibodies to tumor necrosis factor-α and interferon-α. *Journal of Dermatological Science*, **56**, 163–167.

30 Papini, M., Bruni, P.L. & Gaspari, A.A. (1996) Cutaneous reactions to recombinant cytokine therapy [5]. *Journal of the American Academy of Dermatology*, **35**, 1021–1022.

31 Funk, J., Langeland, T., Schrumpf, E. & Hanssen, L.E. (1991) Psoriasis induced by interferon-α. *British Journal of Dermatology*, **125**, 463–465.

32 Parodi, A., Semino, M., Gallo, R. & Rebora, A. (1993) Bullous eruption with circulating pemphigus-like antibodies following interferon-alpha therapy. *Dermatology (Basel, Switzerland)*, **186**, 155–157.

33 Dutcher, J.P., Fisher, R.I. & Weiss, G. (1997) Outpatient Subcutaneous interleukin-2 and interferon-alpha for metastatic renal cell carcinoma: five-year follow-up of the Cytokine Working Group study. *Cancer Journal From Scientific American*, **3**, 157–162.

34 Ridolfi, R., Maltoni, R., Riccobon, A., Flamini, E. & Amadori, D. (1992) Evaluation of toxicity in 22 patients treated with subcutaneous interleukin-2, alpha-interferon with and without chemotherapy. *Journal of Chemotherapy*, **4**, 394–398.

35 Atzpodien, J., Kirchner, H., De Mulder, P. *et al.* (1993) Subcutaneous recombinant interleukin-2 and a-interferon in patients with advanced renal cell carcinoma: results of a multicenter phase II study. *Cancer Biotherapy*, **8**, 289–300.

36 Thomson Reuters. Interferon alfa-2b adverse effects: common. Available from: http://www.micromedexsolutions.com/ (accessed 5 May 2013).

37 UpToDate. Interferon alfa 2b adverse reactions. Available from: www.uptodate.com/index (accessed 10 April 2013).

38 Sangster, G., Kaye, S.B., Calman, K.C. & Toy, J.L. (1983) Cutaneous vasculitis associated with interferon. *European Journal of Cancer and Clinical Oncology*, **19**, 1647–1649.

39 Camisa, C. (2009) Psoriasis: papulosquamous skin disease. Disease Management Project. Cleveland Clinic, OH.

40 Dow, L.W., Raimondi, S.C., Culbert, S.J., Ochs, J., Kennedy, W. & Pinkel, D.P. (1991) Response to alpha-interferon in children with Philadelphia chromosome- positive chronic myelocytic leukemia. *Cancer*, **68**, 1678–1684.

41 Lexicomp Online. Aldesleukin introduction, AFHS essentials. Available from: http://online.lexi.com/crlsql/servlet/crlonline (accessed 10 April 2013).

42 Lexicomp Online. Aldesleukin stability: actions. Available from: http://online.lexi.com/crlsql/servlet/crlonline (accessed 10 April 2013).

43 Chodorowska, G., Czelej, D. & Niewiedziol, M. (2003) Interleukin-2 and its soluble receptor in selected drug-induced cutaneous reactions. *Annales Universitatis Mariae Curie-Sklodowska. Sectio D: Medicina*, **58**, 7–13.

44 Mier, J.W., Aronson, F.R., Numerof, R.P., Vachino, G. & Atkins, M.B. (1988) Toxicity of immunotherapy with interleukin-2 and lymphokine-activated killer cells. *Pathology and Immunopathology Research*, **7**, 459–476.

45 Reichert, T.E., Watkins, S., Stanson, J., Johnson, J.T. & Whiteside, T.L. (1998) Endogenous IL-2 in cancer cells: a marker of cellular proliferation. *Journal of Histochemistry and Cytochemistry*, **46**, 603–611.

46 Wiener, J.S., Tucker, J.A. Jr. & Walther, P.J. (1992) Interleukin-2-induced dermatotoxicity resembling toxic epidermal necrolysis. *Southern Medical Journal*, **85**, 656–659.

47 Kruit, W.H.J., Goey, S.H., Monson, J.R.T. *et al.* (1991) Clinical experience with the combined use of recombinant interleukin-2 (IL2) and interferon alfa-2a (IFNα) in metastatic melanoma. *British Journal of Haematology, Supplement*, **79**, 84–86.

48 Sundin, D.J. & Wolin, M.J. (1998) Toxicity management in patients receiving low-dose aldesleukin therapy. *Annals of Pharmacotherapy*, **32**, 1344–1352.

49 Blessing, K., Park, K.G.M., Heys, S.D., King, G. & Eremin, O. (1992) Immunopathological changes in the skin following recombinant interleukin-2 treatment. *Journal of Pathology*, **167**, 313–319.

50 Segura Huerta, A.A., Tordera, P., Cercós, A.C., Yuste, A.L., López-Tendero, P. & Reynés, G. (2002) Toxic epidermal necrolysis associated with interleukin-2. *Annals of Pharmacotherapy*, **36**, 1171–1174.

51 O'Reilly, F., Feldman, E., Yang, J., Hwu, P. & Turner, M.L. (2003) Recurring cutaneous eruption in a patient with metastatic renal cell carcinoma being treated with high-dose interleukin 2. *Journal of the American Academy of Dermatology*, **48**, 602–604.

52 Jones, M., Philip, T., Palmer, P. *et al.* (1993) The impact of interleukin-2 on survival in renal cancer: a multivariate analysis. *Cancer Biotherapy*, **8**, 275–288.

53 Gaspari, A.A., Lotze, M.T., Rosenberg, S.A., Stern, J.B. & Katz, S.I. (1987) Dermatologic changes associated with interleukin 2 administration. *Journal of the American Medical Association*, **258**, 1624–1629.

54 Daily Med. Proleukin (aldesleukin) injection, powder, lyophilized, for solution. Available from: http://dailymed.nlm.nih.gov/dailymed/drugInfo.cfm?id=23439)accessed 10 April 2013).

55 US Food and Drug Administration. Aldesleukin: drug details original approval. Available from: http://www.accessdata.fda.gov/scripts/cder/drugsatfda/ (accessed 10 April 2013).

56 US Food and Drug Administration. Aldesleukin: label and approval history. Available from: http://www.accessdata.fda.gov/scripts/cder/drugsatfda/ (accessed 10 April 2013).

57 Thomson Reuters. Aldesleukin clinical applications: therapeutic uses. Available from: http://www.micromedexsolutions.com/ (accessed 5 May 2013).

58 Thomson Reuters. Aldesleukin clinical applications: dosing and indications – FDA labeled indications. Available from: http://www.micromedexsolutions.com/ (accessed 5 May 2013).

59 Wolkenstein, P., Chosidow, O., Wechsler, J. et al. (1993) Cutaneous side effects associated with interleukin 2 administration for metastatic melanoma. *Journal of the American Academy of Dermatology*, **28**, 66–70.

60 Cork, M.J., Keohane, S.G., Gawkrodger, D.J., Hancock, B.W., Sheridan, E. & Bleehen, S.S. (1997) Cytokine dermatosis: reactivation of eczema during interleukin-2 infusion. *British Journal of Dermatology*, **136**, 644–645.

61 Vial, T. & Descotes, J. (1992) Clinical toxicity of interleukin-2. *Drug Safety*, **7**, 417–433.

62 Kolitz, J.E. & Mertelsmann, R. (1991) The immunotherapy of human cancer with Interleukin 2: present status and future directions. *Cancer Investigation*, **9**, 529–542.

63 Siegel, J.P. & Puri, R.K. (1991) Interleukin-2 toxicity. *Journal of Clinical Oncology*, **9**, 694–704.

64 Rosenberg, S.A., Yang, J.C., Topalian, S.L. et al. (1994) Treatment of 283 consecutive patients with metastatic melanoma or renal cell cancer using high-dose bolus interleukin 2. *Journal of the American Medical Association*, **271**, 907–913.

65 Hofmann, M., Audring, H., Sterry, W. & Trefzer, U. (2005) Interleukin-2-associated bullous drug dermatosis. *Dermatology (Basel, Switzerland)*, **210**, 74–75.

66 Yamamoto, T. & Tsuboi, R. (2008) Interleukin-2-induced seborrhoeic dermatitis-like eruption [7]. *Journal of the European Academy of Dermatology and Venereology*, **22**, 244–245.

67 Rosenberg, S.A., Lotze, M.T. & Muul, L.M. (1987) A progress report on the treatment of 157 patients with advanced cancer using lymphokine-activated killer cells and interleukin-2 or high-dose interleukin-2 alone. *New England Journal of Medicine*, **316**, 889–897.

68 Thomson Reuters. Aldesleukin cautions: adverse reactions. Available from: http://www.micromedexsolutions.com/ (accessed 5 May 2013).

69 Higuchi, C.M., Thompson, J.A., Petersen, F.B., Buckner, C.D. & Fefer, A. (1991) Toxicity and immunomodulatory effects of interleukin-2 after autologous bone marrow transplantation for hematologic malignancies. *Blood*, **77**, 2561–2568.

70 Sano, T., Saijo, N., Sasaki, Y. et al. (1988) Three schedules of recombinant human interleukin-2 in the treatment of malignancy: side effects and immunologic effects in relation to serum level. *Japanese Journal of Cancer Research*, **79**, 131–143.

71 Dummer, R., Miller, K., Eilles, C. & Burg, G. (1991) The skin: an immunoreactive target organ during interleukin-2 administration? *Dermatologica*, **183**, 95–99.

72 Marolda, R., Belli, F., Prada, A. et al. (1987) A phase I study of recombinant interleukin 2 in melanoma patients: toxicity and clinical effects. *Tumori*, **73**, 575–584.

73 Sondel, P.M., Kohler, P.C., Hank, J.A. et al. (1988) Clinical and immunological effects of recombinant interleukin 2 given by repetitive weekly cycles to patients with cancer. *Cancer Research*, **48**, 2561–2567.

74 Thompson, J.A., Lee, D.J., Lindgren, C.G. et al. (1988) Influence of dose and duration of infusion of interleukin-2 on toxicity and immunomodulation. *Journal of Clinical Oncology*, **6**, 669–678.

75 Fyfe, G., Fisher, R.I., Rosenberg, S.A., Sznol, M., Parkinson, D.R. & Louie, A.C. (1995) Results of treatment of 255 patients with metastatic renal cell carcinoma who received high-dose recombinant interleukin-2 therapy. *Journal of Clinical Oncology*, **13**, 688–696.

76 West, W.H., Tauer, K.W. & Yannelli, J.R. (1987) Constant-infusion recombinant interleukin-2 in adoptive immunotherapy of advanced cancer. *New England Journal of Medicine*, **316**, 898–905.

77 Sosman, J.A., Kohler, P.C., Hank, J. et al. (1988) Repetitive weekly cycles of recombinant human interleukin-2: responses of renal carcinoma with acceptable toxicity. *Journal of the National Cancer Institute*, **80**, 60–63.

78 Urba, W.J., Steis, R.G., Longo, D.L. et al. (1990) Immunomodulatory properties and toxicity of interleukin 2 in patients with cancer. *Cancer Research*, **50**, 185–192.

79 Stein, R.C., Malkovska, V., Morgan, S. et al. (1991) The clinical effects of prolonged treatment of patients with advanced cancer with lose-dose subcutaneous interleukin 2. *British Journal of Cancer*, **63**, 275–278.

80 Staunton, M.R., Scully, M.C., Le Boit, P.E. & Aronson, F.R. (1991) Life-threatening bullous skin eruptions during interleukin-2 therapy. *Journal of the National Cancer Institute*, **83**, 56–57.

81 Rosenberg, S.A., Lotze, M.T., Yang, J.C. et al. (1989) Experience with the use of high-dose interleukin-2 in the treatment of 652 cancer patients. *Annals of Surgery*, **210**, 474–485.

82 Fellner, M.J. (1993) Drug-induced bullous pemphigoid. *Clinics in Dermatology*, **11**, 515–520.

83 Meropol, N.J., Porter, M., Blumenson, L.E. et al. (1996) Daily subcutaneous injection of low-dose interleukin 2 expands natural killer cells in vivo without significant toxicity. *Clinical Cancer Research*, **2**, 669–677.

84 Wagner, R.F. Jr. & Sanchez, R.L. (1991) Presentation of sebaceous carcinoma and dermatofibrosarcoma protuberans subsequent to intralesional interferon alfa-2b for the treatment of in situ squamous cell carcinoma [10]. *Archives of Dermatology*, **127**, 272.

85 Thomas, R. & Stea, B. (2002) Radiation recall dermatitis from high-dose interferon alfa-2b [4]. *Journal of Clinical Oncology*, **20**, 355–357.

86 UpToDate. Aldesleukin adverse effects. Available from: www.uptodate.com/index (accessed 10 April 2013).

87 Lexicomp Online. Aldesleukin cautions. Available from: www.online.lexi.com (accessed 10 April 2013).

Appendix 22.1 Incidence of dermatologic adverse events to biotherapies (interferon-a2a, interferon-a2b, interleukin 2).

Drug name (Trade)	Dermatologic adverse events			
	Cutaneous and subcutaneous		**Hair**	**Mucous membranes**
Interferon-α2b (Intron A)	Rashes (≤25%) [37] (5–23%) [22]: • Generalized [22] (%NR) • Erythematous [13,24] (≤5%) [37] • Erythema multiforme (≤5%) [37] • Pruritus [5,13,22,23] (≤11%) [37] • Purpura [13] (≤5%) [37] • Maculopapular [13,24] (≤5%) [37] • Unspecified type [13] (%NR) • Urticaria [23,24] (≤5%) [37] • Xerosis [13] (≤10%) [37] Psoriasis: • General [22,27,29,31] (%NR) • Exacerbation [13,24,27,28] (≤5%,) [37] • *De novo* [13,24,26,28] (%NR) Autoimmune blistering eruptions • Paraneoplastic pemphigus [13] (%NR) • Bullous eruption pemphigus [32] (%NR) Angioedema [23] (≤5%) [37] Cellulitis (≤5%) [37] Cutaneous vascular lesions [13] (%NR) Cutaneous vasculitis [28,38] (%NR) Development of vesicopapules [13] (%NR) Dermatitis (<8%) [37] Dermatofibrosarcoma protuberans [84] (%NR) Eosinophilic fasciitis [13] (%NR) Eczema (≤5%) [37] Herpes (≤5%) [37]: • Labiales [13] (%NR) • Recurrence [23] (%NR) Leukocytoplastic vasculitis [22] (%NR) Pityriasis versicolor [23] (3%) [23] Radiation recall dermatitis [85] (%NR) Raynaud phenomenon [23] (30%) [23] Sebaceous carcinoma [84] (%NR) Seborrheic dermatitis [23] (9%) [23] Skin lesions [40] (10%) [40] Steven–Johnson syndrome (≤5%) [37] Systemic lupus erythematosus [13] (≤5%) [22,37] Toxic epidermal necrolysis (≤5%) [37] Vitiligo [13,22,23] (3%) [23] Lichen planus [22,30] (%NR) Photosensitivity (≤5%) [37]	Injection site reactions (≤20%) [22,37]: • Necrosis [13,28] (≤5%) [37] • Erythema [22,28] (%NR) • Eczematous reaction [23] (39%) [23] • Induration [14,22] (%NR) • Hardness [13] (%NR) • Pain/painful (%NR) • Nodules [13,28] (%NR) • Deep tissue necrosis [13] (%NR) • Swelling [13] (%NR) • Ulceration [28] (%NR) • Anasarca [13] (≤10%) [37]	Alopecia [13,22–25] (≤38%) [36,37] Excessive eyelash growth [24] (%NR) Hair discoloration [23] (19%) [23] Pohl–Pinkus hair constriction [23] (%NR) Telogen effluvium [25,28] (20–30%) [25]	Xerostomia [13,23] (≤28%) [37] Buccal aphthous ulcer [23] (3%) [23] Stomatitis (≤5%) [37]

(Continued)

Drug name (Trade)	Dermatologic adverse events			
	Cutaneous and subcutaneous		Hair	Mucous membranes
Interleukin -2 (Aldesleukin)	Rash: • General [49,69,70,72,74–78] (20–100%) [69,70,74,76–78] • Erythema [48,49,51–53,59,61,63,65,66,69–71,79](50–100%) [49,52,53,70] • Erythema nodosum [50] (%NR) • Erythematous macular eruption [44,46,50,51,53,62,71,73] (30–100%) [50,62,71,73] • Pruritus [44,46,48–53,59,61–67,70,71,73,75,80,81](20–100%) [50,53,62,71,73] • Burning [44,50,51,53,59,61,63] (100%) [53] • Urticaria [59,73,77] (4%) [77] (<1%) [86] • Xerosis [48,59,65] (%NR) • Desquamation/scaling [44,48,49,53,59,62,63,69,73,80] (60–100%) [63,73] • Purpura or petechiae [59,61] (%NR) Bacterial infection: • *Staphylococcus aureus* [44,48,63] (%NR) • *Staphylococcus epidermis* [48,63] (%NR) Dermatitis: • Exfoliative [44,46,49,53,59,63,80] (4–100%) [49,53,59] • Pruritic [50] (%NR) • Spongiotic [80] (%NR) Iodinated radiographic contrast media skin allergy: • Pruritus [48] (%NR) • Rash [48] (%NR) • Edema [48,61] (%NR) Exacerbation of psoriasis [44,49,53,59–61,63] (10%) [53] Cellulitis (<1%) [86,87] Icterus [53] (%NR) Multifocal fixed drug eruption [51] (%NR) Necrotic lesions [59] (%NR) Photosensitivity [49] (10%) [49] Recurrence of eczema [60] (%NR) Seborrheic dermatitis [66] (%NR) Vitiligo [87] (%NR)	Capillary leak syndrome [14,51,53,59–63] (%NR) Dermatomyositis [63] (%NR) Edema [51–53,59,64] [61,62,65–67], (1–60%) [52,64,67] Scleroderma (<1%) [86] Stevens–Johnson syndrome (<1%) [86,87] Toxic epidermal necrolysis [46,50,78] (%NR) Bullous eruption (<1%) [87]: • Pemphigoid [80,82] (4%) [82] (<1%) [86] • Pemphigus vulgaris [65] (%NR) • Life-threatening eruption [46,50,51,61,80] (2%) [80] • Autoimmune bullous dermatosis [65] (%NR) • Linear IgA bullous dermatosis [65] (%NR) • Tense blisters [59,71,80] (%NR) Injection site reaction: • Cellulitis [87] (%NR) • Nodules [48] (%NR) • Induration [48,83] (%NR) • Erythema [79,83] (25%) [79] • Pruritus [79] (100%) [79] • Pain [83] (%NR) • Necrosis [81] (<1%) [81,87]		Alopecia [44] (%NR) Telogen effluvium [53,61] (10%) [53]	Aphthous ulcers [51] (%NR) Dry eyes [48] (%NR) Glossitis [44,53,59,61] (30%) [53] Mucositis [44,52,61,81] (<10%) [52,81] Painful erosions in buccal mucosa [59] (%NR) Stomatitis [63,75,76] (12–25%) [75,76]

%NR, percentage not reported.

23 Monoclonal Antibodies

Caroline Robert

Dermatology Department, Cancer Institute Gustave Roussy, Villejuif, France

Introduction

Several monoclonal antibodies (mAbs) are available to treat various cancers (Table 23.1). They are of various origins and can be differentiated by their suffix. The first mAbs produced originated from hybridomas between human myeloma cells and murine splenocytes. The murine mAbs suffix is -omab. However, the use of murine mAbs in humans resulted in their rapid removal from the blood, the occurrence of systemic inflammatory effects, and the production of human anti-mouse antibodies (HAMA). In an effort to overcome these obstacles, approaches using recombinant DNA have been explored since the late 1980s. Mouse DNA encoding the binding portion of a mAb was merged with human antibody-producing DNA in living cells, and chimeric (-ximab, 65% human) and humanized (-zumab, 95% human) mAbs have been produced. Later, scientists targeted the creation of "fully" human antibodies (-mumab) to avoid some of the adverse events (AEs) of humanized and chimeric antibodies.

Monoclonal antibody drugs that are used in cancer have three main mechanisms of action:

1. They can make cells more visible to the immune system by attaching to a specific protein expressed on a specific cell type. It is the case for example of rituximab (Rituxan®) which binds CD20 expressed on B cells and facilitates their destruction by the immune system.

2. mAbs can bind growth signal ligands or receptors and block signal transmission. This is the case for bevacizumab (Avastin®) and cetuximab (Erbitux®) which block vascular endothelial growth factor (VEGF) and epidermal growth factor receptor (EGFR), respectively.

3. mAbs can be used as vectors to deliver radiations or cytotoxic drugs or toxins to cancer cells. Ibritumomab (Zevalin®), approved for non-Hodgkin lymphoma, combines a monoclonal antibody

with radioactive particles. Gemtuzumab (Mylotarg®), which has been approved for the treatment of a certain type of acute myelogenous leukemia, is a mAb attached to a potent toxin and kills leukemic cells by delivering the toxin to the cells.

Some AEs of mAbs are generic, resulting from the molecular nature of the drugs, independently of their targets. These events are represented by hypersensitivity and infusion reactions. Their clinical presentation is not different from one mAb to another, although some mAbs are more frequently associated with infusion reactions than others. Other AEs are more specific of a considered mAb and usually result from the pharmacologic action of a given drug. In these cases, the symptoms can vary according to the target that is affected (Figure 23.1).

Effects linked to the nature of the mAbs

Clinical manifestations and mechanisms

Infusion reactions (e.g., pruritus, urticaria, rash, angioedema, hypotension, bronchospasm, and hypotension) can be seen with almost any mAb [1,2]. The exact mechanism of mAb-induced infusion reactions is not always clear. Hypersensitivity reactions classically result from immunoglobulin E (Ig-E) mediated release of histamine, leukotrienes, and prostaglandins from mast cells and basophils. The National Cancer Institute's Common Terminology Criteria for Adverse Events (NCI-CTCAE) distinguishes between allergic reactions and an acute reaction caused by cytokine release (Table 23.2). However, in the case of mAb-associated infusion reactions, specific IgE have rarely been found, and skin tests are not routinely performed. Chimeric and humanized mAbs could, in theory, elicit human antichimeric antibodies (HACAs) and human antihuman antibodies (HAHAs), respectively. However, no correlation could be demonstrated between infusion reactions and the level of HACAs or HAHAs [1].

Dermatologic Principles and Practice in Oncology: Conditions of the Skin, Hair, and Nails in Cancer Patients, First Edition. Edited by Mario E. Lacouture.
© 2014 John Wiley & Sons, Inc. Published 2014 by John Wiley & Sons, Inc.

Table 23.1 Monoclonal antibodies used in cancer.

Mab name	Trade name	Target	Cancer treated	Date of FDA approval
Rituximab	Rituxan	CD20	NHL	1997
Trastuzumab	Herceptin	HER2/neu	Breast	1998
Gemtuzumab ozogamicin	Mylotarg	CD33	AML	2000 on hold since June 2010
Alemtuzumab	Campath	CD52	CLL	2001
Ibritumomab Tiuxetan	Zevalin	CD20	NHL	2002
Tositumamab*	Bexxar	CD20	NHL	2003
Cetuximab	Erbitux	EGFR	CRC	2004
			H&NC	2006
Bevacizumab	Avastin	VEGF-A	CRC, NSCLC, breast, glioblastoma, RCC	2004–2009
Panitumumab	Vectibix	EGFR	CRC	2006
Ofatumumab	Arzerra	CD20	CLL	2009
Ipilimumab	Yervoy	CTLA4	Melanoma	2011

ALM, acute myeloid leukemia; CLL, chronic lymphocytic leukemia; CRC, colorectal cancer; FDA, United States Food and Drug Administration; NHL, non-Hodgkin lymphoma; NSCLC, nonsmall cell lung cancer; RCC, renal cell cancer.

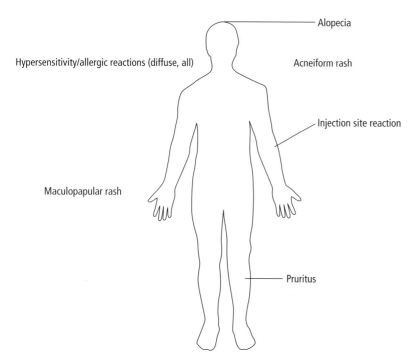

Alopecia

Hypersensitivity/allergic reactions (diffuse, all)

Acneiform rash

Injection site reaction

Maculopapular rash

Pruritus

Figure 23.1 Location of monoclonal antibody induced dermatologic adverse events.

The clinical manifestations of infusion reactions can be mild to moderate, with flushing, rash, fever, rigors, chills, dyspnea, and mild hypotension (grades 1 and 2). Severe reactions (grades 3 and 4) can be associated with severe bronchospasms and hypotension.

The incidence of mAb-associated infusion reactions is quite high for grade 1 and 2 reactions, especially during the first infusions: 77% with rituximab, 40% with trastuzumab, almost 20% with cetuximab, and 5% with the fully humanized panitumumab [1]. Grade 3 and 4 reactions are rare: less than 10% with rituximab, 3% with cetuximab, and less than 1% with trastuzumab [1].

The timing of the infusion reaction varies with the agents. More frequently, it occurs during the first infusions. Cetuximab-associated severe reactions occur during the first infusion in 90% of the cases. However, delayed reactions are also seen. For example, rituximab induces infusion reactions in 77%, 30%, and 14% of cases during the first, fourth, and eighth infusions, respectively [2] (Figure 23.2).

Table 23.2 National Cancer Institute Common Terminology Criteria for Adverse Events version 4.0 (NCI-CTCAE v.4) for allergic reactions, anaphylaxis, and cytokine release syndrome.

Adverse event	Grade				
	1	**2**	**3**	**4**	**5**
Allergic reaction	Transient flushing or rash, drug fever <39°C (>100°F); intervention not indicated	Intervention or infusion interruption indicated; responds promptly to symptomatic treatment (e.g., antihistamines, NSAIDs, narcotics); prophylactic medications indicated for ≤24 hours	Prolonged (e.g., not rapidly responsive to symptomatic medication and/or brief interruption of infusion); recurrence of symptoms following initial improvement; hospitalization indicated for clinical sequelae (e.g., renal involvement, pulmonary infiltrate)	Life-threatening consequences; urgent intervention indicated	Death
Anaphylaxis	–	–	Symptomatic bronchospasm with or without urticaria; parenteral intervention indicated, allergy-related edema/angioedema; hypotension	Life-threatening consequences; urgent intervention indicated	Death
Cytokine release syndrome	Mild reaction, infusion interruption not indicated; intervention not indicated	Therapy or infusion interruption indicated but responds promptly to symptomatic treatment (e.g., antihistamines, NSAIDs, narcotics, IV fluids); prophylactic medications indicated for ≤24 hours	Prolonged (e.g., not rapidly responsive to symptomatic medication and/or brief interruption of infusion); recurrence of symptoms following initial improvement; hospitalization indicated for clinical sequelae (e.g., renal involvement, pulmonary infiltrate)	Life-threatening consequences; pressor or ventilator support indicated	Death

A semi-colon indicates "or" within the description of the grade. A single dash (–) indicates a grade is not available. Not all grades are appropriate for all AEs. Therefore, some AEs are listed with fewer than five options for grade selection.

Management

Prevention

Relying on pharmacologic prophylaxis with antihistamines is recommended. This is usually the case for cetuximab and alemtuzumab. Patients should be monitored during and after all infusions, especially the first one. Patients should be asked to report any symptom during or after the infusion. As hypersensitivity reactions are unpredictable, immediate resuscitation measures should be available including emergency drugs: epinephrine, corticosteroids IV bronchodilatators, and oxygen.

Treatment

When a reaction occurs, the infusion should be stopped and symptomatic measures administered. Patients should be monitored until symptoms resolve. In most cases, patients who present with a mild to moderate infusion reaction during the first exposure of a mAb will tolerate retreatment with premedication using antihistamines and corticosteroids as well as a reduction of the infusion rate by half.

Rechallenge is not recommended for patients who present with a severe infusion reaction (grade 3 or 4). However, the decision to rechallenge a patient has to be made based on the analysis of the benefit : risk ratio on an individual basis.

Desensitization protocols can induce temporary tolerance and have yielded successful results with trastuzumab, for example (for additional information see Chapter 33)[3].

AEs caused by the function of the mAb

Cetuximab (Erbitux®) and panitumumab (Vectibix®) block the function of EGFR (EGFR; HER1). They both induce multiple and sometimes explosive dermatologic manifestations that are directly linked to the inhibition of EGFR. These skin AEs are very similar to the ones observed with small molecules inhibiting the intracellular kinase portion of the receptor, like erlotinib or afatinib. The main symptoms are a papulopustular acneiform rash, hair modifications, xerosis, paronychia, and mucositis. The skin manifestations of EGFR inhibitors are important because these drugs are now routinely used in diverse cancers and can be used for long periods of time. The resulting skin modifications are often painful, both physically and psychologically, and they frequently impact patients' quality of life as well as compliance to treatment. They have to be managed carefully. Information and education of the patient are key elements. These AEs are not treated in details here but are covered in another chapter of this book (see Chapter 17).

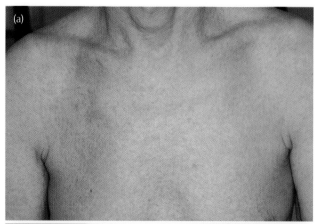

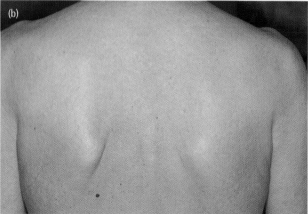

Figure 23.2 (a,b) Rituximab-induced maculopapular rash grade 1.

Bevacizumab (Avastin®) is a chimeric mouse-human mAb binding to VEGF and preventing it from binding to the VEGF receptor (VEGFR). Its toxicity profile is very different from the one of VEGFR inhibitors like sorafenib or sunitinib. The latter induce multiple and frequent AEs (see Chapter 18). Bevacizumab can nevertheless be associated with dermatologic AEs such as pruritus and nonspecific rashes, reported in 20% and 49% of patients, respectively [4,5].

Because of its potent antiangiogenic effect, bevacizumab inhibits scar formation and enhances bleeding [6]. This delay in wound healing is not restricted to skin wounds. Thus, to avoid bleeding and surgery complications, a delay of at least 5 weeks between bevacizumab treatment and invasive surgery procedures is mandatory [7]. Bevacizumab is also associated with a significantly increased risk of venous and arterial thrombosis [8,9].

Trastuzumab (Herceptin®) is a humanized IgG1-κ mAb targeting the HER2 receptor. It is not associated with specific skin toxicities, as opposed to HER1 (EGFR) inhibitors, which induce multiple and very frequent dermatologic AEs. In a first-line monotherapy study, alopecia was reported in 7% and rash in 20% of patients treated with trastuzumab [10].

A case of inflammatory skin rash with tufted hair folliculitis was recently reported but the attribution to trastuzumab was not confirmed [11].

Several mAbs target the CD20 molecule that is found on the surface of normal and malignant B lymphocytes. They can be combined with radioisotopes. Their use is not associated with significant dermatologic AEs.

Rituximab (Rituxan®) is a chimeric human-murine anti-CD20 mAb. Rare cases of severe mucocutaneous reactions have been described with the use of rituximab: paraneoplastic pemphigus, Stevens–Johnson syndrome (n = 18 cases reported to the US MedWatch database www.Asco.org/ASCOv2/Meetings/Abstracts), lichenoid or vesiculobullous dermatitis, and toxic epidermal necrolysis (TEN) [12]. Readministration is not recommended after a severe mucocutaneous reaction.

Ibritumomab tiuxetan (Zevalin®) is a murine IgG1κ mAb directed against the CD20 antigen associated with tiutexan, a linker-chelator with a high affinity for ^{90}Y and ^{111}In. Because of the binding of the radioactive isotopes, this drug is considered radio-immunotherapy. It is used in patients with B lymphomas after treatment with rituximab. As with rituximab, some rare cases of severe and sometimes fatal mucocutaneous reactions have been reported in post-marketing experience (drug monography): erythema multiforme, Steven–Johnson syndrome, TEN. Ibritumomab tiutexan should not be reintroduced after a severe (grade 3–4) mucocutaneous reaction.

Tositumomab (Bexxar®) is a radioimmunotherapeutic agent, a murine antihuman CD20 mAb covalently bound to the radioisotope iodine^{131}. It is used in the treatment of advanced follicular non-Hodgkin lymphoma. It is associated with an increased risk of infection, and can therefore be associated with various bacterial, viral, or fungal skin infections but does not induce specific skin reactions.

Alemtuzumab (MabCampath® or Campath®) is a humanized anti-CD52 mAb. CD52 is expressed on mature lymphocytes, therefore use of this mAb induces lymphocyte destruction. Alemtuzumab results in a nonspecific rash in 21% of patients (NCI-CTCAE grade 3 in 4%) [13]. However, its main AEs are linked to the immunosuppression resulting from the profound lymphopenia induced by the treatment.

Immunosuppression can increase the risk of transfusion-associated graft-versus-host disease, which can be associated with skin manifestations. Therefore, patients treated with alemtuzumab should receive only irradiated blood, unless immediate transfusion is necessary. Infectious complications with bacterial, viral (e.g., herpes zoster in 1.2–18% of patients), or fungal organisms are frequent and can also have skin manifestations. Anti-infective prophylaxis with cotrimoxazole and famciclovir is recommended to minimize the risk of opportunistic infections.

In a series of nine patients, injection site reactions with erythema, edema, pruritus, and pain occurring with subcutaneous injections, especially during the first 24 hours of therapy and persisting until the fourth administration, were the most common dermatologic AEs. One of these patients developed a generalized dermatitis at the completion of therapy, which improved after steroids. Premedication with antihistamines and acetaminophen is recommended to minimize the intensity of site reactions.

Gemtuzumab ozogamicin (Mylotarg®) is a humanized anti-CD33 IgG4κ mAb that is conjugated with the cytotoxic antitumor antibiotic calicheamicin. It is indicated in the treatment of acute myeloid leukemia. It has not demonstrated any specific dermatologic AEs besides injection site reactions. However, its use is not currently approved in the United States. Indeed, although it was approved in 2000 under an FDA accelerated approval program, the confirmatory trial failed to demonstrate any benefit of the drug in addition to chemotherapy. This trial even reported an increased number of deaths among the patients receiving the gemtuzumab. Because of these recent concerns about the drug safety, gemtuzumab is presently not available to new patients (since June 2010) and a new drug application will have to be submitted to the FDA before gemtuzumab can be prescribed again in the United States.

Anti-CTLA-4 antibody: Ipilimumab

Drug and mechanism of action

Ipilimumab has received approval based on the efficacy it demonstrated in the treatment of patients with metastatic melanoma. Indeed, ipilimumab is the first drug to demonstrate a significant improvement of overall survival in patients with metastatic melanoma [14].

CTLA-4 (cytotoxic T-lymphocyte-associated antigen) is expressed on the surface of several lymphocyte subtypes. It decreases the nonspecific immune responses by downregulating the costimulation interaction between CD80 and CD86 (also called B7-1 and B7-2) on antigen-presenting cells and CD28 on lymphocytes. CTLA-4 binds to CD80/86 with much stronger affinity than CD28 and arrests lymphocyte stimulation. The anti-CTLA-4 antibody, ipilimumab (Yervoy; Bristol-Myers Squibb®), inhibits this brake and thus induces a nonspecific stimulation of the immune system. This new immunotherapy is associated with AEs that are different from usual anticancer therapies. Indeed, patients exhibit signs related to hyperfunctioning of the immune system, with clinical and biologic signs of autoimmunity.

The most frequent affected tissues are skin, digestive tract, liver, and endocrine glands. The most frequent AE is diarrhea, found in 40–50% of cases. It may be associated with severe colitis and even colonic perforation (less than 1% of cases). Autoimmune-like hepatitis has been observed in 3–7% of cases, as well as endocrinopathies, dysthyroidism, or pituitary insufficiency in 5–10% of patients. The skin is the most commonly affected organ, but the manifestations are usually moderate and rarely impact treatment continuation.

Skin manifestations

The dermatologic AEs reported are pruritus in 20–26.5% of patients, and a nonspecific rash in 22–46.5% of patients, with grade 3 eruptions in 1–4.2% of cases [15]. Several types of cutaneous manifestations have been reported. Diffuse maculopapular eruptions, can appear 1–2 weeks after the initiation of treatment and usually regress within a few weeks to several months. Biopsy specimens of anti-CTLA-4 associated rash revealed dermal edema and perivascular cell infiltrates containing CD4+ and CD8+ lymphocytes [16–19], or eosinophils [18,19].

In 20 patients treated with anti-CTLA-4 antibodies with or without an antitumor vaccination, a moderate erythematous eruption was observed in 13 patients and biopsies revealed mononuclear infiltrates composed of CD4+ and CD8+ and T-regulatory lymphocytes in the superficial dermis, with changes in the basement membrane reminiscent of the cutaneous eruptions of lupus erythematosus [20]. In a series of 63 consecutive patients, eight (12%) developed dermatologic AEs that could be attributed to ipilimumab. The rash consisted of well-defined pruritic erythematous scaly papules–plaques on the trunk and extensor surfaces of the extremities, especially the legs. Severe alopecia developed in one patient. Histologic analysis showed a perivascular CD4+-predominant T-cell infiltrate with eosinophils in the dermis, and mild spongiosis. Eosinophilia was also found in patients with rash.

In five biopsy specimens of nonspecific erythematous eruptions, lymphocytic infiltrates were found in close association to distressed melanocytes, which would indicate a treatment-induced antimelanocytic immunologic effect [17]. Symptomatic treatment with topical or oral corticosteroids and oral antihistamines often results in resolution.

Two cases of TEN have been reported in randomized trials. In both cases the patients were concomitantly receiving other drugs known to be capable of causing TEN. Vitiligo is reported in several studies concerning small cohorts of patients [16,19, 21]. The exact frequency of this AE is unknown. Thus, the skin AEs of ipilimumab are very common but are usually mild to moderate and do not prevent the continuation of treatment. They appear to be related to immunoallergic mechanisms and a cytotoxic effect directed against normal or malignant melanocytes is sometimes found.

Conclusions

Monoclonal antibodies are useful drugs to treat various forms of cancers. All of these events can be associated with immediate or delayed AEs related to immunoallergic reactions, such as hypersensitivity reactions, or to cytokine releases. Therefore, these drugs must be used with caution, especially during the first infusion. Well-designed protocols for prevention and treatment of these infusion reactions are available; however, in rare cases, severe reactions can occur and jeopardize drug readministration.

In addition to injection site reactions that can occur with any mAb, these drugs can also give rise to skin manifestations resulting from their pharmacologic actions and from the spectrum of their molecular targets. For most of the mAbs used in the clinic, specific dermatologic AEs are rare and usually mild to moderate with the

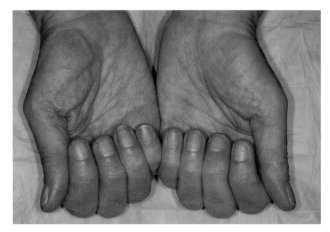

Figure 23.3 Trastuzumab-induced brittle nails grade 2. Photo courtesy of Dr. Mario E. Lacouture.

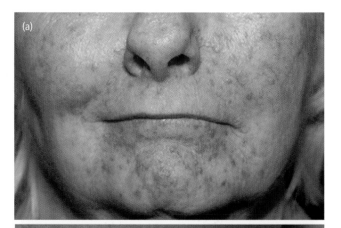

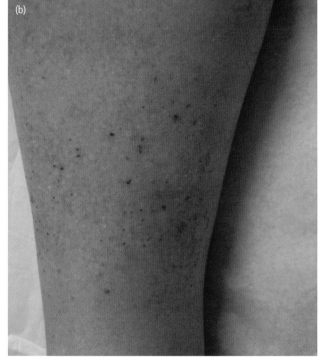

Figure 23.4 (a,b) Ipilimumab-induced rash and pruritus grade 1. Photo courtesy of Dr. Mario E. Lacouture.

exception of mAbs targeting EGFR (e.g., cetuximab and panitumumab) which induce frequent and sometimes severe skin, hair, and nail manifestations (see Figure 23.3 and 23.4) Ipilimumab, which is a new nonspecific immunotherapy blocking CTLA-4 approved for the treatment of metastatic melanoma and is associated with various immune-related events including numerous dermatologic AEs.

References

1 Lenz, H.J. (2007) Management and preparedness for infusion and hypersensitivity reactions. *The Oncologist*, **12**, 601–609.

2 Calogiuri, G., Ventura, M.T., Mason, L. *et al.* (2008) Hypersensitivity reactions to last generation chimeric, humanized [correction of umanized] and human recombinant monoclonal antibodies for therapeutic use. *Current Pharmaceutical Design*, **14**, 2883–2891.

3 Brennan, P.J., Rodriguez Bouza, T., Hsu, F.I., Sloane, D.E. & Castells, M.C. (2009) Hypersensitivity reactions to mAbs: 105 desensitizations in 23 patients, from evaluation to treatment. *Journal of Allergy and Clinical Immunology*, **124**, 1259–1266.

4 Escudier, B., Pluzanska, A., Koralewski, P. *et al.* (2007) Bevacizumab plus interferon alfa-2a for treatment of metastatic renal cell carcinoma: a randomised, double-blind phase III trial. *Lancet*, **370**, 2103–2111.

5 Robert, C. (2007) Cutaneous side effects of antiangiogenic agents. *Bulletin Du Cancer*, **94** (Spec No), S260–S264.

6 Thornton, A.D., Ravn, P., Winslet, M. & Chester, K. (2006) Angiogenesis inhibition with bevacizumab and the surgical management of colorectal cancer. *British Journal of Surgery*, **93**, 1456–1463.

7 Gounant, V., Milleron, B., Assouad, J. *et al.* (2009) Bevacizumab and invasive procedures: practical recommendations. *Revue Des Maladies Respiratoires*, **26**, 221–226.

8 Zangari, M., Fink, L.M., Elice, F., Zhan, F., Adcock, D.M. & Tricot, G.J. (2009) Thrombotic events in patients with cancer receiving antiangiogenesis agents. *Journal of Clinical Oncology*, **27**, 4865–4873.

9 Nalluri, S.R., Chu, D., Keresztes, R., Zhu, X. & Wu, S. (2008) Risk of venous thromboembolism with the angiogenesis inhibitor bevacizumab in cancer patients: a meta-analysis. *Journal of the American Medical Association*, **300**, 2277–2285.

10 Vogel, C.L., Cobleigh, M.A., Tripathy, D., Gutheil, J.C., Harris, L.N., Fehrenbacher, L., Slamon, D.J., Murphy, M., Novotny, W.F., Burchmore, M., Shak, S., Stewart, S.J. (2001) First-line Herceptin monotherapy in metastatic breast cancer. *Oncology*. **61** Suppl2:37–42. Review. PubMed PMID: 11694786.

11 Rosman, I.S. & Anadkat, M.J. (2010) Tufted hair folliculitis in a woman treated with trastuzumab. *Targeted Oncology*, **5**, 295–296.

12 Scheinfeld, N. (2006) A review of rituximab in cutaneous medicine. *Dermatology Online Journal*, **12**, 3.

13 Keating, M.J., Cazin, B., Coutré, S., Birhiray, R., Kovacsovics, T., Langer, W., *et al.* (2002) Campath-1H treatment of T-cell prolymphocytic leukaemia in patients for whom at least one prior chemotherapy regimen has failed. *J Clin Oncol* **20**:205–13.

14 Hodi, F.S., O'Day, S.J., McDermott, D.F. *et al.* (2010) Improved survival with ipilimumab in patients with metastatic melanoma. *New England Journal of Medicine*, **363**, 711–723.

15 Robert, C. & Ghiringhelli, F. (2009) What is the role of cytotoxic T lymphocyte-associated antigen 4 blockade in patients with metastatic melanoma? *The Oncologist*, **14**, 848–861.

16 Attia, P., Phan, G.Q., Maker, A.V. *et al.* (2005) Autoimmunity correlates with tumor regression in patients with metastatic melanoma treated with anti-cytotoxic T-lymphocyte antigen-4. *Journal of Clinical Oncology*, **23**, 6043–6053.

17 Hodi, F.S., Mihm, M.C., Soiffer, R.J. *et al.* (2003) Biologic activity of cytotoxic T lymphocyte-associated antigen 4 antibody blockade in previously vaccinated metastatic melanoma and ovarian carcinoma patients. *Proceedings of the National Academy of Sciences of the United States of America*, **100**, 4712–4717.

18 O'Mahony, D., Morris, J.C., Quinn, C. *et al.* (2007) A pilot study of CTLA-4 blockade after cancer vaccine failure in patients with advanced malignancy. *Clinical Cancer Research*, **13**, 958–964.

19 Phan, G.Q., Yang, J.C., Sherry, R.M. *et al.* (2003) Cancer regression and autoimmunity induced by cytotoxic T lymphocyte-associated antigen 4 blockade in patients with metastatic melanoma. *Proceedings of the National Academy of Sciences of the United States of America*, **100**, 8372–8377.

20 Hodi, F.S., Butler, M., Oble, D.A. *et al.* (2008) Immunologic and clinical effects of antibody blockade of cytotoxic T lymphocyte-associated antigen 4 in previously vaccinated cancer patients. *Proceedings of the National Academy of Sciences of the United States of America*, **105**, 3005–3010.

21 Ribas, A., Camacho, L.H., Lopez-Berestein, G. *et al.* (2005) Anti-tumor activity in melanoma and anti-self responses in a phase I trial with the anti-cytotoxic T lymphocyte-associated antigen 4 monoclonal antibody CP-675,206. *Journal of Clinical Oncology*, **23**, 8968–8977.

24 Endocrine Agents

Katherine Szyfelbein Masterpol[1], Maura Dickler[2] and Mario E. Lacouture[3]

[1]Department of Dermatology, Boston University School of Medicine, Boston, MA, USA
[2]Department of Medicine, Memorial Sloan-Kettering Cancer Center, New York, NY, USA
[3]Dermatology Service, Memorial Sloan-Kettering Cancer Center, New York, NY, USA

Introduction

The endocrine agents used in oncology include estrogen receptor modulators and downregulators, aromatase inhibitors, luteinizing hormone-releasing hormone agonists, antiandrogens, androgens, estrogen, somatostatin analogs, and progestational agents. These therapies generally have a low reported incidence of dermatologic adverse events (AEs). For those that have dermatologic AEs documented in the literature, the reactions tend to be vaguely described. Furthermore, it is difficult to ascertain the true prevalence of such AEs as the trials and studies often use these agents in combination or in comparison with other agents, not always with placebo. In addition, the incidence of cutaneous symptoms in control groups are often high and need to be taken into account when interpreting elevated treatment group rates. Overall, cutaneous AEs that have been reported have included hot flashes, hyperhidrosis, pruritus, allergic reactions, injection site reactions, and alopecia (Figure 24.1).

Selective estrogen receptor modulators

The sex hormone estrogen is important for many physiologic processes. Stimulation of breast ductal epithelium by estrogen, however, can contribute to the development and progression of breast cancer, and treatments designed to block estrogen's effects are important options for the prevention and treatment of breast cancer (Table 24.1). Tamoxifen and other selective estrogen receptor modulators (SERMs) bind the estrogen receptor (ER) and antagonize the proliferative effects of estrogen in normal breast tissue and breast tumors. However, these drugs also have stimulatory estrogenic effects depending on the target tissue, and therefore tamoxifen and other drugs in this class (raloxifene,

toremifene) are referred to as SERMs. SERMs bind the ER, alter receptor conformation, and facilitate binding of co-regulatory proteins that activate or repress transcriptional activation of estrogen target genes.

Tamoxifen was developed more than three decades ago and is approved by the US Food and Drug Administration (FDA) for the prevention and treatment of breast cancer. Tamoxifen is effective for all stages of breast cancer including ductal carcinoma in situ (AJCC Stage 0) and early stage invasive breast cancer (AJCC Stages I–III); in this setting tamoxifen is referred to as "adjuvant therapy," and follows breast surgery and radiation. Tamoxifen is also used for patients with AJCC Stage IV locally advanced and metastatic breast cancer. The standard dose is 20 mg orally once daily, and in the adjuvant setting tamoxifen is typically administered for 2.5 years (and then followed by an aromatase inhibitor) or 5 years.

Tamoxifen's most frequent cutaneous AE is flushing. This flushing may be constituted by hot flashes accompanied by eccrine sweating [1]. It is known that the effects of estrogen deprivation, as in postmenopausal states, include hot flashes. As tamoxifen antagonizes the ER in the central nervous system, the effect is to induce hot flashes and mimic an estrogen-deprived state [2]. This AEs is common, with a large trial of 3094 tamoxifen-treated women having a 40.9% incidence of hot flashes [3]. Another trial of 2338 tamoxifen-treated women reported 38.6% of patients having hot flashes, with the majority (819/903 patients) being grade 1 or 2 toxicities [4]. In this trial, sweating was also reported independently from hot flashes and 17.7% experienced sweating, with the vast majority (359/413) reporting grade 1 or 2 symptoms [4]. A trial of 3988 women on tamoxifen showed 38% incidence of hot flashes, all of grade 1 or 2 severity [5]. However, it is important to mention that larger trials do not always have placebo comparisons and may only report "prespecified adverse events." A smaller study evaluating toxicity

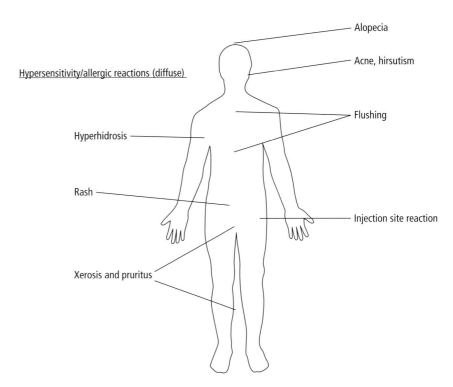

Figure 24.1 Anatomic location of dermatologic adverse events to endocrine agents.

Table 24.1 Classification of endocrine agents.

ER modulators	
ER antagonist/agonist	Tamoxifen
Selective ER modulators	Toremifene
	Raloxifene

Aromatase inhibitors	
Nonsteroidal	Anastrozole
	Letrozole
Steroidal	Exemestane
Estrogen receptor downregulator	Fulvestrant
Luteinizing-hormone releasing hormone agonist	Leuprolide
Antiandrogens	Flutamide
	Bicalutamide
	Nilutamide
Androgen	Fluoxymesterone
Estrogen	Estradiol
Somatostatin analog	Octreotide
Progestational agents	Megestrol
	Medroxyprogesterone acetate

ER, estrogen receptor.

reported 67.2% (43/64) of tamoxifen-treated patients having hot flashes at 6 months, compared to 45.4% at baseline (prior to therapy) and 45.4% in the placebo group [6]. The 6-month evaluation was the only statistically significant time point. However, at 3, 6, and 12 month evaluations, 20%, 20.3%, and 13.3% of tamoxifen-treated patients reported severe hot flashes compared to none at baseline and 3%, 7.6%, and 3.1% of placebo-treated patients [6].

Alopecia has rarely been reported with tamoxifen treatment. In a study with 189 patients, 1.1% of women exhibited alopecia (unspecified type) [7]. Though tamoxifen is not infrequently cited in the literature as causing cutaneous vasculitis, this has not been substantiated in any major trials using tamoxifen, but rather is based on case reports [8].

Other estrogen receptor modulators include toremifene and raloxifene. Toremifene is indicated for the treatment of postmenopausal women with ER+ or unknown metastatic breast cancer. Raloxifene is indicated for the prevention and treatment of osteoporosis as well as to reduce the risk of invasive breast cancer in postmenopausal women. Toremifene and raloxifene have not been reported to cause any significant cutaneous AEs other than hot flashes. In a large trial, 9.7% of patients on 60 mg/day raloxifene and 11.6% on 120 mg/day experienced hot flashes compared to 6.4% on placebo [9]. Another study of 601 women showed no significant difference between 60 mg/day raloxifene compared to placebo with regards to incidence of hot flashes (26.3 vs. 22.7%) [10]. Toremifene was shown in one trial to have 15% of 20 patients experience hot flashes of a grade 1–2 nature [11].

Estrogen receptor downregulators

Fulvestrant is an estrogen receptor antagonist that causes degradation of the ER. Due to this unique mechanism of action, fulvestrant does not have the ER-mediated agonistic effects that are seen with tamoxifen. Fulvestrant is indicated for ER+ metastatic breast cancer in postmenopausal women. It is administered intramuscularly, typically at 250 or 500 mg on days 1, 15, 29, and then monthly for maintenance.

Fulvestrant is well tolerated from a dermatologic perspective. It is associated with hot flashes, with an incidence of 21% (89/423) of patients in one trial [12] and as low as 8.3% (30/361; 500 mg dose) and 6.1% (23/374; 250 mg dose) in another trial [13], nearly all representing grade 1 or 2 severity. A study using a loading dose regimen of fulvestrant in patients who had been on prior aromatase inhibitor therapy for breast cancer demonstrated 8.8% of 351 patients had hot flashes [14]. Of 101 patients being treated with high dose fulvestrant, 7.9% experienced hot flashes [15]. In the same study, fulvestrant was associated with hyperhidrosis in 4% of patients [15]. Fulvestrant has also been reported to cause bromhidrosis in 8% of patients in a study of 26 women. The two patients affected had a grade 1 toxicity [16].

Injection site reactions have been reported in 2.3% (8 of 351 patients) of patients in one trial [14] and 13.6% (49/361) of patients on 500 mg dosing in a another trial [13]. This local injection-site reaction is dependent on method and volume of injection [12], with more frequent reaction seen with two separate smaller volume injections [17]. Alopecia has been rarely reported with fulvestrant, the prior mentioned study of 351 patients stated 2.3% had alopecia, the type and morphology of which was not specified [14]. Vaginitis was reported in 0.3% (1/374) of patients on 250 mg dosing [13].

Aromatase inhibitors

Aromatase inhibitors are a family of steroidal and nonsteroidal agents that prevent the synthesis of estrogenic compounds without impacting the synthesis of other adrenal steroids. Exemestane, anastrozole, and letrozole are third generation aromatase inhibitors that are superselective in nature and result in dermatologic AEs (Figure 24.2, Figure 24.3, and Figure 24.4).

Exemestane is a steroidal type aromatase inhibitor that irreversibly inactivates the aromatase enzyme [13]. Exemestane is usually dosed orally at 25 mg/day. It is indicated to treat advanced breast cancer in postmenopausal women whose disease has progressed after tamoxifen treatment. It is also used as adjuvant therapy in postmenopausal women with ER+ early stage breast cancer after 2–3 years of tamoxifen (for a total of 5 years of adjuvant therapy).

The cutaneous AEs of these agents can partially be explained by their suppression of plasma estrogen levels to undetectable levels in postmenopausal women. Exemestane has been associated with hot flashes, hyperhidrosis, alopecia, hypertrichosis, and acneiform rash [18]. Overall, the incidence of hot flashes with exemestane has ranged 6.9–41.3% in various trials [4, 7, 14, 18–20]. In a large study of 2320 patients on exemestane, 41.3% were reported to have hot flashes, with the majority of patients

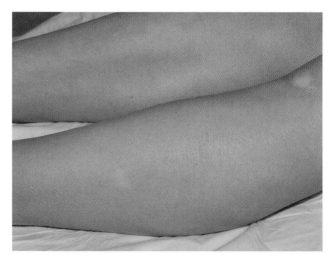

Figure 24.2 Anastrozole-induced dry skin grade 1.

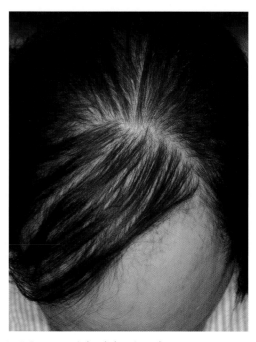

Figure 24.3 Exemestane-induced alopecia grade 1.

(861/957) experiencing grade 1 or 2 symptoms [4]. This study did not report any alopecia, hyperhidrosis, or other cutaneous AEs. In multiple smaller studies (ranging from 80 to 340 patients), alopecia has been reported in 1–1.5% [14, 18, 19] and hypertrichosis in 1% (grade 2) of women [18]. Incidence of acneiform rash was 3% (2/80) in one such study [18].

Skin rash of unspecified or "allergic" type has been reported in <1–2% of patients in multiple small studies, requiring some patients to withdraw from the studies [19, 21, 22].

Anastrozole is a nonsteroidal aromatase inhibitor that reversibly inhibits the aromatase enzyme. It is usually orally dosed at 1 mg/day and is indicated for treatment of ER+ or unknown locally advanced or metastatic breast cancer in postmenopausal women either as first-line endocrine therapy or following tamoxifen,

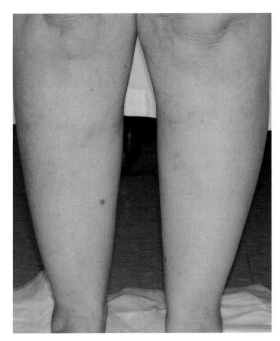

Figure 24.4 Tamoxifen-induced leg edema grade 2.

and as adjuvant treatment of early stage ER+ breast cancer in postmenopausal women.

Hot flashes have been reported in 7.9–39% of patients taking anastrozole [12, 15, 23]. A large trial of 3092 women cited an incidence of 35.7% compared to 40.9% in the tamoxifen comparison group [3]. Hyperhidrosis was seen in 4% of 103 patients in one trial [15]. In a trial of 50 patients on anastrozole with placebo, 10% of patients experienced skin rash (not specified), 10% had pruritus, 2% reported dry skin, and 2% had an exfoliative rash [24]. None of these AEs led to discontinuation of the drug. Mouth and vaginal dryness were each associated with anastrozole in 1.4% of 53 women. It may be important to note that the use of gefitinib along with anastrozole in the treatment arm may have resulted in over-reporting of adverse events on the anastrozole-only control arm.

Allergy/cutaneous toxicity/skin rash, otherwise unspecified, grades 1–4 were noted in 7.5% of 387 patients compared to 1.7% of 469 in the "no further treatment group" [23]. In the same trial, hair loss, unspecified type, grades 1–3 was seen in 9% of the anastrozole group (2.1% in comparison group) [23].

Letrozole is a nonsteroidal aromatase inhibitor with a similar mechanism of action to anastrozole. Letrozole is indicated as adjuvant therapy in postmenopausal women with ER+ early stage breast cancer; as extended adjuvant therapy of early stage breast cancer after 5 years of tamoxifen; for advanced breast cancer with disease progression after antiestrogen therapy; and for ER+ or unknown locally advanced or metastatic breast cancer. It is also used off-label for ovarian cancer. Typical dosing of letrozole is 2.5 mg by mouth once daily.

Letrozole, similar to anastrozole, is associated with hot flashes. One large trial of 3975 patients reported a 33.5% incidence of hot flashes, all grade 1 and 2 [5]; however, there was no placebo comparison group. In a follow-up study to this trial, specifically evaluating toxicity and relation to age, 59% of 834 patients aged 60–69 years old on letrozole experienced hot flashes compared to 52% on placebo. This was the only age group with a statistically significant higher incidence than placebo in this study [25]. Less frequently, letrozole has been associated with night sweats, alopecia, pruritus, xerosis, nail changes, and exanthema. Alopecia was reported in the previous trial in 5% of the same 60–69 year old age group compared to 3% on placebo; likewise only this age group had a statistically significant increased incidence [25]. The incidence of sweating in any of the letrozole groups was not significantly increased compared to placebo [25]. In a trial of 2572 patients on letrozole, 58% experienced hot flashes (grades 1–3) compared to 54% on placebo (statistically significant). Alopecia (grades 1–2) was noted in 5% of the letrozole group compared to 3% of placebo. Sweating was not a statistically significant event [26]. In a study of 624 patients on letrozole with placebo, compared to letrozole with lapatinib, hot flashes were seen in 14% (grades 1–2), alopecia in about 7% (grades 1 and 2), pruritus in approximately 9% (grades 1–3), dry skin in <5% (grades 1 and 2), nail disorder <1%, and rash of unspecified nature in 13% (grades 1 and 2) [27]. There are a few case reports of erythema nodosum occurring in patients on letrozole, but this skin condition has not been reported in any major trials [28].

Luteinizing hormone-releasing hormone agonist

Leuprolide is a luteinizing hormone-releasing hormone (LHRH) agonist, which causes androgen deprivation in men and estrogen deprivation in women [29]. It is a peptide analog of LHRH and is 50–100 times more potent than the natural occurring hormone. It is indicated for palliative treatment of advanced prostate cancer and is used off-label for treatment of breast cancer. It can be administered intramuscularly or subcutaneously. The subcutaneous dosing ranges from 1 mg daily to 7.5 mg monthly, 22.5 mg every 3 months, 30 mg every 4 months or 45 mg every 6 months. The intramuscular dosing is usually 7.5 mg monthly, 22.5 mg every 3 months, or 30 mg every 4 months.

A trial of 160 male patients reported 45% of patients experienced hot flashes, 3.8% had hyperhidrosis, 4.4% displayed injection-site irritation, 1.3% injection-site bruising, and 1.3% injection-site erythema. In this trial, one case developed a "skin rash with blisters" [29]. Leuprolide is cited as causing or exacerbating drug-induced lupus, and this appears to be based upon rare case reports [30]. Reports are emerging of leuprolide potentially causing a psoriasiform exanthem [31].

Antiandrogens

Flutamide is an antiandrogen that has been used in the treatment of prostate cancer for over three decades. Initially, flutamide increases follicle stimulating hormone (FSH) and luteinizing hormone (LH) levels thereby raising estrogen and testosterone levels, but then after a period of time receptor desensitization occurs and testosterone diminishes to castration levels. Flutamide is indicated for metastatic prostate cancer in combination with LHRH agonists. Usual dose is 250 mg orally three times daily.

Flutamide has also been associated with hot flashes [32, 33]. It has also been associated with photosensitivity, though not in any of the major trials. Cases have been described where patients developed a papulovesicular erythema or scaling in a sun-exposed distribution 2–5 months after beginning flutamide therapy. In five cases, the eruption resolved within days to weeks of discontinuation of flutamide. One recurrence was seen upon rechallenge with the drug. The reaction is postulated to be of a photoallergic nature [34–36]. Additional reports of photosensitizing reactions with flutamide have been classified as a pseudoporphyria [37–39]. Other than discontinuing the drug in order to avoid such a photosensitizing effect, patients should be advised to avoid direct sunlight and use sun-protective clothing and sunscreens, especially those containing physical sunscreen agents such as titanium oxide and zinc oxide. Antihistamines and topical corticosteroids may be of help to alleviate symptoms of such reactions. In severe cases, systemic corticosteroids may be needed.

Bicalutamide is a nonsteroidal type antiandrogen, another therapy option for metastatic prostate cancer that is used in conjunction with an LHRH agonist. It is typically dosed at 50 mg orally once per day.

It has primarily been associated with hot flashes in terms of cutaneous AEs. Of 320 patients on bicalutamide in one study, 13.1% developed hot flashes [40]. Another trial reported 23% of 55 patients experienced hot flashes; however, adverse events were irrespective of relation to therapy [41]. A larger trial of 1627 patients treated with bicalutamide and "standard of care" (radical prostatectomy and radiotherapy) showed an incidence of 10.9% compared to 6.6% for the standard care only group [42].

Androgens

Fluoxymesterone is an anabolic steroid with highly androgenic properties. It may act on prolactin or estrogen receptors or production. In oncology, it is infrequently used for palliation in breast cancer. It is administered orally. Given its androgenic effects, the cutaneous effects may include acne/furunculosis and hirsutism. In one study, fluoxymesterone being used for cancer-related cachexia caused hirsutism in 5% of study patients; however, there was no placebo group for comparison [43].

Estrogen

Estrogens modulate the secretion of LH, gonadotropins, and FSH by the pituitary gland. Estradiol is the major intracellular form of estrogen in humans. Prior to the onset of menopause, the secretion of estradiol increases. In postmenopausal women, estrogen replacement can be used to reduce elevated levels of the prior mentioned hormones. Estradiol can be administered intramuscularly, orally, transdermally (patch), intravaginally, or topically as a gel, emulsion, spray, or cream. It can be used for palliation in breast cancer and prostate cancer as well as for vasomotor symptoms of menopause.

Estrogen (estradiol) has not been reported with significant or major cutaneous AEs. There is a commonly cited association of estrogens with erythema nodosum based generally on multiple case reports [44]. Erythema nodosum can be seen in the setting of oral contraceptive use and pregnancy. It is classically characterized by tender erythematous nodules on the lower legs, most often on the extensor surfaces. It can be treated with pain control with nonsteroidal anti-inflammatory agents or prednisone if needed. Furthermore, estrogen has been cited as being associated with melasma; however, the literature shows no clear association of estradiol or estrogen itself with melasma, but rather oral contraceptives containing progestins, and thus an association does not appear to have been established.

Progestational agents

Progestational agents include megestrol acetate, a commonly used progestin. It is produced by dehydrogenation of medroxy-progesterone acetate and is administered orally. It has been used for palliation of endometrial and breast carcinomas, as well as for treatment of acne and hirsutism in females. It has been associated with hot flashes and rarely with skin exanthem. An analysis of two phase III trials of megestrol acetate versus anastrozole showed 8% of 253 patients on megestrol acetate experienced hot flashes [45]. Two of 89 patients on megestrol acetate were noted to have grade 1 rash, otherwise unspecified [46]. A study of 58 patients on high dose megestrol reported one patient with grade 3 "rash," one patient with grade 1 sweating, and one patient with grade 3 ecchymoses [47]. A phase II trial of 36 patients on high dose megestrol reported grade 1 alopecia in four patients [48]. Megestrol has also been reported to cause hirsutism. One study using megestrol for cancer-related cachexia, 7% of patients reported hirsutism, but there was no placebo group for comparison [43]. Many other larger trials do not report any cutaneous toxicities with megestrol [49–51]. It is important to note that trials are not always designed to evaluate for such potential cutaneous effects, therefore none may be observed or reported.

Medroxyprogesterone acetate has been used orally for treatment of secondary amenorrhea and dysfunctional uterine bleeding and for treatment of endometriosis. In oncology, it has been used for endometrial cancers in an off-label fashion. It is available orally and in subcutaneous or intramuscular formulations. It has been cited in the literature of being associated with acne; however, this appears to be based on case reports.

Somatostatin analog

Somatostatin is a hormone secreted by the paracrine cells in the gastrointestinal tract and has the ability to inhibit various gastrointestinal processes. It inhibits numerous other hormones involved in the gastrointestinal system including serotonin, secretin, insulin, gastrin, glucagon, and vasoactive intestinal polypeptide (VIP). Octreotide acetate is a synthetic peptide that maintains the biologic activity of the hormone somatostatin. It is more potent and stable in circulation than is the natural hormone. In oncology, octreotide is indicated for carcinoid tumors and VIPomas. It can be administered intravenously, subcutaneously, or as an intramuscular depot injection. Its dosing depends on the indication for which it is being used.

Octreotate is another somatostatin analog. Octreotide has not been documented in studies to have major cutaneous AEs [52–56]. In a study of 85 patients of whom 42 were assigned to treatment with octreotide, octreotide was not documented to have any AEs on the skin, mucosa, hair, or nails [52]. A larger study using octreotide to treat obesity in 172 patients also did not report any adverse cutaneous events [53]. Similarly, additional studies of 15 [54] and 28 patients [55] did not report any cutaneous AEs. Though some studies using octreotide only reported AEs of grade 3 or higher, it is difficult to assess if mild cutaneous effects may exist [57]. Indeed, multiple (over 10) case reports have been published on alopecia observed with octreotide and octreotate treatment and this may be an underreported finding [58–62]. In a study of 35 patients, octreotate was associated with "mild hair loss" in 17 patients. Of note, hair regrowth was observed at follow-up 3 and 6 months after final administration of the drug [63]. In a series of three patients being treated for acromegaly with octreotide, diffuse nonscarring and reversible alopecia was noted, beginning as early as 3 months into treatment and reversing soon after drug discontinuation [58]. In terms of nail changes, there appears to be only one case report of Beau lines associated with octreotide therapy [64].

Conclusions

Dermatologic AEs to endocrine agents appear to be underreported, likely because of their insidious nature and the simultaneous use of other agents. Moreover, many of these AEs develop over long periods of time, which may explain the lack of their capture in some trials. Most AEs are mild to moderate in severity, but their impact on quality of life commands attention, especially because people receive these agents for long periods of time, which makes these events chronic in nature. Recent studies have shown that the persistence and adherence to hormonal therapies may be as low as 50%, underscoring the importance of minimizing any event that would negatively impact patients' willingness to receive therapy.

References

1 Wilkin, J.K. (1992) Flushing reactions in the cancer chemotherapy patient: the lists are longer but the strategies are the same. *Archives of Dermatology*, **128** (10), 1387–1389.

2 Hall, G. & Phillips, T.J. (2005) Estrogen and skin: the effects of estrogen, menopause, and hormone replacement therapy on the skin. *Journal of the American Academy of Dermatology*, **53** (4), 555–568; quiz 569–572.

3 Howell, A., Cuzick, J., Baum, M. *et al.*; ATAC Trialists' Group (2005) Results of the ATAC (Arimidex, Tamoxifen, Alone or in Combination) trial after completion of 5 years' adjuvant treatment for breast cancer. *Lancet*, **365** (9453), 60–62.

4 Coombes, R.C., Kilburn, L.S., Snowdon, C.F. *et al.*; Intergroup Exemestane Study (2007) Survival and safety of exemestane versus tamoxifen after 2–3 years' tamoxifen treatment (Intergroup Exemestane Study): a randomised controlled trial. *Lancet*, **369** (9561), 559–570.

5 Thürlimann, B., Keshaviah, A., Coates, A.S. *et al.*; Breast International Group (BIG) 1-98 Collaborative Group (2005) A comparison of letrozole and tamoxifen in postmenopausal women with early breast cancer. *New England Journal of Medicine*, **353** (26), 2747–2757.

6 Love, R.R., Cameron, L., Connell, B.L. & Leventhal, H. (1991) Symptoms associated with tamoxifen treatment in postmenopausal women. *Archives of Internal Medicine*, **151** (9), 1842–1847.

7 Paridaens, R.J., Dirix, L.Y., Beex, L.V. *et al.* (2008) Phase III study comparing exemestane with tamoxifen as first-line hormonal treatment of metastatic breast cancer in postmenopausal women: the European Organisation for Research and Treatment of Cancer Breast Cancer Cooperative Group. *Journal of Clinical Oncology*, **26** (30), 4883–4890.

8 Drago, F., Arditi, M. & Rebora, A. (1990) Tamoxifen and purpuric vasculitis. *Annals of Internal Medicine*, **112** (12), 965–966.

9 Cummings, S.R., Eckert, S., Krueger, K.A. *et al.* (1999) The effect of raloxifene on risk of breast cancer in postmenopausal women: results from the MORE randomized trial. Multiple Outcomes of Raloxifene Evaluation. *Journal of the American Medical Association*, **281** (23), 2189–2197.

10 Delmas, P.D., Bjarnason, N.H., Mitlak, B.H. *et al.* (1997) Effects of raloxifene on bone mineral density, serum cholesterol concentrations, and uterine endometrium in postmenopausal women. *New England Journal of Medicine*, **337** (23), 1641–1647.

11 Perry, J.J., Berry, D.A., Weiss, R.B., Hayes, D.M., Duggan, D.B. & Henderson, I.C. (1995) High dose toremifene for estrogen and progesterone receptor negative metastatic breast cancer: a phase II trial of the Cancer and Leukemia Group B (CALGB). *Breast Cancer Research and Treatment*, **36** (1), 35–40.

12 Robertson, J.F., Osborne, C.K., Howell, A. *et al.* (2003) Fulvestrant versus anastrozole for the treatment of advanced breast carcinoma in postmenopausal women: a prospective combined analysis of two multicenter trials. *Cancer*, **98** (2), 229–238.

13 Di Leo, A., Jerusalem, G., Petruzelka, L. *et al.* (2010) Results of the CONFIRM phase III trial comparing fulvestrant 250 mg with fulvestrant 500 mg in postmenopausal women with estrogen receptor-positive advanced breast cancer. *Journal of Clinical Oncology*, **28** (30), 4594–4600.

14 Chia, S., Gradishar, W., Mauriac, L. *et al.* (2008) Double-blind, randomized placebo controlled trial of fulvestrant compared with exemestane after prior nonsteroidal aromatase inhibitor therapy in postmenopausal women with hormone receptor-positive, advanced

breast cancer: results from EFECT. *Journal of Clinical Oncology*, **26** (10), 1664–1670.

15 Robertson, J.F., Llombart-Cussac, A., Rolski, J. *et al.* (2009) Activity of fulvestrant 500 mg versus anastrozole 1 mg as first-line treatment for advanced breast cancer: results from the FIRST study. *Journal of Clinical Oncology*, **27** (27), 4530–4535.

16 Argenta, P.A., Thomas, S.G., Judson, P.L. *et al.* (2009) A phase II study of fulvestrant in the treatment of multiply-recurrent epithelial ovarian cancer. *Gynecologic Oncology*, **113** (2), 205–209.

17 Wilkes, G.M. & Barton-Burke, M. (2009) *Oncology Nursing Drug Handbook*. Jones and Bartlett Publishers, Boston, MA.

18 Mlineritsch, B., Tausch, C., Singer, C. *et al.*; Austrian Breast, Colorectal Cancer Study Group (ABCSG) (2008) Exemestane as primary systemic treatment for hormone receptor positive post-menopausal breast cancer patients: a phase II trial of the Austrian Breast and Colorectal Cancer Study Group (ABCSG-17). *Breast Cancer Research and Treatment*, **112** (1), 203–213.

19 Kvinnsland, S., Anker, G., Dirix, L.Y. *et al.* (2000) High activity and tolerability demonstrated for exemestane in postmenopausal women with metastatic breast cancer who had previously failed on tamoxifen treatment. *European Journal of Cancer*, **36** (8), 976–982.

20 Lønning, P.E., Bajetta, E., Murray, R. *et al.* (2000) Activity of exemestane in metastatic breast cancer after failure of nonsteroidal aromatase inhibitors: a phase II trial. *Journal of Clinical Oncology*, **18** (11), 2234–2244.

21 Falandry, C., Debled, M., Bachelot, T. *et al.* (2009) Celecoxib and exemestane versus placebo and exemestane in postmenopausal metastatic breast cancer patients: a double-blind phase III GINECO study. *Breast Cancer Research and Treatment*, **116** (3), 501–508.

22 Mustacchi, G., Mansutti, M., Sacco, C. *et al.* (2009) Neo-adjuvant exemestane in elderly patients with breast cancer: a phase II, multicentre, open-label, Italian study. *Annals of Oncology*, **20** (4), 655–659.

23 Jakesz, R., Greil, R., Gnant, M. *et al.*; Austrian Breast and Colorectal Cancer Study Group (2007) Extended adjuvant therapy with anastrozole among postmenopausal breast cancer patients: results from the randomized Austrian Breast and Colorectal Cancer Study Group Trial 6a. *Journal of the National Cancer Institute*, **99** (24), 1845–1853. Erratum in: *Journal of the National Cancer Institute*, 2008; **100**(3), 226.

24 Cristofanilli, M., Valero, V., Mangalik, A. *et al.* (2010) Phase II, randomized trial to compare anastrozole combined with gefitinib or placebo in postmenopausal women with hormone receptor-positive metastatic breast cancer. *Clinical Cancer Research*, **16** (6), 1904–1914.

25 Muss, H.B., Tu, D., Ingle, J.N. *et al.* (2008) Efficacy, toxicity, and quality of life in older women with early-stage breast cancer treated with letrozole or placebo after 5 years of tamoxifen: NCIC CTG intergroup trial MA.17. *Journal of Clinical Oncology*, **26** (12), 1956–1964.

26 Goss, P.E., Ingle, J.N., Martino, S. *et al.* (2005) Randomized trial of letrozole following tamoxifen as extended adjuvant therapy in receptor-positive breast cancer: updated findings from NCIC CTG MA.17. *Journal of the National Cancer Institute*, **97** (17), 1262–1271.

27 Johnston, S., Pippen, J. Jr., Pivot, X. *et al.* (2009) Lapatinib combined with letrozole versus letrozole and placebo as first-line therapy for postmenopausal hormone receptor-positive metastatic breast cancer. *Journal of Clinical Oncology*, **27** (33), 5538–5546.

28 Jhaveri, K., Halperin, P., Shin, S.J. & Vahdat, L. (2007) Erythema nodosum secondary to aromatase inhibitor use in breast cancer patients: case reports and review of the literature. *Breast Cancer Research and Treatment*, **106** (3), 315–318.

29 Marberger, M., Kaisary, A.V., Shore, N.D. *et al.* (2010) Effectiveness, pharmacokinetics, and safety of a new sustained-release leuprolide acetate 3.75-mg depot formulation for testosterone suppression in patients with prostate cancer: a Phase III, open-label, international multicenter study. *Clinical Therapeutics*, **32** (4), 744–757.

30 Wiechert, A., Tüting, T., Bieber, T., Haidl, G. & Wenzel, J. (2008) Subacute cutaneous lupus erythematosus in a leuprorelin-treated patient with prostate carcinoma. *British Journal of Dermatology*, **159** (1), 231–233.

31 Efran, G., Rifaioglu, E.N., Kulac, M. *et al.* (2013) Precipitation and exacerbation of psoriasiform eruption due to leuprolide acetate. *Journal of Dermatology*, **40** (1), 54–55.

32 Susser, W.S., Whitaker-Worth, D.L. & Grant-Kels, J.M. (1999) Mucocutaneous reactions to chemotherapy. *Journal of the American Academy of Dermatology*, **40** (3), 367–398; quiz 399-400.

33 Prussick, R. (1996) Adverse cutaneous reactions to chemotherapeutic agents and cytokine therapy. *Seminars in Cutaneous Medicine and Surgery*, **15** (4), 267–276.

34 Fujimoto, M., Kikuchi, K., Imakado, S. & Furue, M. (1996) Photosensitive dermatitis induced by flutamide. *British Journal of Dermatology*, **135** (3), 496–497.

35 Leroy, D., Dompmartin, A. & Szczurko, C. (1996) Flutamide photosensitivity. *Photodermatology, Photoimmunology and Photomedicine*, **12** (5), 216–218.

36 Moraillon, I., Jeanmougin, M., Manciet, J.R., Revuz, J. & Bagot, M. (1991) Photoallergic reaction induced by flutamide. *Photodermatology, Photoimmunology and Photomedicine*, **8** (6), 264–265.

37 Schmutz, J.L., Barbaud, A. & Tréchot, P. (1999) Flutamide and pseudoporphyria [Article in French]. *Annales de Dermatologie et de Venereologie*, **126** (4), 374.

38 Mantoux, F., Bahadoran, P., Perrin, C., Bermon, C., Lacour, J.P. & Ortonne, J.P. (1999) Flutamide-induced late cutaneous pseudoporphyria [Article in French]. *Annales de Dermatologie et de Venereologie*, **126** (2), 150–152.

39 Borroni, G., Brazzelli, V., Baldini, F. *et al.* (1998) Flutamide-induced pseudoporphyria. *British Journal of Dermatology*, **138** (4), 711–712.

40 Iversen, P., Tyrrell, C.J., Kaisary, A.V. *et al.* (2000) Bicalutamide monotherapy compared with castration in patients with nonmetastatic locally advanced prostate cancer: 6.3 years of followup. *Journal of Urology*, **164** (5), 1579–1582.

41 Kucuk, O., Fisher, E., Moinpour, C.M. *et al.* (2001) Phase II trial of bicalutamide in patients with advanced prostate cancer in whom conventional hormonal therapy failed: a Southwest Oncology Group study (SWOG 9235). *Urology*, **58** (1), 53–58.

42 McLeod, D.G., See, W.A., Klimberg, I. *et al.* (2006) The bicalutamide 150 mg early prostate cancer program: findings of the North American trial at 7.7-year median followup. *Journal of Urology*, **176** (1), 75–80.

43 Loprinzi, C.L., Kugler, J.W., Sloan, J.A. *et al.* (1999) Randomized comparison of megestrol acetate versus dexamethasone versus fluoxymesterone for the treatment of cancer anorexia/cachexia. *Journal of Clinical Oncology*, **17** (10), 3299–3306.

44 Salvatore, M.A. & Lynch, P.J. (1980) Erythema nodosum, estrogens, and pregnancy. *Archives of Dermatology*, **116** (5), 557–558.

45 Buzdar, A., Jonat, W., Howell, A. *et al.* (1996) Anastrozole, a potent and selective aromatase inhibitor, versus megestrol acetate in postmenopausal women with advanced breast cancer: results of overview analysis of two phase III trials. Arimidex Study Group. *Journal of Clinical Oncology*, **14** (7), 2000–2011.

46 Russell, C.A., Green, S.J., O'Sullivan, J. *et al.* (1997) Megestrol acetate and aminoglutethimide/hydrocortisone in sequence or in combination as second-line endocrine therapy of estrogen receptor-positive metastatic breast cancer: a Southwest Oncology Group phase III trial. *Journal of Clinical Oncology*, **15** (7), 2494–2501.

47 Lentz, S.S., Brady, M.F., Major, F.J., Reid, G.C. & Soper, J.T. (1996) High-dose megestrol acetate in advanced or recurrent endometrial carcinoma: a Gynecologic Oncology Group Study. *Journal of Clinical Oncology*, **14** (2), 357–361.

48 Wilailak, S., Linasmita, V. & Srisupundit, S. (2001) Phase II study of high-dose megestrol acetate in platinum-refractory epithelial ovarian cancer. *Anti-Cancer Drugs* **12** (9), 719–724.

49 Loprinzi, C.L., Michalak, J.C., Schaid, D.J. *et al.* (1993) Phase III evaluation of four doses of megestrol acetate as therapy for patients with cancer anorexia and/or cachexia. *Journal of Clinical Oncology*, **11** (4), 762–767.

50 Fietkau, R., Riepl, M., Kettner, H., Hinke, A. & Sauer, R. (1997) Supportive use of megestrol acetate in patients with head and neck cancer during radio(chemo)therapy. *European Journal of Cancer*, **33** (1), 75–79.

51 Ansfield, F.J., Kallas, G.J. & Singson, J.P. (1982) Clinical results with megestrol acetate in patients with advanced carcinoma of the breast. *Surgery, Gynecology and Obstetrics*, **155** (6), 888–890.

52 Rinke, A., Müller, H.H., Schade-Brittinger, C. *et al.* (2009) Placebo-controlled, double-blind, prospective, randomized study on the effect of octreotide LAR in the control of tumor growth in patients with metastatic neuroendocrine midgut tumors: a report from the PROMID Study Group. *Journal of Clinical Oncology*, **27** (28), 4656–4663.

53 Lustig, R.H., Greenway, F., Velasquez-Mieyer, P. *et al.* (2006) A multicenter, randomized, double-blind, placebo-controlled, dose-finding trial of a long-acting formulation of octreotide in promoting weight loss in obese adults with insulin hypersecretion. *International Journal of Obesity (2005)*, **30** (2), 331–341.

54 Grozinsky-Glasberg, S., Kaltsas, G., Gur, C. *et al.* (2008) Long-acting somatostatin analogues are an effective treatment for type 1 gastric carcinoid tumours. *European Journal of Endocrinology*, **159** (4), 475–482.

55 Giustina, A., Bonadonna, S., Bugari, G. *et al.* (2009) High-dose intramuscular octreotide in patients with acromegaly inadequately controlled on conventional somatostatin analogue therapy: a randomised controlled trial. *European Journal of Endocrinology*, **161** (2), 331–338.

56 Rinke, A., Muller, H., Schade-Brittinger, C. *et al.* (2009) Placebo-controlled, double-blind, prospective, randomized study of the effect of octreotide LAR in the control of tumor growth in patients with metastatic neuroendocrine midgut tumors: a report from the PROMID study group. *Journal of Clinical Oncology*, **27** (15S), 4508.

57 Hisanaga, T., Shinjo, T., Morita, T. *et al.* (2010) Multicenter prospective study on efficacy and safety of octreotide for inoperable malignant bowel obstruction. *Japanese Journal of Clinical Oncology*, **40** (8), 739–745.

58 Lami, M.C., Hadjadj, S. & Guillet, G. (2003) Hair loss in three patients with acromegaly treated with octreotide. *British Journal of Dermatology*, **149** (3), 655–656.

59 Jo¨nsson, A. & Manhem, P. (1991) Octreotide and loss of scalp hair. *Annals of Internal Medicine*, **115**, 913.

60 O'Keefe, J.D.S., Peterson, M.E. & Fleming, C.R. (1994) Octreotide as an adjunct to home parenteral nutrition in the management of permanent endojejunostomy syndrome. *Journal of Parenteral and Enteral Nutrition*, **18**, 26–34.

61 Nakauchi, Y., Kumon, Y., Yamasaki, H. (1995) Scalp hair loss caused by octreotide in a patient with acromegaly: a case report. *Endocrine Journal*, **42**, 385–389.

62 Vecht, J., Lamers, C.B. & Masclee, A.A. (1999) Long-term results of octreotide-therapy in severe dumping syndrome. *Clinical Endocrinology*, **51**, 619–624.

63 Kwekkeboom, D.J., Bakker, W.H., Kam, B.L. *et al.* (2003) Treatment of patients with gastro-entero-pancreatic (GEP) tumours with the novel radiolabelled somatostatin analogue [177Lu-DOTA(0),Tyr3] octreotate. *European Journal of Nuclear Medicine and Molecular Imaging*, **30** (3), 417–422.

64 Gregoriou, S., Chiolou, Z. & Rigopoulos, D. (2009) Beau's lines after octreotide therapy. *Clinical and Experimental Dermatology*, **34** (8), e1020–e1021.

65 Coates, A.S., Keshaviah, A., Thürlimann, B. *et al.* (2007) Five years of letrozole compared with tamoxifen as initial adjuvant therapy for postmenopausal women with endocrine-responsive early breast cancer: update of study BIG 1-98. *Journal of Clinical Oncology*, **25** (5), 486–492.

Appendix 24.1 Incidence of dermatologic adverse events to endocrine therapies.

Drug name (Trade)				Dermatologic adverse events			
				Cutaneous and subcutaneous			Hair
Tamoxifen	Injection site reaction	Rash	Xerosis/ pruritus	Hyperhidrosis 5–9% (grade 1/2) [7]	Hot flashes 37–67.2% (placebo as high as 45.4%) (grade 1–2) [3, 6, 7]	Panniculitis/erythema nodosum/vasculitis Vasculitis Case reports	Alopecia 1.1% [7]
Toremifene					Hot flashes 15% (grade 1–2) [11]		*(Continued)*

Drug name (Trade)	Dermatologic adverse events						Hair
	Cutaneous and subcutaneous						**Hair**
Raloxifene					Hot flashes 9.7–11.6 % depending on dose (6.4% in placebo) [9]		
Fulvestrant	Injection site reaction 2.3–13.6% [13, 14]			Hyperhidrosis 4% [15] Bromhidrosis 8% [16]	Hot flashes 6.1–21% [12–15]		Alopecia 2.3% [12]
Exemestane		Rash Acneiform 3% [18] Unspecified <1% [19, 21, 22]		Hyperhidrosis 4.2–10.4% [7, 20]	Hot flashes 6.9–41.3% [4, 7, 14, 18–20]		Alopecia 1.5–2.5% [14, 18, 20] Hypertrichosis 1% [18]
Anastrozole		Rash Unspecified 7.5–10% [23, 24] Exfoliative 2% [24]	Xerosis 2% [24] Pruritus 10% [24]	Hyperhidrosis 4% [15]	Hot flashes 7.9–39% [3, 12, 15, 23]		Alopecia 9% [23]
Letrozole		Rash Unspecified 13% [27]	Xerosis <5% [27] Pruritus 9% [27]		Hot flashes 32.8–59% (placebo as high as 54%) [25, 26, 65]	Erythema nodosum Case reports	Alopecia 5–7% (3% placebo) [25–27]
Leuprolide	Injection site reaction 4.4% irritation 1.3% erythema [29]	Rash <1% [29]		Hyperhidrosis 3.8% [29]	Hot flashes 45% [29]		
Bicalutamide					Hot flashes 10.9–23% [40–42]		
Fluoxymegesterone							Hirsutism 5% [43]
Estrogen						Erythema nodosum Case reports	
Megestrol		Rash Unspecified 1% [46] Bruising <1%		Hyperhidrosis <1% [47]	Hot flashes 8% [45]		Alopecia 10% [48] Hirsutism 7% [43]

25 Agents for the Management of Hematologic Reactions

Mee-young Lee and Caroline C. Kim

Cutaneous Oncology Program, Department of Hematology Oncology, Beth Israel Deaconess Medical Center, Boston, MA, USA

Introduction

Oncology patients frequently develop hematologic changes as a result of their underlying malignancy or adverse events (AEs) from their therapies. Common medications used to support oncologic patients for the treatment of anemia are: epotein alfa (Epogen®, Procrit®), darbopoetin (Aranesp®); neutropenia: granulocyte colony-stimulating factors (G-CSF), granulocyte–macrophage colony-stimulating factor(GM-CSF): filgrastim (Neupogen®), pegfilgrastim (Neulasta®), sargramostim (Leukine®); thrombocytopenia: oprelvekin (Neumega®); and for anticoagulation: low molecular weight heparin and warfarin (Table 25.1). It is not common for dermatologic AEs to occur with these medications. This chapter discusses the presentation and management of dermatologic AEs of these therapies for the complete care of the oncology patient (Figure 25.1).

Erythropoietic growth factors: epotein alfa and darbopoetin alfa

Erythropoietic growth factors such as epotein alfa and darbopoetin alfa are widely used for chemotherapy-induced anemia or anemia after bone marrow transplantation. Both drugs are recombinant glycoproteins that bind to the erythropoietin receptor to induce erythropoiesis [1]. Epotein alfa and darbopoetin alfa are given subcutaneously or intravenously, and tend to be tolerated well with minimal systemic AEs. Hypertension, headache, arthralgia, clotting at the injection site, allergic reactions, seizures, and thrombotic events have been reported [2–4]. In oncology patients on chemotherapy, fever, diarrhea, nausea, vomiting, and edema are more commonly observed [5].

Dermatologic AEs

Cutaneous AEs from erythropoietin are uncommon and occur as case reports [3]. These are injection site erythema and pain, and, rarely, mild and transient rash or urticaria. Use of cold compresses may be helpful for injection site tenderness or redness. Antihistamines can be helpful for urticaria. Case reports have also described in the dialysis-dependent population, including increased hair growth on the extremities and widespread eczema that resolved upon discontinuation of the drug [3,6].

Granulocyte colony-stimulating factors and granulocyte–macrophage colony-stimulating factors

Iatrogenic neutropenia secondary to chemotherapy and bone marrow transplant conditioning, as well as idiopathic neutropenia are commonly treated with G-CSF or GM-CSF, which have mild AEs. G-CSF such as filgrastim (Neupogen®) and pegfilgrastim (Neulasta®), and GM-CSF such as sargramostim (Leukine®) are synthetic recombinant colony-stimulating factors that bind to the G-CSF and GM-CSF receptors, respectively, increasing proliferation and differentiation of neutrophils (G-CSF) and granulocytes and macrophages (GM-CSF) [3,7,8]. Evidence suggests that these agents decrease the risk of infection in the setting of febrile neutropenia, and accelerate myeloid recovery in patients receiving antineoplastic therapy. All three agents are given subcutaneously or intravenously, and are tolerated well by patients. Both G-CSF and GM-CSF can cause transient bone pain given the locations of bone marrow. GM-CSF can also cause dyspnea, chest pain, nausea, hypoxemia, diaphoresis, anaphylaxis, syncope, alopecia, and flushing. These AEs are often dose-limiting [8,9]. They are managed effectively by discontinuation of therapy

Dermatologic Principles and Practice in Oncology: Conditions of the Skin, Hair, and Nails in Cancer Patients, First Edition. Edited by Mario E. Lacouture.
© 2014 John Wiley & Sons, Inc. Published 2014 by John Wiley & Sons, Inc.

or dose reductions. GM-CSF is associated with fever, nausea, fatigue, headache, bone pain, chills, myalgia, and injection site reactions. Other AEs include diarrhea, anorexia, arthralgia, transient skin rashes and pruritus in less than 1% of patients, facial flushing, capillary leak, thrombotic events, hypotension, conjunctivitis, and hydrocephalus [10].

Dermatologic AEs

Common cutaneous complications of G-CSF and GM-CSF include phlebitis when given intravenously, injection site erythema that can be treated with cold compresses, and pruritic wheals (Table 25.2). In addition, there have been case reports of folliculitis, and transient skin eruptions and pruritus [3]. These clinical issues resolve rapidly after discontinuation of therapy [10]. G-CSF and GM-CSF are also associated with the exacerbation of pre-existing

chronic and acute inflammatory conditions such as leukocytoclastic vasculitis and psoriasis [2,3]. GM-CSF is also been reported to be associated with necrotizing vasculitis [11]. Cessation of the drug is the foremost effective treatment in the management of these AEs. Topical and systemic steroids may be considered in severe cases, but may not be necessary in less severe cases as these AEs resolve with discontinuation of the drug.

Neutrophilic dermatoses can rarely be precipitated with administration of G-CSF and GM-CSF. Sweet syndrome (acute febrile neutrophilic dermatosis) is characterized by the sudden onset of fever, leukocytosis, and tender erythematous edematous well-demarcated papules and plaques, and is known to be precipitated by G-CSF and GM-CSF (Figure 25.2). The lesions may be pseudovesicular or pseudopustular, or even bullous or ulcerative. Oral or eye involvement can also occur, and arthralgia or arthritis can present in 33–62% of cases [12]. Histologically, there is a dense perivascular neutrophilic infiltration of the skin, and leukocytoclasis can be seen. The etiology is unknown, although it is presumed to be caused by any type of reaction that leads to stimulation of a cascade of cytokines which precipitate neutrophil activation [10,13]. It is likely that G-CSF and/or GM-CSF directly stimulates neutrophilic involvement in Sweet syndrome via upregulation of neutrophil function and release of cytokines. Interestingly, it has been reported that patients who develop Sweet syndrome were found to have increased GM-CSF level in their serum, suggesting the role of GM-CSF endogenously [13,14]. A skin biopsy is needed to confirm the diagnosis of Sweet syndrome. Once a confirmed diagnosis is made, the growth factor can be modified, and systemic corticosteroids are the treatment of choice. Prednisone or prednisolone is usually used at an initial dose of 0.5–1.5 mg/kg/day, then tapered over at least 2–4 weeks. Fever and malaise usually respond readily to this treatment, and

Table 25.1 Classification of hematopoietic and platelet growth factors.

Granulocyte colony-stimulating factors	
	Filgrastim
	Pegfilgrastim (PEGylated filgastrim)
Granulocyte–macrophage colony-stimulating factor	Sargramostin
Thrombopoietic growth factor	Oprelvekin (interleukin-11)
Erythrocyte growth factor	Erythropoietin alfa
	Daropoetin alfa

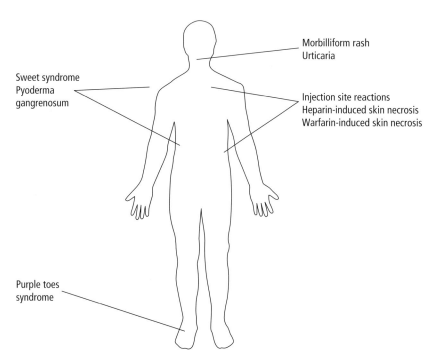

Sweet syndrome
Pyoderma gangrenosum

Morbilliform rash
Urticaria

Injection site reactions
Heparin-induced skin necrosis
Warfarin-induced skin necrosis

Purple toes
syndrome

Figure 25.1 Anatomic location of dermatologic adverse events to agents for the management of hematologic reactions.

Table 25.2 Dermatologic adverse events to hematopoietic and platelet growth factors.

Agents	Classification	Adverse events	Dermatologic adverse events
Erythropoietin and darbopoetin alfa	Erythrocyte growth factor	Nausea 11% [58]	Erythema 7% [58]
		Headache 16% [58]	Injection site irritations 7% [58]
		Hypertension 24% [58]	
		Arthralgia 11% [58]	
GM-CSF (sargramostim)	GM-CSF	Fever 81% [59][a]	Injection site erythema [12,59]
		Nausea 58% [59][a]	Generalized morbilliform eruption [12]
		Fatigue	Folliculitis [12]
		Headache	Exacerbation of pre-existing chronic and acute inflammatory conditions [12]
		Bone pain	Neutrophilic dermatoses [12]
		Chills	Bullous pyoderma gangrenosum seronegative epidermolysis bullosa acquisita (case reports) [12], exacerbation of cutaneous vasculitis (leukocytoclastic) [12]
		Myalgia	Necrotizing vasculitis [12][b]
G-CSF (filgrastim and pegfilgrastim)	G-CSF	Dyspnea	Phlebitis >1% [60,61][c]
		Chest pain	Injection site erythema pruritic wheals >1% [60,61][c]
		Nausea	Folliculitis >1% [60,61][c]
		Hypoxemia	Generalized morbilliform eruption >1% [60,61][c]
		Diaphoresis	Exacerbation of preexisting chronic and acute inflammatory conditions >1% [60,61][c]
		Anaphylaxis	Neutrophilic dermatoses (Sweet syndrome, pyoderma gangrenosum) >1% [60,61][c]
		Syncope	
		Anecdotal alopecia	
		Flushing	
Oprelvekin (Neumega or IL-11)	Platelet growth factor	Edema 41% [62]	Injection irritation 17% [62]
		Dyspnea 33% [62]	Morbilliform eruption 17% [62]
		Pleural effusions 7% [62]	
		Conjunctival injection 13% [62]	
		Atrial arrhythmia 14% [62]	

G-CSF, granulocyte colony-stimulating factor; GM-CSF, granulocyte–macrophage colony-stimulating factor.

[a]AML patients receiving GM-CSF.

[b]No specific percentages were indicated. General skin reactions were recorded as 33–62%.

[c]No life-threatening or serious adverse events were noted in clinical trials.

skin lesions resolve typically over the next 1–4 weeks [15,16]. A high potency topical steroid and intralesional injections of steroids to affected lesions have also been shown to be effective for mild cases, or as an adjunct to systemic treatment [17–19]. Other systemic therapeutic options that have been reported in the literature include nonsteroidal anti-inflammatory drugs such as indomethacin, and potassium iodide, cyclosporine, doxycycline, dapsone, colchicine, clofazamine, and pentoxifylline [12,15,16,20–22].

Likely through a similar mechanism of neutrophilic activation and cytokine release, pyoderma gangrenosum has also been associated with G-CSF and GM-CSF [10]. Pyoderma gangrenosum is characterized by a painful papule, pustule, nodule, or bulla, which progresses to a necrotic ulcer with a purulent base and overhanging erythematous border. Ulcerations may occur after trauma or injury to the skin. A skin biopsy should be performed for diagnosis and this typically shows massive neutrophilic infiltration. Infection and malignancy should be ruled out.

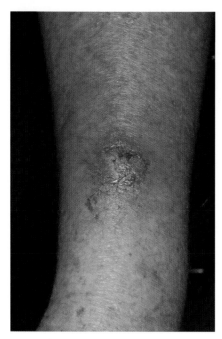

Figure 25.2 Sweet syndrome to granulocyte–macrophage colony-stimulating factor(GM-CSF).

G-CSF/GM-CSF therapy should be discontinued immediately and systemic corticosteroids are recommended. Alternative anti-inflammatory medications may also be considered if corticosteroids are not used.

Platelet growth factors

Oprelvekin (Neumega®) is a thrombopoietic growth factor approved by the US Food and Drug Administration (FDA) for prevention of severe thrombocytopenia following myelosuppressive chemotherapy regimen in nonmyeloid malignancies, which is well tolerated by patients [23]. It is administered subcutaneously or intravenously after chemotherapy. Common AEs are edema, dyspnea, pleural effusions, conjunctival injection, and, in some patients, cardiac arrhythmia associated with fluid retention [24]. These AEs can be managed medically with diuresis [24].

Dermatologic AEs

Reported dermatologic AEs of oprelvekin include a transient rash, as well as conjunctival injection, both of which resolve when the drug is discontinued, and injection site irritation. Cold compresses may be helpful for injection site reactions.

Anticoagulation agents

Venous thromboembolism (VTE) is a well-known complication for oncology patients who are hospitalized and for those who are

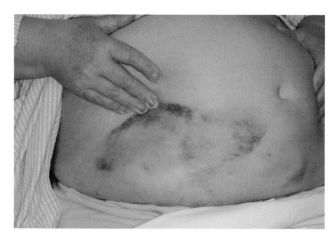

Figure 25.3 Injection site reaction to low molecular weight heparin.

receiving antineoplastic therapy [25–28]. Of oncology patients, 4–20% will have risk of developing VTE [28]. Both deep-vein thrombosis (DVT) and pulmonary embolism (PE) are included in VTE diagnosis [26]. There are multiple etiologies for this increased risk of thrombosis in oncology patients such as the release of procoagulation factors by tumors, decreased fibrinolytic activity, and extrinsic venous compression by the tumor. Other factors include increased catheterizations, surgical procedures, antineoplastic therapies, and fatigue-induced sedentary lifestyle [26,29]. Therefore, thrombosis prophylaxis for oncology patients and managing those with VTE is a critical component of patient care.

Low molecular weight heparin

Heparin is a naturally occuring polysaccharide of varying molecular weights, which inhibits coagulation via activation of antithrombin to inhibition of factor Xa. Low molecular weight heparin (LMWH) consists of only short molecular chains, and can be given subcutaneously with once-daily dosing. LMWH inhibits coagulation mainly via blocking factor Xa. It is reported to have fewer AEs than heparin, and has other advantages such as increased bioavailability, a more predictable anticoagulant response than heparin, and it does not require frequent blood work to monitor its level except in cases of renal dysfunction. AEs include hemorrhage, nausea, vomiting, dizziness, osteoporosis, heparin-induced thrombocytopenia (HIT), hepatitis, and hypoaldosteronism. LMWHs are widely used as standard of care for prophylaxis and management for thromboembolic complications in oncology patients who are at high risk for thrombosis.

Dermatologic AEs

Dermatologic AEs of LMWHs documented up to this date are injection site erythema (Figure 25.3), hypersensitivity rash, alopecia, local and distant skin necrosis from the injection site, and two cases describing a bullous pemphigoid-like eruption [30,31]. These AEs can occur immediately or within the first week of treatment, and resolve with discontinuation of LMWH [32]. Topical and systemic corticosteroids may be considered.

Heparin-induced necrosis is a rare complication of LMWH therapy, either at the local injection site or distant location, caused by thrombosis of the superficial vasculature. One variant, HIT, is associated with thrombocytopenia with a decrease in platelet count of greater than 50% or to levels less than 100 000 and paradoxical thrombosis, likely secondary to an antibody-platelet-heparin complex leading to an activation of the coagulation cascade and microthrombosis of dermal vessels [33]. HIT occurs in 1–4% of those who are being treated with either IV or subcutaneous unfractionated heparin therapy but with lower risk in LMWHs (0–0.8%) [34]. Heparin-induced necrosis presents on average 7 days after starting therapy. Redness, pain, and swelling rapidly evolve to become blisters and necrosis [32]. A biopsy may reveal epidermal necrosis and thrombotic occlusion of small blood vessels in the dermis [35]. The mainstay of treatment of heparin-induced necrosis is to discontinue LMWH immediately to avoid potentially fatal complications, and to perform a systemic work-up to identify the cause of heparin reaction and to exclude other causes of skin necrosis [36,37]. Conservative wound care with cleaning and dressings should be initiated to areas of skin loss with treatment for any related pain. Depending on the severity, surgical intervention and reconstructive surgery may be required [33,38,39]. If further anticoagulation is required, various skin tests can be performed to determine appropriate therapy for the patient.

Warfarin

Warfarin (Coumadin®) is the most common oral anticoagulant used in patient care. Warfarin inhibits vitamin K_1-2,3 epoxide reductase which prevents vitamin K from being reduced to its active form. Therefore, hepatic synthesis of the vitamin K-dependent coagulation factors II, VII, IX, and X and the anticoagulant proteins C and S is inhibited. Some 3–4 days of therapy may be needed before complete response to warfarin is achieved because previously synthesized and circulating coagulation factors must first be depleted. The duration of anticoagulant effect after a single dose is usually around 5–7 days. Warfarin is metabolized in the liver by hepatic cytochrome P-450 (CYP) isoenzymes. Serious systemic AEs of warfarin include hemorrhagic complications, cholesterol embolus syndrome, and hypersensitivity in 5–11% of patients [40]. After serious AEs, an alternative long-term anticoagulant may be considered for the patient, such as LMWH or a synthetic factor Xa inhibitor, fondaparinux.

Dermatologic AEs

Cutaneous AEs of warfarin occur less frequently than hemorrhagic complications, and include urticaria [41], morbilliform eruption [42], and livedo reticularis [43]. Discontinuation of warfarin is the mainstay of treatment along with antihistamines and/or topical steroids if the patient is symptomatic.

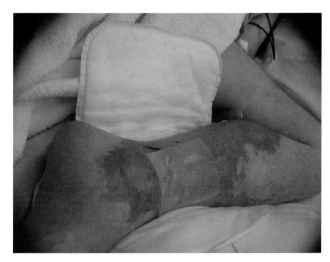

Figure 25.4 Warfarin necrosis: large purpuric patch with retiform edges and central areas of breakdown on lower extremity of patient found to have widespread thromboses after starting warfarin.

Purple toes syndrome has also been described as an uncommon AE of warfarin therapy [44–46]. Purple toes syndrome has been described as an acute onset of painful or burning bilateral violaceous discoloration of the toes and sides of the feet, which blanches with pressure and may fade when the patient is supine, occurring around 3–8 weeks after starting warfarin therapy. The etiology is not well understood; however, it is hypothesized that warfarin may either damage the cutaneous vessels directly, or interfere with the healing of ulcerated atherosclerotic plaques, leading to widespread cholesterol embolization and cyanosis of the skin [46]. A biopsy may reveal cholesterol microemboli. Warfarin therapy should be discontinued as this syndrome may portend a risk for widespread cholesterol emboli, and an alternative anticoagulant should be considered.

Warfarin-induced skin necrosis (WISN) is a rare, unusual, but well-described sequela of warfarin therapy (Figure 25.4) [47–49]. WISN occurs in approximately 0.01–0.1% of the patients receiving anticoagulation therapy and at this time around 200 cases have been reported [50,51]. WISN usually appears within the first 3–6 days of therapy, although there are cases of late onset, and it tends to occur more often in obese middle-aged women [50–53]. Clinically, WISN may initially present with an area of paraesthesia on the skin followed by a well-demarcated painful purpuric edematous area which evolves into hemorrhagic bulla and necrosis (Figure 25.1) [53]. The spectrum of tissue damage can range from self-limited superficial tissue loss to extensive necrosis to the subcutaneous tissue. Histopathology findings in WISN reveal fibrin and thrombi in small dermal vessels with no evidence of inflammatory infiltration [50,51,53–55]. The pathophysiology of WISN is unclear to date although one theory is that warfarin causes direct toxicity to the cutaneous capillaries, causing rupture, thrombosis, and tissue necrosis. Another theory is that patients with WISN may have an inherited hypercoagulable state, such as protein C and protein S deficiencies as well as antithrombin deficiency, factor V Leiden mutation, and lupus [50–53,55]. Work-up of the patient should differentiate WISN from purpura fulminans, necrotizing fasciitis, calciphylaxis, cryoglobulinemia (types II and III), cholesterol microemboli, pressure ulcers, heparin-induced skin necrosis, and inflammatory breast carcinoma [39,51,53,55].

There is no consensus for treatment of WISN; however, discontinuation of warfarin, initiation of intravenous heparin, fresh frozen plasma, and subcutaneous vitamin K should be considered initially to attempt to reverse the effects of warfarin [32,40,50,51,53,55]. Purified protein C concentrate may also be considered for patients who are deficient. WISN may progress despite discontinuation of warfarin, however, and management involves topical therapies including topical antibiotics such as silver sulfadiazine and special dressings including impregnated gauzes and hydrogels [56]. More than 50% of cases need surgical intervention including flaps and grafts to close large defects, debridement, and amputations [57]. Patients need to be carefully evaluated for future long-term anticoagulation therapy, and options may include LMWH or insertion of inferior vena cava filters. Clinicians may consider restarting warfarin, as some cases have been reported of patients with WISN without any further problems. However, this should be done with caution with monitoring for signs of recurrence. Preventative measures for WISN include continuing heparin until the International normalized ratio (INR) is near the therapeutic range with warfarin therapy, using standard or low dose warfarin.

References

1 Macdougall, I.C. (2002) Optimizing the use of erythropoietic agents: pharmacokinetic and pharmacodynamic considerations. *Nephrology, Dialysis, Transplantation*, **17** (Suppl. 5), 66–70.

2 Gaspari, A.A., Zalka, A.D. *et al.* (1997) Successful treatment of a generalized human papillomavirus infection with granulocyte-macrophage colony-stimulating factor and interferon gamma immunotherapy in a patient with a primary immunodeficiency and cyclic neutropenia. *Archives of Dermatology*, **133** (4), 491–496.

3 Asnis, L.A. & Gaspari, A.A. (1995) Cutaneous reactions to recombinant cytokine therapy. *Journal of the American Academy of Dermatology*, **33** (3), 393–410, quiz 410–412.

4 Ellis, J.D., Munro, P. & McGettrick, P. (1994) Blindness with a normal erythrocyte sedimentation rate in giant cell arteritis. *British Journal of Hospital Medicine*, **52** (7), 358–359.

5 Warkentin, T.E. & Greinacher, A. (2004) Heparin-induced thrombocytopenia: recognition, treatment, and prevention: the Seventh ACCP Conference on Antithrombotic and Thrombolytic Therapy. *Chest*, **126** (3 Suppl.), 311S–337S.

6 Wakefield, P.E., James, W.D., Samlaska, C.P. & Meltzer, M.S. (1990) Colony-stimulating factors. *Journal of the American Academy of Dermatology*, **23** (5 Pt 1), 903–912.

7 Weisbart, R.H., Gasson, J.C. & Golde, D.W. (1989) Colony-stimulating factors and host defense. *Annals of Internal Medicine*, **110** (4), 297–303.

8 Martin, L., Comalada, M., Marti, L. *et al.* (2006) Granulocyte-macrophage colony-stimulating factor increases L-arginine transport through the induction of CAT2 in bone marrow-derived macrophages. *American Journal of Physiology: Cell Physiology*, **290** (5), C1364–C1372.

9 Khoury, H., Adkins, D., Brown, R. *et al.* (2000) Adverse side-effects associated with G-CSF in patients with chronic myeloid leukemia undergoing allogeneic peripheral blood stem cell transplantation. *Bone Marrow Transplantation*, **25** (11), 1197–1201.

10 Johnson, M.L. & Grimwood, R.E. (1994) Leukocyte colony-stimulating factors: a review of associated neutrophilic dermatoses and vasculitides. *Archives of Dermatology*, **130** (1), 77–81.

11 Farmer, K.L., Kurzrock, R., Gutterman, J.U. & Duvic, M. (1990) Necrotizing vasculitis at granulocyte-macrophage-colony-stimulating factor injection sites. *Archives of Dermatology*, **126** (9), 1243–1244.

12 von den Driesch, P. (1994) Sweet's syndrome (acute febrile neutrophilic dermatosis). *Journal of the American Academy of Dermatology*, **31** (4), 535–556, quiz 557–560.

13 Lesuer, A., Palangie, A., Khanlou, N., Bouscary, D. & Jondeau, K. (1997) Sweet's syndrome associated with G-CSF treatment. *European Journal of Dermatology*, **7** (5), 375–376.

14 Kawakami, T., Ohashi, S., Kawa, Y. *et al.* (2004) Elevated serum granulocyte colony-stimulating factor levels in patients with active phase of Sweet syndrome and patients with active Behcet disease: implication in neutrophil apoptosis dysfunction. *Archives of Dermatology*, **140** (5), 570–574.

15 Fett, D.L., Gibson, L.E. & Su, W.P. (1995) Sweet's syndrome: systemic signs and symptoms and associated disorders. *Mayo Clinic Proceedings*, **70** (3), 234–240.

16 von den Driesch, P., Steffan, C., Zöbe, A. & Hornstein, O.P. (1994) Sweet's syndrome: therapy with cyclosporin. *Clinical and Experimental Dermatology*, **19** (3), 274–277.

17 Cohen, P.R. (2007) Sweet's syndrome: a comprehensive review of an acute febrile neutrophilic dermatosis. *Orphanet Journal of Rare Diseases*, **2**, 34.

18 Cohen, P.R. (2009) Neutrophilic dermatoses: a review of current treatment options. *American Journal of Clinical Dermatology*, **10** (5), 301–312.

19 Cohen, P.R. & Kurzrock, R. (2002) Sweet's syndrome: a review of current treatment options. *American Journal of Clinical Dermatology*, **3** (2), 117–131.

20 Jeanfils, S., Joly, P., Young, P., Le Corvaisier-Pieto, C., Thomine, E. & Lauret, P. (1997) Indomethacin treatment of eighteen patients with Sweet's syndrome. *Journal of the American Academy of Dermatology*, **36** (3 Pt 1), 436–439.

21 Suehisa, S., Tagami, H., Inoue, F., Matsumoto, K. & Yoshikuni, K. (1983) Colchicine in the treatment of acute febrile neutrophilic dermatosis (Sweet's syndrome). *British Journal of Dermatology*, **108** (1), 99–101.

22 Joshi, R.K., Atukorala, D.N., Abanmi, A., al Khamis, O. & Haleem, A. (1993) Successful treatment of Sweet's syndrome with doxycycline. *British Journal of Dermatology*, **128** (5), 584–586.

23 Rust, D.M., Wood, L.S. & Battiato, L.A. (1999) Oprelvekin: an alternative treatment for thrombocytopenia. *Clinical Journal of Oncology Nursing*, **3** (2), 57–62.

24 Smith, J.W. 2nd (2000) Tolerability and side-effect profile of rhIL-11. *Oncology (Williston Park, NY)*, **14** (9 Suppl. 8), 41–47.

25 Coleman, R. & MacCallum, P. (2010) Treatment and secondary prevention of venous thromboembolism in cancer. *British Journal of Cancer*, **102** (Suppl. 1), S17–S23.

26 Khorana, A.A. (2007) The NCCN Clinical Practice Guidelines on Venous Thromboembolic Disease: strategies for improving VTE prophylaxis in hospitalized cancer patients. *The Oncologist*, **12** (11), 1361–1370.

27 Khorana, A.A., Francis, C.W., Culakova, E., Kuderer, N.M. & Lyman, G.H. (2007) Thromboembolism is a leading cause of death in cancer patients receiving outpatient chemotherapy. *Journal of Thrombosis and Haemostasis*, **5** (3), 632–634.

28 Lyman, G.H., Khorana, A.A., Falanga, A. *et al.* (2007) American Society of Clinical Oncology guideline: recommendations for venous thromboembolism prophylaxis and treatment in patients with cancer. *Journal of Clinical Oncology*, **25** (34), 5490–5505.

29 Connie, M.H.F., Yarbro, H. & Goodman, M. (eds), *Cancer Nursing: Principles and Practice*, 6th edn, p. 1879. Jones and Bartlett, Sudbury.

30 Trautmann, A. & Seitz, C.S. (2010) The complex clinical picture of side effects to anticoagulation. *Medical Clinics of North America*, **94** (4), 821–834, xii–iii.

31 Dyson, S.W., Lin, C. & Jaworsky, C. (2004) Enoxaparin sodium-induced bullous pemphigoid-like eruption: a report of 2 cases. *Journal of the American Academy of Dermatology*, **51** (1), 141–142.

32 Bircher, A.J., Harr, T., Hohenstein, L. & Tsakiris, D.A. (2006) Hypersensitivity reactions to anticoagulant drugs: diagnosis and management options. *Allergy*, **61** (12), 1432–1440.

33 Handschin, A.E., Trentz, O., Kock, H.J. & Wanner, G.A. (2005) Low molecular weight heparin-induced skin necrosis: a systematic review. *Langenbeck's Archives of Surgery*, **390** (3), 249–254.

34 Menajovsky, L.B. (2005) Heparin-induced thrombocytopenia: clinical manifestations and management strategies. *American Journal of Medicine*, **118** (Suppl. 8A), 21S–30S.

35 Gibson, G.E., Coughlan, J., Wilson, A.J., Garrett, C.R. & Gertz, M.A. (1997) Skin necrosis secondary to low-molecular weight heparin in a patient with antiphospholipid antibody syndrome. *Journal of the American Academy of Dermatology*, **37** (5 Pt 2), 855–859.

36 Singh, S., Verma, M., Bahekar, A. *et al.* (2007) Enoxaparin-induced skin necrosis: a fatal outcome. *American Journal of Therapeutics*, **14** (4), 408–410.

37 Wutschert, R., Piletta, P. & Bounameaux, H. (1999) Adverse skin reactions to low molecular weight heparins: frequency, management and prevention. *Drug Safety*, **20** (6), 515–525.

38 Harenberg, J., Hoffmann, U., Huhle, G., Winkler, M. & Bayerl, C.. (2001) Cutaneous reactions to anticoagulants: recognition and management. *American Journal of Clinical Dermatology*, **2** (2), 69–75.

39 Harenberg, J., Zimmermann, R., Schwarz, F. & Kübler, W. (1983) Treatment of heparin-induced thrombocytopenia with thrombosis by new heparinoid. *Lancet*, **1** (8331), 986–987.

40 Koda-Kimble, M.A. & Young, Y.L. (eds) (1992) *Applied Therapeutics: The Clinical Use of Drugs*, 5th edn, Applied Therapeutics Inc., Vancouver.

41 Sheps, S.G. & Gifford, R.W. Jr (1959) Urticaria after administration of warfarin sodium. *American Journal of Cardiology*, **3** (1), 118–120.

42 Kwong, P., Roberts, P., Prescott, S.M. & Tikoff, G. (1978) Dermatitis induced by warfarin. *Journal of the American Medical Association*, **239** (18), 1884–1885.

43 Park, S., Schroeter, A.L., Park, Y.S. & Fortson, J. (1993) Purple toes and livido reticularis in a patient with cardiovascular disease taking coumadin: cholesterol emboli associated with coumadin therapy. *Archives of Dermatology*, **129** (6), 777–780.

44 Feder, W. & Auerbach, R. (1961) "Purple toes": an uncommon sequela of oral coumarin drug therapy. *Annals of Internal Medicine*, **55**, 911–917.

45 Moldveen-Geronimus, M. & Merriam, J.C. Jr (1967) Cholesterol embolization: from pathological curiosity to clinical entity. *Circulation*, **35** (5), 946–953.

46 Hyman, B.T., Landas, S.K., Ashman, R.F., Schelper, R.L. & Robinson, R.A. (1987) Warfarin-related purple toes syndrome and cholesterol microembolization. *American Journal of Medicine*, **82** (6), 1233–1237.

47 Flood, E., Redish, M.H., Bociek, S.J. & Shapiro, S. (1943) Thrombophlebitis migrans disseminate: report of a case which gangrene of the breast occurred: observations on the therapeutic use of dicumarol (3, 3¢methylenebis(4-hydroxycoumarin)). *New York State Journal of Medicine*, **43**, 1121–1124.

48 Verhagen, H. (1954) Local haemorrhage and necrosis of the skin and underlying tissues, during anti-coagulant therapy with dicumarol or dicumacyl. *Acta Medica Scandinavica*, **148**, 435–437.

49 Kipen, C.S. (1961) Gangrane of the breast: a complication of anticoagulant therapy. Report of two cases. *New England Journal of Medicine*, **265**, 638–640.

50 Chan, Y.C., Valenti, D., Mansfield, A.O. & Stansby, G. (2000) Warfarin induced skin necrosis. *British Journal of Surgery*, **87** (3), 266–272.

51 Nazarian, R.M., Van Cott, E.M., Zembowicz, A. & Duncan, L.M. (2009) Warfarin-induced skin necrosis. *Journal of the American Academy of Dermatology*, **61** (2), 325–332.

52 Essex, D.W., Wynn, S.S. & Jin, D.K. (1998) Late-onset warfarin-induced skin necrosis: case report and review of the literature. *American Journal of Hematology*, **57** (3), 233–237.

53 Beitz, J.M. (2002) Coumadin-induced skin necrosis. *Wounds*, **14** (6), 217–220.

54 Ng, T. & Tillyer, M.L. (2001) Warfarin-induced skin necrosis associated with Factor V Leiden and protein S deficiency. *Clinical and Laboratory Haematology*, **23** (4), 261–264.

55 Roujeau, J.C. & Stern, R.S. (1994) Severe adverse cutaneous reactions to drugs. *New England Journal of Medicine*, **331** (19), 1272–1285.

56 Timmons, J. (2000) Dressing selection for the treatment of coumarin necrosis. *Nursing Standard*, **14** (49), 66–70.

57 Cheng, A., Scheinfeld, N.S., McDowell, B. & Dokras, A.A. (1997) Warfarin skin necrosis in a postpartum woman with protein S deficiency. *Obstetrics and Gynecology*, **90** (4 Pt 2), 671–672.

58 Henke, M., Laszig, R., Rübe, C. *et al.* (2003) Erythropoietin to treat head and neck cancer patients with anaemia undergoing radiotherapy: randomized, double-blind, placebo-controlled trial. *Lancet*, **362**, 1255–1260.

59 Leukine® (sargramostim) [package insert]. (2007) Seattle, Wash: Bayer HealthCare Pharmaceuticals Inc.

60 American Society of Clinical Oncology (1994) Recommendations for the use of hematopoietic colony-stimulating factors: evidence-based, clinical practice guidelines. *Journal of Clinical Oncology*, **12** (11), 2471–2508.

61 Neupogen® (filgrastim) prescription information provided by Amgen. Available at: http://pi.amgen.com/united_states/neupogen/neupogen_pi_hcp_english.pdf (accessed 12 April 2013).

62 Du, X. & Williams, D. (1997) Interleukin 11: review of molecular, cell biology and clinical use. *Blood*, **89** (11), 3897–3908.

26 Radiation-Induced Skin Reactions

Rebecca K.S. Wong[1] and Zahra Kassam[2]

[1]Radiation Oncology, University of Toronto; Princess Margaret Hospital, University Health Network, Toronto, Canada
[2]Radiation Medicine Program at the Stronach Regional Cancer Centre, Southlake Regional Health Centre, Newmarket, ON, Canada

Introduction

Radiation-induced skin reaction, or radiation dermatitis, is a common adverse event (AE) of radiation treatment [1]. The pathophysiology and management approach is different for acute and late reactions. Acute reactions can range from erythema, dry and moist desquamation, to ulceration. Late reactions can include telangiectasia, atrophy, fibrosis, and edema. A commonly accepted definition for acute reaction is that which occurs within 90 days of radiation exposure [2]. Acute dermatitis changes in a previously irradiated area can also occur remote from radiotherapy, triggered by drugs, and is referred to as radiation recall dermatitis [3].

In contemporary radiotherapy practice, due to the use of megavoltage radiotherapy with its skin-sparing properties, acute radiation skin reactions are typically mild, especially for patients undergoing radiotherapy for deep-seated tumors. However, it can be severe and dose limiting in patients where superficial structures or the skin itself is intentionally included in the higher dose volumes. Prevention is one of the key strategies for the management of radiation skin reactions (Figure 26.1). Once an acute reaction is observed, additional management strategies are aimed at minimizing symptoms, facilitating healing, and preventing secondary complications. While these general principles are well established, clinical practices for the prevention and management of acute radiation skin reaction is quite variable. This is predominantly due to the relatively weak evidence upon which to base clinical practice. In a recent North American trial conducted in 2000–2002 on the prevention of radiation-induced dermatitis, where the control arm is "institutional preference," 14 different products were declared [4].

In this chapter we first describe the clinical manifestations and underlying pathophysiology of radiation skin reactions. Second, we discuss factors that affect the severity of acute skin reactions:

patient factors (comorbid, genetic conditions) and treatment factors (systemic agents and technical aspects of radiotherapy). Third, primary tumor sites where moderate to severe acute skin reaction are commonly encountered in the curative use of radiotherapy are described. Finally, a systematic review of interventions for the prevention and management of acute radiation skin reaction is presented. The management of late radiation-induced skin reaction is discussed in Chapter 32.

Clinical features and pathophysiology

The earliest clinical manifestation of skin reaction from radiation exposure is faint erythema. This is followed by dry and moist desquamation and, in more severe cases, ulceration and necrosis of the full thickness of the epidermis and dermis. This can be associated with edema, bleeding, and can be complicated by superadded infection. Hair loss will typically accompany mild to severe skin reactions. Subjectively, tightness and burning can occur, but the most common descriptors are itching and pain. Pathologically, acute irradiation of the skin results in a perivascular inflammatory infiltrate around dilated blood vessels with swelling and sloughing of epithelial cells and growth arrest [5]. This can be followed by obstruction of arterioles by fibrin thrombi and edema, manifesting as tender edematous erythema and moist desquamation. Disruption of the epithelial basement membrane increases the risk of superadded infection, with *Staphyloccocus aureus* [6] infections being present, especially in severe reactions.

After the acute phase, some patients are left with hypo- or hyperpigmentation. After higher doses, telangiectasia, atrophy, fibrosis, and edema can occur. In severe cases, ulcers and skin breakdown with superadded infections can occur. Alopecia and reduced sebacous glands typically accompanies these changes. Pathologically, dermis and subcutaneous adipose tissue are

Dermatologic Principles and Practice in Oncology: Conditions of the Skin, Hair, and Nails in Cancer Patients, First Edition. Edited by Mario E. Lacouture.
© 2014 John Wiley & Sons, Inc. Published 2014 by John Wiley & Sons, Inc.

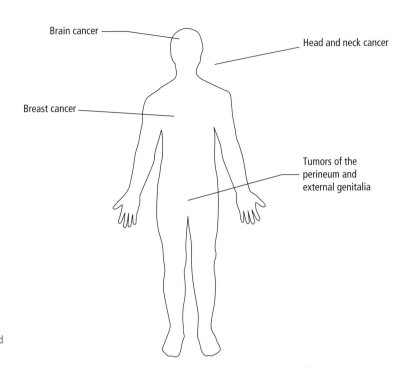

Figure 26.1 Anatomic location of radiation dermatitis will depend on area receiving radiation. The most common tumor sites associated with radiation dermatitis are shown.

Table 26.1 Acute radiation dermatitis grading system (RTOG [2], modified RTOG [10], CTCAE v.4 [105]).

Name	0	1	2	3	4
RTOG [2]	No change over baseline	Follicular, faint or dull erythema, epilation, dry desquamation, decreased sweating	Tender or bright erythema, patchy moist desquamation, moderate edema	Confluent moist desquamation other than skin folds, pitting edema	Ulceration, hemorrhage necrosis
Modified RTOG [10]	None	Dryness	Moderate flaking	Severe flaking	Patchy moist, desquamation
CTCAE V4.0 [105]	No change over baseline	Faint erythema or dry desquamation	Moderate to brisk erythema; patchy moist desquamation, mostly confined to skin folds and creases; moderate edema	Moist desquamation other than skin folds andcreases; bleeding induced by minor trauma or abrasion	Life-threatening consequences; skin necrosis or ulceration of full thickness dermis; spontaneous bleeding from involved site; skin graft indicated

A semi-colon indicates "or" within the description of the grade.

replaced by atypical fibroblasts and fibrous tissue. A reduction in the population of dermal fibroblasts and reabsorption of collagen will manifest as skin atrophy. Eccentric myointimal proliferation of the small arteries and arterioles may progress to thrombosis or obstruction, increasing the risk of skin breakdown [5]. It has not been demonstrated that the development of severe early reactions predicts whether there will be long-term effects.

Classification of acute radiation-induced dermatitis
Acute radiation-induced dermatitis varies in severity. This can be described both in terms of pathologic changes, observed clinical changes, or subjective patient reported outcomes including symptoms, function, and quality of life. The ability to classify

these consistently is important both in terms of clinical care and quality assurance, and for facilitating research [7].

The Radiation Therapy Oncology Group (RTOG) and Common Terminology Criteria for Adverse Events version 4 (CTCAE v.4) dermatology/skin AE criteria or, more specifically, the descriptors used within these scales, are commonly used (Table 26.1) [8, 9]. The scales are similar, briefly, based on visual inspection of the skin using a four-point ordinal scale (0. no change; 4, ulceration and necrosis), with minor differences in the descriptors used for each category. While these scales cover the full spectrum of acute skin changes, they are relatively insensitive in detecting more subtle changes. Modifications expanding on the grading classification below moist desquamation (Grade 2), sometimes referred to as "modified RTOG," where 0 is no change and 4 is patchy moist desquamation, is also commonly seen in clinical trials [10]. Quality of life scales provide another dimension towards the description of skin toxicities [11]. Commonly used scales in radiation-induced dermatitis trials include generic tools such as SF-36 [12] and dermatology-specific tools such as Skindex [13].

Objective measures of skin reactions such as spectrophotometry, Doppler studies, and digital photography [14] have also been used in more recent clinical trials. Reflectance spectrophotometry measures the peak value of reflectance, which is then expressed as a percentage deviation from the pre-irradiated skin [15]. Laser Doppler perfusion measures changes in skin perfusion as a result of acute radiation changes [16]. Digital photographs should be taken under ambient light and temperature conditions. It is relatively easy and accurate, useful for storing information on skin reactions, and allows for comparison at a later stage, making it particularly useful in clinical trials [17]. When combined with computerized image analysis digital photographs can be used to measure subtle changes in skin color. Color image analysis utilizes red, green, and blue coordinates which can then be used to define skin redness or erythema index [17]. While the objectiveness of these measures provide a clear methodologic advantage, limitations exist for their widespread use. In patients with severe skin reactions, and crust formation, spectophotometry and to a lesser extent Doppler studies become less reliable measures. The complexity and cost remain barriers for their use in a clinical setting, and these tools are typically reserved for selected research studies. Arguably, for pragmatic trials, patient reported outcomes are the most important outcome measures for the study of acute radiation skin toxicities.

Modulating factors for acute radiation dermatitis

The range of acute skin reactions following similar courses of radiotherapy (dose fractionation, target volumes) can vary as a result of patient and treatment factors (Figure 26.2). Important patient factors include comorbidities (diabetes, hypertension, collagen vascular diseases, smoking) and inherent genetic susceptibility. Important treatment factors include the use of combined modalities (such as chemotherapy and/or biologics) and choice of radiotherapy techniques. Knowledge of these factors can help clinicians anticipate AEs, or plan radiotherapy to minimize toxicities where appropriate.

Patient factors
Genetic susceptibility and medical comorbidities
A number of rare inherited syndromes, including ataxia-telangectasia, Nijmegen breakage syndrome, DNA ligase IV deficiency, and Fanconi anemia [18], have long been known to be associated with increased radiosensitivity, sometimes with severe and fatal responses to radiation at doses as low as 3 Gy. In recent

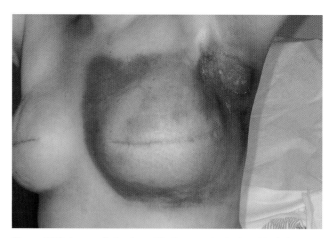

Figure 26.2 Acute radiation dermatitis, Common Terminology Criteria for Adverse Events version 4 (CTCAE v.4) grade 3. Photo courtesy of Dr Mario Lacouture.

years, the concept that variability in normal tissue reactions also has a genetic basis with an inherited complex trait is actively being investigated through radiogenomics, in which the study of the genetic variants associated with clinical normal tissue sensitivity has been described in recent years [19]. For example, *IL2RB2* and *ABCA1* genes were found to be associated with higher probability of radiation-induced dermatitis based on an analysis involving 3000 Japanese patients and genotyping of over 3000 single-nucleotide polymorphisms (SNPs) covering 494 genes [20]. P53 and P21 genetic polymorphisms, important in cell cycle regulation for response to ionizing radiation, were found to have some correlation with acute AEs among 446 breast cancer patients in Germany [21]. Existing studies have explored a range of hypotheses and employed differing methodologies. Improved understanding of these factors could guide better patient selection and individualization of therapies.

Collagen vascular diseases including rheumatoid arthritis, systemic lupus erythematosus, scleroderma, dermatomyositis, Sjögren syndrome, and mixed connective tissue disorder have traditionally been viewed as relative contraindications to radiotherapy. The potential mechanisms hypothesized include the additive effect of microvascular injury between collagen vascular disease and radiotherapy, and the increased fibrosis mediation by growth factors and cytokines [22]. Initial concern for increased radiation-induced toxicities associated with connective tissue disorders were highlighted by case reports [23]. However, larger retrospective series have not shown a definite increased risk of acute toxicity [24].

Diabetes and hypertension, both common within the cancer population, can lead to pathophysiologic changes including occlusive microvascular change, and altered blood viscosity, contributing to end organ damage (nephropathy, neuropathy, cardiovascular disease) and impaired wound healing. Both diabetes and hypertension are factors expected to increase radiation acute toxicities. Data in support of this relationship are more plentiful for late effects and less well demonstrated for acute effects [25]. Other factors that may contribute to an increase in acute toxicities or delay in healing include smoking, age, history of skin cancer, large bra size, weight >165 lbs, infection in the treated area, treatment in areas of poor vascular supply (e.g., chronic edema) [26]. While a high level of evidence is lacking to support a clear causative relationship of acute radiation toxicities and these risk factors and comorbidities, heightened awareness for the risk of developing toxicities and the need for best supportive measures is prudent.

Treatment-related factors
Cytotoxic therapy, biologics, and radiation skin reactions

The use of combined chemotherapy and radiation treatment has led to improved outcomes in the curative management of many cancers such as head and neck, lung, gynecologic, gastrointestinal, and central nervous system tumors. This is often accomplished with heightened toxicities including acute radiation skin reaction. For example, a randomized comparison of radiation and chemoradiation for anal cancer found overall radiation dermatitis in 76% for radiation alone versus 93% for chemoradiation [27]. In contrast, a three-arm randomized trial in advanced larynx cancer found similar (7–10%) Grade 3–4 skin toxicities for patients receiving radiation alone, concurrent chemoradiotherapy, and sequential chemoradiotherapy [28]. For radiotherapy to primary cancers in which skin toxicities are already moderate to severe and potentially dose limiting, the adoption of combination regimens means a greater treatment toxicity burden [29].

The combination of biologic agents and radiotherapy could result in additive, or synergistic interactions and this is under investigation in many cancer sites. It is hypothesized that this is due to interference with DNA repair pathways for epidermal growth factor receptor (EGFR) inhibitors, and preventing repair of sublethal radiation damage for vascular endothelial growth factor receptor (VEGFR) inhibitors [30]. Preclinical data supported this radiosensitizing effect for both EGFR and VEGFR inhibitors. Two randomized trials in head and neck cancers comparing cetuximab and radiotherapy with radiotherapy alone did not confirm an increase in the radiation dermatitis [31]. However, retrospective case series, as well as a quantitative meta-analysis of toxicity in patients receiving radiotherapy and EGFR inhibitor in phase I–III trials (with increased power to detect a difference should one exist) [32] estimated an increase risk of high grade (Grade 3–4) radiation dermatitis with adding cetuximab to radiation therapy with a relative risk of 2.38 (95% CI 1.8–3.2, $p < 0.001$). A recent consensus report by an advisory panel for Merck provided recommendations on skin toxicity secondary to biologics and radiotherapy, using various anecdotal strategies similar to acute dermatitis resulting from radiotherapy alone [33]. Until more evidence is available, heightened awareness represents a sound strategy, as there are no studies investigating the management of radiation dermatitis in the setting of EGFR inhibitors.

Radiation recall is a relatively rare but well-recognized phenomenon [34]. It is characterized by the reappearance of

Table 26.2 Agents associated with radiation recall in the skin [36, 106].

Cytotoxics
Actinomycin D
Bleomycin
Capecitabine
Cisplatin [106]
Cyclophosphamide [108]
Dacarbazine
Doxorubicin
Edatrexate
Erlotinib [109]
Etoposide
5-Fluorouracil
Gemcitabine
Hydroxyurea
Melphalan
Methotrexate
Oxaliplatin
Pemetrexed [110]
Taxanes (docetaxol, paclitaxol)
Transtuzamab [41]
Trimetrexate
Vinblastine
Vinorelbine [107]

Antibiotics
Azithromycin [111]
Cefotecan
Gatifloxacin
Tuberculosis treatment [112]

Other
Interferon α2b
Nimesulide [113]
Phentermine
Simvastatin
St. John's wort [39]
Sunlight
Tamoxifen

acute dermatitis changes within the radiation treatment field, occurring days, months, or years after radiation treatment. The longest interval following radiation exposure has been 15 years following administration of doxorubicin treatment [35]. While it can be precipitated by a variety of agents (Table 26.2), cytotoxics such as taxanes and anthracyclines are the most commonly associated [36]. It has also been described with biologic agents such as sorafenib [37] and cetuximab [38], as well as alternative agents such as St. Johns Wort [39]. The mechanism underlying this reaction is poorly understood. A number of hypotheses have been proposed, including vascular damage causing increased permeability and proliferative change; depletion of the epithelial stem cells; sensitization of the epithelial stem cells; and drug hypersensitivity reaction [40]. Cessation of the drug leads to a resolution of the reaction. Treatment is similar to that of radiation dermatitis resulting from radiation treatment. There have been a number of reports of re-exposure of the patient to the drug in question, using reduced doses, or coverage with steroids [41, 42]. In general, there is no need to discontinue the causal drug, as management of the skin with topical steroids usually results in resolution.

Technical radiation factors

Incidence and severity of acute skin reactions can vary significantly because of technical radiation factors including dose fractionation, choice of beam energy, and treatment techniques. In general terms, higher dose, larger treated volume, and greater dose per fraction will lead to greater acute toxicities. Accelerated treatments (use of more than one fraction per day) may result in greater acute toxicities, whereas split course treatments (where a gap is deliberately introduced into the treatment) will cause lower acute toxicities [43]. Megavoltage energy beams (used almost exclusively in contemporary radiotherapy practice) have the advantage of skin sparing effect owing to their differing physical properties. During a bolus, tissue equivalent material placed on the skin is specifically designed to ensure full dose to the skin, in selected situations with an expected increase in skin toxicities. Prior radiotherapy may incur incremental risks of toxicities because radiation repair is imcomplete [44].

Intensity modulated radiotherapy (IMRT) is a newer technique where the intensity of the radiation beams is modulated temporally or spatially, thereby allowing improved targeting of the tumor and sparing of healthy surrounding tissues. This approach is increasingly been used in many different cancers ranging from head and neck cancers to breast, sarcomas, and perineal tumors. Whether local control of tumors is improved and normal tissue toxicity is reduced with this technique is under continued investigation for different tumor sites. A randomized trial has compared IMRT with conventional two-dimensional (2D) radiotherapy in breast cancer and found a lower incidence of acute radiation dermatitis with IMRT when compared with conventional therapy (31% IMRT vs. 48% 2D; $p = 0.002$), although there were no significant differences in pain and quality of life [45]. A second study focusing on late toxicities reported similar advantages [46]. The implementation of IMRT requires significant infrastructure and incremental resources for its optimal delivery. In clinical jurisdictions where ready access to IMRT is available, its cost–benefit becomes the main consideration for its routine use [47].

Special considerations for different anatomic sites

The use of radiation in certain tumors and anatomic locations is associated with significant radiation dermatitis as a result of deliberate inclusion of skin and superficial structures in the high dose region. Six primary cancer sites are discussed including skin, brain, head and neck, breast, perineal cancers (e.g., anal canal, vulva, penile tumors), and extremity soft tissue sarcomas (STS). Typical radiotherapy dose fractionation and target volumes and anticipated toxicities are discussed.

Skin

Radiotherapy is a curative treatment option, typically for primary lesions where surgery would potentially have poor functional and cosmetic results or in a postoperative setting for patients with poor risk factors (e.g., positive margins). Typical dose fractionations ranged from 35 Gy in five fractions to 66 Gy in 33 fractions. As the target volume includes the skin and subcutaneous tissues, all patients will experience some degree of acute radiation dermatitis. Radiation treatment around the eye region may also lead to radiation-induced conjunctivitis and mucositis.

Brain

Whole brain radiotherapy to modest doses (e.g., 30 Gy in 10 fractions) is commonly recommended for the treatment or prophylaxis against brain metastases (e.g., small cell lung cancer). Partial brain radiotherapy to higher doses (e.g., 50 Gy in 25 fractions) is recommended for patients with primary brain tumors. Hair loss is one of the most emotive AE in cancer therapy, and a significant feature in cranial irradiation. Doses used in palliative and prophylactic whole brain radiation most commonly cause temporary alopecia, which occurs approximately 2–3 weeks after radiation exposure and usually resolves within 2–3 months after completion of radiotherapy, while higher doses as used in the curative setting can cause permanent alopecia. Kondziolka et al. [48] report hair loss in 88% of patients following palliative whole brain radiation with total regrowth in 24%. Lawenda et al. [49] studied 26 patients receiving higher doses (30.6–63 Gy in 1.5–2.0 Gy fractions), describing a 50% risk of developing permanent alopecia with doses of 43 Gy (95% CI 33–50 Gy) in 30 fractions. While complex skin-sparing technique with efficacy in reducing alopecia has been described [50], the possibility of underdosing the meninges and the technical treatment burden on the patient means these approaches remain experimental.

Head and neck

Radiation with or without chemotherapy and surgery is an important modality for the curative treatment of head and neck cancers. A high incidence of acute skin toxicity is typically observed as high doses (e.g., 50–70 Gy in 25–35 fractions) targeting the primary and local regional nodes is typically employed. Many studies have been published using IMRT techniques in head and neck cancers showing promising evidence of the benefits of IMRT in survival and varying acute and late toxicity outcomes [51], although this remains to be confirmed in a randomized trial setting [52, 53].

Breast

Radiotherapy to the breast is generally recommended following lumpectomy, and to the chest wall and locoregional nodal areas (axilla, supraclavicular fossa) in the post-mastectomy setting for patients with poor risk features. Doses delivered are 50 Gy in 25 fractions or its equivalent. The axillary fold, the inframammary fold, and the nipple are particularly sensitive to radiation injury.

About one-third of patients will experience significant acute skin toxicity [54]. A randomized trial demonstrated reduced incidence of moist desquamation (31% IMRT group vs. 48%; $p = 0.002$) with the use of IMRT techniques compared with standard wedge-based techniques [45].

Soft tissue sarcoma

STS are typically located in the extremities (approximately 60%) although they can also occur in other areas including the head and neck region, the trunk and the retroperitoneum. Preoperative or postoperative radiotherapy in combination with surgery is the mainstay of curative therapy in extremity sarcoma. Because of the high propensity of local recurrence, treatment volumes are typically large, with margins of 4–5 cm longitudinally and 2–3 cm radially on the gross disease or tumor bed, calling for high doses in the order of 50–70 Gy in 25–35 fractions. The surgical scar, biopsy sites, drain sites, and regions of superficial involvement are usually included, requiring bolus to ensure adequate skin dose. In a randomized trial comparing preoperative with postoperative radiotherapy, acute skin toxicity of grade 2 or greater was lower (36%) compared with 68% in the postoperative setting ($p < 0.0001$) [55]. IMRT is expected to provide better normal tissue sparing, with supportive evidence in single arm studies [56].

Tumors of the perineum and external genitalia

Tumors involving the perineal area include anal, vulvar, and penile cancers. They share many similarities in terms of acute radiation toxicities. The target area typically includes the primary tumor, involving the perianal and external genitalia skin, and the inguinal nodal areas that are included either because of gross nodal spread or prophylactic treatment for nodal regions at risk. As a result the external genitalia and perianal region are frequently exposed to high doses, with associated dose-limiting toxicities. The use of a combination of chemotherapy and radiotherapy, increasingly used as part of standard practice for anal, and vulva cancers, is associated with increased toxicities. In a randomized study comparing radiotherapy with chemoradiotherapy in 585 patients with anal cancer, all-grade acute skin toxicity was reported in 76% and 93%, respectively, while severe acute skin toxicities were observed in 39% and 50% of patients, respectively [27]. As in other clinical areas, single-arm studies would suggest skin toxicities can be reduced when IMRT techniques are used [57]. In penile cancers, bolus to ensure full skin dose is uniformly required. Skin toxicity affects all patients and may be substantial [58]. In the setting of interstitial brachytherapy, moist desquamation is maximal at 2–3 weeks after implant, but complete healing might take up to 2–3 months [59].

Management

Interventions designed to minimize the effect of radiation dermatitis can be categorized into preventive and treatment strategies, and further divided into topical versus systemic. Our group published an evidence-based guideline in 2004. In this section, we conduct an update of the systematic review [60].

Methods of the systematic review
Literature search

An updated literature search was conducted to supplement the findings from our previous work [60]. This consisted of an electronic Medline search for the period 2004 to August 2010 using the same search strategy as previously. A search for non-English language articles (previously excluded) was also conducted for the previous search period (1980 to April 2004). The search strategy employed MeSH terms and keywords designed to optimize the identification of randomized trials, guidelines, and systematic reviews on radiation dermatitis. Reference list for relevant articles were reviewed. Conference proceedings of the American Society of Clinical Oncology were conducted for the time period 2004–2010. The National Guidelines Clearinghouse [61] was searched for existing practice guidelines. We did not search specifically for nonpublished articles.

Study eligibility

Only randomized trials were included. Trials designed to examine the effect of interventions compared with control (placebo, open controls, or alternative active strategies) for the prevention or management of radiation-induced dermatitis were included. Degree of skin reaction needed to be evaluated using a validated skin toxicity scale. Only published articles were included.

Synthesizing the evidence

Studies were grouped separately based on treatment or prevention trials, and topical or systemic strategies. Toxicty grade ≥2 or its equivalent (moist desquamation) was our primary outcome of interest. Other outcomes collated included pain and itch intensity where feasible.

Study quality was assessed through a number of characteristics including randomization method, unit of randomization, accounting for all patients, and outcome assessment.

Results

Three general systematic reviews [60, 62, 63], one on the effect of aloe vera [64], one on acute radiation dermatitis, one on complementary therapy on cancer toxicity [65], two consensus guidelines from British Columbia and Ontario [62, 66], and one consensus guideline on the management of skin toxicities for EGFR inhibitors [33] were identified. A Cochrane review on this topic is under preparation [67]. A total of 37 randomized controlled trials [4, 10, 54, 68–101], with 31 prevention [4, 10, 54, 68–73, 76–95] and seven treatment trials [4, 96–101] (one trial tested sequential prevention and treatment interventions [4]) formed our evidence base.

Prevention

Washing practices

Historically, patients undergoing radiotherapy were recommended not to wash the area, nor to use soap or deodorants. Three trials (304 patients) [10, 68, 69] challenged this practice and compared washing with no washing during radiation therapy. There were fewer patients with a maximum toxicity grade of ≥ 2 in one trial (36% vs. no washing 56%, $p = 0.04$) [68] when washing was permitted, while others found a trend in favor of washing [10, 69]. Given the important psychosocial benefit of allowing patients to maintain their normal healthcare routine, the practice of allowing washing with water and mild soap is generally accepted as standard clinical practice.

Topical steroids

Four trials (181 patients) [70–73] compared topical steroids with either no treatment [70, 71], an emollient [72], or dexpathenol (a vitamin B5 preparation) [73]. While all four studies were performed on breast cancer patients, the study by Omidvari et al. [70] differed significantly by employing orthovoltage radiation. This older technology has no skin-sparing effect and is expected to result in much greater skin toxicities. In this study, the authors observed maximum toxicity grade 4 in 1/15, 2/17, and 0/19 of patients receiving no treatment, petroleum, and betamethasone, respectively, suggesting a positive benefit with the use of prophylactic steroids.

Of the remaining three studies, two [71, 72] examined the role of steroids against no treatment [71] and an emollient diprobase [72] in contemporary breast radiotherapy practice. There was a trend in support of steroids in reducing either the maximum toxicity grade (maximum grade ≥ 2; 4/30 steroid, 11/30 no treatment; $p = 0.04$) [71], or the intensity of skin erythema over time (maximum grade = moist desquamation; 4/24 steroid, 10/25 no treatment) [72]. Schmuth et al. [73] compared treatment with methylprednisolone with dexpanthenol, an emollient, and found a trend in favor of methylprednisolone in reducing significant (Grade ≥ 4, scale 0–15) radiation dermatitis ($p < 0.05$), and some suggestion of benefit in quality of life.

While all of these studies suffer significantly from inadequate sample size, there appears to be a consistent trend in support of topical steroids for reducing the severity of skin reaction in patients undergoing radiotherapy. This is frequently used in clinical practice.

Trolamine (Biafine®)

Trolamine is a nonsteroidal anti-inflammatory thought to function via early recruitment of macrophages and stimulation of granulation tissue. Three trials (n = 506) [4, 54, 74] compared trolamine with no treatment [74], best supportive care [54], or institutional preference [4] as controls. Collectively, there was no significant benefit demonstrable with trolamine. A single trial compared trolamine as the control arm with calendula and is discussed below (see Other agents).

Aloe vera

Three randomized trials compared aloe vera with use of aqueous cream, mild soap, or no treatment (n = 375) [76–78]. No significant benefit was found. A systematic review arrived at a similar conclusion [64].

Sulfacrate and its derivatives

Sulfacrate, better known for its gastric protectant effect, is expected to have an angiogenic effect and increase blood flow. Perhaps mediated via growth factors of the skin, it may stimulate the regenerative processes.

Three randomized trials were identified (476 patients) [79–81, 93], with two using the patient as their own control. In the later two studies, different halves of the patient's treatment area were randomized to sulfacrate versus base cream [79] or placebo [80] involving 50 breast and 60 head and neck patients, respectively. Maiche et al. [79] found a significant benefit with sulfacrate in the proportion of patients experiencing moist desquamation, Evensen et al. [79] found no difference but a trend for a detrimental effect. Wells et al. [80] compared sulfacrate with an aqueous control with no treatment control in 366 patients receiving radiotherapy to head and neck, breast, or anorectum but found no significant difference. The predominantly negative result would suggest no role for this class of agent outside a clinical trial setting.

Hyaluronic acid or hyaluronic acid-based combination (MAS065D: Xclair)

Hyaluronic acid (HA) is a natural polymer belonging to the sulfated glycosaminoglycans class and represents the main component of the dermis extracellular matrix. It stimulates fibrin development, neutrophilous granulocytes, and macrophage phagocytic mobility and activity, and stimulates fibroblast proliferation and therefore the healing process. MAS065D contains multiple agents among which HA is considered one of its key ingredients. Three studies employed a double blind design comparing HA alone [82] or MAS065D [83, 84] with placebo [83] or vehicle [83, 84]. The largest study (n = 152) found the proportion of patients experiencing moist desquamation was 4% HA vs. 15% in the control group ($p = 0.035$) [82]. The two smaller studies testing the combination preparation found conflicting results. Leonardi et al. (n = 40) [84] reported at least moist desquamation in 9% vs. 89% ($p < 0.0001$) while no significant difference was found by Primavera et al. (n = 20) [83]. These results suggest potential effect and the need for further study in this agent.

Dexpanthenol

Dexpanthenol (Bepanthen®) is the alcohol analog of pantothenic acid (vitamin B5), and is thus a provitamin of B5. It is a moisturizer and emollient. A single study compared it with no cream [85].

No significant benefit was observed. Two trials using dexpanthenol as the control arm, where it was compared with steroids [73] and Theta Cream [86] are discussed in the respective sections.

Other agents

A number of other agents have each been tested through a single randomized trial. These include ascorbic acid [87], combination preparations including Raygel (glutathione and anthocyanins) [88], and Theta Cream (CMGulcan, Hydroxyprolisilan C, matrixyl) [86]. Almond oil was compared with camomile cream in one study [89]. There is no convincing evidence in support of efficacy for any of these agents.

A single trial (n = 254), using a single blind design, compared trolamine, the control arm, against calendula (a marigold extract) in patients undergoing breast radiotherapy [75]. The proportion of patients experiencing Grade ≥2 toxicity was 41% calendula vs. 63% trolamine ($p < 0.001$). Benefit was also seen in maximum pain score. Adherence to the application of ointment was lower for calendula, however (84% vs 92%; $p = 0.047$), perhaps related to the consistency of the ointment.

Systemic therapy

Oral proteolytic enzymes

Oral proteolytic enzymes, including papain, trypsin, and cymotrypsin are packaged together as the enzyme combination Wobe-Mugos E. It is intended to act through its analgesic and anti-inflammatory effects. Three randomized controlled trials compared oral enzymes with no treatment [90–92]. In all three studies ≥Grade 2 skin reaction or maximum toxicity grade were all significantly lower. However, none of the studies were blinded and further evaluation with stringent methodology would serve to evaluate its role towards reducing radiotherapy toxicity.

Others

Single trials examined the efficacy of oral sucralfate [93], zinc [94], and pentoxyphylline [95]. No significant benefit was observed for oral sucralfate, although there is some suggestion for a favorable effect for zinc and pentoxyphylline. Additional studies are warranted.

Treatment

Dressings

Four randomized controlled trials were identified within this strategy [96–99]. One small study (21 patients) compared moisture vapor permeable dressing (Tegaderm®) with hydrous lanolin gauze dressing [96]. The former consist of a thin polyurethane layer covered with a hypoallergenic adhesive to allow it to stay in place. It is intended to maintain a moist environment which protects the skin allowing for wound healing to take place. The remaining three studies compared hydrocolloid dressing with gentian violet [97, 99] or dry dressing [98] as the control arm. Hydrocolloid dressings create a moist protected environment to encourage wound healing. Historically, gentian violet has been used for management of open wound because of its antibacterial and drying effect although this is seldom used in contemporary practice.

Mak *et al.* [97] counted wound area as the unit for analysis while patients were the unit of randomization, substantially weakening the randomized design. Macmillan *et al.*'s study [98] consisted of a double randomization first to evaluate prophylactic sucralfate [81] and then managing moist desquamation when it occurs. Mak *et al.* [97] and Macdonald *et al.* [104] observed a detrimental effect for hydrogel, although only the latter was statistically significant, while Gollins *et al.* [99] found a significant benefit. The methodologic limitations of these trials would mean the role of hydrocolloid dressings for established radiation-induced moist desquamation remains controversial.

Others

Single small randomized trials have been conducted on sulcrafate cream for moist desquamation [100], composite strategies comparing a cream-based regimen with a powder-based regimen for the various stages of radiation dermatitis as the patient progressed through radiotherapy [101], and trolamine introduced at the onset of itching [4] have been conducted. None of these found any significant difference between the study and control groups.

Summary of findings

The adoption of washing with water or mild soap is supported by randomized trials. The use of topical prophylactic steroids appears to have a positive effect on the incidence of severe radiation dermatitis and symptoms of itching and burning [102, 103]. There is some suggestion for efficacy with topical calendula cream, hyaluronic acid-based combinations, oral zinc, and pentoxyphylline, which deserves further study.

There is no evidence to support the prophylactic use of trolamine, aloe vera, sulfacrate and its derivatives, dexpanthenol, ascorbic acid, combination preparations, almond oil, and camomile cream for the prevention of acute radiation dermatitis. Similarly, there is no evidence in support for superiority for any specific treatment intervention although the types of interventions investigated were limited.

Conclusions

Acute radiation dermatitis is a common AE, particularly in tumors where skin or superficial structures need to be included in the higher dose target, and can represent a dose-limiting toxicity. The intensity of the radiation toxicity is expected to be increase when treatment is combined with systemic agents such as chemotherapy and biologics. In addition to known clinical factors, genetic susceptibility accounting for variants in acute toxicities is under investigation. The use of IMRT techniques has the potential for reducing acute toxicities and evidence is building in different clinical areas. The use of water and mild soap for care as part of skin care is encouraged. Prophylactic steroids have shown some evidence in reducing severe toxicities. Secondary infections with *Staphylococcus areus* appear to be associated with severe toxicity, so antimicrobial treatment should be considered in this situation. Other promising agents include calendula cream and hyaluronic acid-based combinations, oral zinc and pentoxyphylline, which deserve further study.

References

1 Balter, S., Hopewell, J.W., Miller, D.L., Wagner, L.K. & Zelefsky, M.J. (2010) Fluoroscopically guided interventional procedures: a review of radiation effects on patients' skin and hair. *Radiology*, **254**, 326–341.

2 Radiation Therapy Oncology Group. (2010) RTOG acute toxicity criteria. http://www.rtog.org/members/toxicity/acute.html (accessed 17 July 2013)

3 Ristic, B. & Ristic, B. (2004) Radiation recall dermatitis. *International Journal of Dermatology*, **43**, 627–631.

4 Elliott, E.A., Wright, J.R., Swann, R.S. *et al.* (2006) Phase III Trial of an emulsion containing trolamine for the prevention of radiation dermatitis in patients with advanced squamous cell carcinoma of the head and neck: results of Radiation Therapy Oncology Group Trial 99-13. *Journal of Clinical Oncology*, **24**, 2092–2097.

5 Hymes, S.R., Strom, E.A., Fife, C., Hymes, S.R., Strom, E.A. & Fife, C. (2006) Radiation dermatitis: clinical presentation, pathophysiology, and treatment 2006. *Journal of the American Academy of Dermatology*, **54**, 28–46.

6 Hill, A., Hanson, M., Bogle, M.A., Duvic, M. Severe radiation dermatitis is related to Staphylococcus aureus. *Am J Clin Oncol*. 2004 Aug;27(4):361–3. PubMed PMID: 15289728

7 López, E., Núñez, M.I., Guerrero, M.R. *et al.* (2002) Breast cancer acute radiotherapy morbidity evaluated by different scoring systems. *Breast Cancer Research and Treatment*, **73**, 127–134.

8 Trotti, A., Byhardt, R., Stetz, J. *et al.* (2000) Common toxicity criteria: version 2.0. an improved reference for grading the acute effects of cancer treatment: impact on radiotherapy. *International Journal of Radiation Oncology, Biology, Physics*, **47**, 13–47.

9 Cox, J.D., Stetz, J. & Pajak, T. (1995) Toxicity Criteria of the Radiation Therapy Oncology Group(RTOG) and the European Organization for Research and Treatment of Cancer(EORTC). *International Journal of Radiation Oncology, Biology, Physics*, **31**, 1341–1346.

10 Westbury, C., Hines, F., Hawkes, E., Ashley, S. & Brada, M. (2000) Advice on hair and scalp care during cranial radiotherapy: a prospective randomized trial. *Radiotherapy and Oncology*, **54**, 109–116.

11 Both, H., Essink-Bot, M.L., Busschbach, J. & Nijsten, T. (2007) Critical review of generic and dermatology-specific health-related quality of life instruments. *Journal of Investigative Dermatology*, **127**, 2726–2739.

12 http://www.sf-36.org/tools/SF36.shtml (accessed 17 July 2013)

13 Chren, M.M., Lasek, R.J., Quinn, L.M., Mostow, E.N. & Zyzanski, S.J. (1996) Skindex, a quality-of-life measure for patients with skin disease: reliability, validity, and responsiveness. *Journal of Investigative Dermatology*, **107**, 707–713.

14 Nystrom, J., Geladi, P., Lindholm-Sethson, B., Rattfelt, J., Svensk, A.C. & Franzen, L. (2004) Objective measurements of radiotherapy-induced erythema. *Skin Research and Technology*, **10**, 242–250.

15 Taylor, S., Westerhof, W., Im, S. & Lim, J. (2006) Noninvasive techniques for the evaluation of skin color. *Journal of the American Academy of Dermatology*, **54**, S282–S290.

16 Amols, H.I., Goffman, T.E., Komaki, R. & Cox, J.D. (1988) Acute radiation effects on cutaneous microvasculature: evaluation with a laser Doppler perfusion monitor. *Radiology*, **169**, 557–560.

17 Setaro, M. & Sparavigna, A. (2002) Quantification of erythema using digital camera and computer-based colour image analysis: a multicentre study. *Skin Research and Technology*, **8**, 84–88.

18 Pollard, J.M. & Gatti, R.A. (2009) Clinical radiation sensitivity with DNA repair disorders: an overview. *International Journal of Radiation Oncology, Biology, Physics*, **74**, 1323–1331.

19 Andreassen, C.N. & Alsner, J. (2009) Genetic variants and normal tissue toxicity after radiotherapy: a systematic review. *Journal of the European Society for Therapeutic Radiology and Oncology*, **92**, 299–309.

20 Isomura, M., Oya, N., Tachiiri, S. *et al.* (2008) IL12RB2 and ABCA1 genes are associated with susceptibility to radiation dermatitis. *Clinical Cancer Research*, **14**, 6683–6689.

21 Tan, X.L., Popanda, O., Ambrosone, C.B. *et al.* (2006) Association between TP53 and p21 genetic polymorphisms and acute side effects of radiotherapy in breast cancer patients. *Breast Cancer Research and Treatment*, **97**, 255–262.

22 Morris, M.M. & Powell, S.N. (1997) Irradiation in the setting of collagen vascular disease: acute and late complications. *Journal of Clinical Oncology*, **15**, 2728–2735.

23 Ransom, D.T. & Cameron, F.G. (1987) Scleroderma: a possible contra-indication to lumpectomy and radiotherapy in breast carcinoma. *Australasian Radiology*, **31**, 317–318.

24 Pinn, M.E., Gold, D.G., Petersen, I.A., Osborn, T.G., Brown, P.D. & Miller, R.C. (2008) Systemic lupus erythematosus, radiotherapy, and the risk of acute and chronic toxicity: the Mayo Clinic Experience. *International Journal of Radiation Oncology, Biology, Physics*, **71**, 498–506.

25 Herold, D.M., Hanlon, A.L. & Hanks, G.E. (1999) Diabetes mellitus: a predictor for late radiation morbidity. *International Journal of Radiation Oncology, Biology, Physics*, **43**, 475–479.

26 Porock, D., Nikoletti, S. & Cameron, F. (2004) The relationship between factors that impair wound healing and the severity of acute radiation skin and mucosal toxicities in head and neck cancer. *Cancer Nursing*, **27**, 71–78.

27 UKCCCR Anal Cancer Trial Working Party. UK Co-ordinating Committee on Cancer Research (1996) Epidermoid anal cancer: results from the UKCCCR randomised trial of radiotherapy alone versus radiotherapy, 5-fluorouracil, and mitomycin.. *Lancet*, **348**, 1049–1054.

28 Forastiere, A.A., Goepfert, H., Maor, M. *et al.* (2003) Concurrent chemotherapy and radiotherapy for organ preservation in advanced laryngeal cancer. *New England Journal of Medicine*, **349**, 2091–2098.

29 Wilson, G.D., Bentzen, S.M. & Harari, P.M. (2006) Biologic basis for combining drugs with radiation. *Seminars in Radiation Oncology*, **16**, 2–9.

30 Harari, P.M. & Huang, S.M. (2004) Combining EGFR inhibitors with radiation or chemotherapy: will preclinical studies predict clinical

results? *International Journal of Radiation Oncology, Biology, Physics*, **58**, 976–983.

31 Bonner, J.A., Harari, P.M., Giralt, J. *et al.* (2006) Radiotherapy plus cetuximab for squamous-cell carcinoma of the head and neck. *New England Journal of Medicine*, **354**, 567–578.

32 Tejwani, A., Wu, S., Jia, Y. (2009) Increased risk of high-grade dermatologic toxicities with radiation plus epidermal growth factor receptor inhibitor therapy. *Cancer*, **115**, 1286–1299.

33 Bernier, J., Bonner, J., Vermorken, J.B. *et al.* (2008) Consensus guidelines for the management of radiation dermatitis and coexisting acne-like rash in patients receiving radiotherapy plus EGFR inhibitors for the treatment of squamous cell carcinoma of the head and neck. *Annals of Oncology*, **19**, 142–149.

34 Azria, D., Larbouret, C., Cunat, S. *et al.* (2005) Letrozole sensitizes breast cancer cells to ionizing radiation. *Breast Cancer Research*, **7**, R156–R163.

35 Burdon, J., Bell, R., Sullivan, J. & Henderson, M. (1978) Adriamycin-induced recall phenomenon 15 years after radiotherapy. *Journal of the American Medical Association*, **239**, 931.

36 Azria, D., Magne, N., Zouhair, A. *et al.* (2005) Radiation recall: a well recognized but neglected phenomenon. *Cancer Treatment Reviews*, **31**, 555–570.

37 Chung, C., Dawson, L.A., Joshua, A.M. & Brade, A.M. (2010) Radiation recall dermatitis triggered by multi-targeted tyrosine kinase inhibitors: sunitinib and sorafenib. *Anti-Cancer Drugs*, **21**, 206–209.

38 Law, A.B. & Junor, E.J. (2009) Chemotherapy-induced recall of cetuximab and radiation skin reaction. *Clinical Oncology)*, **21**, 77–78.

39 Putnik, K., Stadler, P., Schafer, C. & Koelbl, O. (2006) Enhanced radiation sensitivity and radiation recall dermatitis (RRD) after hypericin therapy: case report and review of literature. *Radiation Oncology*, **1**, 32.

40 Camidge, R. & Price, A. (2001) Characterizing the phenomenon of radiation recall dermatitis. *Journal of the European Society for Therapeutic Radiology and Oncology*, **59**, 237–245.

41 Shrimali, R.K., McPhail, N.J., Correa, P.D., Fraser, J. & Rizwanullah, M. (2009) Trastuzumab-induced radiation recall dermatitis: first reported case. *Clinical Oncology*, **21**, 634–635.

42 Camidge, D.R. & Kunkler, I.H. (2000) Docetaxel-induced radiation recall dermatitis and successful rechallenge without recurrence. *Clinical Oncology*, **12**, 272–273.

43 Bentzen, S.M., Saunders, M.I. & Dische, S. (2002) From CHART to CHARTWEL in non-small cell lung cancer: clinical radiobiological modelling of the expected change in outcome. *Clinical Oncology*, **14**, 372–381.

44 Sher, D.J., Haddad, R.I., Norris, C.M. Jr. *et al.* (2010) Efficacy and toxicity of reirradiation using intensity-modulated radiotherapy for recurrent or second primary head and neck cancer. *Cancer*, **15**, 4761–4768.

45 Pignol, J.P., Olivotto, I., Rakovitch, E. *et al.* (2008) A multicenter randomized trial of breast intensity-modulated radiation therapy to reduce acute radiation dermatitis. *Journal of Clinical Oncology*, **26**, 2085–2092.

46 Donovan, E., Bleakley, N., Denholm, E. *et al.* (2007) Randomised trial of standard 2D radiotherapy (RT) versus intensity modulated radiotherapy (IMRT) in patients prescribed breast radiotherapy. *Radiotherapy and Oncology*, **82**, 254–264.

47 Haffty, B.G., Buchholz, T.A., McCormick, B., Haffty, B.G., Buchholz, T.A. & McCormick, B. (2008) Should intensity-modulated radiation therapy be the standard of care in the conservatively managed breast cancer patient? *Journal of Clinical Oncology*, **26**, 2072–2074.

48 Kondziolka, D., Niranjan, A., Flickinger, J.C. & Lunsford, L.D. (2005) Radiosurgery with or without whole-brain radiotherapy for brain metastases: the patients' perspective regarding complications. *American Journal of Clinical Oncology*, **28**, 173–179.

49 Lawenda, B.D., Gagne, H.M., Gierga, D.P. *et al.* (2004) Permanent alopecia after cranial irradiation: dose-response relationship. *International Journal of Radiation Oncology, Biology, Physics*, **60**(3), p. 879–887.

50 Roberge, D., Parker, W., Niazi, T.M. & Olivares, M. (2005) Treating the contents and not the container: dosimetric study of hair-sparing whole brain intensity modulated radiation therapy. *Technology in Cancer Research and Treatment*, **4**, 567–570.

51 Staffurth, J. (2010) A review of the clinical evidence for intensity-modulated radiotherapy. *Clinical Oncology*, **22**, 643–657.

52 Kam, M.K., Leung, S.F., Zee, B. *et al.* (2007) Prospective randomized study of intensity-modulated radiotherapy on salivary gland function in early-stage nasopharyngeal carcinoma patients. *Journal of Clinical Oncology*, **25**, 4873–4879.

53 Pow, E.H., Kwong, D.L., McMillan, A.S. *et al.* (2006) Xerostomia and quality of life after intensity-modulated radiotherapy vs. conventional radiotherapy for early-stage nasopharyngeal carcinoma: initial report on a randomized controlled clinical trial. *International Journal of Radiation Oncology, Biology, Physics*, **66**, 981–991.

54 Fisher, J., Scott, C., Stevens, R. *et al.* (2000) Randomized phase III study comparing Best Supportive Care to Biafine as a prophylactic agent for radiation-induced skin toxicity for women undergoing breast irradiation: Radiation Therapy Oncology Group (RTOG) 97-13. *International Journal of Radiation Oncology, Biology, Physics*, **48**, 1307–1310.

55 O'Sullivan, B., Davis, A.M., Turcotte, R. *et al.* (2002) Preoperative versus postoperative radiotherapy in soft-tissue sarcoma of the limbs: a randomised trial. *Lancet*, **359**, 2235–2241.

56 Alektiar, K.M., Hong, L., Brennan, M.F., Della-Biancia, C. & Singer, S. (2007) Intensity modulated radiation therapy for primary soft tissue sarcoma of the extremity: preliminary results. *International Journal of Radiation Oncology, Biology, Physics*, **68**, 458–464.

57 Saarilahti, K., Arponen, P., Vaalavirta, L. & Tenhunen, M. (2008) The effect of intensity-modulated radiotherapy and high dose rate brachytherapy on acute and late radiotherapy-related adverse events following chemoradiotherapy of anal cancer. *Journal of the European Society for Therapeutic Radiology and Oncology*, **87**, 383–390.

58 Zouhair, A., Coucke, P.A., Jeanneret, W. *et al.* (2001) Radiation therapy alone or combined surgery and radiation therapy in squamous-cell carcinoma of the penis? *European Journal of Cancer*, **37**, 198–203.

59 Crook, J.M., Jezioranski, J., Grimard, L., Esche, B. & Pond, G. (2005) Penile brachytherapy: results for 49 patients. *International Journal of Radiation Oncology, Biology, Physics*, **62**, 460–467.

60 Bolderston, A., Lloyd, N.S., Wong, R.K., Holden, L., Robb-Blenderman, L.; Supportive Care Guidelines Group of Cancer Care Ontario Program in Evidence-Based Care. (2006) The prevention and management of acute skin reactions related to radiation therapy: a systematic review and practice guideline. *Supportive Care in Cancer*, **14**, 802–817.

61 National Guidelines Clearinghouse. Available from: http://www.guideline.gov/about/index.aspx (accessed on 13 April 2013).

62 McQuestion, M. & McQuestion, M. (2006) Evidence-based skin care management in radiation therapy. *Seminars in Oncology Nursing*, **22**, 163–173.

63 Wickline, M.M. & Wickline, M.M. (2004) Prevention and treatment of acute radiation dermatitis: a literature review. *Oncology Nursing Forum*, **31**, 237–247.

64 Richardson, J., Smith, J.E., McIntyre, M., Thomas, R. & Pilkington, K. (2005) Aloe vera for preventing radiation-induced skin reactions: a systematic literature review. *Clinical Oncology*, **17**, 478–484.

65 Kassab, S., Cummings, M., Berkovitz, S., van Haselen, R. & Fisher, P. (2009) Homeopathic medicines for adverse effects of cancer treatments. *Cochrane Database of Systematic Reviews*, **15**, CD004845.

66 Nystedt, K.E., Hill, J.E., Mitchell, A.M. *et al.* (2005) The standardization of radiation skin care in British Columbia: a collaborative approach. *Oncology Nursing Forum*, **32**, 1199–1205.

67 Chan, R., Webster, J., Battistutta, D., Chung, B. & Brooks, L. (2010) Interventions for preventing and managing radiation-induced skin reactions in cancer patients. *Cochrane Database of Systematic Reviews*, **5**, CD008522..

68 Roy, I., Fortin, A. & Larochelle, M. (2001) The impact of skin washing with water and soap during breast irradiation: a randomized study. *Radiotherapy and Oncology*, **58**, 333–339.

69 Campbell, I.R. & Illingworth, M.H. (1992) Can patients wash during radiotherapy to the breast or chest wall? A randomized controlled trial. *Clinical Oncology*, **4**, 78–82.

70 Omidvari, S., Saboori, H., Mohammadianpanah, M. *et al.* (2007) Topical betamethasone for prevention of radiation dermatitis. *Indian Journal of Dermatology, Venereology and Leprology*, **73**, 209.

71 Shukla, P.N., Gairola, M., Mohanti, B.K. & Rath, G.K. (2006) Prophylactic beclomethasone spray to the skin during postoperative radiotherapy of carcinoma breast: a prospective randomized study. *Indian Journal of Cancer*, **43**, 180–184.

72 Bostrom, A., Lindman, H., Swartling, C., Berne, B. & Bergh, J. (2001) Potent corticosteroid cream (mometasone furoate) significantly reduces acute radiation dermatitis: results from a double-blind, randomized study. *Radiotherapy and Oncology*, **59**, 257–265.

73 Schmuth, M., Wimmer, M.A., Hofer, S. *et al.* (2002) Topical corticosteroid therapy for acute radiation dermatitis: a prospective, randomized, double-blind study. *British Journal of Dermatology*, **146**, 983–991.

74 Fenig, E., Brenner, B., Katz, A. *et al.* (2001) Topical Biafine and Lipiderm for the prevention of radiation dermatitis: a randomized prospective trial. *Oncology Reports*, **8**, 305–309.

75 Pommier, P., Gomez, F., Sunyach, M.P., D'Hombres, A., Carrie, C. & Montbarbon, X. (2004) Phase III randomized trial of Calendula officinalis compared with trolamine for the prevention of acute dermatitis during irradiation for breast cancer. *Journal of Clinical Oncology*, **22**, 1447–1453.

76 Williams, M.S., Burk, M., Loprinzi, C.L. *et al.* (1996) Phase III double-blind evaluation of an aloe vera gel as a prophylactic agent for radiation-induced skin toxicity. *International Journal of Radiation Oncology, Biology, Physics*, **36**, 345–349.

77 Olsen, D.L., Raub, W. Jr, Bradley, C. *et al.* (2001) The effect of aloe vera gel/mild soap versus mild soap alone in preventing skin reactions in patients undergoing radiation therapy. *Oncology Nursing Forum*, **28**, 543–547.

78 Heggie, S., Bryant, G.P., Tripcony, L. *et al.* (2002) A Phase III study on the efficacy of topical aloe vera gel on irradiated breast tissue. *Cancer Nursing*, **25**, 442–451.

79 Maiche, A., Isokangas, O.P. & Gröhn, P. (1994) Skin protection by sucralfate cream during electron beam therapy. *Acta Oncologica*, **33**, 201–203.

80 Evensen, J.F., Bjordal, K., Jacobsen, A.B., Lokkevik, E. & Tausjo, J.E. (2001) Effects of Na-sucrose octasulfate on skin and mucosa reactions during radiotherapy of head and neck cancers: a randomized prospective study. *Acta Oncologica*, **40**, 751–755.

81 Wells, M., Macmillan, M., Raab, G. *et al.* (2004) Does aqueous or sucralfate cream affect the severity of erythematous radiation skin reactions? A randomised controlled trial. *Radiotherapy and Oncology*, **73**, 153–162.

82 Liguori, V., Guillemin, C., Pesce, G.F., Mirimanoff, R.O. & Bernier, J. (1997) Double-blind, randomized clinical study comparing hyaluronic acid cream to placebo in patients treated with radiotherapy. *Radiotherapy and Oncology*, **42**, 155–161.

83 Primavera, G., Carrera, M., Berardesca, E., Pinnaro, P., Messina, M. & Arcangeli, G. (2006) A double-blind, vehicle-controlled clinical study to evaluate the efficacy of MAS065D (XClair), a hyaluronic acid-based formulation, in the management of radiation-induced dermatitis. *Cutaneous and Ocular Toxicology*, **25**, 165–171.

84 Leonardi, M.C., Gariboldi, S., Ivaldi, G.B. *et al.* (2008) A double-blind, randomised, vehicle-controlled clinical study to evaluate the efficacy of MAS065D in limiting the effects of radiation on the skin: interim analysis. *European Journal of Dermatology*, **18**, 317–321.

85 Lokkevik, E., Skovlund, E., Reitan, J.B., Hannisdal, E. & Tanum, G. (1996) Skin treatment with bepanthen cream versus no cream during radiotherapy: a randomized controlled trial. *Acta Oncologica*, **35**, 1021–1026.

86 Roper, B., Kaisig, D., Auer, F., Mergen, E. & Molls, M. (2004) Theta-Cream versus Bepanthol lotion in breast cancer patients under radiotherapy: a new prophylactic agent in skin care? *Strahlentherapie und Onkologie*, **180**, 315–322.

87 Halperin, E.C., Gaspar, L., George, S., Darr, D. & Pinnell, S. (1993) A double-blind, randomized, prospective trial to evaluate topical vitamin C solution for the prevention of radiation dermatitis. CNS Cancer Consortium. *International Journal of Radiation Oncology, Biology, Physics*, **26**, 413–416.

88 Miko Enomoto, T., Johnson, T., Peterson, N., Homer, L., Walts, D. & Johnson, N. (2005) Combination glutathione and anthocyanins as an alternative for skin care during external-beam radiation. *American Journal of Surgery*, **189**, 627–630, discussion 630–631.

89 Maiche, A.G., Grohn, P. & Maki-Hokkonen, H. (1991) Effect of chamomile cream and almond ointment on acute radiation skin reaction. *Acta Oncologica*, **30**, 395–396.

90 Kaul, R., Mishra, B.K., Sutradar, P., Choudhary, V. & Gujral, M.S. (1999) The role of Wobe-Mugos in reducing acute sequele of radiation in head and neck cancers: a clinical phase-III randomized trial. *Indian Journal of Cancer*, **36**, 141–148.

91 Gujral, M.S., Patnaik, P.M., Kaul, R. *et al.* (2001) Efficacy of hydrolytic enzymes in preventing radiation therapy-induced side effects in patients with head and neck cancers. *Cancer Chemotherapy and Pharmacology*, **47** (Suppl.), S23–S28.

92 Dale, P.S., Tamhankar, C.P., George, D. & Daftary, G.V. (2001) Co-medication with hydrolytic enzymes in radiation therapy of uterine cervix: evidence of the reduction of acute side effects. *Cancer Chemotherapy and Pharmacology*, **47** (Suppl.), S29–S34.

93 Lievens, Y., Haustermans, K., Van den Weyngaert, D. *et al.* (1998) Does sucralfate reduce the acute side-effects in head and neck cancer

treated with radiotherapy? A double-blind randomized trial. *Radiotherapy and Oncology*, **47**, 149–153.

94 Lin, L.C., Que, J., Lin, L.K. & Lin, F.C. (2006) Zinc supplementation to improve mucositis and dermatitis in patients after radiotherapy for head-and-neck cancers: a double-blind, randomized study. *International Journal of Radiation Oncology, Biology, Physics*, **65**, 745–750.

95 Aygenc, E., Celikkanat, S., Kaymakci, M. Aksaray, F. & Ozdem, C. (2004) Prophylactic effect of pentoxifylline on radiotherapy complications: a clinical study. *Otolaryngology: Head and Neck Surgery*, **130**, 351–356.

96 Shell, J.A., Stanutz, F. & Grimm, J. (1986) Comparison of moisture vapor permeable (MVP) dressings to conventional dressings for management of radiation skin reactions. *Oncology Nursing Forum*, **13**, 11–16.

97 Mak, S.S., Molassiotis, A., Wan, W.M., Lee, I.Y. & Chan, E.S. (2000) The effects of hydrocolloid dressing and gentian violet on radiation-induced moist desquamation wound healing. *Cancer Nursing*, **23**, 220–229.

98 Macmillan, M.S., Wells, M., MacBride, S., Raab, G.M., Munro, A. & MacDougall, H. (2007) Randomized comparison of dry dressings versus hydrogel in management of radiation-induced moist desquamation. *International Journal of Radiation Oncology, Biology, Physics*, **68**, 864–872.

99 Gollins, S., Gaffney, C., Slade, S. & Swindell, R. (2008) RCT on gentian violet versus a hydrogel dressing for radiotherapy-induced moist skin desquamation. *Journal of Wound Care*, **17**, 268–270.

100 Delaney, G., Fisher, R., Hook, C. & Barton, M. (1997) Sucralfate cream in the management of moist desquamation during radiotherapy. *Australasian Radiology*, **41**, 270–275.

101 Schreck, U., Paulsen, F., Bamberg, M. & Budach, W. (2002) Intraindividual comparison of two different skin care conceptions in patients undergoing radiotherapy of the head-and-neck region. Creme or powder? *Strahlentherapie und Onkologie*, **178**, 321–329.

102 Neben-Wittich, M.A., Atherton, P.J., Schwartz, D.J., Sloan, J.A., Griffin, P.C., Deming, R.L., Anders, J.C., Loprinzi, C.L., Burger, K.N., Martenson, J.A., Miller, R.C. Comparison of Provider-Assessed and Patient-Reported Outcome Measures of Acute Skin Toxicity During a Phase III Trial of Mometasone Cream Versus Placebo During Breast Radiotherapy: The North Central Cancer Treatment Group (N06C4). *Int J Radiat Oncol Biol Phys.* 2010 Sep 30. [Epub ahead of print] PubMed PMID: 20888137.

103 Miller, R.C., Schwartz, D.J., Sloan, J.A., Griffin, P.C., Deming, R.L., Anders, J.C., Stoffel, T.J., Haselow, R.E., Schaefer, P.L., Bearden, J.D. 3rd, Atherton, P.J., Loprinzi, C.L., Martenson, J.A. Mometasone Furoate Effect on Acute Skin Toxicity in Breast Cancer Patients Receiving Radiotherapy: A Phase III Double-Blind, Randomized Trial from the North Central Cancer Treatment Group N06C4. *Int J Radiat Oncol Biol Phys.* 2010 Aug 26. [Epub ahead of print] PubMed PMID: 20800381; PubMed Central PMCID: PMC2995007.

104 Macdonald, O.K., Kruse, J.J., Miller, J.M. *et al.* (2009) Proton beam radiotherapy versus three-dimensional conformal stereotactic body radiotherapy in primary peripheral, early-stage non-small-cell lung carcinoma: a comparative dosimetric analysis. *International Journal of Radiation Oncology, Biology, Physics*, **75**, 950–958.

105 Common Terminology Criteria for Adverse Events (CTCAE) and Common Toxicity Criteria (CTC) (2010) Available from: http://ctep.cancer.gov/protocolDevelopment/electronic_applications/ctc.htm (accessed 17 July 2013) (accessed on October 2010).

106 Fitzgerald, T.J., Jodoin, M.B., Tillman, G. *et al.* (2008) Radiation therapy toxicity to the skin. *Dermatologic Clinics*, **26**, 161–172, ix.

107 Zhu, Z.F., Fan, M. & Fu, X.L. (2010) Radiation recall with vinorelbine and cisplatin. *Onkologie*, **33**, 107–109.

108 Borroni, G., Vassallo, C., Brazzelli, V. *et al.* (2004) Radiation recall dermatitis, panniculitis, and myositis following cyclophosphamide therapy: histopathologic findings of a patient affected by multiple myeloma. *American Journal of Dermatopathology*, **26**, 213–216.

109 Dauendorffer, J.N. & Dupuy, A. (2009) Radiation recall dermatitis induced by erlotinib. *Journal of the American Academy of Dermatology*, **61**, 1086.

110 Barlesi, F., Tummino, C., Tasei, A.M. & Astoul, P. (2006) Unsuccessful rechallenge with pemetrexed after a previous radiation recall dermatitis. *Lung Cancer (Amsterdam, Netherlands)*, **54**, 423–425.

111 Vujovic, O. (2010) Radiation recall dermatitis with azithromycin. *Current Oncology*, **17**, 119–121.

112 Extermann, M., Vogt, N., Forni, M. & Dayer, P. (1995) Radiation recall in a patient with breast cancer treated for tuberculosis. *European Journal of Clinical Pharmacology*, **48**, 77–78.

113 Ng, A.W., Wong, F.C., Tung, S.Y. & S. K.O. (2007) Nimesulide: a new trigger of radiation recall reaction. *Clinical Oncology*, **19**, 364–365.

Appendix 26.1 Summary of prophylactic and treatment randomized trials.

PROPHYLAXIS				Intervention	No	Scale	Criteria	Proportion/ scores	p value
TOPICAL									
Washing practices									
Roy [68]	2001	Breast	Study	Washing	50	RTOG	(>Grade 2)	18/50	0.04
			Control	No washing	50			28/50	
Westbury [10]	2000	Brain	Study	Washing	54	Mod RTOG	Grade 4 at week 6	1/54	ns
			Control	No washing	55			1/55	
Campbell [69]	1992	Breast	Study 1	Washing with soap and water	32	Mod RTOG	Grade 4 at week 8	0.45 (no bolus) 0.45 (with bolus)	<0.05
			Study 2	Washing with water	35			0.45 (no bolus) 0.8 (with bolus)	<0.05
			Control	No washing	28			1.1 (no bolus) 1.45 (with bolus)	
Topical steroids									
Omidvari [70]	2007	Breast orthovoltage	Study	Betamethasone 0.1%	19	RTOG	>Grade 2	17/19	na
			Control1	Petrolatum	17			17/17	
			Control 2	None	15			14/15	
Shukla [71]	2006	Breast	Study	Beclomethasone spray 200 µg bid	30	RTOG	>Grade 2	4/30	0.04
			Control	None	30			11/30	
Bostrom [72]	2001	breast	Study	Mometasone + emollient (diprobase)	24	1–6			0.011 for trend over time
			Control	Placebo + emollient (diprobase)	25			10/25	
Schmuth [73]	2002		Study 1	0.5% dexpathenol	11	0–15		data not shown	<0.05, for patients with score ±4 (max 15)
			Study 2	0.1% methylprednisolon	10				
Trolamine									
Fenig [74]	2000	breast	Study	Trolamine	25	RTOG	Grade 3–4	6 (25%)	0.98 (nurses)
			control1	Lipiderm	24			5 (23%)	
			control 2	No treatment	25			6 (25%)	
Fisher [54]	2000	Breast	Study	Trolamine	83	RTOG	≥Grade 2	27 (41%)	0.77
			Control	Best supportive care	89			26 (35%)	

PROPHYLAXIS		Type of patients		Intervention	No	Scale	Criteria	Proportion/ scores	p value
Elliott [4]	2006	H+N	Study 1	Prevention	166	RTOG	≥Grade 2	131/166 (79%)	ns
			Study 2	Intervention	175			135/175 (77%)	
			Control	Institutional preference	165			130/165 (79%)	
Pommier [75]	2004	breast	Study 1	Trolamine	128	RTOG	≥Grade 2	63%	<0.001
			Study 2	Calendula	126			42%	
Aloe vera									
Williams Trial 1 [76]	1996	Breast	Study	Aloe vera	97	0–3		20%	0.36
			Control	Placebo	97			20%	
Willaims Trial 2 [76]	1996	Breast	Study	Aloe vera	54			28%	0.31
			Control	No treatment	53			32%	
Olsen [77]	2001	Misc	Study	Aloe vera + mild soap	33	0–4		Time to erythema	0.95
			Control	Mild soap	40				
Heggie [78]	2002	Breast	Study	Aloe vera cream	107	Descriptors	≥1% moist desquamation	35/107	0.35
			Control	Aqueous cream	101			27/101	
Sulfacrate									
Maiche [79]	1994	Breast	Study	Sucralfate cream (7%)	50	0–4 scale	Gradw 2 week 5	17/50;34%	<0.05
			Control	Base cream				35/50; 70%	
Evensen [80]	2001	H+N	Study	Topical na sucrose octasulfate to skin and oral rinse	60	Mod RTOG	≥Grade 3 Mean desquamation score	19/60 (31%) 0.82 ± 0.47	0.02
			Control	Placebo				10/60 (27%) 0.72 ± 0.46	
Wells [81]	2004	Misc (H+N, breast, anorectum)	Study	Sucralfate cream	122	Mod RTOG		1.24	0.41
			Control 1	Aqueous cream	120			1.29	
			Control 2	No cream	124			1.31	
Hyaluronic acid alone or combination									
Liguori [82]	1997	Misc (H+N, breast, pelvis)	Study	Hyaluronic acid 0.2%	70	0–5 scale	≥3	4.1% (3/70)	0.035
			Control	Placebo	64			15% (10/64)	

(Continued)

PROPHYLAXIS		Type of patients		Intervention	No	Scale	Criteria	Proportion/ scores	p value
Primavera [83]	2006	Breast	Study	Xclair	20				ns
			Control	Vehicle					
Leonardi [84]	2008	Breast	Study	Xclair	22	NCI CTC	≥Grade	2 2/22 (9%)	<0.0001
			Control	Vehicle	18			16/18 (89%)	
Dexpathenol									
Lokkevik [85]	1996		Study	Dexpanthenol	79	Mod RTOG	Grade 4	10/79	ns
			Control	No cream				14/79	
Schmuth [73]	2002			See steroids					
Roper [86]				See Thetacream					
Ascorbic acid									
Halperin [87]	1993	brain	Study	Ascorbic acid	84	0–4		–	0.1
			Control	Placebo					
Raygel									
Miko Enomoto [88]	2005	breast	Study	Glutathione, anthocyanins	15	Unclear		–	ns
			Control	Placebo	15			–	
Theta cream									
Roper [86]	2004	breast	Study	CM Glucan, Hydroxyprolisilan C Matrixyl	10	Unclear		–	ns
			Control		10			–	
Almond oil & camomile cream									
Maiche [89]	1991	breast	Study	Chamomile cream	50	0–3	Grade 3	8%	ns
			Control	Almond oil				6%	
Calendula									
Pommier [75]	2004	See Trolamine section							
SYSTEMIC									
Oral proteolytic enzymes									
Kaul [90]	1999	H+N	Study	WM enzymes	25	EORTC 0–4	≥Grade 2	28%	na
			Control	No treatment	25			84%	
Gujral [91]	2001	H+N	Study	WM enzymes	53	RTOG	Mean max toxicity	1.23 (SD 0.75)	<0.0001
			Control	No treatment	47			2.39 (SD 1.1)	
Dale [92]	2001	Cervix	Study	WM enzymes	60	RTOG	Mean max toxicity	0.97 (SD0.82)	<0.001
			Control	No treatment	60			1.68 (SD 0.87)	

PROPHYLAXIS		Type of patients		Intervention	No	Scale	Criteria	Proportion/ scores	p value
Sulcrafate									
Leivens [93]	1998	H+N	Study	Sulcrafate 1 g x6/ day	50	0–6	Mean	2.5 ± 1.2	ns
			Control	Placebo	38			2.3 ± 1.3	
Zinc									
Lin [94]	2006	H+N	Study	Zinc 25 mg x3/day	49	RTOG	Severity of dermatitis	(Data as time curves only)	0.003
			Control	Placebo	48				
Pentoxyphylline									
Aygenic [95]	2004	H+N	Study	Pentoxifylline 400 mg tid	40	1–5		2.6	>0.05
			Control	Placebo	38			2.55	
TREATMENT									
Dressings									
Shell [96]	1986	Misc H+N, Breast, esoph, lung	Study	Moisture vapor pemeable (Tegarderm®) changed q 3–5 days	10	Time to wound healing		9 days	na
			Control	Hydrous lanolin gauze dressing Changed daily	11			24 days	
Mak [97]	2000	Pred Nasopharynx	Study	Hydrocolloid dressing	21 (33 wounds)	Time to wound healing		11.4 days (range 4–22)	ns
			Control	Gentian violet	18 (32 wounds)			11.7days (range 6–19)	
MacMillan [98]	2007	Misc H+N, Breast, anorectum	Study	Hydrogel dressing	185 (58 Grade 2)	Time to wound healing		Median 10 days	
			Control	Dry dressing	181 (42 Grade 2)			8 days	HR 0.64 (95%CI 0.4 ± 1) p = 0.043
Golllins [99]	2008	H+N or breast	Study	Hydrogel dressing	14	Time to wound healing		Median 12 days	
			Control	Gentian violet (0.5%)	16			>30 days	HR 7.95 (95% CI 2.2–27) p = 0.002

(Continued)

PROPHYLAXIS		Type of patients		Intervention	No	Scale	Criteria	Proportion/ scores	p value
Sulcrafate									
Delaney [100]	1997	Misc H+N, breast, other	Study	Sulcralfate 10% in sorbolene cream	20	Time to wound healing		Median 14.8 days	0.86
			Control	Sorbolene cream	19			14.2 days	
Composite strategies									
Schreck [101]	2002		Study	Cream-based regimen	12				ns
			Control	Power-based regimen					
Trolamine									
Elliott [4] (also in prophylaxis)	2006	H+N	Study 1	Prevention	166	RTOG	≥Grade 2	131/166 (79%)	
			Study 2	Intervention	175			135/175 (77%)	
			Control	Institutional preference	165			130/165 (79%)	

27 Hematopoietic Stem Cell Transplantation and Graft Versus Host Disease

Stephanie W. Hu[1] and Jonathan Cotliar[2]

[1]Ronald O. Perelman Department of Dermatology, New York University School of Medicine, New York, NY, USA
[2]Robert H. Lurie Comprehensive Cancer Center, Northwestern University Feinberg School of Medicine, Chicago, IL, USA

Introduction

Hematopoietic stem cell transplantation (HSCT) is a therapeutic intervention utilized primarily for hematologic and lymphoid cancers. It also provides the best chance for a cure for several autoimmune and many genetic diseases, and as such has become an important therapeutic option for various malignant and nonmalignant conditions. Indications for its use have expanded, especially among older patients, and novel strategies including donor leukocyte infusions, nonmyeloablative conditioning, and umbilical cord blood (UCB) transplantation have emerged [1]. The number of allogeneic HSCTs has risen to more than 25 000 procedures undertaken annually. The growing importance of this treatment modality and increasing numbers of patients presenting with its acute and chronic complications render understanding of HSCT-related dermatologic adverse events (AEs) even more crucial. This chapter summarizes several dermatologic complications of HSCT, with particular attention to graft versus host disease (GVHD).

Indications for and methods of hematopoietic stem cell transplantation

Hematopoietic stem cells give rise to primitive progenitors that produce less-differentiated precursors which, in turn, continuously synthesize mature blood cells. These original stem cells have the unique capacity to produce some daughter cells that retain stem cell properties, capable of providing a lifelong source of blood cells rather than becoming specialized. Cancers, including those of hematopoietic origin, arise from malignant stem cells that usually originate from normal stem cells but have retained the mechanism for self-renewal. For example, most leukemic cells have a limited capacity for proliferation and are continuously replenished by leukemic stem cells.

Chemotherapy used to treat cancers acts predominantly on proliferating cells. Normal and malignant stem cells, however, are quiescent and therefore insensitive to therapy. Thus, while the lethal doses of total-body irradiation and chemotherapy given in preparation for HSCT can destroy a tumor almost completely, the stem cells are often spared, allowing the cancer to recur. However, even these cells maintain their susceptibility to immunologically active donor cells received during HSCT, which initiate immune reactions related to histocompatibility. The severity of the reaction depends on the degree of incompatibility, which is determined by the binding of small peptides from degraded proteins to polymorphic class I and II human leukocyte antigen (HLA) cell-surface glycoproteins and their presentation to T lymphocytes by the antigen-presenting cells of the body. Graft rejection occurs when recipient T cells recognize foreign donor antigens; GVHD and graft versus tumor/leukemia (GVT/GVL) effects arise when donor T cells recognize recipient antigens. In the setting of hematologic malignancies, a delicate balance exists between the harmful consequences of GVHD and the benefits of donor lymphocyte attack on recipient malignant cells (GVT/GVL).

Preparative regimens

Prior to transplantation, a preparative regimen is given with the goal of eradicating cancer and, in allogeneic transplantation, to induce the immunosuppression that permits donor cell engraftment. This preparative regimen can also enhance the antitumor immune response by causing a breakdown of tumor cells, which results in an inundation of tumor antigens into the system, all of which can be recognized by antigen-presenting cells. This can lead to the proliferation of the latter, which immunologically trigger the demise of residual cancer by attacking the surviving malignant cells and eliminating them [2].

Source of stem cells

Hematopoietic stem cells were first obtained by repeated aspiration of the bone marrow in the posterior iliac crests while the donor was under general or local anesthesia [3]. Peripheral blood stem cells (PBSC) have now largely replaced marrow for autologous and most allogeneic transplantations, as it constantly cycles between continuous detachment of marrow stem cells, their entry into the circulation, and their eventual return to the marrow, rendering it a convenient source of such cells. Unfortunately, PBSC also contain more T cells than bone marrow does, thus increasing the incidence [4] and prolong the course [5] of GVHD in allogeneic transplantation. The number of CD34$^+$ stem cells (a cell-surface molecule used as a surrogate marker for estimating PBSC), can be increased by mobilizing them from the marrow with granulocyte colony-stimulating factor (G-CSF), which causes neutrophil proliferation and protease release, leading to degradation of the anchoring proteins tethering stem cells to the marrow stroma [6]. When G-CSF is given after chemotherapy, the mobilization of CD34$^+$ cells is increased; in addition, combining G-CSF and plerixafor (AMD3100) is superior to administering G-CSF alone in mobilizing CD34$^+$ cells, with the latter agent functioning as a small-molecule reversible inhibitor of the CXC chemokine receptor 4 (CXCR4), a receptor on CD34$^+$ cells that mediates the adhesion of CD34$^+$ cells to marrow [7].

Autologous stem cell transplantation is now used more often than allotransplantation. As this technique does not typically induce GVHD (recent studies have challenged this paradigm), it can be used in older patients. Mortality is considerably lower with autotransplantation than with allotransplantation, but the absence of GVT activity in autotransplantation reduces its efficacy. Indeed, the failure to eradicate cancer in the autologous transplant patient is the primary cause of relapse, and the contamination of the graft with the patient's own tumor cells also contributes [8]. Unfortunately, survival does not appear to improve with the eradication of tumor cells from autografts, immunologically or with the use of other techniques [9].

If transplantation is urgent or if suitable donors are not found, umbilical cord blood can be used. This source is rich in hematopoietic stem cells and is easily and safely procured, but also limited in supply. It is collected immediately after birth and then frozen. While infection is common during the post-transplant course because hematologic and immunologic reconstitution is slow in transplanted cord blood, cord blood as a source of stem cells can be advantageous in several respects. Its transplantation requires less stringent HLA matching than is required for that of adult peripheral blood or marrow, and mismatched cord blood cells are less likely to cause GVHD, without losing the GVT effect [10]. The results are thus better with fewer HLA mismatches and greater numbers of CD34$^+$ cells [10]. Additionally, when the first graft contains few cells, the use of additional grafts from different donors can allow for improvement of the engraftment [11].

Type of donor

Less than 30% of patients undergoing HSCT have HLA-identical siblings. Thus, the recruitment of other donor types has been an important advance in the field. High rates of engraftment failure and GVHD initially accompanied transplantation involving a haploidentical donor using stem cells from parents, siblings, or children of patients with only one identical HLA haplotype. The complications that ensued caused death soon after transplantation, but technical advances have improved outcomes over the past decade [12], with increased harnessing of the ability to improve the chances of engraftment and reduce the risk of GVHD; in patients with acute myeloid leukemia, the concept of alloreactivity has even allowed the reduction of the rates of relapse [13].

Today, HSCT results in more cures and remissions than alternative treatments but remains a significant cause of morbidity and mortality. Although the mortality rate is less than 2% for some autologous transplantations and less than 10% for some allogeneic transplantations, complications related to transplantation resulting in death continue to occur in nearly 40% of patients with advanced cancer who undergo allogeneic transplantation [14]. The safety of transplantation may be enhanced by reducing the toxicity of the preparative regimen and selecting the appropriate donor. In addition, it is critical that the appropriate use of HSCT be accompanied by full knowledge of its outcome and likely complications.

Complications of HSCT

Early complications of HSCT include mucositis, hepatic veno-occlusive disease [15–19], transplantation-related lung injury [20, 21], transplantation-related infections [22], and acute GVHD. Delayed effects include chronic GVHD [23], reduced fertility in both men and women [24, 25], impaired growth and development in children [26], and an increased frequency of secondary cancers [27, 28]. Other conditions that have been reported following transplantation include hypothyroidism, sexual problems, depression, and anxiety [29].

Early cutaneous complications

Mucositis is an important problem after HSCT, developing and requiring treatment in 70–80% of patients. In the short term, it is the most common complication of myeloablative preparative regimens. Methotrexate, one of the typical agents used as GVHD prophylaxis in HSCT patients, compounds this mucositis early after allotransplantation. Oropharyngeal mucositis is painful and can involve the supraglottic area, necessitating intubation for adequate management. Intestinal mucositis causes nausea, cramping, and diarrhea, which may entail parenteral nutrition as a supportive measure. A recombinant human keratinocyte growth factor, palifermin, reduces the incidence of oral mucositis after autologous transplantation, with only 20% of patients in the palifermin group developing grade 4 oral mucositis, compared with 62% in the placebo group ($p < 0.001$) [30].

Acute graft versus host disease

Pathogenesis

Despite technical advances, GVHD remains the most frequent and serious complication following allogeneic HSCT, and limits the broader application of this important therapy. In 1966, Billingham [31] formulated three conditions required for the development of GVHD:

1. The graft must contain immunologically competent cells;
2. The recipient must express tissue antigens different from those in the transplant donor; and
3. The patient must be incapable of mounting an effective response against the transplanted cells.

It is now clear that the immunologically competent cells are in fact T cells, and that GVHD can develop in various clinical settings when tissues containing T cells (blood products, bone marrow, and solid organs) are transferred from one person to another, the latter being unable to eradicate those cells [32, 33].

Allogeneic HSCT is the most common setting for the development of GVHD, which arises when donor T cells respond to genetically defined proteins on host cells as a result of mismatches between major or minor histocompatibility antigens between the donor and recipient, in an environment in which immunoablative chemotherapy or radiation had previously eliminated host cell function. The most important proteins are HLAs, which are highly polymorphic and are encoded by the major histocompatibility complex (MHC) on the short arm of chromosome 6 [34, 35]. The incidence of GVHD is directly related to the degree of mismatch between HLA proteins [36, 37]; while donors and recipients are matched at HLA A, B, C, and DRB1 in an ideal setting, mismatches can be tolerated for umbilical cord blood grafts.

Despite full HLA matching between a patient and donor, however, the incidence of acute GVHD ranges 26–32% in recipients of sibling donor grafts, and 42–52% in recipients of unrelated donor grafts [38]. The frequency of this phenomenon is likely related to genetic differences that lie outside the HLA loci, or "minor" histocompatibility antigens (HA). These are immunogenic peptides derived from polymorphic proteins presented on the cell surface by MHC molecules [39], and it has been shown that some HAs, such as HY and HA-3, are expressed on all tissues and are targets for both GVHD and GVT, whereas other HAs, such as HA-1 and HA-2, are expressed abundantly on hematopoietic cells (including leukemic cells) and may induce a greater GVT effect with less GVHD [39, 40].

Other than the degree of HLA disparity, risk factors for the development of GVHD include older donor and recipient ages [41–44], donor and recipient gender disparity (with multiparous female donors imparting particularly high risk) [44, 45], advanced malignant condition at time of transplantation [45, 46], cytomegalovirus status of donor and host, intensity of the transplant conditioning regimen, donor HLA type [44], donor hematopoietic cell source [4, 47, 48], and the specific GVHD prophylactic regimen used. The impact of donor and recipient polymorphisms in cytokine genes that have been shown to contribute to the development of GVHD has been examined as a risk factor for GVHD [49]. These gene polymorphisms include tumor necrosis factor α (TNF-α), interleukin 10 (IL-10), and interferon-γ (IFN-γ) variants, and have been associated with GVHD, though not in all cases [50–52]. Additionally, other significant features such as the presence of a sterile environment (via gut decontamination) and certain favorable HLA haplotypes likely contribute to GVHD development. However, distinct risk models may be required for each disease, as risk factors for acute GVHD differ by condition [46].

Acute GVHD is mediated by donor lymphocytes infused into the recipient (along with the infused stem cell graft), in whom they encounter tissues damaged by the cumulative effects of the underlying disease, prior infections, and the transplant conditioning regimen [53]. These damaged tissues produce proinflammatory cytokines and chemokines, which increase expression of key receptors on antigen-presenting cells. This increased expression enhances presentation of polypeptide proteins (i.e., HAs) to the donor cells and creates an environment that promotes the activation and proliferation of the very inflammatory cells that mediate GVHD. Thus, GVHD reflects an exaggerated response of the normal immune mechanisms that involve donor T cells, as well as multiple innate and adaptive cells and mediators within the recipient.

Recent studies have shown that a GVHD-like syndrome may be possible following autologous transplantation [54]. The underlying mechanism involves a failure to re-establish tolerance to self, which can lead to systemic autoimmunity that may exacerbate or even mimic GVHD. Two major factors underlie the induction of autologous GVHD: the disruption of thymic-dependent immune reconstitution and the failure to re-establish peripheral self-tolerance [54].

Clinical manifestations

GVHD is characterized by specific derangements of the skin, liver, gastrointestinal tract, and, rarely, other organs. The form of GVHD typically occurring early after transplantation is referred to as acute GVHD, while a later form with different clinical characteristics has been termed chronic GVHD. For practical purposes, the two forms were originally distinguished by time of onset: acute was considered to occur in less than 100 days after transplantation, and chronic in more than 100 days [55]. However, a clear distinction between acute and chronic forms of GVHD as originally described can no longer be delineated, given the alterations in the recipient's relative level of immunosuppression that occur with increased use of nonmyeloablative conditioning and employment of donor lymphocyte infusions. These factors can delay or hasten the clinical appearance of acute GVHD, rendering traditional diagnostic guidelines inadequate. In 2005, a

National Institutes of Health (NIH) working group sought to standardize the definitions of acute and chronic GVHD (Table 27.1), mindful of those factors that can produce such clinical variability among transplant patients [56].

After high-intensity (conventional) conditioning, acute GVHD generally occurs within 14–42 days of stem cell infusion. A "hyperacute" form of GVHD can occur in patients with severe HLA mismatch from donor, and in patients whose T-cell-rich transplants were received without or with inadequate GVHD prophylaxis [57]. Hyperacute GVHD is manifested by high fever, a more severe cutaneous component (generalized erythema with desquamation), in addition to hepatitis and intestinal symptoms. This form of GVHD typically occurs within the first 2 weeks after stem cell infusion and may be rapidly fatal.

In patients receiving routine GVHD prophylaxis, such as a combination of cyclosporine and methotrexate, the median onset of GVHD is 21–25 days after transplantation; *in vitro* T-cell depletion of the graft, however, can delay the onset [58]. The "engraftment syndrome" occurs when a less ominous combination of fever, morbilliform eruption, and fluid retention arises in the first 1–2 weeks after stem cell infusion comprise. This complication may be seen with either allogeneic or autologous transplantation and is related to cytokine production as the graft begins to function, but divergent from the "cytokine storm" [49] believed to have a role in acute GVHD, in that there is no concomitant T-cell-mediated tissue damage. In most patients, engraftment syndrome typically presents earlier than does acute GVHD, and responds rapidly to corticosteroids [59].

Acute GHVD normally develops at, or near, the time of engraftment; the time of onset depends, in part, on the conditioning regimen, with a peak incidence of around 30 days after myeloablative transplantation, and later in the setting of reduced-intensity regimens or delayed engraftment of UCB-derived stem cells. The skin is generally the first and most commonly affected organ, and can be the only target organ in acute GVHD (Figure 27.1). Initially, a sensation of skin pain or itching may occur, but GVHD may also be asymptomatic. The earliest cutaneous manifestations of acute GVHD may be prominent palmar erythema and erythematous to violaceous discoloration of the face and ears. Diffuse patchy erythema with follicular prominence can ensue, followed by a more generalized morbilliform eruption. In severe cases, the exanthema can progress to a diffuse erythroderma with bullae formation, a positive Nikolsky sign, and desquamation that resembles Stevens–Johnson syndrome and toxic epidermal necrolysis. Involvement of the mucous membranes, particularly the conjunctivae, can occur, making these features of acute GVHD difficult to differentiate from conditioning-related mucositis [60] as well as oral herpes simplex viral infection. Acral erythema, a mimicker of acute GVHD, may also present with painful palmar and plantar lesions; however, this entity is related to conditioning chemotherapy and usually occurs in the second week following HSCT and can resemble a second-degree burn [61].

Recently, the term toxic erythema of chemotherapy has been proposed as a descriptive diagnosis to encompass the spectrum

Table 27.1 NIH Classification of Acute and Chronic GVHD.

		Symptoms post HSCT or DLI	Presence of acute features	Presence of chronic features
Classic acute	Acute GVHD	≤100 days	Yes	No
Persistent, Recurrent, Late-onset acute		>100 days	Yes	No
Classic chronic	Chronic GVHD	No time limit	No	Yes
Overlap syndrome		No time limit	Yes	Yes

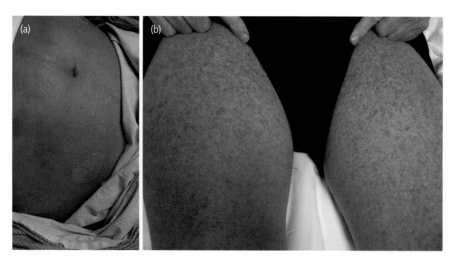

Figure 27.1 (a, b) Acute graft versus host disease (GVHD).

of cutaneous toxicities seen in response to a multitude of chemotherapeutic medications including cytarabine, anthracyclines, taxanes, and methotrexate, whether an HSCT is to follow or not [62]. Confusion with regards to nomenclature of these reactions has been rampant, as the term acral erythema has previously been referred to as acral erythrodysesthesia syndrome, hand-foot syndrome, and palmar-plantar erythema to name just a few. Such variability in monikers, even when describing the same clinical entity, has led to difficulty in the interpretation of literature and standardization of diagnosis and treatment by physicians who care for patients that develop these toxicities. Toxic erythema of chemotherapy also incorporates previously distinct diagnoses such as neutrophilic eccrine hidradenitis, flexural erythematous eruption, epidermal dysmaturation and Burgdorf reaction. The unifying factor, despite the variability in the clinical presentation of toxic erythema of chemotherapy, is that the underlying pathologic process is driven by the likelihood that there is a higher relative concentration of these toxic agents (or their metabolites), at eccrine-rich anatomic sites. These sites (axillae, groin, palms, soles), and the skin changes that involve them, reflect this process, as many of these seemingly distinct clinical entities, have identical histologic features when biopsied.

The skin involvement in acute GVHD is staged according to the extent of body surface area involved (Table 27.2). Similar staging is incorporated to describe the extent of liver and intestinal GVHD, and has prognostic relevance when used to provide overall grading of acute GVHD (Table 27.3).

Diagnosis

The diagnosis of acute GVHD can be readily made on clinical grounds alone in the patient who presents with classic skin lesions, diarrhea, and a rising serum bilirubin concentration within the first 100 days following transplantation. In most cases, however, the diagnosis is less straightforward because the clinical

symptoms, laboratory abnormalities, and histologic features can be mimicked by other clinical entities, which must be excluded; for example, similar cutaneous findings can be seen as a rash or hand-foot syndrome caused by myeloablative regimens, maculopapular drug reactions, and even viral exanthema (Table 27.4). As with mimickers of acute cutaneous GVHD, other causes of diarrhea (bacterial, parasitic, viral infections) and increasing total bilirubin (hepatic veno-occlusive disease, infection, hepatotoxicity of medications) must be considered, and may need to be confirmed via intestinal or hepatic biopsy. Unfortunately, in patients with neutropenia and thrombocytopenia, tissue biopsies of the gut and liver have safety implications, and results can be equivocal even in those patients where acute GVHD is highly suspected [63, 64].

Skin biopsy, the gold standard by which cutaneous disease is diagnosed under normal conditions, has questionable utility in the early post-transplant course of the HSCT patient. One previous study that investigated concordance among three pathologists who blindly evaluated tissue sections from patients considered to have clinical suspicion of acute GVHD, compared with those from patients who were not suspected to have GVHD, showed no differences between these groups in terms of histopathologic characteristics. A consensus among the three pathologists was reached in only 31% of the slides, illustrating the difficulty of formulating conclusions with regards to the etiology of skin eruptions seen in transplant recipients [65]. A similar study employed two blinded dermatopathologists asked to retrospectively interpret skin biopsies from patients without acute GVHD from those with acute GVHD (both cohorts presenting with skin eruptions early after HSCT), using 16 histologic parameters. No single parameter could accurately distinguish between these two groups and the authors concluded that skin biopsy in this setting was of limited utility when trying to confirm acute GVHD or when attempting to differentiate drug eruptions and viral exanthema from acute GVHD [66]. More recently, a retrospective study designed to determine the value of skin biopsies in the management of suspected GVHD within 30 days of allogeneic HSCT found that biopsy findings correlated poorly

Table 27.2 Clinical staging of acute graft-versus-host disease.

STAGE	SKIN	LIVER	GUT
1	Rash <25% BSA	Total bilirubin 2.0–2.9 mg/dL	Diarrhea 0.5–1 L/day or Persistent nausea/emesis with +gut biopsy
2	Rash 25–50% BSA	Total bilirubin 3.0–5.8 mg/dL	Diarrhea 1–1.5 L/day
3	Rash >50% BSA	Total Bilirubin 5.9–14.9 mg/dL	Diarrhea >1.5 L/day
4	Generalized erythema with bullae and/or desquamation	Total bilirubin >14.9 mg/dL	Severe abdominal pain or ileus

Table 27.3 Clinical grading of acute graft-versus-host disease.

GRADE	SKIN STAGE	LIVER STAGE	GUT STAGE
I (Mild)	1-2	0	0
II (Moderate) and	3 or	1 or	1
III (Severe)	0-3 and	2-3 or	2-4
IV (Life-threatening)	4 or	4 or	0-4 + Grade 4 skin or liver

Table 27.4 Differential diagnosis of morbilliform eruption after hsct.

Disease	Onset	Clinical Presentation	Histopathology	Treatment
Eruption of Lymphocyte Recovery	Within 21 days after chemotherapy	Early- erythema hands/feet/face, Morbilliform	Vacuolar change, Necrotic keratinocytes	Self-limited
Hyperacute GVHD	Within 14 days after HSCT	Early- erythema hands/feet/face, Morbilliform	Vacuolar change, Necrotic keratinocytes	Systemic steroids
Acute GVHD	Variable within 1 month after HSCT	Early- erythema hands/feet/face, Morbilliform	Vacuolar change, Necrotic keratinocytes	Systemic steroids
Toxic Erythema of Chemotherapy	Pre-transplant-21 days after HSCT	hands/feet/face Flexural	Vacuolar change, Necrotic keratinocytes, Eccrine squamous syringometaplasia	Self-limited
Viral exanthem	Anytime	Morbilliform	Non-specific	Antivirals
Morbilliform drug eruption	Anytime	Morbilliform	Non-specific Eosinophils +/−	Withdraw inciting medication

Table 27.5 Histologic grading of acute cutaneous graft-versus-host disease.

Grade I	Grade II	Grade III	Grade IV
Focal or diffuse vacuolar change	Grade I plus necrotic keratinoyctes	Grade II plus Subepidermal clefting	Complete effacement of epidermis

with the clinical severity of skin eruptions suggestive of acute GVHD soon after HSCT [67]. Lastly, some authors even go as far to conclude that skin biopsy need not even be performed within 3 weeks after HSCT as a means to confirm or exclude acute GVHD [68].

Despite the various shortcomings of a skin biopsy, histologic confirmation may still be of benefit to corroborate a clinical impression of acute GVHD. The histologic criteria for the diagnosis of acute cutaneous GVHD were established in 1974 and are still in use today (Table 27.5) [69]. Lymphocytic interface dermatitis with vacuolar degeneration, disorganization of epiderma cell maturation, and necrotic/apoptotic keratinoyctes are the major features of acute GVHD. Focal or diffuse spongiosis may be seen, with lymphocytes in proximity to the necrotic keratinoyctes, referred to as "satellite cell necrosis." This feature has been considered illustrative of the pathogenesis of GVHD, demonstrating an activated donor lymphocyte in the act of recognizing a host cell. In more severe forms, clefting of the basal cell layer results in separation of the dermo-epidermal junction, correlating with a clinical vesicle or bulla. Anecdotal data suggest that the presence of eosinophils is not useful to distinguish between GVHD and a drug-induced rash [70].

Direct immunofluorescence labeling of skin has demonstrated granular deposits of IgM and/or C3, similar to a lupus band test, in 39% of biopsy specimens from patients with acute GVHD, whereas this pattern was seen in only 11% of HSCT recipients without GHVD [71]

Many studies have been conducted to determine which lymphocyte subpopulations are found in the skin of patients with acute GVHD. Unfortunately, the results seem to be in conflict with each other [72–84]. The infiltrate is composed of T cells, but both CD4+ and CD8+ subsets have been shown to predominate [72–84]. Tregs are also found in greater quantities in skin of patients with GVHD, although FOXP3+ cells correlated with less severe GVHD and response to anti-GVHD therapy [85].

In recent years, plasma and urine proteomics have shown promise in enabling early diagnosis of acute GVHD [86–89]. It has been proposed that a panel of plasma biomarkers including IL-2-receptor-α, TNF receptor-1, IL-8, and hepatocyte growth factor can confirm the diagnosis of acute GVHD at the onset of clinical symptoms and provide prognostic information independent of GVHD severity [90]. Additional experience with these techniques is required before they can be applied widely to the clinical discrimination of patients with and without GVHD. Another group, using a large-scale quantitative proteomic discovery procedure, validated elafin as a critical surrogate protein in acute GVHD via enzyme-linked immunosorbent assay using samples from 492 patients [91]. They found that elafin, an alarm antiprotease secreted in response to IL-1 and TNF-α, was overexpressed in GVHD skin biopsies. In addition, plasma concentrations of elafin were significantly higher at the onset of skin GVHD, correlated with the eventual maximum grade of GVHD, and were associated with a greater risk of death.

Until absolute criteria for the diagnosis of acute GVHD can be developed and validated, the differential diagnosis of recent

HSCT recipients with an acute morbilliform skin eruption must always include toxic erythema of chemotherapy, drug eruptions, viral exanthema, and the eruption of lymphocyte recovery. The presence of extracutaneous involvement can help support the diagnosis of acute GVHD, but is frequently absent or may mimic, and be unrelated to, GVHD. In most cases, physicians must weigh the risk : benefit ratio of introducing further immunosuppressive treatment (systemic steroids) to patients already at risk of developing severe infections or a recurrence of their primary disease, when the diagnosis of acute GVHD may be elusive.

Prevention

Prevention of acute GVHD is an integral component in the management of patients undergoing allogeneic HSCT. This is achieved primarily through the use of pharmacologic GVHD prophylaxis. The most widely used regimen following full-intensity conditioning includes a combination of a calcineurin inhibitor (cyclosporine, tacrolimus) with a brief course of methotrexate (MTX). Since its initial implementation in 1986 [92], several clinical trials in matched sibling transplants after myeloablative conditioning chemotherapy have shown the superiority of this regimen in reducing GVHD incidence and improving survival compared with either agent alone [37, 93–95]; a recent systemic review and meta-analysis showed the relative risk of developing acute GVHD in patients receiving MTX and cyclosporine to be 0.52 (95% CI 0.39–0.7), compared with cyclosporine alone [95]. Large randomized studies comparing tacrolimus-MTX with cyclosporine-MTX have demonstrated a reduced incidence of Grade II–IV acute GHVD with tacrolimus (overall and relapse-free survival rates for the tacrolimus and cyclosporine arms at 2 years was 54% versus 50% ($p = 0.46$) and 47% versus 42% ($p = 0.58$), respectively), but no overall survival advantage [94, 96]. Calcineurin inhibitors interfere with the activation and expansion of donor T cells, and are very effective in the prevention of GVHD but need to be taken over a long period of time and are associated with significant AEs, such as nephrotoxicity.

For higher risk groups or groups receiving nonconventional grafts (such as mismatched donors, older patients, and those receiving reduced-intensity regimens), the best prophylaxis is less well-established, often requiring more intensive immunosuppression [96]. A commonly used GVHD prophylactic regimen following reduced-intensity conditioning includes a combination of a calcineurin inhibitor (i.e., cyclosporine, tacrolimus) with mycophenolate mofetil (MMF) instead of MTX. In a prospective randomized trial, patients who received MMF experienced significantly less severe mucositis (21 vs. 65%, $p = 0.008$) and more rapid neutrophil engraftment (11 vs. 18 days, $p < 0.001$) than those who received MTX [97]. Although the optimal prophylactic regimen following reduced-intensity HSCT remains to be established, MMF has been shown to be safe in this context [98–102]. In UCB transplants, MMF is also often preferred to MTX because of its advantageous toxicity profile with respect to neutropenia and mucositis.

Many centers have attempted to decrease the risk of GVHD using *ex vivo* T-cell depletion. Despite significant reductions in the incidence and severity of GVHD, T-cell depletion has not achieved wide acceptance because of high rates of graft rejection, life-threatening infections, and leukemia relapse [103–114]. Newer cytokine-based approaches such as antithymocyte globulin, anti-TNF-α agents (infliximab, etanercept), or anti-IL-2 receptor antibody (daclizumab) are being employed to neutralize the conditioning-induced epithelial tissue damage that leads to acute GVHD. However, these techniques are not yet firmly established for clinical use and may have a more important role in the treatment of steroid-refractory acute GVHD [115].

Treatment

The standard therapy of isolated acute cutaneous GVHD of less than 50% body surface area of involvement (≤grade II) includes topical application of potent corticosteroids or tacrolimus [116]. The first-line treatment of significant acute (≥grade II) or chronic GVHD consists of high doses of systemic corticosteroids (1–3 mg/kg/day), sometimes given as a bolus [117, 118]. Most centers treat grade II–IV acute GVHD by continuing prophylactic immunosuppression as previously discussed, and adding methylprednisolone at 2–2.5 mg/kg/day. Starting doses can range from 1 to >20 mg/kg/day [119]. In general, 40–50% of patients have an overall response to systemic corticosteroids [120]. The steroid can be tapered after control of GVHD; a rapid steroid taper over 86 days was found to be just as effective as a slow taper over 147 days with regard to preventing flares of GVHD or development of chronic GVHD [121]. There is no compelling evidence to support the use of higher doses of steroids, as a few studies have shown that patients who responded to high-dose methylprednisolone (20–50 mg/kg/day) generally flared after dose reduction, and a number of patients in these studies ultimately succumbed to opportunistic infections [122, 123].

Regardless of the dose of steroids, the initial response of the patient to this therapy is very predictive of future severity of GVHD and other transplant complications [120]. Patients remaining refractory to systemic corticosteroids are treated with salvage therapy, in which no specific approach has been established as standard of care.

Chronic graft versus host disease
Pathogenesis

Chronic GVHD is the major cause of late nonrelapse death following allogeneic HSCT [124], usually as a consequence of infection (in fact, the risk of infection is higher in patients with chronic GVHD), cachexia, or liver dysfunction [125]. It remains the most common problem in long-term survivors of HSCT, and is associated with decreased quality of life and impaired physical and functional status [126].

The disease develops after a mean delay of onset of 4 months after HLA-identical sibling transplantation and 4 months after unrelated donor transplantation [127], but manifestations resembling chronic GVHD can appear as early as day 40 following transplantation. Its incidence has increased with the wider availability of PBSC and the increased age of transplant recipients. Currently, the incidence of chronic GVHD ranges from 30% in recipients of fully histocompatible sibling donor transplants to 60–70% in recipients of mismatched and unrelated donors. Other factors that likely increase the development of chronic GVHD include prior acute GVHD, older recipient age, female donor (multiparous, in particular) with a male recipient, and use of PBSC [126].

In contrast to that of acute GVHD, the pathophysiology of chronic GVHD is not as well delineated. Chronic GVHD is a complex multisystem disorder with myriad manifestations that involve several organ systems, all linked by the characteristics of immune dysregulation, immunodeficiency, impaired organ function, and decreased survival [128]. Alloreactive T cells have been implicated in the pathogenesis, and most immunohistochemical studies have shown that CD8+ lymphocytes predominate [129, 130]; in addition, autoreactivity has been suggested as an additional etiology of chronic GVHD [131, 132].

As might be expected, chronic GVHD has been associated with beneficial GVT effects [133]. Multivariate analyses have shown that the presence of chronic GVHD is the most significant factor correlated to a reduced risk of leukemia relapse [134]; this antileukemic effect increases with the severity of chronic GHVD.

Clinical manifestations

The diagnosis of chronic GVHD is based on the extent of organ involvement (mild, moderate, severe), laboratory data, and histopathologic confirmation of involved tissue rather than the time of onset post-transplant. Historically, the most commonly utilized staging system adopted a classification of "limited" (localized skin involvement with or without limited hepatic dysfunction) versus "extensive" (generalized skin involvement or limited disease plus eye, oral, liver, or other target organ involvement) disease [125].

Chronic GVHD may present as acute GHVD that evolves into chronic GVHD (progressive type; 32% of cases), may develop following a variable symptom-free period in patients who experienced an acute GVHD episode (quiescent or interrupted type, 36% of cases), or may occur *de novo* (30% of cases). An overlap syndrome is recognized in which clinical features of both chronic GVHD and acute GHVD coexist, including an erythematous skin rash, nausea, vomiting, diarrhea, and liver dysfunction [56].

The skin is involved in almost all cases of chronic GVHD, and the oral mucosa in 90% (Figure 27.2) [135]. Mucous membrane involvement can manifest as oral or conjunctival dryness and lichenoid oral GVHD (mimicking lichen planus) appears as lacy white patches or plaques along with erosions or ulcerative lesions of the lips, tongue, or buccal regions. Dental caries and periodontitis/gingivitis may also occur. Cutaneous lesions often present with either of two forms: lichenoid or sclerodermoid. Both can develop spontaneously or may be triggered by several events: UV irradiation, physical trauma, herpes zoster (reactiva-

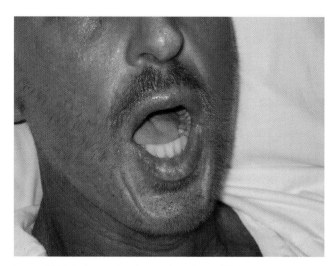

Figure 27.2 Oral mucosal graft versus host disease (GVHD).

tion of varicella zoster virus), and even *Borrelia* infections. Lichenoid lesions usually occur early in the course of chronic GVHD and are easily recognized [136, 137]. These lesions are erythematous or violaceous, scaly papules or plaques that can coalesce into larger, confluent areas. The periorbital region, ears, dorsal aspects of the hands and forearms, trunk, palms, and soles are typically affected sites. In some cases, lichenoid papules can occur around hair follicles. Less typically, the lesions may appear vesicular, and if present on the hands, can resemble dyshidrotic eczema. Lichenoid chronic GVHD can also affect the nails, with development of onychatrophia (when fully grown nail, shrinks in its size and falls off) and pterygium (skin growth over the nail plate), and the genital region, with a risk of phimosis in males and vaginal strictures in women. Recently, lichenoid chronic GVHD restricted to a dermatome has been reported [138].

Chronic GVHD can also present with sclerodermoid lesions, which usually develop later in the course of disease (Figure 27.3) [139]. These appear as indurated sclerotic shiny white–yellow plaques with poorly circumscribed borders, and may be associated with areas of hyperpigmentation or poikiloderma. Sclerodermoid chronic GVHD can remain localized or become generalized, which may be disabling. On the extremities, severe sclerodermoid chronic GVHD can cause the skin to adhere to deeper tissues, which may lead to leg ulcers. As a consequence of entrapment of the nerve endings from bound-down skin, peripheral axonal neuropathy at the same site as the cutaneous sclerosis has been reported in the legs of individuals with chronic GVHD [140]. When sclerodermatous plaques are located over the joints, the fibrosis can involve the ligaments, causing retraction. Cutaneous adnexal involvement with various nail changes, alopecia (scarring and nonscarring), and impairment of sweating are also common. Of note, acrosclerosis and Raynaud phenomenon are uncommon in chronic sclerodermatous GVHD, in contrast to systemic sclerosis. Bullous sclerodermoid chronic GVHD has also been described [141].

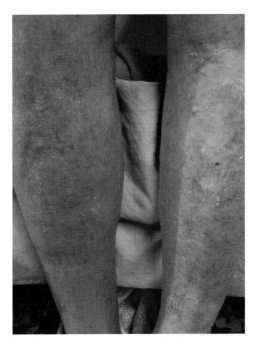

Figure 27.3 Chronic graft versus host disease (GVHD).

Unlike the staging/grading of acute GVHD, chronic GVHD has no correlative metric to relate symptoms and prognosis [125]. Most authors recommend the use of the Karnofsky scale, which measures an individual's ability to perform activities of daily living [142].

Diagnosis and differential diagnosis

Because the clinical manifestations of chronic GVHD are variable and involve multiple organs and sites, at least one distinctive manifestation of chronic GVHD is required for diagnosis. When confronted with the possibility of cutaneous chronic GVHD, the presence of other visceral involvement may be important to ascertain. In addition to mucocutaneous disease, chronic GVHD may lead to liver disease that resembles primary biliary cirrhosis with obstructive jaundice, diarrhea, and malabsorption. Bronchiolitis obliterans, polymyositis, and peripheral entrapment neuropathy are not uncommon. Definitive diagnosis of chronic GVHD requires excluding other possible etiologies of visceral organ dysfunction such as infection, drug toxicity, and malignancy.

Histologic examination of involved tissue is also vital in the diagnosis of chronic GVHD. Lichenoid lesions microscopically resemble those skin lesions of acute GVHD, with a lymphocytic infiltrate in the superficial dermis and moderate exocytosis of inflammatory cells into the epidermis; the dermal infiltrate may be perineural. The epidermis is thickened with acanthosis, parakeratosis, and hypergranulosis, with a variable degree of keratinocyte necrosis that may feature satellite cell necrosis.

Sclerodermoid chronic GHVD lesions have marked epidermal atrophy with linearization of the dermo-epidermal junction, destruction of adnexal structures, and superficial collagen fibrosis.

Keratinoyctes are small, flattened, and contain a high amount of melanin. Necrotic keratinoyctes are few and found in the basal cell layer if present [143]. In 86% of skin biopsy specimens from patients with chronic GVHD, direct immunofluorescence reveals granular IgM deposits at the dermo-epidermal junction [71].

Prevention

Although prevention of acute GVHD has improved during the past three decades, no effective prophylaxis regimen exists for chronic GVHD. Management of chronic GVHD is guided by a multidisciplinary approach to treatment, including adjustment of immunosuppressive medications and aggressive supportive care.

Treatment

Definitive treatment of chronic GVHD and a consensus with regard to optimal treatment regimens remains elusive. The choice of treatment is affected by the prior use of prophylactic agents and the history of therapies used to treat acute GVHD in an individual patient. Generally, treatment of chronic GVHD is less intense and less aggressive than that used for acute GVHD, but may require a prolonged duration and a multiagent approach. Physical therapy may be necessary for patients with severe sclerodermoid chronic GVHD in order to maintain flexibility and range of motion of extremities. In addition, transplant patients with chronic GVHD are at increased risk for the development of secondary malignancies, particularly oral squamous cell carcinoma and melanoma [144, 145]. Dermatologists thus have a critical role in the prolonged monitoring of these patients.

The most widely used first-line therapy for patients with chronic GVHD is a combination of systemic corticosteroids and a calcineurin inhibitor. The recently published NIH guidelines recommend this treatment if three or more organs are involved, or if any single organ has severe involvement [144]. Generally, prednisone at a dose of 1 mg/kg/day is given in combination with cyclosporine for a length of time depending on disease severity (usually 9–12 months). In severe GVHD and/or sclerodermatous disease that is refractory to standard treatment, alternating cyclosporine (12 mg/kg/day) and systemic corticosteroids (1 mg/kg/day) may be beneficial [139]. Cyclophosphamide, methotrexate, or azathioprine represent alternatives if first-line therapy fails. The NIH Working Group defines failure of initial therapy or requirement of additional secondary therapy as follows:

1. Progression of chronic GVHD despite optimal first-line therapy (including >1 mg/kg/day of prednisolone for 2 weeks); or
2. No improvement after 4–8 weeks of sustained therapy; or
3. Inability to taper corticosteroid dose [56].

Chronic immunosuppressive regimens, particularly those containing systemic steroids, often result in life-threatening infectious complications. Many second-line therapies for chronic GVHD have been studied, including extracorporeal photopheresis (ECP), MMF, and rituximab, but none has achieved widespread acceptance. ECP has been successfully applied in chronic GVHD, with consistently high complete responses in up to 80% of patients with cutaneous manifestations and significant improvement in sclerodermatous skin involvement [146, 147].

Treatment regimens utilizing MMF are under current investigation. While MMF showed initial promise, a multicenter placebo-controlled randomized trial showed that the addition of MMF to the initial systemic treatment regimen for chronic GVHD did not show any benefit [115]. Other approaches, including anti-TNF-α and anti-CD20 antibodies, pentostatin, and sirolimus are currently being studied [148]; thalidomide has also been used in steroid-refractory chronic GVHD, with 14 of 37 patients (38%) responding to thalidomide (1 complete, 13 partial) in a study by Browne *et al.* [149], including 10 of 21 children (46%) and 4 of 16 adults (25%). Finally, early reports in steroid-refractory severe acute GVHD suggest some efficacy with the use of mesenchymal stem cells. Whether these beneficial effects have a role in the treatment of chronic GVHD, and whether they will persist over time, necessitates further investigation [150, 151].

References

1 Welniak, L.A., Blazar, B.R. & Murphy, W.J. (2007) Immunobiology of allogeneic hematopoietic stem cell transplantation. *Annual Review of Immunology*, **25**, 139–170.

2 Lake, R.A. & Robinson, B.W. (2005) Immunotherapy and chemotherapy: a practical partnership. *Nature Reviews: Cancer*, **5**, 397–405.

3 Anderlini, P., Rizzo, J.D., Nugent, M.L., Schmitz, N., Champlin, R.E. & Horowitz, M.M. (2001) Peripheral blood stem cell donation: an analysis from the International Bone Marrow Transplant Registry (IBMTR) and European Group for Blood and Marrow Transplant (BMT) databases. *Bone Marrow Transplantation*, **27**, 689–692.

4 Cutler, C., Giri, S., Jeyapalan, S., Paniagua, D., Viswanathan, A. & Antin, J.H. (2001) Acute and chronic graft-versus-host disease after allogeneic peripheral-blood stem-cell and bone marrow transplantation: a meta-analysis. *Journal of Clinical Oncology*, **19**, 3685–3691.

5 Stewart, B.L., Storer, B., Storek, J. *et al.* (2004) Duration of immunosuppressive treatment for chronic graft-versus-host disease. *Blood*, **104**, 3501–3506.

6 Levesque, J.-P., Liu, F., Simmons, P.J. *et al.* (2004) Characterization of hematopoietic progenitor mobilization in protease-deficient mice. *Blood*, **104**, 65–72.

7 Flomenberg, N., Devine, S., DiPersio, J.F. *et al.* (2005) The use of AMD3100 plus G-CSF for autologous hematopoietic progenitor cell mobilization is superior to G-CSF alone. *Blood*, **106**, 1867–1874.

8 Brenner, M.K., Rill, D., Moen, R.C. *et al.* (1993) Gene-marking to trace origin of relapse after autologous bone-marrow transplantation. *Lancet*, **341**, 85–86.

9 Stewart, A.K., Vescio, R., Schiller, G. *et al.* (2001) Purging of autologous peripheral-blood stem cells using CD34 selection does not improve overall or progression-free survival after high-dose chemotherapy for multiple myeloma: results of a multicenter randomized controlled trial. *Journal of Clinical Oncology*, **19**, 3771–3779.

10 Wagner, J.E., Barker, J., DeFor, T.E. *et al.* (2002) Transplantation of unrelated donor umbilical cord blood in 102 patients with malignant and nonmalignant diseases: influence of CD34 cell dose and HLA disparity on treatment-related mortality and survival. *Blood*, **100**, 1611–1618.

11 Barker, J.N., Weisdorf, D.J., DeFor, T.E. *et al.* (2005) Transplantation of 2 partially HLA-matched umbilical cord blood units to enhance engraftment in adults with hematologic malignancy. *Blood*, **105**, 1343–1347.

12 Aversa, F., Tabilio, A., Velardi, A. *et al.* (1998) Treatment of high-risk acute leukemia with T-cell-depleted stem cells from related donors with one fully mismatched HLA haplotype. *New England Journal of Medicine*, **339**, 1186–1193.

13 Ruggeri, L., Capanni, M., Urbani, E. *et al.* (2002) Effectiveness of donor natural killer cell alloreactivity in mismatched hematopoietic transplants. *Science*, **295**, 2097–2100.

14 Copelan, E.A. (2006) Hematopoietic stem-cell transplantation. *New England Journal of Medicine*, **354**, 1813–1826.

15 DeLeve, L.D., Shulman, H. & McDonald, G.B. (2002) Toxic injury to hepatic sinusoids: sinusoidal obstruction syndrome (veno-occlusive disease). *Seminars in Liver Disease*, **22**, 27–42.

16 Kallianpur, A.R., Hall, L., Yadav, M. *et al.* (2005) The hemochromatosis C282Y allele: a risk factor for hepatic veno-occlusive disease after hematopoietic stem cell transplantation. *Bone Marrow Transplantation*, **35**, 1155–1164.

17 Srivastava, A., Poonkuzhali, B., Shaji, R.V. *et al.* (2004) Glutathione S-transferase M1 polymorphism: a risk factor for hepatic venoocclusive disease in bone marrow transplantation. *Blood*, **104**, 1574–1577.

18 Bornhauser, M., Storer, B., Slattery, J.T. *et al.* (2003) Conditioning with fludarabine and targeted busulfan for transplantation of allogeneic hematopoietic stem cells. *Blood*, **102**, 820–826.

19 Hogan, W.J., Maris, M. & Storer, B. *et al.* (2004) Hepatic injury after nonmyeloablative conditioning followed by allogeneic hematopoietic cell transplantation: a study of 193 patients. *Blood*, **103**, 78–84.

20 Cooke, K.R. & Yanik, G. (2004) Acute lung injury after allogeneic stem cell transplantation: is the lung a target of acute graft-versus-host disease? *Bone Marrow Transplantation*, **34**, 753–765.

21 Yanik, G., Hellerstedt, B., Custer, J. *et al.* (2002) Etanercept (Enbrel) administration for idiopathic pneumonia syndrome after allogeneic hematopoietic stem cell transplantation. *Journal of the American Society for Blood and Marrow Transplantation*, **8**, 395–400.

22 Meyers, J.D., Flournoy, N. & Thomas, E.D. (1982) Nonbacterial pneumonia after allogeneic marrow transplantation: a review of ten years' experience. *Reviews of Infectious Diseases*, **4**, 1119–1132.

23 Tivol, E., Komorowsk, R. & Drobyski, W.R. (2005) Emergent autoimmunity in graft-versus-host disease. *Blood*, **105**, 4885–4891.

24 Dann, E.J., Epelbaum, R., Avivi, I. *et al.* (2005) Fertility and ovarian function are preserved in women treated with an intensified regimen of cyclophosphamide, adriamycin, vincristine and prednisone (Mega-CHOP) for non-Hodgkin lymphoma. *Human Reproduction*, **20**, 2247–2249.

25 Lass, A., Akagbosu, F. & Brinsden, P. (2001) Sperm banking and assisted reproduction treatment for couples following cancer treatment of the male partner. *Human Reproduction Update*, **7**, 370–377.

26 Sanders, J.E., Guthrie, K., Hoffmeister, P.A., Woolfrey, A.E., Carpenter, P.A. & Appelbaum, F.R. (2005) Final adult height of patients who received hematopoietic cell transplantation in childhood. *Blood*, **105**, 1348–1354.

27 Curtis, R.E., Rowlings P., Deeg, H.J. *et al.* (1997) Solid cancers after bone marrow transplantation. *New England Journal of Medicine*, **336**, 897–904.

28 Krishnan, A., Bhatia, S., Slovak, M.L. *et al.* (2000) Predictors of therapy-related leukemia and myelodysplasia following autologous transplantation for lymphoma: an assessment of risk factors. *Blood*, **95**, 1588–1593.

29 Syrjala, K.L., Langer, S., Abrams, J.R., Storer, B.E. & Martin, P.J. (2005) Late effects of hematopoietic cell transplantation among 10-year adult survivors compared with case-matched controls. *Journal of Clinical Oncology*, **23**, 6596–6606.

30 Spielberger, R., Stiff, P., Bensinger, W. *et al.* (2004) Palifermin for oral mucositis after intensive therapy for hematologic cancers. *New England Journal of Medicine*, **351**, 2590–2598.

31 Billingham, R.E. (1966) The biology of graft-versus-host reactions. *Harvey Lectures*, **62**, 21–78.

32 Korngold, R. & Sprent, J. (1987) Purified T cell subsets and lethal graft-versus-host disease in mice. In: R.P. Gale and R.E. Champlin (eds), *Progress in Bone Marrow Transplant*, pp. 213–218. Alan R. Liss, Inc., New York.

33 Kernan, N.A., Collins, N., Juliano, L.L., Cartagena, T., Dupont, B. & O'Reilly, R.J. (1986) Clonable T lymphocytes in T cell-depleted bone marrow transplants correlate with development of graft-v-host disease. *Blood*, **68**, 770–773.

34 Petersdorf, E.W., Longton, G., Anasetti, C. *et al.* (1995) The significance of HLA-DRB1 matching on clinical outcome after HLA-A, B, DR identical unrelated donor marrow transplantation. *Blood*, **86**, 1606–1613.

35 Krensky, A.M., Weiss, A., Crabtree, G., Davis, M.M. & Parham, P. (1990) T-lymphocyte-antigen interactions in transplant rejection. *New England Journal of Medicine*, **322**, 510–517.

36 Loiseau, P., Busson, M., Balere, M.L. *et al.* (2007) HLA Association with hematopoietic stem cell transplantation outcome: the number of mismatches at HLA-A, -B, -C, -DRB1, or -DQB1 is strongly associated with overall survival. *Journal of the American Society for Blood and Marrow Transplantation*, **13**, 965–974.

37 Ratanatharathorn, V., Nash, R., Przepiorka, D. *et al.* (1998) Phase III study comparing methotrexate and tacrolimus (prograf, FK506) with methotrexate and cyclosporine for graft-versus-host disease prophylaxis after HLA-identical sibling bone marrow transplantation. *Blood*, **92**, 2303–2314.

38 Report, Center for International Blood and Marrow Transplant Research (CIBMTR) Progress, January-December 2008.

39 Goulmy, E., Schipper, R., Pool, J. *et al.* (1996) Mismatches of minor histocompatibility antigens between HLA-identical donors and recipients and the development of graft-versus-host disease after bone marrow transplantation. *New England Journal of Medicine*, **334**, 281–285.

40 Bleakley, M. & Riddell, S.R. (2004) Molecules and mechanisms of the graft-versus-leukemia effect. *Nature Reviews: Cancer*, **4**, 371–380.

41 Weisdorf, D., Hakke, R., Blazar, B. *et al.* (1991) Risk factors for acute graft-versus-host disease in histocompatible donor bone marrow transplantation. *Transplantation*, **51**, 1197–1203.

42 Eisner, M.D. & August, C. (1995) Impact of donor and recipient characteristics on the development of acute and chronic graft-versus-host disease following pediatric bone marrow transplantation. *Bone Marrow Transplantation*, **15**, 663–668.

43 Martin, P., Bleyzac, N., Souillet, G. *et al.* (2003) Clinical and pharmacological risk factors for acute graft-versus-host disease after

paediatric bone marrow transplantation from matched-sibling or unrelated donors. *Bone Marrow Transplantation*, **32**, 881–887.

44 Gale, R.P., Bortin, M.M., van Bekkum, D.W. *et al.* (1987) Risk factors for acute graft-versus-host disease. *British Journal of Haematology*, **67**, 397–406.

45 Nash, R.A., Pepe, M., Storb, R. *et al.* (1992) Acute graft-versus-host disease: analysis of risk factors after allogeneic marrow transplantation and prophylaxis with cyclosporine and methotrexate. *Blood*, **80**, 1838–1845.

46 Hahn, T., McCarthy, P.J. Jr., Zhang, M.J. *et al.* (2008) Risk factors for acute graft-versus-host disease after human leukocyte antigen-identical sibling transplants for adults with leukemia. *Journal of Clinical Oncology*, **26**, 5728–5734.

47 Vigorito, A.C., Azevedo, W., Marques, J.F. *et al.* (1998) A randomised, prospective comparison of allogeneic bone marrow and peripheral blood progenitor cell transplantation in the treatment of haematological malignancies. *Bone Marrow Transplantation*, **22**, 1145–1151.

48 Eapen, M., Rubenstein, P., Zhang, M.J. *et al.* (2007) Outcomes of transplantation of unrelated donor umbilical cord blood and bone marrow in children with acute leukaemia: a comparison study. *Lancet*, **369**, 1947–1954.

49 Antin, J.H. & Ferrara, J. (1992) Cytokine dysregulation and acute graft-versus-host disease. *Blood*, **80**, 2964–2968.

50 Cavet, J., Middleton, P., Segall, M., Noreen, H., Davies, S.M. & Dickinson, A.M. (1999) Recipient tumor necrosis factor-alpha and interleukin-10 gene polymorphisms associate with early mortality and acute graft-versus-host disease severity in HLA-matched sibling bone marrow transplants. *Blood*, **94**, 3941–3946.

51 Lin, M.T., Storer, B., Martin, P.J. *et al.* (2003) Relation of an interleukin-10 promoter polymorphism to graft-versus-host disease and survival after hematopoietic-cell transplantation. *New England Journal of Medicine*, **349**, 2201–2210.

52 Dickinson, A.M. & Charron, D. (2005) Non-HLA immunogenetics in hematopoietic stem cell transplantation. *Current Opinion in Immunology*, **17**, 517–525.

53 Ferrara, J.L. & Deeg, H. (1991) Graft-versus-host disease. *New England Journal of Medicine*, **324**, 667–674.

54 Hess, A.D. (2010) Reconstitution of self-tolerance after hematopoietic stem cell transplantation. *Immunologic Research*, **47**, 143–152.

55 Glucksberg, H., Storb, R., Fefer, A. *et al.* (1974) Clinical manifestations of graft-versus-host disease in human recipients of marrow from HL-A-matched sibling donors. *Transplantation*, **18**, 295–304.

56 Filipovich, A.H., Weisdorf, D., Pavletic, S. *et al.* (2005) National Institutes of Health consensus development project on criteria for clinical trials in chronic graft-versus-host disease: I. Diagnosis and staging working group report. *Journal of the American Society for Blood and Marrow Transplantation*, **11**, 945–956.

57 Rowlings, P.A., Przepiorka, D., Klein, J.P. *et al.* (1997) IBMTR Severity Index for grading acute graft-versus-host disease: retrospective comparison with Glucksberg grade. *British Journal of Haematology*, **97**, 855–864.

58 Antin, J.H., Bierer, B., Smith, B.R. *et al.* (1991) Selective depletion of bone marrow T lymphocytes with anti-CD5 monoclonal antibodies: effective prophylaxis for graft-versus-host disease in patients with hematologic malignancies. *Blood*, **78**, 2139–2149.

59 Spitzer, T.R. (2001) Engraftment syndrome following hematopoietic stem cell transplantation. *Bone Marrow Transplantation*, **27**, 893–898.

60 Johnson, M.L. & Farmer, E. (1998) Graft-versus-host reactions in dermatology. *Journal of the American Academy of Dermatology*, **38**, 369–392.

61 Crider, M.K., Jansen, J., Norins, A.L. & McHale, M.S. (1986) Chemotherapy-induced acral erythema in patients receiving bone marrow transplantation. *Archives of Dermatology*, **122**, 1023–1027.

62 Bolognia, J.L., Cooper, D.L. & Glusac, E.J. (2008) Toxic erythema of chemotherapy: a useful clinical term. *Journal of the American Academy of Dermatology*, **59** (3), 524–529.

63 Washington, K. & Jagasia, M. (2009) Pathology of graft-versus-host disease in the gastrointestinal tract. *Human Pathology*, **40** (7), 909–917.

64 Quaglia, A., Duarte, R., Patch, D., Ngianga-Bakwin, K. & Dhillon, A.P. (2007) Histopathology of graft versus host disease of the liver. *Histopathology*, **50** (6), 727–738.

65 Sale, G., Lerner, K., Barker, E., Shulman, H. & Thomas, E. (1977) The skin biopsy in the diagnosis of acute graft-versus-host disease in man. *American Journal of Pathology*, **89**, 621–636.

66 Kohler, S., Hendrickson, M.R., Chao, N.J. & Smoller, B.R. (1997) Value of skin biopsies in assessing prognosis and progression of acute graft-versus-host disease. *American Journal of Surgical Pathology*, **21** (9), 988–996.

67 Zhou, Y., Barnett, M. & Rivers, J.K. (2000) Clinical significance of skin biopsies in the diagnosis and management of graft-vs-host disease in early postallogeneic bone marrow transplantation. *Archives of Dermatology*, **136**, 717–721.

68 Kuykendall, T.D. & Smoller, B.R. (2003) Lack of specificity in skin biopsy specimens to assess for acute graft-versus-host disease in initial 3 weeks after bone-marrow transplantation. *Journal of the American Academy of Dermatology*, **49** (6), 1081–1085.

69 Lerner, K.G., Kao, G., Strob, R., Buckner, C.D., Clift, R.A. & Thomas, E.D. (1974) Histopathology of graft-versus-host reaction (GVHR) in human recipients of marrow from HLA-matched sibling donors. *Transplantation Proceedings*, **6**, 367–371.

70 Marra, D.E., McKee, P. & Nghiem, P. (2004) Tissue eosinophils and the perils of using skin biopsy specimens to distinguish between drug hypersensitivity and cutaneous graft-versus-host disease. *Journal of the American Academy of Dermatology*, **51**, 543–546.

71 Tsoi, M., Storb, R., Jones, E. *et al.* (1978) Deposition of IgM and complement at the dermoepidermal junction in acute and chronic cutaneous graft-vs-host disease in man. *Journal of Immunology*, **120**, 1485–1492.

72 Gilliam, A., Whitaker-Menezes, D., Korngold, R. & Murphy, G. (1996) Apoptosis is the predominant form of epithelial target cell injury in acute experimental graft versus host disease. *Journal of Investigative Dermatology*, **107**, 377–383.

73 Elliott, C., Sloane, J., Pallett, C. & Sanderson, K. (1988) Cutaneous leukocyte composition after human allogeneic bone marrow transplantation: relationship to marrow purging, histology, and clinical rash. *Histopathology*, **12**, 1–16.

74 Acevedo, A., Aramburu, J., Lopez, J., Fernandez-Herrera, J., Fernandez-Ranada, J. & Lopez-Botet, M. (1991) Identification of natural killer (NK) cells in lesions of human cutaneous graft-versus-host disease: expression of a novel NK-associated surface antigen (Kp43) in mononuclear infiltrates. *Journal of Investigative Dermatology*, **97**, 659–666.

75 Paller, S., Nelson, A., Steffen, L., Gottschalk, L. & Kaiser, H. (1988) T-lymphocyte subsets in the lesional skin of allogeneic and autologous bone marrow transplant patients. *Archives of Dermatology*, **124**, 1795–1801.

76 Volc-Platzer, B., Rappersberger, K., Mosberger, I. *et al.* (1988) Sequential immunohistologic analysis of the skin following allogeneic bone marrow transplantation. *Journal of Investigative Dermatology*, **91**, 162–168.

77 Sviland, L., Pearson, A., Green, M.A. *et al.* (1991) Immunopathology of early graft-versus-host disease – a prospective study of skin, rectum, and peripheral blood in allogeneic and autologous bone marrow transplant recipients. *Transplantation*, **52**, 1029–1036.

78 Sloane, J., Thomas, J., Imrie, S., Easton, D. & Powles, R. (1984) Morphological and immunohistological changes in the skin in allogeneic bone marrow recipients. *Journal of Clinical Pathology*, **37**, 919–930.

79 Kay, V., Neumann, P., Kersey, J. *et al.* (1984) Identity of immune cells in graft-versus-host disease in the skin: analysis using monoclonal antibodies by indirect immunofluorescence. *American Journal of Pathology*, **116**, 436–440.

80 Lever, R., Turbitt, M., Mackie, R. *et al.* (1986) A prospective study of the histological changes in the skin in patietns receiving bone marrow transplants. *British Journal of Dermatology*, **114**, 161–170.

81 Dreno, B., Milpied, N., Harousseau, J. *et al.* (1986) Cutaneous immunological studies in diagnosis of acute graft-versus-host disease. *British Journal of Dermatology*, **114**, 7–15.

82 Atkinson, K., Munro, V., Vasak, E. & Biggs, J. (1986) Mononuclear cell subpopulations in the skin defined by monoclonal antibodies after HLA-identical sibling marrow transplantation. *British Journal of Dermatology*, **114**, 145–160.

83 Girolomoni, G., Pincelli, C., Zambruno, G. *et al.* (1991) Immunohistochemistry of cutaneous graft-versus-host disease after allogeneic bone marrow transplantation. *Journal of Dermatology*, **18**, 314–323.

84 Leskinen, R., Taskinen, E., Volin, L., Ruutu, T. & Hayry, P. (1992) Immunohistology of skin and rectum biopsies in bone marrow transplant recipients. *Acta Pathologica, Microbiologica, et Immunologica Scandinavica*, **100**, 1115–1122.

85 Fondi, C., Nozzoli, C., Benemei, S. *et al.* (2009) Increase in FOXP3+ regulatory T cells in GVHD Skin biopsies is associated with lower disease severity and treatment response. *Journal of the American Society for Blood and Marrow Transplantation*, **15**, 938–947.

86 Lunn, R.A., Sumar, N., Bansal, A.S. & Treleaven, J. (2005) Cytokine profiles in stem cell transplantation: possible use as a predictor of graft-versus-host disease. *Hematology*, **10**, 107–114.

87 Srinivasan, R., Daniels, J., Fusaro, V. *et al.* (2006) Accurate diagnosis of acute graft-versus-host disease using serum proteomic pattern analysis. *Experimental Hematology*, **34**, 796–801.

88 Wissinger, E.M., Schiffer, E., Hertenstein, B. *et al.* (2007) Proteomic patterns predict acute graft-versus-host disease after allogeneic hematopoietic stem cell transplantation. *Blood*, **109**, 5511–5519.

89 Hori, T., Naishiro, Y., Sohma, H. *et al.* (2008) CCL8 is a potential molecular candidate for the diagnosis of graft-versus-host disease. *Blood*, **118**, 4403–4412.

90 Paczesny, S., Krijanovski, O.I., Braun, T.M. *et al.* (2009) A biomarker panel for acute graft-versus-host disease. *Blood*, **113**, 273–278.

91 Paczesny, S., Braun, T., Levine, J.E. *et al.* (2010) Elafin is a biomarker of graft-versus-host disease of the skin. *Science Translational Medicine*, **2**, 13ra2.

92 Storb, R., Deeg, H., Whitehead, J. *et al.* (1986) Methotrexate and cyclosporine alone for prophylaxis of acute graft versus host disease

after marrow transplantation for leukemia. *New England Journal of Medicine*, **314**, 729–735.

93 Hiraoka, A., Ohashi, Y., Okamoto, S. *et al.* (2001) Phase III study comparing tacrolimus (FK506) with cyclosporine for graft-versus-host disease prophylaxis after allogeneic bone marrow transplantation. *Bone Marrow Transplantation*, **28**, 181–185.

94 Horowitz, M.M., Przepiorka, D., Bartels, P. *et al.* (1999) Tacrolimus vs. cyclosporine immunosuppression: results in advanced-stage disease compared with historical controls treated exclusively with cyclosporine. *Journal of the American Society for Blood and Marrow Transplantation*, **5**, 180–186.

95 Ram, R., Gafter-Gvili, A., Yeshurun, M., Paul, M., Raanani, P. & Shpilberg, O. (2009) Prophylaxis regimens for GVHD: systematic review and meta-analysis. *Bone Marrow Transplantation*, **43**, 643–653.

96 Nash, R.A., Antin, J., Karanes, C. *et al.* (2000) Phase 3 study comparing methotrexate and tacrolimus with methotrexate and cyclosporine for prophylaxis of acute graft-versus-host disease after marrow transplantation from unrelated donors. *Blood*, **96**, 2062–2068.

97 Bolwell, B., Sobecks, R., Pohlman, B. *et al.* (2004) A prospective randomized trial comparing cyclosporine and short course methotrexate with cyclosporine and mycophenolate mofetil for GVHD prophylaxis in myeloablative allogeneic bone marrow transplantation. *Bone Marrow Transplantation*, **34**, 621–625.

98 Bornhauser, M., Schuler, U., Pörksen, G. *et al.* (1999) Mycophenolate mofetil and cyclosporine as graft-versus-host disease prophylaxis after allogeneic blood stem cell transplantation. *Transplantation*, **67**, 499–504.

99 Mohty, M., de Lavallade, H., Faucher, C. *et al.* (2004) Mycophenolate mofetil and cyclosporine for graft-versus-host disease prophylaxis following reduced intensity conditioning allogeneic stem cell transplantation. *Bone Marrow Transplantation*, **34**, 527–530.

100 Kasper, C., Sayer, H., Mügge, L.O. *et al.* (2004) Combined standard graft-versus-host disease (GvHD) prophylaxis with mycophenolate mofetil (MMF) in allogeneic peripheral blood stem cell transplantation from unrelated donors. *Bone Marrow Transplantation*, **33**, 65–69.

101 Vogelsang, G.B. & Arai, S. (2001) Mycophenolate mofetil for the prevention and treatment of graft-versus-host disease following stem cell transplantation: preliminary findings. *Bone Marrow Transplantation*, **27**, 1255–1262.

102 Niederwieser, D., Maris, M., Shizuru, J.A. *et al.* (2003) Low-dose total body irradiation (TBI) and fludarabine followed by hematopoietic cell transplantation (HCT) from HLA-matched or mismatched unrelated donors and postgrafting immunosuppression with cyclosporine and mycophenolate mofetil (MMF) can induce durable complete chimerism and sustained remissions in patients with hematological diseases. *Blood*, **101**, 1620–1629.

103 Marmont, A.M., Horowitz, M., Gale, R.P. *et al.* (1991) T-cell depletion of HLA-identical transplants in leukemia. *Blood*, **78**, 2120–2130.

104 Martin, P.J., Hansen, J., Torok-Storb, B. *et al.* (1988) Graft failure in patients receiving T cell-depleted HLA-identical allogeneic marrow transplants. *Bone Marrow Transplantation*, **3**, 445–456.

105 O'Reilly, R.J. (1992) T-cell depletion and allogeneic bone marrow transplantation. *Seminars in Hematology*, **29**, 20–26.

106 Kottaridis, P.D., Milligan, D.W., Chopra, R. *et al.* (2001) In vivo CAMPATH-1H prevents GvHD following nonmyeloablative stem-cell transplantation. *Cytotherapy*, **3**, 197–201.

107 Bacigalupo, A., Lamparelli, T., Bruzzi, P. *et al.* (2001) Antithymocyte globulin for graft-versus-host disease prophylaxis in transplants from unrelated donors: 2 randomized studies from Gruppo Italiano Trapianti Midollo Osseo (GITMO). *Blood*, **98**, 2942–2947.

108 Reddy, P. & Ferrara, J. (2003) Immunobiology of acute graft-versus-host disease. *Blood*, **17**, 187–194.

109 Hill, G.R. & Ferrara, J. (2000) The primacy of the gastrointestinal tract as a target organ of acute graft-versus-host disease: rationale for th euse of cytokine shields in allogeneic bone marrow transplantation. *Blood*, **95**, 2754–2759.

110 Xun, C.Q., Thompson, J., Jennings, C.D., Brown, S.A. & Widmer, M.B. (1994) Effect of total body irradiation, busulfan-cyclophosphamide, or cyclophosphamide conditioning on inflammatory cytokine release and development of acute and chronic graft-versus-host disease in H-2-incompatible transplanted SCID mice. *Blood*, **83**, 2360–2367.

111 Couriel, D.R., Saliba, R., Giralt, S. *et al.* (2004) Acute and chronic graft-versus-host disease after ablative and nonmyeloablative conditioning for allogeneic hematopoietic transplantation. *Journal of the American Society for Blood and Marrow Transplantation*, **10**, 178–185.

112 Choi, S.W., Kitko, C., Braun, T. *et al.* (2008) Change in plasma tumor necrosis factor receptor 1 levels in the first week after myeloablative allogeneic transplantation correlates with severity and incidence of GVHD and survival. *Blood*, **112**, 1539–1542.

113 Matzinger, P. (2002) The danger model: a renewed sense of self. *Science*, **296**, 301–305.

114 Shlomchik, W.D., Couzens, M., Tang, C.B. *et al.* (1999) Prevention of graft versus host disease by inactivation of host antigen-presenting cells. *Science*, **285**, 412–415.

115 Chao, N.J., Holler, E. & Deeg, H.J. (2005) Prophylaxis and treatment of acute graft-versus-host disease. In: J.L.M. Ferrara, K.R. Cooke & H.J. Deeg (eds), *Graft-vs.-Host Disease*, 3rd ed., pp. 459–479. Dekker, New York.

116 Peñas, P.F., Fernández-Herrera, J. & García-Diez, A. (2004) Dermatologic treatment of cutaneous graft versus host disease. *American Journal of Clinical Dermatology*, **5**, 403–416.

117 Couriel, D., Caldera, H., Champlin, R. & Komanduri, K. (2004) Acute graft-versus-host disease: pathophysiology, clinical manifestations, and management. *Cancer*, **101**, 1936–1946.

118 Higman, M.A. & Vogelsang, G.B. (2004) Chronic graft versus host disease. *British Journal of Haematology*, **125**, 435–454.

119 Ruutu, T., Niederwieser, D., Gratwohl, A. & Apperley, J.F. (1997) A survey of the prophylaxis and treatment of acute GVHD in Europe: a report of the European Group for Blood and Marrow, Transplantation (EBMT), Chronic Leukemia Working Party of the EBMT. *Bone Marrow Transplantation*, **19**, 759–764.

120 Saliba, R.M., de Lima, M., Giralt, S. *et al.* (2007) Hyperacute GVHD: risk factors, outcomes, and clinical implications. *Blood*, **109**, 2751–2758.

121 Hings, I.M., Filipovich, A., Miller, W.J. *et al.* (1993) Prednisone therapy for acute graft-versus-host disease: short- versus long-term treatment: a prospective randomized trial. *Transplantation*, **56**, 577–580.

122 Bacigalupo, A., van Lint, M., Frassoni, F. *et al.* (1983) High dose bolus methylprednisolone for the treatment of acute graft versus host disease. *Blut*, **46**, 125–132.

123 Kanojia, M.D., Anagnostou, A., Zander, A.R. *et al.* (1984) High-dose methylprednisolone treatment for acute graft-versus-host disease

after bone marrow transplantation in adults. *Transplantation*, **37**, 246–249.

124 Socié, G., Stone, J., Wingard, J.R. *et al.* (1999) Long-term survival and late deaths after allogeneic bone marrow transplantation. Late Effects Working Committee of the International Bone Marrow Transplant Registry. *New England Journal of Medicine*, **341**, 14–21.

125 Shulman, H., Sullivan, K., Weiden, P.L. *et al.* (1980) Chronic graft-versus-host syndrome in man: a long-term clinicopathologic study of 20 Seattle patients. *American Journal of Medicine*, **69**, 204–217.

126 Lee, S.J., Vogelsang, G. & Flowers, M.E. (2003) Chronic graft-versus-host disease. *Journal of the American Society for Blood and Marrow Transplantation*, **9**, 215–233.

127 Lee, S.J., Klein, J., Barrett, A.J. *et al.* (2002) Severity of chronic graft-versus-host disease: association with treatment-related mortality and relapse. *Blood*, **100**, 406–414.

128 Pavletic, S.Z., Smith, L., Bishop, M.R. *et al.* (2005) Prognostic factors of chronic graft-versus-host disease after allogeneic blood stem-cell transplantation. *American Journal of Hematology*, **78**, 265–274.

129 Tsoi, M., Storb, R., Dobbs, S., Medill, L. & Thomas, D. (1980) Cell-mediated immunity to non-HLA antigens of the host by donor lymphocyts in patients with chronic graft-versus-host disease. *Journal of Immunology*, **125**, 2258–2262.

130 Bunjes, D., Theobald, M., Nierle, T., Arnold, R. & Heimpel, H. (1995) Presence of host-specific interleukin 2-secreting T helper cell precursors correlates closely with active primary and secondary chronic graft-versus-host disease. *Bone Marrow Transplantation*, **15**, 727–732.

131 Graze, P. & Gale, R.P (1979) Chronic graft-versus-host disease: a syndrome of disordered immunity. *American Journal of Medicine*, **66**, 611–620.

132 Anasetti, C., Rybka, W., Sullivan, K., Banaji, M. & Slichter, S. (1989) Graft-versus-host disease is associated with autoimmune-like thrombocytopenia. *Blood*, **73**, 1054–1058.

133 Weiden, P.L., Flournoy, N., Sanders, J.E., Sullivan, K.M. & Thomas, E.D. (1981) Antileukemic effect of graft-versus-host disease contributes to improved survival after allogeneic marrow transplantation. *Transplantation Proceedings*, **13**, 248–251.

134 Weiden, P., Sullivan, K., Flournoy, N., Storb, R. & Thomas, E. (1981) The Seattle marrow transplant team: antileukemic effect of chronic graft-versus-host disease: contribution to improved survival after allogeneic marrow transplantation. *New England Journal of Medicine*, **304**, 1529–1533.

135 Schubert, M.M., Sullivan, K., Morton, T.H. *et al.* (1984) Oral manifestations of chronic graft-v-host disease. *Archives of Internal Medicine*, **144**, 1591–1595.

136 Saurat, J., Gluckman, E., Bussel, A., Didierjean, L. & Puissant, A. (1975) The lichen planus-like eruption after bone marrow transplantation. *British Journal of Dermatology*, **92**, 675–681.

137 Touraine, R., Revuz, J., Dreyfus, B., Rochant, H. & Mannoni, P. (1975) Graft versus host reaction and lichen planus. *British Journal of Dermatology*, **92**, 589.

138 Beers, B., Kalish, R., Kaye, V. & Dahl, M. (1993) Unilateral linear lichenoid eruption after bone marrow transplantation: an unmasking of tolerance to an abnormal keratinocyte clone? *Journal of the American Academy of Dermatology*, **28**, 888–892.

139 Chosidow, O., Bagot, M., Vernant, J., Touraine, R., Cordonnier, C. & Revuz, J. (1992) Sclerodermatous chronic graft versus host disease. *Journal of the American Academy of Dermatology*, **26**, 49–55.

140 Aractingi, S., Socié, G., Deergie, A., Dubertret, L. & Gluckman, E. (1993) Localized scleroderma-like lesions on the legs in bone marrow transplant recipients: association with polyneuropathy in the same distribution. *British Journal of Dermatology*, **129**, 201–203.

141 Moreno, J.C., Valverde, F., Martinez, F. *et al.* (2003) Bullous scleroderma-like changes in chronic graft-versus-host disease. *Journal of the European Academy of Dermatology and Venereology*, **17**, 200–203.

142 Akpek, G., Zahurak, M.L., Piantadosi, S. *et al.* (2001) Development of a prognostic model for grading chronic graft-versus-host disease. *Blood*, **97**, 1219–1226.

143 Shulman, H., Sale, G., Lerner, K. *et al.* (1978) Chronic cutaneous graft-versus-host disease in man. *American Journal of Pathology*, **91**, 545–570.

144 Rizzo, J.D., Curtis, R., Socié, G. *et al.* (2009) Solid cancers after allogeneic hematopoietic cell transplantation. *Blood*, **113**, 1175–1183.

145 Curtis, R.E., Rowlings, P., Deeg, J. *et al.* (1997) Solid cancers after bone marrow transplantation. *New England Journal of Medicine*, **336**, 897–904.

146 Greinix, H.T., Volc-Platzer, B., Rabitsch, W. *et al.* (1998) Successful use of extracorporeal photochemotherapy in the treatment of severe acute and chronic graft-versus-host disease. *Blood*, **92**, 3098–3104.

147 Seaton, E.D., Szydlo, R., Kanfer, E., Apperley, J.F. & Russell-Jones, R. (2003) Influence of extracorporeal photopheresis on clinical and laboratory parameters in chronic graft-versus-host disease and analysis of predictors of response. *Blood*, **102**, 1217–1223.

148 Akpek, G., Via, C.S. & Vogelsang, G. (2005) Clinical spectrum and therapeutic approaches to chronic graft-vs-host disease. In: J.L.M. Ferrara, K.R. Cooke & H.J. Deeg (eds), *Graft-versus-Host Disease*, pp. 595–650. Dekker, New York.

149 Browne, P.V., Weisdorf, D., Defor, T. *et al.* (2000) Response to thalidomide therapy in refractory chronic graft-versus-host disease. *Bone Marrow Transplantation*, **26**, 865–869.

150 Le Blanc, K., Rasmusson, I., Sundberg, B. *et al.* (2004) Treatment of severe acute graft-versus-host disease with third party haploidentical mesenchymal stem cells. *Lancet*, **363**, 1439–1441.

151 Ringdén, O., Uzunel, M., Rasmusson, I. *et al.* (2006) Mesenchymal stem cells for treatment of therapy-resistant graft-versus-host disease. *Transplantation*, **81**, 1390–1397.

28 Extravasation Reactions

Seppo W. Langer

Department of Oncology, Copenhagen University Hospital – Rigshospitalet, Copenhagen, Denmark

Introduction

Extravasation describes the unintended leakage of a drug from a vessel into the surrounding tissues or the unintended instillation of a drug directly into the perivascular tissues. In a broader sense, the term also refers to the resulting tissue damage (i.e., the extravasation reaction; Figure 28.1). The signs and symptoms range from mild discomfort and irritation, with sparse objective clinical findings, to large, progressive, long-lasting, and devastating necrosis, which may ultimately be fatal. Key points of extravasation reactions are as follow:

• Extravasation reactions may be devastating;
• Extravasation is largely preventable;
• International guidelines for prevention and treatment are available; and documentation and aftercare is mandatory.

Accidental extravasation is one of the most feared complications of chemotherapy administration. The percentage of adult patients affected by symptomatic extravasation reactions ranges between 0.1% and 6% [1]. Cancer patients generally have a higher risk as a result of repetitive infusions into fragile veins, with the highest prevalence in peripheral IV infusions. The reported ratio of extravasations from central ports versus peripheral veins varies from very few to more than 25%. Accordingly, the use of implanted venous access ports may decrease but do not eliminate the risk [2–5]. The consequences of extravasations from a centrally inserted catheter may be more serious. The incidence of extravasations has decreased over the years, which is probably because of a markedly increased awareness of the complication, more intensive surveillance during infusions, better infusion remedies and technique, and better training of healthcare professionals [4,6].

Chemotherapeutic agents can broadly be divided into three categories according to their cutaneous extravasation reactions:
drugs that produce vesicant reactions ("vesicants"), irritation ("irritants"), and the more or less neutral (Table 28.1). This division is somewhat arbitrary and can vary with increasing clinical experience. Vesicants can cause ulceration and necrosis, with the most important vesicants being the anthracyclines (e.g., doxorubicin, epirubicin, and daunorubicin; Figure 28.2 and 28.3), antineoplastic antibiotics (e.g., mitomycin C and dactinomycin), and the vinca alkaloids (e.g., vinorelbine and vincristine; Figure 28.4). Irritants can cause an inflammatory reaction; the platinum compounds (e.g., cisplatin and carboplatin), the taxanes (e.g., docetaxel and paclitaxel), and the topoisomerase I inhibitors (e.g., irinotecan and topotecan) belong in this category [7]. However, an irritant drug can have vesicant properties depending on the concentration, volume, and diluents [7]. Conversely, a small extravasation of a vesicant drug does not necessarily result in blistering and necrosis. The distinction between these categories is therefore fluid.

Risk factors

Risk factors can be divided into three main categories:
1. *Patient-associated factors:* include small, damaged, sclerosed, and fragile veins, lymphedema, obesity, polyneuropathy, prior radiation, and impaired consciousness.
2. *Medication-related factors:* large volume and duration of infusions, high concentration, hypersensitivity, and vesicant properties.
3. *Iatrogenic risk factors:* poor infusion technique, improper cannulas, insufficient training, and lack of patient information.
In the event of an extravasation, the risk of extensive damage depends on whether prompt action is taken. Every institution should have clear instructions for immediate action during an extravasation.

Dermatologic Principles and Practice in Oncology: Conditions of the Skin, Hair, and Nails in Cancer Patients, First Edition. Edited by Mario E. Lacouture.
© 2014 John Wiley & Sons, Inc. Published 2014 by John Wiley & Sons, Inc.

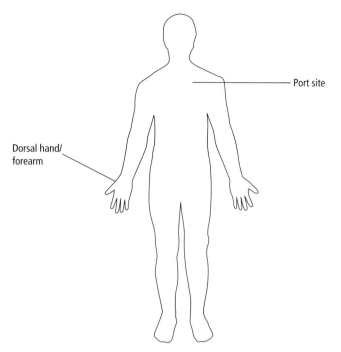

Figure 28.1 Anatomic location of extravasation reactions.

Table 28.1 Examples of chemotherapeutic agents that may cause vesicant and irritant extravasation reactions.

Vesicants	Irritants
DNA binding agents	Carboplatin
Anthracyclines	Cisplatin*
Daunorubicin	Cyclophosphamide
Doxorubicin	Dacarbazine
Epirubicin	Docetaxel*
Idarubicin	Etoposide
Amrubicin	Fluorouracil
Nonanthracyclines	Ifosfamide
Dactinomycin	Irinotecan
Mechlorethamine	Liposomal anthracyclines*
Mitomycin C	Melphalan
Trabectedin	Mitoxantrone*
	Oxaliplatin*
Non-DNA binding agents	Paclitaxel*
Vincristine	Streptozocin*
Vinblastine	Topotecan
Vindesine	
Vinorelbine	

*Some of the irritants may also be weak vesicants.

Clinical features

The clinical course will depend on drug volume and concentration, the anatomic location, and especially the vesicant potential.

Extravasations occur more easily from small veins on dorsal hands, and may spread to the fingers, thereby complicating the clinical course and the treatment. The drug volume that diffuses into the perivascular tissue from an extravasation in the antecubital fossa or in centrally inserted catheters can be significant before the extravasation is noted. The symptoms of irritant extravasation includes edema, pain, warmth, discomfort, erythema, and tenderness. Some irritants and vesicants (e.g., the vinca alkaloids) produce phlebitis, hyperpigmentation, and sclerosis along the vein. The symptoms and signs often resolve within days to weeks, and long-term sequelae are rare.

Clinical hallmarks of vesicant extravasations are acute pain, swelling, erythema, and intense burning or tingling [6,8,9]. Infiltration from a centrally placed catheter may present as shoulder pain and can have a delayed onset. Blistering may develop immediately or within days after the extravasation followed by induration, discoloration, and, in severe cases, signs of tissue destruction. The slowly growing ulceration that appears after weeks to months may invade deep structures such as tendons and joints [10–15]. The protracted healing process can extend over several months. The presence of necrotic tissue is a risk factor for bacterial colonization which can aggravate the extravasation reaction in immunocompromised cancer patients. A high index of suspicion for a secondary infection should be considered, especially when discharge, edema, and warmth are

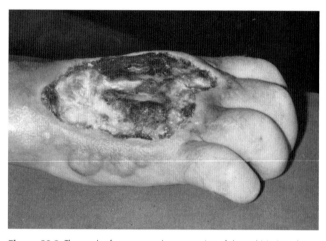

Figure 28.2 The result of an untreated extravasation of doxorubicin into the dorsum of the hand.

present. Scar formation can lead to long-term cosmetic and functional deficits. Treatment delay, termination of further planned chemotherapy, and even death from wound complications may be the ultimate outcome. Grading is carried out using the Common Terminology Criteria for Adverse Events Version 4 (Table 28.2):

Grade 1: not applicable;

Grade 2: erythema with associated symptoms (e.g., edema, pain, induration, phlebitis);

Grade 3: ulceration or necrosis; severe tissue damage; operative intervention indicated;

Grade 4: life-threatening consequences or urgent intervention indicated;
Grade 5: death.

Pathophysiology and dermatopathology

Many of the drugs with the highest vesicant potential bind to nucleic acids (Table 28.1). The protracted course of the tissue damage and the progressive ulceration is probably due to anthracyclin recycling as it intercalates into DNA. Extravasated anthracyclines are likely continuously released from necrotic cells, thereby enabling damage to adjacent healthy tissue (endocytolysis). The persistence of vesicant anthracyclines has been demonstrated by high performance liquid chromatography (HPLC) of biopsies from chronic extravasation ulcers [16–18]. Additional cellular toxicity results from free radical formation and peroxidation of the cell membrane. Conversely, alkylating agents are consumed during the DNA binding processes and subsequently inactivated by enzyme repair systems. Hence, direct cytotoxicity gradually decreases as agents are cleared from tissues. The antineoplastic toxicity of vinca alkaloids and the taxanes are tubulin mediated,

but do not explain the reactions that show elements of direct cellular damage, inflammation, and hypersensitivity.

Histologic examinationss have shown that inflammation is not a central part of anthracycline extravasation reactions. Instead, the morphology is more analogous to that seen in erythema multiforme, toxic epidermal necrolysis (TEN), and graft versus host disease (GVHD), with necrosis of the epidermis and vessel damage [19,20].

Treatment

Extravasation is a preventable condition, and it is recommended that international guidelines for both prevention and treatment are implemented [21,22]. In the event of an extravasation, a stepwise action must betaken: the infusion is stopped, the affected

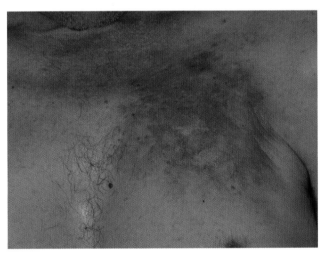

Figure 28.3 Vesicant extravasation from an implanted port. Photo courtesy of Mario E Lacouture MD.

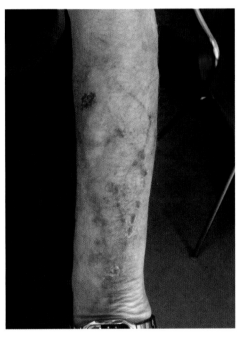

Figure 28.4 Extravasation reaction along the veins of a forearm with impaired venous flow after vinorelbine infusion.

Table 28.2 Grading of extravasation reactions. Administration site conditions category of Common Terminology Criteria for Averse Events (CTCAE) Version 4.0.

CTCAE v4.0 AE term	Grade 1	Grade 2	Grade 3	Grade 4	Grade 5
Infusion site extravasation	–	Erythema with associated symptoms (e.g., edema, pain, induration, phlebitis)	Ulceration or necrosis; severe tissue damage; operative intervention indicated	Life-threatening consequences; urgent intervention indicated	Death

AE, adverse event.
A semi-colon indicates "or" within the description of the grade. A single dash (–) indicates a grade is not available. Not all grades are appropriate for all AEs.
Therefore, some AEs are listed with fewer than five options for grade selection.

Table 28.3 Recommended and often used acute antidotes in extravasation injuries.

	ONS	EONS
Alkylating agents	Sodium thiosulfate SC	–
Vinca alkaloids	Hyaluronidase SC	Hyaluronidase SC*
Nonanthracycline antibiotics	–	Topical DMSO*
Anthracyclines	Dexrazoxane IV (Totect(®))	Dexrazoxane IV (Savene(®))
Taxanes	–	Hyaluronidase SC*

EONS, Guidelines from the European Oncology Nursing Society [21]; IV, intravenous; ONS, Guidelines from the Oncology Nursing Society [22];SC, subcutaneous.
Intermittent cooling is recommended as immediate treatment except in extravasation of vinca alkaloids, where local heating is recommended instead.
*Marks frequently used treatments where further studies are recommended due to lack of evidence.

Examples of treatment schedules
Hyaluronidase: 1–6 mL of a 150 units/mL solution is injected SC into the area of extravasation. Often 1 mL of solution is used for each milliliter of extravasated drug.
Sodium thiosulfate: 4 mL of 10% sodium thiosulfate is mixed with 6 mL of sterile water producing a 1/6 molar solution which is injected SC. A dose example is 2 mL for each milligram of extravasated mechlorethamine.
DMSO: A solution of 50–100% is applicated topically every 2–8 hours for up to 14 days.
Dexrazoxane: Treatment is started within 6 hours of the extravasation. Intravenous infusion of 1000 mg/m² on days 1 and 2, and 500 mg/m² on day 3 of the prepared solution.

limb elevated, and the affected area clearly marked. The demarcation is important to ensure documentation and in case surgery is needed. The next treatment step is drug-dependent: with a nonvesicant, intermittent cooling and observation is often sufficient. Symptomatic treatment of itching, scaling, and superficial phlebitis may be indicated. With a vesicant extravasation, the agent should be either dispersed or localized and neutralized with an antidote (Table 28.3). Dispersal seems the most logical approach with non-DNA binding compounds such as the vinca alkaloids. Conversely, the DNA-binding vesicants, such as the anthracyclines, mitomycin C, nitrogen mustard, and trabectedin may require localization and neutralization with an antidote. Topical cooling can serve as pain relief, but heating is recommended with vinca alkaloids.

There are no uniform guidelines for the surgical treatment of extravasations, although traditionally anthracycline and mitomycin C extravasations would result in surgery to remove the

tissue-bound drug [8,23–26]. The timing of the intervention is controversial (i.e., early versus late surgery). Surgical excision often requires wide margins; after removal of the necrotic tissues, skin grafting may be necessary. Surgical margins for anthracycline extravasation can be guided by fluorescence microscopy [27–29]. However, after the introduction of dexrazoxane as a specific antidote in anthracycline extravasation, the need for surgery has decreased. Surgical intervention is indicated in a vesicant extravasation when necrosis occurs despite pharmacologic treatment or when progressive necrosis develops in an untreated extravasation. Various liposuction procedures and surgical wash out procedures (SWOP) using multiple incisions and saline flushing have been used in selected cases of large vesicant extravasations [30,31]. No controlled biopsy-proven studies have been conducted to demonstrate their efficacy in anthracycline extravasations.

Antidotes in chemotherapeutic drug extravasations

The list of nonsurgical treatments that have been used empirically in anthracycline extravasations is very long. Frequently used strategies include topical dimethyl sulfoxide (DMSO), topical and intralesional hyaluronidase, and corticosteroids [32–36]. The rationale for their use includes free radical scavenging, skin permeability alterations, enhanced anthracycline absorption, and anti-inflammatory properties. Treatment with dexrazoxane (Totect®) is recommended and is the only licensed drug for this indication [21,22]. Dexrazoxane is administered IV immediately after the extravasation and for the following 2 days. Its clinical efficacy was demonstrated in multinational prospective trials after extensive preclinical studies [37–39]. In 80 analyzed patients, extravasation was confirmed by fluorescence-positive biopsies in 57 assessable patients. The median values of the affected skin areas were 24 and 39 cm² in the two studies, respectively. Eleven patients had areas of extravasation exceeding 75 cm². Dexrazoxane was administered as an intravenous infusion over 1–2 hours; 1000 mg/m² was given within 6 hours after the extravasation injury, 1000 mg/m² 24 hours later, and 500 mg/m² another 24 hours later. After dexrazoxane treatment, only 1 of the 57 assessable patients, a patient with an extravasation area >250 cm², required surgery. Seventy percent of the patients had no sequelae at all, and two-thirds of all patients were able to continue their scheduled chemotherapy without any postponement. These results were confirmed in a small pharmacokinetic study, in which six patients with biopsy-verified anthracycline extravasations also achieved excellent treatment results. Topical application of DMSO may have a beneficial effect in small (grade 1) anthracycline extravasations, but the lack of a biopsy-verified diagnosis and detailed information in published cases makes it very hard to conclude whether real benefit has been obtained [36]. The concomitant use of topical DMSO and IV dexrazoxane is not recommended. Inflammation is not a core feature in acute or late anthracycline extravasation injuries, and neither clinical nor experimental studies support the use of topical or subcutaneous treatment with corticosteroids [20,40].

In animal experiments, local cooling actually increased the toxicity of vinca alkaloids, while hot packs tended to limit the skin damage. This principle has translated into clinical practice, partly because the treatment strategy relies on dispersion rather than localization [6,21,22]. Dispersion and dilution of vinca alkaloid extravasation drugs with saline or hyaluronidase in combination with hot packs may be a relevant treatment option in large extravasations. Hyaluronidase has not been tested in controlled clinical trials and is not commercially available in all countries. Mitomycin C is a vesicant drug that can produce very large, distant, and delayed ulcerations. According to several reports, the toxicity of mitomycin C can be reduced by topical application of 99% DMSO [35–38]. DMSO is not available in all countries, especially not at high concentrations. Recently, trabectedin was recognized as a vesicant drug [41]. There is no known antidote to trabectedin extravasation, and so far no clinical experience with, for example, hyaluronidase or DMSO. Mechlorethamine produces extremely severe and prolonged skin ulceration after extravasation. Intralesional injection of sodium thiosulfate has shown antidotal effect in animal experiments [42]. Therefore, in humans the recommendation in case of nitrogen mustard extravasation is an immediate subcutaneous administration of sodium thiosulfate solution. However, clinical studies in humans have not been carried out, and sodium thiosulfate is not readily available in all institutions. Taxanes have been reported to cause tissue damage after extravasation, paclitaxel in particular. Conservative management usually results in complete recovery, and the taxanes are normally considered to be predominantly irritant and only mildly vesicant [43,44]. Intradermal hyaluronidase diluted in saline treatment has been adopted in some institutions as standard treatment but is generally not recommended.

Aftercare

The initial treatment of chemotherapeutic extravasation cannot stand alone. A clinical follow-up program is mandatory, especially in the management of vesicant extravasations. Many patients receiving chemotherapy are immunocompromised and the extravasation reactions are therefore at risk of being additionally aggravated by infection in the sloughing tissues, which occurs quite frequently. Antibiotic treatment should therefore be started on clinical suspicion of an infection in the extravasation site. Long-term sequelae of vesicant extravasations or the surgical treatment thereof can generate scarring, nerve and muscle damage that leads to functional deficits and significant cosmetic changes. Accordingly, clinical documentation in the follow-up period may be an important support for the patient, especially if the extravasation gives rise to an insurance case.

References

1 Schrijvers, D.L. (2003) Extravasation: a dreaded complication of chemotherapy. *Annals of Oncology*, **14** (Suppl. 3), 26–30.

2 Lemmers, N.W., Gels, M.E., Sleijfer, D.T. *et al.* (1996) Complications of venous access ports in 132 patients with disseminated testicular cancer treated with polychemotherapy. *Journal of Clinical Oncology*, **14** (11), 2916–2922.

3 Shetty, P.C., Mody, M.K., Kastan, D.J. *et al.* (1997) Outcome of 350 implanted chest ports placed by interventional radiologists. *Journal of Vascular and Interventional Radiology*, **8** (6), 991–995.

4 Langstein, H.N., Duman, H., Seelig, D., Butler, C.E. & Evans, G.R. (2002) Retrospective study of the management of chemotherapeutic extravasation injury. *Annals of Plastic Surgery*, **49** (4), 369–374.

5 Langer, S.W. (2008) Treatment of anthracycline extravasation from centrally inserted venous catheters. *Oncology Reviews*, **2** (2), 114–116.

6 Schulmeister, L. (2007) Extravasation management. *Seminars in Oncology Nursing*, **23** (3), 184–190.

7 Berghammer, P., Pøhnl, R., Baur, M. & Dittrich, C. (2001) Docetaxel extravasation. *Supportive Care in Cancer*, **9** (2), 131–134.

8 Larson, D.L. (1982) Treatment of tissue extravasation by antitumor agents. *Cancer*, **49** (9), 1796–1799.

9 Seyfer, A.E. & Solimando, D.A. Jr. (1983) Toxic lesions of the hand associated with chemotherapy. *Journal of Hand Surgery*, **8** (1), 39–42.

10 Laughlin, R.A., Landeen, J.M. & Habal, M.B. (1979) The management of inadvertent subcutaneous adriamycin infiltration. *American Journal of Surgery*, **137** (3), 408–412.

11 Preuss, P. & Partoft, S. (1987) Cytostatic extravasations. *Annals of Plastic Surgery*, **19** (4), 323–329.

12 Linder, R.M., Upton, J. & Osteen, R. (1983) Management of extensive doxorubicin hydrochloride extravasation injuries. *Journal of Hand Surgery*, **8** (1), 32–38.

13 Bowers, D.G. Jr & Lynch, J.B. (1978) Adriamycin extravasation. *Plastic and Reconstructive Surgery*, **61** (1), 86–92.

14 Rudolph, R., Stein, R.S. & Pattillo, R.A. (1976) Skin ulcers due to adriamycin. *Cancer*, **38** (3), 1087–1094.

15 Reilly, J.J., Neifeld, J.P. & Rosenberg, S.A. (1977) Clinical course and management of accidental adriamycin extravasation. *Cancer*, **40** (5), 2053–2056.

16 Ignoffo, R.J. & Friedman, M.A. (1980) Therapy of local toxicities caused by extravasation of cancer chemotherapeutic drugs. *Cancer Treatment Reviews*, **7** (1), 17–27.

17 Garnick, M., Khetarpal, V. & Luce, J.K. (1981) Persistence of anthracycline levels following dermal and subcutaneous adriamycin extravasation. *Proceedings of the American Association for Cancer Research*, **22**, 173.

18 Sonneveld, P., Wassenaar, H.A. & Nooter, K. (1984) Long persistence of doxorubicin in human skin after extravasation. *Cancer Treatment Reports*, **68** (6), 895–896.

19 Bhawan, J., Petry, J. & Rybak, M.E. (1989) Histologic changes induced in skin by extravasation of doxorubicin (adriamycin). *Journal of Cutaneous Pathology*, **16** (3), 158–163.

20 Thougaard, A.V., Langer, S.W., Hainau, B. *et al.* (2010) A murine experimental anthracycline extravasation model: pathology and study

of the involvement of topoisomerase II alpha and iron in the mechanism of tissue damage. *Toxicology*, **269** (1), 67–72.

21 Wengström, Y., Margulies, A. & European Oncology Nursing Society Task Force (2008) European oncology Nursing Society extravasation guidelines. *European Journal of Oncology Nursing*, **12** (4), 357–361.

22 Polovich, M., Whitford, J.M. & Olsen, M. (2009) *Chemotherapy and Biotherapy Guidelines and Recommendations for Practice*, 3rd ed., Oncology Nursing Society, Pittsburg, PA.

23 Pitkänen, J., Asko-Seljavaara, S., Gröhn, P., Sundell, B., Heinonen, E. & Appelqvist, P. (1983) Adriamycin extravasation: surgical treatment and possible prevention of skin and soft-tissue injuries. *Journal of Surgical Oncology*, **23** (4), 259–262.

24 Larson, D.L. (1985) What is the appropriate management of tissue extravasation by antitumor agents? *Plastic and Reconstructive Surgery*, **75** (3), 397–405.

25 Loth, T.S. & Eversmann, W.W. Jr (1991) Extravasation injuries in the upper extremity. *Clinical Orthopaedics and Related Research*, **272**, 248–254.

26 Heitmann, C., Durmus, C. & Ingianni, G. (1998) Surgical management after doxorubicin and epirubicin extravasation. *Journal of Hand Surgery*, **23** (5), 666–668.

27 Duray, P.H., Cuono, C.B. & Madri, J.A. (1986) Demonstration of cutaneous doxorubicin extravasation by rhodamine-filtered fluorescence microscopy. *Journal of Surgical Oncology*, **31** (1), 21–25.

28 Dahlström, K.K., Chenoufi, H.L. & Daugaard, S. (1990) Fluorescence microscopic demonstration and demarcation of doxorubicin extravasation. Experimental and clinical studies. *Cancer*, **65** (8), 1722–1726.

29 Andersson, A.P. & Dahlstrøm, K.K. (1993) Clinical results after doxorubicin extravasation treated with excision guided by fluorescence microscopy. *European Journal of Cancer*, **29A** (12), 1712–1714.

30 Fleming, A., Butler, B. & Gault, D. (1999) Surgical management after doxorubicin and epirubicin extravasation. *Journal of Hand Surgery*, **24** (3), 390.

31 Steiert, A., Hille, U., Burke, W. *et al.* (2010) Subcutaneous wash-out procedure (SWOP) for the treatment of chemotherapeutic extravasations. *Journal of Plastic, Reconstructive and Aesthetic Surgery*, **64**, 240–247..

32 Lawrence, H.J., Walsh, D., Zapotowski, K.A., Denham, A., Goodnight, S.H. & Gandara, D.R. (1989) Topical dimethylsulfoxide may prevent tissue damage from anthracycline extravasation. *Cancer Chemotherapy and Pharmacology*, **23** (5), 316–318.

33 Ludwig, C.U., Stoll, H.R., Obrist, R. & Obrecht, J.P. (1987) Prevention of cytotoxic drug induced skin ulcers with dimethyl sulfoxide (DMSO) and alpha-tocopherole. *European Journal of Cancer and Clinical Oncology*, **23** (3), 327–329.

34 Olver, I.N., Aisner, J., Hament, A., Buchanan, L., Bishop, J.F. & Kaplan, R.S. (1988) A prospective study of topical dimethyl sulfoxide for treating anthracycline extravasation. *Journal of Clinical Oncology*, **6** (11), 1732–1735.

35 Bert Bertelli, G., Gozza, A., Forno, G.B. *et al.* (1995) Topical dimethylsulfoxide for the prevention of soft tissue injury after extravasation of vesicant cytotoxic drugs: a prospective clinical study. *Journal of Clinical Oncology*, **13** (11), 2851–2855.

36 Langer, S.W., Sehested, M. & Jensen, P.B. (2009) Anthracycline extravasation: a comprehensive review of experimental and clinical treatments. *Tumori*, **95** (3), 273–282.

37 Langer, S.W., Sehested, M. & Jensen, P.B. (2000) Treatment of anthracycline extravasation with dexrazoxane. *Clinical Cancer Research*, **6** (9), 3680–3686.

38 Langer, S.W., Sehested, M. & Jensen, P.B. (2001) Dexrazoxane is a potent and specific inhibitor of anthracycline induced subcutaneous lesions in mice. *Annals of Oncology*, **12** (3), 405–410.

39 Mouridsen, H.T., Langer, S.W., Buter, J. *et al.* (2007) Treatment of anthracycline extravasation with Savene (dexrazoxane): results from two prospective clinical multicentre studies. *Annals of Oncology*, **18** (3), 546–550.

40 Langer, S.W., Thougaard, A.V., Sehested, M. & Jensen, P.B. (2006) Treatment of anthracycline extravasation in mice with dexrazoxane with or without DMSO and hydrocortisone. *Cancer Chemotherapy and Pharmacology*, **57** (1), 125–128.

41 Theman, T.A., Hartzell, T.L., Sinha, I. *et al.* (2009) Recognition of a new chemotherapeutic vesicant: trabectedin (ecteinascidin-743) extravasation with skin and soft tissue damage. *Journal of Clinical Oncology*, **27** (33), e198–e200.

42 Owen, O.E., Dellatorre, D.L., Van Scott, E.J. & Cohen, M.R. (1980) Accidental intramuscular injection of mechlorethamine. *Cancer*, **45** (8), 2225–2226.

43 Raymond, E., Cartier, S., Canuel, C. *et al.* (1995) Extravasation of paclitaxel (Taxol). [In French] *Revue de Medecine Interne*, **16** (2), 141–142.

44 Ascherman, J.A., Knowles, S.L. & Attkiss, K. (2000) Docetaxel (Taxotere) extravasation: a report of five cases with treatment recommendations. *Annals of Plastic Surgery*, **45** (4), 438–441.

29 Topical Anticancer Therapies

Patricia L. Myskowski

Dermatology Service, Memorial Sloan-Kettering Cancer Center; Department of Dermatology, Weill Cornell Medical College, New York, NY, USA

Recent years have witnessed the successful development of topical pharmacologic agents useful in the management of malignancies in the skin. The most commonly treated conditions are the nonmelanoma skin cancers (basal cell carcinoma, Bowen disease or squamous cell carcinoma *in situ*, and the latter's precursor, actinic keratosis; AK), cutaneous T-cell lymphoma (specifically mycosis fungoides; MF) and Kaposi sarcoma. Many of these agents have potent therapeutic effects, but may be accompanied by severe irritant, allergic, or other long-term adverse events (AEs) (Figure 29.1). For organizational purposes, these topical agents are divided and discussed under the headings of topical chemotherapy, retinoids, biologic response modifiers, and corticosteroids. A summary of these agents, and some of their uses in cutaneous oncology, is shown in Table 29.1. The cutaneous AEs of these drugs are shown in Table 29.2.

Topical chemotherapy

Carmustine

Carmustine (1,3-bis-(2-chloroethyl-)-1-nitrosourea; BCNU) is an alkylating agent used in systemic cancer therapy since the 1960s. Topical carmustine solution, 2–4 mg/mL (0.02–0.04%) in an alcoholic vehicle, has been used for patients with limited patch/plaque MF (skin only disease, stage IA–IB) [1–3]. In a long-term analysis of 188 patients followed for 36 months, 91% of T1 patients and 62% of stage T2 patients were maintained successfully with topical carmustine (BCNU) [3].

Clinical features

The primary cutaneous reaction of topical carmustine in these patients was erythema, developing 4–8 weeks into treatment, and often accompanied by a "burning" sensation and tenderness [1,2]. Erythema was accentuated in body folds (groin and axillae),

but not the hands and face. Dark-skinned patients manifested hyperpigmention more commonly [2].

Irritant or allergic contact dermatitis occurred in approximately 6–10% of patients, the latter confirmed with patch testing using 0.1% solution [2]. Topical BCNU ointment 10 mg/100 g petrolatum) has also been used recently, because it appears to be better tolerated than the solution, but may not be as effective [3].

The most common long-term cutaneous AE of topical carmustine was telangiectasia – transient or permanent – in the treated areas. Although carmustine is a carcinogen, secondary skin cancers related to this agent have been rarely reported [2].

Topical carmustine is absorbed systemically (up to 28% percutaneous absorption) [1–3]. The most frequent dose-limiting AE has been mild bone marrow suppression (7–10% of patients) followed by mild elevations in aspartate transaminase (serum glutamic oxaloacetic transaminase) (AST(SGOT)) [2]. Patients using topical carmustine should have complete blood counts every 2 weeks, and liver function tests every 4 weeks, during and for up to 6 weeks following cessation of treatment [2].

Treatment of choice

Additional episodes of contact dermatitis to topical carmustine have been avoided by successful desensitization in two patients. In those with irritant reactions, less concentrated solutions have used with success. Topical corticosteroids, emollients, and cool water soaks have been used to lessen discomfort [2].

Mechlorethamine

Nitrogen mustard (mechlorethamine) is a bifunctional alkylating agent that interferes with DNA synthesis, which has been used in systemic chemotherapy regimens for various lymphomas [4]. While topical mechlorethamine has also been used successfully in Langerhans cell histiocytosis and cutaneous B-cell lymphoma [5], it is used most commonly in the treatment of early (T1/T2,

Dermatologic Principles and Practice in Oncology: Conditions of the Skin, Hair, and Nails in Cancer Patients, First Edition. Edited by Mario E. Lacouture.

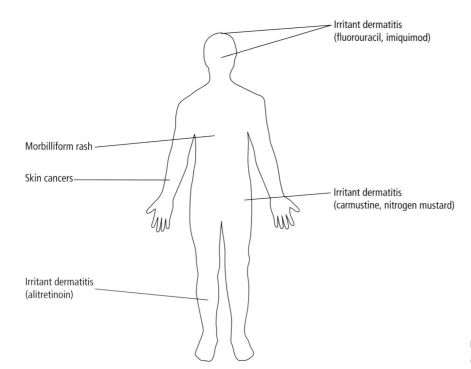

Irritant dermatitis
(fluorouracil, imiquimod)

Morbilliform rash

Skin cancers

Irritant dermatitis
(carmustine, nitrogen mustard)

Irritant dermatitis
(alitretinoin)

Figure 29.1 Anatomic location of topical anticancer therapy-induced adverse events.

Table 29.1 Topical anticancer agents (and treated conditions).

Chemotherapy:
- Carmustine (mycosis fungoides)
- Mechloroethamine (mycosis fungoides, cutaneous B-cell lymphoma, Langerhans cell histiocytosis)
- Fluorouracil[a] (actinic keratoses,[a] basal cell carcinoma,[a] Bowen disease, squamous cell carcinoma)

Retinoids:
- Alitretinoin[a] (Kaposi sarcoma[a])
- Bexarotene[a] (mycosis fungoides/CTCL[a])

Biologic response modifiers:
- Imiquimod[a] (actinic keratoses,[a] basal cell carcinoma,[a] Bowen disease, squamous cell carcinoma, mycosis fungoides)
- Corticosteroids (mycosis fungoides/CTCL, cutaneous B-cell lymphoma)

[a]Approved by US Food and Drug Administration.

patch/plaque) MF [6–8]. In a retrospective study of clinical stage I–III MF patients with topical mechlorethamine treatment, in aqueous solution or ointment, overall response rates of 93% and 72% were seen in T1 and T2 patients, respectively [8]. Topical mechlorethamine was originally prepared by diluting 10–20 mg mechloroethamine in 40–60 mL water, with once daily applications to affected skin areas [6,8]. Topical mechlorethamine does not appear to be systemically absorbed [6].

Clinical features

Cutaneous AEs are common with topical mechlorethamine. Immediate reactions include urticaria (up to 5% of patients) [7]

and, rarely, anaphylaxis [9]. Pruritus and "unmasking" of previously unrecognized areas of MF are common initially. Hyperpigmentation often occurs later [7,8].

Irritant and allergic contact dermatitis are the most common dose-limiting AEs (up to 44%), usually developing during the first 3 months of therapy (Figure 29.2) [4,5]. Irritation occurs in skin folds, the face (up to 25%), and genital area [8]. Acute contact dermatitis develops in 20–80% of patients treated with the aqueous solution of mechlorethamine, but occurs in <10% of patients treated with the ointment preparation [5,6,8].

Late effects of topical mechlorethamine include higher rates of nonmelanoma skin cancer (NMSC) (relative rate (RR) = 7.6), much more so for squamous cell carcinoma (SCC) (RR = 8.6) than basal cell carcinoma (BCC) (RR = 1.8) [10]. Median time of onset for NMSC was 8.3 years after topical mechlorethamine therapy [11].

Treatment of choice

The use of ointment-based topical nitrogen mustard has largely replaced aqueous preparations, because of the lower risk of contact dermatitis. Avoiding application to the skin folds and face is prudent, when possible, because of the high rate of irritation. In addition, topical nitrogen mustard is not usually applied to the genital area because of frequent irritation and possible increased carcinogenic potential in this area [8].

The prevention and treatment of irritant and/or contact dermatitis has remained especially problematic. Concomitant topical corticosteroids and 0.02% aqueous mechlorethamine solution twice weekly were studied but 28% of patients developed severe cutaneous intolerance requiring discontinuation of

Table 29.2 Incidence of dermatologic adverse events (AEs) to topical anticancer therapies.

Drug name	Cutaneous and subcutaneous toxicities (frequency)
Carmustine	Telangiectasia (common)
	Irritant/contact dermatitis (10%) [1,2], contact dermatitis (7%) [2]
Mechlorethamine (nitrogen mustard)	Urticaria (5%) [7]
	Irritation: skin folds (common), face (25%) [8]
	Contact dermatitis: aqueous (20–80%) [6,8], ointment (<10%) [6,8]
	Late: hyperpigmentation, increased risk of BCC & SCC [10,11]
Fluorouracil	Any cutaneous AE (97%) [14]
	Erythema (33–97%) [14]
	Scabbing/crusting (13%) [14]
	Ulceration (4–9%) [14]
	Scarring (9–11%) [14]
	Hyperpigmentation (3%) [14]
Alitretinoin	Rash (69–83%) [20,21]
	Dry skin (10%) [21]
	Ulceration (9%) [21]
Bexarotene	Rash (73%) [24]
	"Sticky skin" (14%) [25]
	Vesiculobullous reaction (6%) [24]
Imiquimod	Erythema (63–100%) [14]
	Edema (3–92%) [14]
	Weeping (69%) [14]
	Scabbing/crusting (52–65%) [14]
	Ulceration (25–27%)
	Vesiculation (3–17%) [14]
	Hypopigmentation (9–67%) [14]
Corticosteroids	Irritant dermatitis (10%) [25]
	Purpura (20%) [25]
	Striae, cutaneous atrophy [25]

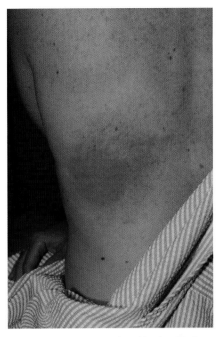

Figure 29.2 Contact dermatitis to topical mechlorethamine. Note central papulovesicles and erythema extending beyond mycosis fungoides patch.

treatment [12]. Desensitization regimens (using weekly aqueous mechlorethamine, 10 mg/1200–1800 mL, with gradual escalation) have shown some success but contact dermatitis may have a beneficial effect on the resolution of MF lesions [6].

Fluorouracil

Fluorouracil (5-fluorouracil) is an antimetabolite that inhibits thymidylate synthase [13], which has long been used systemically in the treatment of solid tumors. The drug is currently available in two slightly different topical preparations of 5% and 0.5% cream. Topical 5% fluorouracil cream is approved by the United States' Food and Drug Administration (FDA) for treatment of AKs and superficial BCC, with the latter being applied twice daily for 3–6 weeks for superficial BCC on the trunk and extremities [13]. Fluorouracil 0.5% cream is also approved by the FDA for the treatment of AKs [14,15]. However, topical fluorouracil has been used off-label for Bowen disease (SCC *in situ*) and SCC [14], especially in patients who are not candidates for more effective surgical therapies (e.g., Mohs surgery) [13]. Topical 0.5% fluorouracil cream is generally used once daily for 4 weeks for AKs [13,16].

Clinical features

Adverse cutaneous reactions are extremely common with topical fluorouracil therapy, with 97% of patients having some untoward cutaneous reaction and 5% of patients discontinuing therapy as a result [14].

Local reactions to daily or twice daily fluorouracil cream generally begin in the first week of therapy [17], are most intense

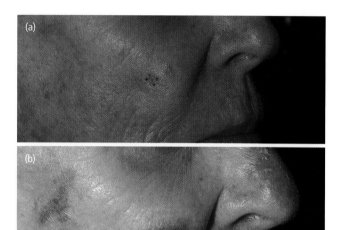

Figure 29.3 Actinic keratoses and topical 0.5% fluorouracil cream: (a) baseline and biopsy site; (b) after 21 daily applications.

at 2–6 weeks into the regimen, and continue throughout therapy (Figure 29.3) [14]. Subclinical AKs within the treated field may also "light up" during therapy. The median duration of acute localized reactions was 16 days post-therapy [17].

The most common cutaneous signs associated with topical fluorouracil therapy are erythema (33–97%), dermatitis (20%), scabbing and crusting (13%), and erosions and ulceration [14]. Associated symptoms include pain (33–50%), pruritus (17%), burning (7%), and stinging (7%) [14]. Post-treatment erythema may persist 6 weeks or more after therapy [14]. Long-term AEs include scarring (9–16%) and hyperpigmentation (3%) [14].

Treatment of choice
Initial efforts to mitigate the adverse reactions of topical fluorouracil cream involved different vehicles (i.e., 5% fluorouracil cream versus a 0.5% fluorouracil microsphere formula; $p < 0.003$) [18]. However, 20% of patients did use concomitant topical steroids [18].

"Rest periods" for a few days, or shortened treatment durations, are often used in patients who cannot tolerate the cutaneous AEs. Application of topical fluorouracil in a less frequent, more prolonged regimen (e.g., 1–2 times a week for 6–7 weeks) [13,16] or shorter periods (1–4 weeks) [17] has been suggested, but equivalent efficacy has not been demonstrated [13,16]. True allergic contact dermatitis is rare [13]. Routine use of topical steroids during therapy is not advocated. Sunblock, emollients, and mild topical steroids may be used for post-treatment erythema.

Retinoids

Systemic retinoids are natural or synthetic analogs of vitamin A, which have earned their place in the armamentarium against hematopoietic malignancies. The topical use in dermatologic malignancies has been primarily limited to cutaneous T-cell lymphoma and Kaposi sarcoma [19–25].

Retinoids are members of the larger superfamily of hormone receptors including glucocorticoid, thyroid hormone, and vitamin D receptors. The retinoid receptors are divided into two intracellular families – retinoid acid receptor (RAR) and retinoid X receptor (RXR) with slightly different functions [6]. Topical retinoids and rexinoids are readily absorbed into skin.

Alitretinoin
Alitretinoin, also known as 9-*cis*-retinoic acid, is a naturally occurring pan-retinoid that activates both RARs and RXRs in the skin [6,19]. In 1999, 0.1% alitretinoin gel was approved by the FDA for treatment of HIV-associated Kaposi sarcoma. In HIV-associated Kaposi sarcoma lesions, clinically significant responses have been reported in 19–37% of treated lesions, versus 11% of controls [19–21]. Treatment-related AEs were limited to the application sites, and related to the frequency of application. The median time to response in patients was 30 days [20]. In addition, topical alitretinoin gel has been used with some benefit in localized lesions of classic Kaposi sarcoma [22,23].

Clinical features
The most common AE of topical alitretinoin gel is a nonspecific rash occurring in 69%, usually during the first month of therapy (Figure 29.4). The AEs of scaling, erythema, and burning are common with all forms of topical retinoids. A typical therapeutic response is flattening of the violaceous lesions of Kaposi sarcoma, accompanied by marked erythema at the treatment site corresponding to the area of application. In one study, 83% of patients noted some rash, and 22% of patients noted pain at the application site. Xerosis was noted in 10% of patients, ulceration in 9%, as well as pruritus, edema, skin discoloration, and hemorrhage. Approximately 9% of patients discontinued alitretinoin due to these adverse reactions [20]. Post-inflammatory hyperpigmentation may develop later in patients with darker skin. As alitretinoin is a teratogen, pregnancy must be avoided in women of childbearing age with Kaposi sarcoma.

Treatment of choice
The usual approach is to reduce the frequency of, or temporarily withhold, the application of topical 0.1% alitretinoin gel. Erythema and scaling generally improve within a few days, and emollients may help. Topical corticosteroids are not routinely used, because of theoretical concern that they could increase the growth of Kaposi sarcoma lesions.

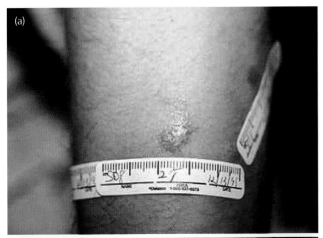

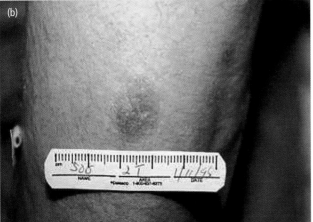

Figure 29.4 Topical alitretinoin 1% gel in HIV-associated Kaposi sarcoma: (a) pretreatment; (b) surrounding erythema and flattening of lesion, after 4 weeks of therapy.

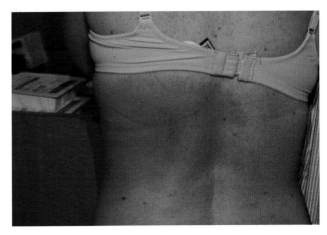

Figure 29.5 Irritant dermatitis from topical bexarotene, extending medially beyond mycosis fungoides patch.

Bexarotene

Bexarotene is a novel synthetic RXR inhibitor that suppresses proliferation, induces apoptosis, and effects cytokine secretion, specifically IL-2, as well as suppressing inflammation [6]. Bexarotene 1% gel was approved by the FDA in 2000 for the treatment of refractory stage IA and IB MF [6,24]. Overall response rates range 44–63%, with complete responses of 8–21% [23,26].

Clinical features

Cutaneous AEs are very common with topical bexarotene. In one study, 87% of patients reported local cutaneous AEs, usually 2–6 weeks into therapy [24]. The most frequent local reactions were "rash" (73%), pruritus (33%), pain (24%), and vesiculobullous lesions (6%), as well as "sticky skin" (14%) [25]. Redness associated with treatment (retinoid erythema) could be confused with the signs of MF (Figure 29.5) [24]. Cutaneous AEs were the most common treatment-limiting toxicity (64%), but were reversible

upon discontinuation of the drug [25]. Abnormal laboratory results included lymphopenia (21%), hypophosphatemia (31%), abnormal glucose levels (37%), and elevated liver function tests (6%) [24]. Complete blood counts and liver functions tests are recommended every 4–6 months, as well as a pregnancy test in women with MF of childbearing age.

Treatment of choice

Cutaneous irritation may be minimized by beginning topical bexarotene 1% gel every other day to limited areas of disease, and slowly increasing to twice daily applications over several weeks, as tolerated. Irritant reactions may be also be ameliorated with class 1 (super-potent) topical corticosteroids, which also have clinical efficacy in MF [27,28]. When evaluating treatment response, many physicians advocate stopping topical bexarotene 1–2 weeks before the patient's visit, to make possible the separation of "retinoid erythema" from residual MF lesions. Patients should avoid excessive sun exposure because of the photosensitizing effects of retinoids.

Bexarotene is a teratogen and rated category X in pregnancy. As retinoids are stored in fat for prolonged periods, and because so many other skin-directed therapies are available for MF, it may be most prudent to avoid topical bexarotene in women of childbearing age who may become pregnant.

Biologic response modifiers

Imiquimod

Imiquimod is a topical immune modulator that activates both the innate and adaptive immune systems [29–32]. Imiquimod activates toll-like receptors 7 and 8, ultimately resulting in a cytokine and chemokine cascade [13,29–32]. Imiquimod 5% is

FDA approved for the treatment of AKs of the face and balding scalp of immunocompetent patients, when applied three times per week for 4 weeks in a total application area of 25 cm² or less [13,16]. A similar regimen has been approved by the FDA for the treatment of superficial BCC with a diameter of 0.5–2 cm on the trunk and extremities (i.e., once daily applications, 5 days per week, for 6–12 weeks) [29]. Clearance rates of 81% were achieved for BCC with at least once daily, at least 5 days per week, applications for 6–12 weeks [14]. Imiquimod has also been used off-label in the treatment of SCC *in situ* (Bowen disease) [14,33,34], invasive SCC [14,35]), nodular [36], facial BCC [37], in patients who are not willing or able to undergo surgery [13] and even MF [38]. Imiquimod has been used in lentigo maligna, especially with extensive lesions on the face of elderly individuals [39], although concerns have been raised about lack of histologic clearing and/or progression or recurrence [13,40]. A 3.75% preparation of topical imiquimod has been approved for the treatment of the treatment of AKs on a balding scalp with two cycles of once daily applications separated by a 2-week rest period [41].

Clinical features

Topical imiquimod is associated with significant local treatment-related reactions in 52–100% of patients [29]. These AEs are related to frequency and schedule of application and increased tumor clearance rates appear associated with more severe local inflammatory reactions [14]. Approximately 3% of patients discontinue imiquimod therapy because of adverse events [14].

Local cutaneous reactions are usually most severe 2–6 weeks into therapy, and may persist for up to 3 months [14]. The most common findings are erythema (63–100%), edema (3–92%), weeping (69%), scabbing/crusting (52–65%), ulceration (25–27%), and vesiculation (3–17%) [14]. Associated symptoms include pruritus (16–67%), burning (6–35%), pain (3–35%), and tenderness (7–20%) [14]. Topical imiquimod is also associated with a number of systemic symptoms, including flu-like syndromes (9%) and headache (6–8%). Long-term (>6 months) AEs include hypopigmentation (9–67%), scarring (15%), hyperpigmentation (2–6%), and scaling. Scaling may last up to 2 years, and hypopigmentation may be permanent [14].

Treatment of choice

Various approaches have been used to avoid or lessen these untoward local reactions, including cycling of therapy in AK [42] and less frequent applications, over longer periods in BCC [13,14,30]; however, cure rates are generally lower with less intensive regimens [13,14,29].

Patients who develop severe reactions usually require temporary discontinuation of the medication for 1–2 weeks. Routine use of topical steroids during therapy is not advocated. Imiquimod heightens photosensitivity [13], so sun exposure should be minimized or avoided. Sunblock and emollients may be used for post-treatment residual erythema. The use of topical imiquimod during pregnancy is not recommended [13].

Corticosteroids

Topical corticosteroids have earned their place in the dermatology armamentarium for a variety of inflammatory disorders, such as psoriasis, atopic dermatitis, and allergic drug reactions, but have also been used with some success in cutaneous malignant disease [6,43]. There are anecdotal reports of the use of topical steroids for the treatment of primary cutaneous B-cell lymphoma lesions [44,45], as well as superpotent topical steroids (clobetasol) to lessen the discomfort of extensive cutaneous metastases of breast cancer [46]. However, by far the most common use for topical corticosteroids has been in the treatment of MF and Sézary syndrome.

Topical corticosteroids are categorized according to their relative potency into seven classes, with class VII being the least potent (e.g., hydrocortisone) and class I being the most potent (e.g., clobetasol and betamethasone diproprionate). These medications are also available in a variety of vehicles, which may affect their tolerability and absorption, including ointments, gels, foams, lotions, and creams. The actions of topical corticosteroids are primarily anti-inflammatory (e.g., inhibition of transcription factors) but they also have vasoconstrictive, immunosuppressive, and antiproliferative properties [43]. Specific effects on lymphocytes include inhibition of adhesion to endothelium and enhanced apoptosis [47]. In many centers, topical corticosteroids, particularly class 1, are the treatment of choice for early MF [6,27,28]. Overall response rates of 90–94% in stage T1 patients (<10% BSA involved with patch or plaque MF) and 80–82% in stage 2 patients (>10% of BSA with patch or plaque MF) have been reported [6,28]. In a larger group of MF patients, overall response rate was 90%. The high potency corticosteroid of choice was clobetasol because of its availability as a generic preparation, its efficacy, and its availability both as a cream and ointment. While the ointment was more effective, the greasy nature of the vehicle often limited patient compliance. Other class 1 steroids that have been used are betamethasone dipropionate 0.05% [6] and mometasone furoate 0.1% [4]. The current National Cancer Comprehensive Network guidelines suggest that symptomatic relief may be obtained, (particularly pruritus), in patients with Sézary syndrome and erythrodermic MF, with the less potent triamcinolone 0.1% ointment because of the large areas involved [48].

Clinical features

AEs are related to prolonged periods of treatment, often much longer than the recommended use of 2 weeks for class 1 topical corticosteroids, site of application, and ratio of body surface area and body weight [43]. In the initial report of 79 patients treated with high potency topical corticosteroids, baseline and monthly serum cortisol levels were obtained during treatment and a reversible depression of serum cortisol levels occurred in 13%. Minor skin irritation was present in two patients, and localized reversible skin atrophy occurred in one patient after long-term

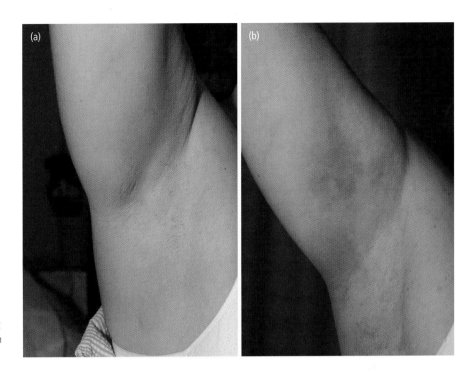

Figure 29.6 Mycosis fungoides: (a) pre treatment with topical corticosteroids; (b) after treatment with corticosteroids, showing striae.

use [28]. In a larger review, approximately 10–20% of patients developed irritant dermatitis or purpura [25]. Cutaneous atrophy and striae may be noted after longer use. In another study, one patient with advanced MF who was treated with a prolonged course of high dose topical corticosteroids developed Cushing syndrome, which was reversible 3 months after stopping the topical therapy [28].

Most adult patients are instructed to apply the topical clobetasol twice a day without any limitation to the total area of skin treated, but elderly patients with extensive disease are usually given a less potent topical steroid (e.g., triamcinolone 0.1% ointment or cream) [43]. Intertriginous sites and skin fold areas treated with the topical steroids are more prone to develop atrophy because of increased absorption and should be monitored carefully. The maximal suggested amount of topical clobetasol is <50 g/week [43]. The prevalence of contact dermatitis to topical corticosteroids is <0.025% and higher with nonhalogenated than with halogenated steroids. The major AEs are atrophic striae, purpura, telangiectasia, and hypopigmentation. Most are reversible on discontinuation except for atrophic striae, which are irreversible (Figure 29.6) [43]. It should be noted that while there are few children with MF, the use of super-potent topical steroids can cause increased and significant systemic absorption in this group, because of their lower ratio of body surface area to body weight, so this is not recommended.

Treatment of choice
Blood tests are not routinely drawn to follow these topical corticosteroids in MF; however, following serum cortisol levels remains controversial [6]. Serum cortisol levels are not routinely

drawn, except perhaps in frail elderly patients with extensive skin involvement [27].

The treatment for most of the AEs of super-potent topical steroids is the discontinuation or, ideally, slow tapering. Rebound dermatosis may occur with abrupt discontinuation and the patient needs to taper the use of topical corticosteroids just as one would taper the use of oral systemic steroids. Most AEs are reversible except for striae. For those patients with suspected allergy to topical corticosteroids, a chemically different compound may be substituted (e.g., betamethasone diproprionate substituted for clobetasol in the case of allergic contact dermatitis occurring paradoxically). Corticosteroid allergy can be diagnosed by patch testing. Other AEs of topical steroids include acneiform eruptions and perioral dermatitis. For this reason, only low potency topical steroids (e.g., hydrocortisone 2.5%, alclometasone 0.05%) should be used on the face. In addition, the application of low potency topical corticosteroids in the periorbital area may result in increased intraocular pressure and glaucoma, so this is also not advocated.

Conclusions

A variety of topical agents have been used over the last few decades to treat various malignancies in the skin. Some of the cutaneous AEs of these agents are inextricably linked to their therapeutic actions, while others may be allergic or irritant in nature. The recognition, prevention, and management of these cutaneous AEs of these agents can allow successful continuation of antineoplastic therapy, and minimize patient discomfort.

References

1 Zackheim, H.S., Epstein, E.H. Jr., McNutt, N.S., Grekin, D.A. & Crain, W.R. (1983) Topical carmustine (BCNU) for mycosis fungoides and related disorders: a 10-year experience. *Journal of the American Academy of Dermatology*, 9, 363–374.

2 Zackheim, H.S., Epstein, E.H. Jr. & Crain, W.R. (1990) Topical carmustine (BCNU) for cutaneous T cell lymphoma: a 15-year experience in 143 patients. *Journal of the American Academy of Dermatology*, 22 (5 Pt 1), 802–810.

3 Zackheim, H.S. (2003) Topical carmustine (BCNU) in the treatment of mycosis fungoides. *Dermatologic Therapy*, 16 (4), 299–302.

4 Prince, H.M., Whittaker, S. & Hoppe, R.T. (2009) How I treat mycosis fungoides and Sezary syndrome. *Blood*, 114 (20), 4337–4353.

5 Sharon, V., Mecca, P.S., Steinherz, P.G., Trippett, T.M. & Myskowski, P.L. (2009) Two pediatric cases of primary cutaneous B-cell lymphoma and review of the literature. *Pediatric Dermatology*, 26, 34–39.

6 Berthelot, C., Rivera, A. & Duvic, M. (2008) Skin directed therapy for mycosis fungoides: a review. *Journal of Drugs in Dermatology*, 7 (7), 655–666.

7 Ramsay, D.L., Meller, J.A. & Zackheim, H.S. (1995) Topical treatment of early cutaneous T-cell lymphoma. *Hematology Oncology Clinics of North America*, 9 (5), 1031–1056.

8 Kim, Y.H., Martinez, G., Varghese, A. & Hoppe, R.T. (Feb 2003) Topical nitrogen mustard in the management of mycosis fungoides: update of the Stanford experience. *Archives of Dermatology*, 139 (2), 165–173.

9 Grunnet, E. (1976) Contact urticaria and anaphylactoid reaction induced by topical application of nitrogen mustard. *British Journal of Dermatology*, 94 (1), 101–103.

10 Vonderheid, E.C., Tan, E.T., Kantor, A.F., Shrager, L., Micaily, B. & Van Scott, E.J. (1989) Long-term efficacy, curative potential, and carcinogenicity of topical mechlorethamine chemotherapy in cutaneous T cell lymphoma. *Journal of the American Academy of Dermatology*, 20 (3), 416–428.

11 Smoller, B.R. & Marcus, R. (1994) Risk of secondary cutaneous malignancies in patients with long-standing mycosis fungoides. *Journal of the American Academy of Dermatology*, 30 (2 Pt 1), 201–204.

12 de Quatrebarbes, J., Esteve, E., Bagot, M. *et al.* (2005) Treatment of early stage mycosis fungoides with twice-weekly applications of mechlorethamine and topical steroids: a prospective study. *Archives of Dermatology*, 141, 1117–1120.

13 Micali, G., Lacarrurubba, F., Dinotta, F., Massimino, D. & Nasca, M.R. (2010) Treating skin cancer with topical cream. *Expert Opinion on Pharmacotherapy*, 11 (9), 1515–1527.

14 Love, W.E., Bernhard, J.D. & Bordeaux, J.S. (2009) Topical imiquimod or fluorouracil therapy for basal and squamous cell carcinoma: a systematic review. *Archives of Dermatology*, 145, 1431–1438.

15 Gross, K., Kircik, L. & Kricorian, G. (2007) 5% 5-Fluorouracil cream for the treatment of small superficial Basal cell carcinoma: efficacy, tolerability, cosmetic outcome, and patient satisfaction. *Dermatologic Surgery*, 33 (4), 433–439, discussion 440.

16 Askew, D.A., Mickan, S.M., Soger, P. & Wilkinson, D. (2009) Effectivenexx of 5-fluorouracil treatment for actinic keratoses: a systemic review of randomized controlled trials. *International Journal of Dermatology*, 48 (48), 453–463.

17 Weiss, J., Menter, A., Hevia, A. *et al.* (2002) Effective treatment of actinic keratoses with 0.5% fluorouracil cream for 1, 2, or 4 weeks. *Cutis: Cutaneous Medicine for the Practitioner*, 70, 22–29.

18 Loven, K., Stein, L., Furst, K. & Levy, S. (2002) Evaluation of the efficacy and tolerability of 0.5% fluorouracil cream and 5% fluorouracil cream applied to each side of the face in patients with actinic keratosis. *Clinical Therapeutics*, 24 (6), 990–1000.

19 Cheng, C., Michaels, J. & Scheinfeld, N. (2008) Alitretinoin: a comprehensive review. *Expert Opinion on Investigational Drugs*, 17 (3), 437–443.

20 Duvic, M., Friedman-Kien, A.E. & Looney, D.J. (2000) Topical treatment of cutaneous lesions of acquired immunodeficiency syndrome-related Kaposi sarcoma using alitretinoin gel: results of phase 1 and 2 trials. *Archives of Dermatology*, 136 (12), 1461–1469.

21 Bodsworth, N.J., Bloch, M., Bower, M., Donnell, D., Yocum, R.; International Panretin Gel KS Study Group. (2001) Phase III vehicle-controlled, multi-centered study of topical alitretinoin gel 0.1% in cutaneous AIDS-related Kaposi's sarcoma. *American Journal of Clinical Dermatology*, 2 (2), 77–87.

22 Rongioletti, F., Zaccaria, E. & Viglizzo, G. (2006) Failure of topical 0.1% alitretinoin gel for classic Kaposi sarcoma: first European experience. *British Journal of Dermatology*, 155 (4), 856–857.

23 Morganroth, G.S. (2002) Topical 0.1% alitretinoin gel for classic Kaposi sarcoma. *Archives of Dermatology*, 138, 542–543.

24 Breneman, D., Duvic, M., Kuzel, T., Yocum, R., Truglia, J. & Stevens, V.J. (2002) Phase 1 and 2 trial of bexarotene gel for skin-directed treatment of patients with cutaneous T-cell lymphoma. *Archives of Dermatology*, 138, 325–332.

25 Heald, P., Mehlmauer, M. & Martin, A.G. (2003) Topical bexarotene therapy for patients with refractory or persistent early-stage cutaneous T-cell lymphoma: results of the phase iii clinical trial. *Journal of the American Academy of Dermatology*, 49, 801–815.

26 Falkson, G. & Schulz, C.J. (1962) Skin changes in patients treated with 5-fluorouracil. *British Journal of Dermatology*, 74, 229–236.

27 Zackheim, H.S. (2003) Treatment of patch-stage mycosis fungoides with topical corticosteroids. *Dermatologic Therapy*, 16 (4), 283–287.

28 Zackheim, H.S., Kashani-Sabet, M. & Amin, S. (1998) Topical corticosteroids for mycosis fungoides. Experience in 79 patients. *Archives of Dermatology*, 134 (8), 949–954.

29 Karve, S.J., Feldman, S.R., Yentzer, B.A., Pearce, D.J. & Balkrishnan, R. (2008) Imiquimod: a review of basal cell carcinoma treatments. *Journal of Drugs in Dermatology*, 7 (1), 1044–1051.

30 Washauer, E. & Warshauer, B.L. (2008) Clearance of basal cell carcinoma and superficial squamous cell carcinomas after imiquimod therapy. *Journal of Drugs in Dermatology*, 7 (5), 447–451.

31 Geisse, J.K., Rich, P., Pandya, A. *et al.* (2002) Imiquimod 5% cream for the treatment of superficial basal cell carcinoma: a double-blind, randomized, vehicle-controlled study. *Journal of the American Academy of Dermatology*, 47 (3), 390–398.

32 Geisse, J., Caro, I., Lindholm, J., Golitz, L., Stampone, P., & Owens, M. (2004) Imiquimod 5% cream for the treatment of superficial basal cell carcinoma: results from two phase III, randomized, vehicle-controlled studies. *Journal of the American Academy of Dermatology*, 50 (5), 722–733.

33 Patel, G.K., Goodwin, R., Chawla, M. *et al.* (2006) Imiquimod 5% cream monotherapy for cutaneous squamous cell carcinoma in situ (Bowen's disease): a randomized, double-blind, placebo-controlled trial. *Journal of the American Academy of Dermatology*, 54 (6), 1025–1032.

34 Rosen, T., Harting, M. & Gibson, M. (2007) Treatment of Bowen's disease with topical 5% imiquimod cream: retrospective study. *Dermatologic Surgery*, **33** (4), 427–431, discussion 431–432.

35 Peris, K., Micantonio, T., Fargnoli, M.C., Lozzi, G.P. & Chimenti, S. (2006) Imiquimod 5% cream in the treatment of Bowen's disease and invasive squamous cell carcinoma. *Journal of the American Academy of Dermatology*, **55** (2), 324–327.

36 Eigentler, T.K., Kamin, A., Weide, B.M. *et al.* (2007) A phase III, randomized, open label study to evaluate the safety and efficacy of imiquimod 5% cream applied thrice weekly for 8 and 12 weeks in the treatment of low-risk nodular basal cell carcinoma. *Journal of the American Academy of Dermatology*, **57** (4), 616–621.

37 Vun, Y. & Siller, G. (2006) Use of 5% imiquimod cream in the treatment of facial basal cell carcinoma: a 3-year retrospective follow-up study. *Australasian Journal of Dermatology*, **47** (3), 169–171.

38 Deeths, M.J., Chapman, J.T., Dellavalle, R.P., Zeng, C. & Aeling, J.L. (2005) Treatment of patch and plaque stage mycosis fungoides with imiquimod 5% cream. *Journal of the American Academy of Dermatology*, **52**, 275–280.

39 Naylor, M.F., Crowson, N., Kuwahara, R. *et al.* (2003) Treatment of lentigo maligna with topical imiquimod. *British Journal of Dermatology*, **149** (Suppl. 66), 66–70.

40 Junkins-Hopkins, J.M. (2009) Imiquimod use in the treatment of lentigo maligna. *Journal of the American Academy of Dermatology*, **61**, 865–867.

41 Gupta, A.K. & Cooper, E.A. (2010) Abramavoitz. Zyclara (imiquimod) cream 3.75%. *Skinmed*, **8** (4), 227–229.

42 Salasche, S.J., Levine, N. & Morrison, L. (2002) Cycle therapy of actinic keratoses of the face and scalp with 5% topical imiquimod cream. An open label trial. *Journal of the American Academy of Dermatology*, **47**, 571–577.

43 Tadicherla, S., Ross, K., Shenefelt, P.D. & Fenske, N.A. (2009) Topical corticosteroids in dermatology. *Journal of Drugs in Dermatology*, **8**, 1093–1105.

44 Amity-Laish, I., Feinmasser, M., Ben-Amitai, D. *et al.* (2009) Juvenile onset of primary low-grade cutaneous B-cell lymphoma. *British Journal of Dermatology*, **161**, 140–147.

45 Hoefnagel, J.J., Vermeer, M.H., Jansen, P.M. *et al.* (2005) Primary cutaneous marginal zone B-cell lymphoma: clinical and therapeutic features in 50 cases. *Archives of Dermatology*, **141**, 1139–1145.

46 Cheville, A. & Gonzales, G.R. (1999) A superpotent topical steroid for constricting breast cancer symptoms. *Journal of Pain and Symptom Management*, **17**, 149–152.

47 Momtaz, P. & Zippin, J.H. (2009) Cutaneous T-cell lymphoma: a review of current therapies and the future therapeutic implications of chemokine biology. *Journal of Drugs in Dermatology*, **8**, 1142–1149.

48 Horwitz, S.M., Olsen, E.A. & Duvic, M. (2008) Review of the treatment of mycosis fungoides and Sézary syndrome: a stage-based approach. *Journal of the National Comprehensive Cancer Network*, **6** (4), 436–442.1.

30 Life-threatening (Serious) Dermatologic Adverse Events

Milan J. Anadkat

Division of Dermatology, Washington University School of Medicine, St. Louis, MO, USA

A reaction should be deemed "serious" (grades > 3) if it results in death, is life-threatening, requires hospitalization or prolongs an existing hospital stay, or results in permanent damage or significant disability [1]. By this definition, approximately 1 in every 1000 inpatients [2], and approximately 2% of all drug reactions identified by physicians [3,4] are considered serious and life-threatening.

Stevens–Johnson syndrome and toxic epidermal necrolysis

Stevens–Johnson syndrome (SJS) is characterized by erosions on at least two mucosal surfaces along with "target-like" cutaneous lesions [5]. A purulent conjunctivitis and a severe necrotic stomatitis are the most typical mucosal findings (Figure 30.1). Cutaneous lesions resemble the target-like lesions of erythema multiforme, with central dusky necrosis and a surrounding rim of erythema. Toxic epidermal necrolysis (TEN) is characterized by extensive erythema and pain of mucosal and cutaneous surfaces that lead to widespread necrosis and exfoliation (Figure 30.2) [6].

There has existed much confusion among authors over the last few decades in delineating SJS and TEN from one another and from their close clinical mimic, erythema multiforme (EM). these entities SJS, TEN, and EM are characterized by target-like lesions clinically and epidermal necrosis histopathologically. For years, a variant of EM known as "EM major" was felt to be synonymous with SJS and TEN [7]. It is now clear and virtually universally accepted, however, that SJS and TEN are entities distinct from EM [8]. Classification amongst these three entities, first proposed in 1993, is based on the characteristics of skin lesions and extent of epidermal detachment [9]. Detachment of less than 10% of the body surface area plus widespread erythematous or purpuric macules or flat atypical target lesions leading to detachment of the epidermis is seen in most instances. SJS is the term when less than 10% of the body surface area is involved, whereas TEN occurs when greater than 30% of the body surface area is affected. When 10–30% body surface area is involved, the term SJS/TEN overlap syndrome should be used. Lastly, a subset termed TEN without spots is used when greater than 10% epidermal detachment is seen, but purpuric or target lesions are absent.

Drug exposure is the primary, and perhaps exclusive, trigger in the development of SJS and TEN [10]. The most frequent culprits are sulfonamide antibiotics, anticonvulsants, nonsteroidal anti-inflammatory drugs (NSAIDs), and allopurinol [11–14]. It is important to recognize that many of these agents are often used in conjunction with anticancer agents.

SJS and TEN resulting from anticancer agents have been sporadically reported in the literature. There have been recent systematic analyses of the association of SJS and TEN specifically to anticancer agents [15,16]. There is also uncertainty whether any potential interaction of various agents may increase the risk for its development. Lastly, there is likely considerable underreporting of these events.

The creation of a TEN-specific severity scoring tool, the SCORTEN ("SCORe of TEN"), has allowed for a more accurate prediction of TEN-associated mortality [17,18]. Seven independent risk factors are equally weighted in determining a score of 0–7 (Table 30.1). Most experts recommend calculating the SCORTEN within 24 hours of admission and also 72 hours after admission for patients with TEN [17,19]. It should be emphasized that a diagnosis of cancer represents one of the SCORTEN criteria, as it independently increases the mortality risk.

In terms of management, discontinuing the offending agent is critical. Skin-directed therapy is encouraged to prevent infection, encourage wound healing, and minimize water loss. Systemic antibiotics should be reserved for culture proven infections, with

Dermatologic Principles and Practice in Oncology: Conditions of the Skin, Hair, and Nails in Cancer Patients, First Edition. Edited by Mario E. Lacouture.
© 2014 John Wiley & Sons, Inc. Published 2014 by John Wiley & Sons, Inc.

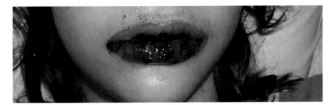

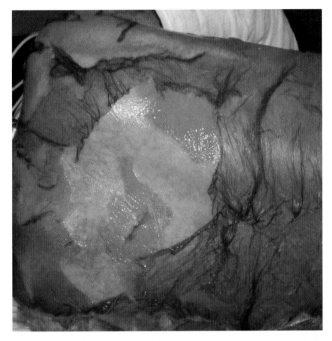

Figure 30.1 Stevens–Johnson syndrome. Photo courtesy of Dr. Milan J. Anadkat.

Figure 30.2 Toxic epidermal necrolysis. Photo courtesy of Dr. Milan J. Anadkat.

Table 30.1 Toxic epidermal necrolysis (TEN) specific severity scoring tool, the SCORTEN ("SCORe of TEN") [17]. Seven independent risk factors, consisting of both clinical and laboratory parameters, are equally weighted in determining a score of 0 to 7. It is recommended calculating the SCORTEN within 24 hours of admission and also 72 hours after admission for patients with TEN [17,19]. A diagnosis of cancer represents one of the SCORTEN criteria, as it independently increases the mortality risk.

Risk factors	
Age (years)	>40
Associated malignancy	yes
Heart rate (beats/min)	>120
Serum BUN (mg/dL)	>27
Involved (detached) body surface area	>10%
Serum bicarbonate (mEq/L)	<20
Serum glucose (mg/dL)	>250

Risk factors	Mortality estimate
0–1	3.2%
2	12.1%
3	35.3%
4	58.3%
5 or more	>90%

BUN, blood, urea, and nitrogen.

prophylactic or empiric use of antimicrobials not recommended. In many cases, granulocyte colony-stimulating factor (G-CSF) is recommended for TEN-associated neutropenia [20–23]. Parenteral fluid, electrolyte, and nutrient resuscitation are often necessary, given that SJS and TEN are considered to be hypercatabolic disease processes [24,25]. Given the need for such specialized services, patients often need to be transferred to a burn unit or intensive care unit familiar with handling either SJS or TEN.

The role of steroids has been the subject of decades of debate [26–34]. Extended duration of therapy (>2 weeks) and initiation of therapy late in the course of disease has been associated with an increased risk of both cutaneous and systemic superinfection [35]. In contrast, short-term therapy (i.e., <5 days) has been shown beneficial for early presentations of TEN [36]. The role of alternate immunosuppressive agents, such as cyclosporine or infliximab, may be beneficial [27,37–48]. Most recently, the use of intravenous gammaglobulin (IVIG) at a dosage of up to 2 g/kg divided over 3–4 days has been proposed [49–54]. While not immunosuppressive or associated with increased infection, conflicting studies exist on the extent of its efficacy [55].

Hypersensitivity reactions

The most common hypersensitivity reactions to chemotherapeutic agents are IgE-mediated, type I allergic reactions characterized by cutaneous signs of urticaria (Figure 30.3), angioedema, pruritus, and flushing. Anaphylaxis is characterized by these cutaneous signs coupled with systemic manifestations such as tachycardia, hypotension, bronchospasm, and abdominal cramping. This life-threatening reaction often appears within minutes of drug exposure, and is traditionally more severe with parenterally administered drugs than oral agents. Anaphylactoid reactions are nonallergic serious reactions that have a striking clinical similarity to anaphylaxis. The major distinction, however, lies in the mechanism. Unlike anaphylaxis, anaphylactoid reactions are not mediated by IgE but rather via direct nonspecific degranulation of mast cells or basophils.

Treatment of anaphylaxis/anaphylactoid reaction consists of drug discontinuation and close monitoring. Systemic corticosteroids and antihistamines are frequently administered. Subcutaneous epinephrine may also be indicated for life-threatening instances. It is recommended to draw a tryptase level

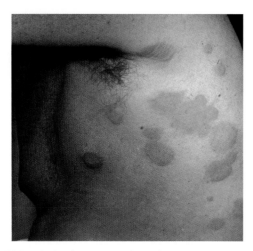

Figure 30.3 Urticaria. Photo courtesy of Dr. Arthur Z. Eisen.

within the first few hours after drug administration to confirm presence of hypersensitivity reaction [56].

Hypersensitivity reactions from anticancer agents pose an obvious dilemma to the treating oncologist, who is forced to balance the risk of withholding potentially life-saving therapy against the risk of administering life-threatening therapy. There are three major options if continued therapy is pursued: premedication, desensitization, or change of therapy. The development of a hypersensitivity rash of any grade, such as type I hypersensitivity reactions, is a biologically independent process from SJS/TEN, and is therefore unrelated and not predictive of the development of SJS/TEN.

The most common chemotherapeutics associated with infusion reactions include platinum compounds (cisplatin, carboplatin, oxaliplatin), taxanes (paclitaxel, docetaxel), l-asparaginase, and epipodophyllotoxins (teniposide, etoposide) [57]. Infusion reactions from these agents are primarily believed to result from sensitivity to the parent compound itself or the infusion solvent. Infusion reactions may also result with newer biologic compounds, specifically monoclonal antibody preparations.

Platinum compounds

Reactions to the platinum compounds are true IgE-mediated type I allergic reactions. The risk of developing a reaction increases precipitously with increasing exposure. In fact, there is a significant increase in the risk of developing a reaction after the sixth infusion of carboplatin, with the peak risk after the eighth infusion (cumulative risk of 19.5%), and a subsequent decrease in risk thereafter [58]. Similarly, the risk for hypersensitivity to oxaliplatin increases after the fifth cycle of therapy [59]. Oxaliplatin reactions are typically milder than carboplatin or cisplatin and are rarely life-threatening, with an annual incidence of hypersensitivity reactions and severe reactions estimated at 13% and 0.5%, respectively [60]. Intradermal skin testing has been shown to be reliable in predicting hypersensitivity reactions to these

compounds, although its availability is limited [61]. However, there is no standard protocol for preventing platinum hypersensitivity. Premedication is not consistently effective. Desensitization has also been inconsistent, but has recently shown promise as an effective strategy for patients who continue to require platinum therapy [62–67].

Taxanes

Hypersensitivity reactions to taxanes are thought to represent anaphylactoid reactions, with clinical features mimicking type I allergic reactions. Most reactions occur after the first or second infusion. The incidence of infusion reactions in early studies with paclitaxel and docetaxel without premedication was estimated up to 30% [68,69]. The rate of severe reactions, by contrast, because of the routine employment of premedication, has been reduced to 2–4% [70]. Slower infusion speeds may also be beneficial, but are typically not necessary when appropriate premedication with corticosteroids and antihistamines are given. Most attribute reactions to paclitaxel to the infusion solvent, Cremophor EL®, which is assumed to directly degranulate mast cells and basophils. Evidence to support this theory lies in the rare incidence of reactions with a newer Cremophor EL-free version of paclitaxel (Abraxane®) [71]. It is still likely that the active taxane itself has some role, however. Some studies have estimated a cross-reactivity to docetaxel in patients sensitive to paclitaxel in up to 90% of patients, despite the fact that docetaxel is formulated with an alternative solvent (polysorbate 80) [72]. It should be noted that docetaxel is also associated with a dose-related capillary leak syndrome characterized by fluid retention (peripheral edema, ascites, and pulmonary effusion) that can be life-threatening [73]. This effect is delayed, and potentially decreased, with corticosteroids [74].

l-asparginase

l-asparginase is an enzyme derived from a bacterium, typically *Escherichia coli*, associated with a high rate of hypersensitivity reactions (35%), with serious anaphylactic reactions affecting less than 10% [75,76,77]. Reactions are believed to by IgE-mediated type I reactions, although some authors feel indirect complement activation may also have a role [78,79]. Intravenous administration is associated with a higher rate of hypersensitivity [57]. Therefore, l-asparaginase is typically given via intramuscular or subcutaneous routes. Other risk factors include prior exposure and greater intervals between doses [76,79]. Desensitization is an effect strategy for patients who experience l-asparaginase hypersensitivity. Switching to a different preparation may also be helpful, especially if derived from an alternative bacterium such as *Erwinia chrysanthemi* or *Erwinia carotovora* [80,81]. Peglyated versions of l-asparaginase are also less reactive [82,83].

Etoposide and teniposide

Etoposide is given in both oral and intravenous forms, with only the latter being associated with hypersensitivity reactions.

Teniposide, available only in intravenous form and dissolved in Cremophor, is estimated with a slightly higher rate of hypersensitivity (etoposide is dissolved in polysorbate 80) [84]. Both immunologic and nonimmunologic mechanisms are assumed to be responsible, with reactions occurring from minutes to days after infusion [84–86]. The overall rate of anaphylaxis is low, estimated at 0.7–14% for these agents, and symptoms are typically mild [85,87]. Cutaneous symptoms are not widely prevalent compared with the more common manifestations of hypotension, bronchospasm, and dyspnea [88,89].

Procarbazine

Procarbazine is an oral agent, which is also frequently mentioned with this class of drugs given its high rate of hypersensitivity (albeit not infusion) reactions. The metabolites of procarbazine, produced at a higher rate in the presence of anticonvulsants, are believed to be the culprit in the development of associated hypersensitivity reactions [90]. Procarbazine is not only associated with typical type I reactions, but has also been reported to cause type III reactions (primarily manifested as allergic alveolitis), fixed drug reactions, morbilliform rash, and TEN [91–96].

Drug rash with eosinophilia and systemic symptoms

Drug rash with eosinophilia and systemic symptoms (DRESS) was originally described in 1959 as "pseudolymphoma," manifesting with erythematous and edematous cutaneous plaques clinically and a lymphocytic infiltrate mimicking lymphoma histopathologically [97]. Over the ensuing decades, this reaction pattern was believed to have two distinct presentations. The first, "hypersensitivity syndrome," was characterized by a rapid onset, fever, lymphadenopathy, hematologic abnormalities, and end organ damage. The second presentation had a more insidious onset, similar cutaneous findings, but without systemic abnormalities. In 1996, the term DRESS was coined by Bocquet et al. [98] to replace the entity formerly referred to as "hypersensitivity syndrome." (Alternate names for DRESS have also been applied including drug-induced delayed multiorgan hypersensitivity syndrome and drug-induced hypersensitivity syndrome [99,100].) The second clinical entity, still referred to pseudolymphoma, was confirmed to be a distinct entity during the same year [101].

The precise mechanism for development of DRESS syndrome is unclear, but is believed to result from altered metabolism of certain drugs and impaired clearance of toxic metabolites. Genetic factors likely have a role in predisposing patients to this syndrome [102,103]. Primary HHV6 infection and HHV6 reactivation have also been implicated in assisting in the development of DRESS syndrome [104–108]. Associated mortality from this syndrome is estimated as high as 10% [98,109,110]. The most widely reported agents to result in DRESS are the aromatic anticonvulsants (phenobarbital, phenytoin, and carbamazepine), sulfonamide antibiotics, and allopurinol [111–120]. Anticancer agents have not been shown to be a consistent culprit in inciting DRESS syndrome. A brief mention of this entity is nonetheless discussed given severity of complications, the rarity of the disease itself, and the frequency with which the above agents are used in conjunction with current chemotherapy regimens.

There exist no universally accepted criteria for making a diagnosis of DRESS [109]. One of the largest prospective analyses to date evaluating DRESS and other life-threatening reactions is being conducted by the European Registry of Severe Cutaneous Adverse Reactions (RegiSCAR) study group [121]. (The predecessor study groups, SCAR and EuroSCAR, evaluated only SJS and TEN.) The goal is to explore for consistent clinical, serologic, tissue, and/or genetic findings. The initial phase of this study was completed in 2007, evaluating hospitalized patients in six countries with severe cutaneous drug reactions.

The proposed criteria for making a diagnosis of DRESS, based on the original definition by Bocquet et al. and the current RegiSCAR study, are summarized in Table 30.2. It is apparent that many cutaneous and noncutaneous findings help the clinician distinguish DRESS from the typical drug eruption. For instance, DRESS typically presents at least 2–6 weeks after exposure to the inciting drug, much later than classic drug reactions [109,122].

Table 30.2 Two proposed diagnostic criteria for drug rash with eosinophilia and systemic symptoms (DRESS).

Criteria for DRESS syndrome – Bocquet et al. [98]. (each criteria must be met)

1. Cutaneous drug eruption

2. Hematologic abnormalities:
(a) Eosinophilia greater than 1.5×10^9 cells/L
or
(b) Presence of atypical lymphocytes

3. Systemic involvement:
(a) Lymphadenopathies greater than 2 cm in diameter
(b) Hepatitis
(c) Interstitial nephritis
(d) Interstitial pneumonia
or
(e) Carditis

RegiSCAR criteria for DRESS syndrome [121] (three of the four criteria required for diagnosis)

Acute rash with fever >38°C
Lymphadenopathy in at least two sites
Involvement of at least one internal organ
Hematologic abnormalities (lymphocytosis, eosinophilia, thrombocytopenia)

In addition to a typical morbilliform exanthem, DRESS is frequently associated with edema, especially over the face and upper extremities [122]. The presence of facial edema is a major clinical distinction separating DRESS from classic drug eruptions.

Systemic symptoms of DRESS are consistently present, but may vary in severity. Fever, lymphadenopathy, and nonspecific arthralgias and arthritis are common [98,109,122–124]. Hematologic abnormalities are characterized by peripheral eosinophilia, which is also often accompanied by circulating atypical lymphocytes [98,100,122]. Visceral involvement may be severe and is the primary cause of DRESS-associated mortality. Liver damage in the form of fulminant hepatitis, detected by significant transaminitis, is the most common form of end organ damage [125,126]. Involvement of the heart, lungs, kidneys, thyroid, and brain has also been reported [2,127–134].

Cutaneous and systemic symptoms may persist for weeks, or even months, after the inciting drug has been removed. Standardized therapeutic regimens do not exist at this time. High dose systemic steroids are generally recommended, and therapy may be prolonged when systemic involvement is severe [135–138]. The use of alternate immunosuppressive agents such as IVIG, mycophenolate mofetil, azathioprine, or cyclosporine is sporadic, supported only by anecdotal reports, and generally reserved for cases requiring prolonged systemic steroid usage as a steroid-sparing agent. The use of *N*-acetylcysteine, a precursor of glutathione, has also been reported recently with some success [139]. It is assumed that the antioxidative effects of *N*-acetylcysteine may counteract the effects of toxic metabolites, especially from anticonvulsants.

Conclusions

Each life-threatening (serious) dermatologic adverse event (AE) discussed in this chapter is distinct, with a unique pathophysiology, and varying recommendations guiding management approaches. Determining the presence of a life-threatening reaction in the oncology patient is frequently challenging. Furthermore, determining which drug is causative in these drug reactions is difficult as most patients are on multiple agents, many of which have been known to cause similar untoward events. Nevertheless, life-threatening (serious) dermatologic AEs require immediate attention and discontinuation of the most likely offending agent.

References

1 US Food and Drug Administration. (2011) What is a serious adverse event? Available at: http://www.fda.gov/safety/medwatch/howtoreport/ucm053087.htm (accessed 16 April 2013).

2 Roujeau, J.C. & Stern, R.S. (1994) Severe adverse cutaneous reactions to drugs. *New England Journal of Medicine*, **331**, 1272–1285.

3 Alanko, K., Stubb, S. & Kauppinen, K. (1989) Cutaneous drug reactions: clinical types and causative agents: a five-year survey of in-patients (1981–1985). *Acta Dermato-Venereologica. Supplementum*, **69**, 223–226.

4 Ives, T.J., Bentz, E.J. & Gwyther, R.E. (1992) Dermatologic adverse drug reactions in a family medicine setting. *Archives of Family Medicine*, **1**, 241–245.

5 Stevens, A.M. & Johnson, F.C. (1922) A new eruptive fever associated with stomatitis and ophthalmia. *American Journal of Diseases of Children*, **24**, 526–533.

6 Lyell, A. (1956) Toxic epidermal necrolysis: an eruption resembling scalding of the skin. *British Journal of Dermatology*, **68**, 355–361.

7 Thomas, B.A. (1950) The so-called Stevens-Johnson syndrome. *British Medical Journal*, **1**, 1393–1397.

8 Assier, H., Bastuji-Garin, S., Revuz, J. & Roujeau, J.C. (1995) Erythema multiforme with mucous membrane involvement and Stevens-Johnson syndrome are clinically different disorders with distinct causes. *Archives of Dermatology*, **131**, 539.

9 Bastuji-Garin, S., Rzany, B., Stern, R.S., Shear, N.H., Naldi, L. & Roujeau, J.C. (1993) Clinical classification of cases of toxic epidermal necrolysis, Stevens-Johnson syndrome, and erythema multiforme. *Archives of Dermatology*, **129**, 92–96.

10 Borchers, A.T., Lee, J.L., Naguwa, S.M., Cheema, G.S. & Gershwin, M.E. (2008) Stevens-Johnson syndrome and toxic epidermal necrolysis. *Autoimmunity Reviews*, **7**, 598–605.

11 Roujeau, J.C., Kelly, J.P., Naldi, L. *et al.* (1995) Medication use and the risk of Stevens-Johnson syndrome or toxic epidermal necrolysis. *New England Journal of Medicine*, **333**, 1600–1607.

12 La Grenade, L., Lee, L., Weaver, J. *et al.* (2005) Comparison of reporting of Stevens-Johnson syndrome and toxic epidermal necrolysis in association with selective COX-2 inhibitors. *Drug Safety*, **28**, 917–924.

13 Mockenhaupt, M., Viboud, C., Dunant, A. *et al.* (2008) Stevens-Johnson syndrome and toxic epidermal necrolysis: assessment of medication risks with emphasis on recently marketed drugs: the EuroSCAR-study. *Journal of Investigative Dermatology*, **128**, 35–44.

14 Halevy, S., Ghislain, P.D., Mockenhaupt, M. *et al.* (2008) Allopurinol is the most common cause of Stevens-Johnson syndrome and toxic epidermal necrolysis in Europe and Israel. *Journal of the American Academy of Dermatology*, **58**, 25–32.

15 Sorrell, J., West, D.P., Bennett, C.L., Raisch, D.W. & Lacouture, M.E. (2009) Life-threatening dermatologic toxicities to cancer drug therapy: an assessment of the published peer-reviewed literature. *Journal of Clinical Oncology*, **27**, 15S (suppl. abstr e20592).

16 Garg, V., Balagula, Y., Raisch, D.W., Anadkat, M.J. & Lacouture, M.E. (2011) Stevens-Johnson syndrome (SJS) and toxic epidermal necrolysis (TEN) in a setting of chemotherapy treatment: an assessment of FDA MedWatch database. *Journal of Clinical Oncology*, 29, (Suppl; abstr. e19519).

17 Bastuji-Garin, S., Fouchard, N., Bertocchi, M., Roujeau, J.C., Revuz, J. & Wolkenstein, P. (2000) SCORTEN: a severity-of-illness score for toxic epidermal necrolysis. *Journal of Investigative Dermatology*, **115**, 149–153.

18 Trent, J.T., Kirsner, R.S., Romanelli, P. & Kerdel, F.A. (2004) Use of SCORTEN to accurately predict mortality in patients with toxic epidermal necrolysis in the United States. *Archives of Dermatology*, **140**, 890–892.

19 Guegan, S., Bastuji-Garin, S., Poszepczynska-Guigne, E., Roujeau, J.C. & Revuz, J. (2006) Performance of the SCORTEN during the

first five days of hospitalization to predict the prognosis of epidermal necrolysis. *Journal of Investigative Dermatology*, **126**, 272–276.

20 de Sica-Chapman, A., Williams, G., Soni, N. & Bunker, C.B. (2010) Granulocyte colony-stimulating factor in toxic epidermal necrolysis (TEN) and Chelsea & Westminster TEN management protocol. *British Journal of Dermatology*, **162** (4), 860–865.

21 Kalyoncu, M., Cimsit, G., Cakir, M. & Okten, A. (2004) Toxic epidermal necrolysis treated with intravenous immunoglobulin and granulocyte colony-stimulating factor. *Indian Pediatrics*, **41** (4), 392–395.

22 Jarrett, P., Rademaker, M., Havill, J. & Pullon, H. (1997) Toxic epidermal necrolysis treated with cyclosporin and granulocyte colony stimulating factor. *Clinical and Experimental Dermatology*, **22** (3), 146–147.

23 Goulden, V. & Goodfield, M.J. (1996) Recombinant granulocyte colony-stimulating factor in the management of toxic epidermal necrolysis. *British Journal of Dermatology*, **135** (2), 305–306.

24 Windle, E.M. (2005) Immune modulating nutrition support for a patient with severe toxic epidermal necrolysis. *Journal of Human Nutrition and Dietetics*, **18** (4), 311–314.

25 Coss-Bu, J.A., Jefferson, L.S., Levy, M.L., Walding, D., David, Y. & Klish, W.J. (1997) Nutrition requirements in patients with toxic epidermal necrolysis. *Nutrition in Clinical Practice*, **12** (2), 81–84.

26 Pasricha, J., Khaitan, B., Shantharaman, R., Mital, A. & Girdhar, M. (1996) Toxic epidermal necrolysis. *International Journal of Dermatology*, **35**, 523–527.

27 Rai, R. & Srinivas, C.R. (2008) Suprapharmacologic doses of intravenous dexamethasone followed by cyclosporine in the treatment of toxic epidermal necrolysis. *Indian Journal of Dermatology, Venereology and Leprology*, **74** (3), 263–265.

28 Araki, Y., Sotozono, C., Inatomi, T. *et al.* (2009) Successful treatment of Stevens-Johnson syndrome with steroid pulse therapy at disease onset. *American Journal of Ophthalmology*, **147** (6), 1004–1011.

29 Kardaun, S.H. & Jonkman, M.F. (2007) Dexamethasone pulse therapy for Stevens-Johnson syndrome/toxic epidermal necrolysis. *Acta Dermato-Venereologica*, **87** (2), 144–148.

30 van der Meer, J.B., Schuttelaar, M.L., Toth, G.G. *et al.* (2001) Successful dexamethasone pulse therapy in a toxic epidermal necrolysis (TEN) patient featuring recurrent TEN to oxazepam. *Clinical and Experimental Dermatology*, **26** (8), 654–656.

31 Engelhardt, S.L., Schurr, M.J. & Helgerson, R.B. (1997) Toxic epidermal necrolysis: an analysis of referral patterns and steroid usage. *Journal of Burn Care and Rehabilitation*, **18** (6), 520–524.

32 Stables, G.I. & Lever, R.S. (1993) Toxic epidermal necrolysis and systemic corticosteroids. *British Journal of Dermatology*, **128** (3), 357.

33 Rzany, B., Schmitt, H. & Schöpf, E. (1991) Toxic epidermal necrolysis in patients receiving glucocorticosteroids. *Acta Dermato-Venereologica*, **71** (2), 171–172.

34 Sherertz, E.F., Jegasothy, B.V. & Lazarus, G.S. (1985) Phenytoin hypersensitivity reaction presenting with toxic epidermal necrolysis and severe hepatitis. Report of a patient treated with corticosteroid "pulse therapy". *Journal of the American Academy of Dermatology*, **12** (1 Pt 2), 178–181.

35 Kim, P.S., Goldfarb, I.W., Gaisford, J.C. & Slater, H. (1983) Stevens-Johnson syndrome and toxic epidermal necrolysis: a pathophysiologic review with recommendations for a treatment protocol. *Journal of Burn Care and Rehabilitation*, **4**, 91–100.

36 Patterson, R., Miller, M., Kaplan, M. *et al.* (1994) Effectiveness of early therapy with corticosteroids in Stevens-Johnson syndrome: experience with 41 cases and a hypothesis regarding pathogenesis. *Annals of Allergy*, **73**, 27–34.

37 Aihara, Y., Ito, R., Ito, S., Aihara, M. & Yokota, S. (2007) Toxic epidermal necrolysis in a child successfully treated with cyclosporin A and methylprednisolone. *Pediatrics International*, **49** (5), 659–662.

38 Hashim, N., Bandara, D., Tan, E. & Ilchyshyn, A. (2004) Early cyclosporine treatment of incipient toxic epidermal necrolysis induced by concomitant use of lamotrigine and sodium valproate. *Acta Dermato-Venereologica*, **84** (1), 90–91.

39 Robak, E., Robak, T., Góra-Tybor, J. *et al.* (2001) Toxic epidermal necrolysis in a patient with severe aplastic anemia treated with cyclosporin A and G-CSF. *Journal of Medicine*, **32** (1–2), 31–39.

40 Arévalo, J.M., Lorente, J.A., González-Herrada, C. & Jiménez-Reyes, J. (2000) Treatment of toxic epidermal necrolysis with cyclosporin A. *Journal of Trauma*, **48** (3), 473–478.

41 Zaki, I., Patel, S., Reed, R. & Dalziel, K.L. (1995) Toxic epidermal necrolysis associated with severe hypocalcaemia, and treated with cyclosporin. *British Journal of Dermatology*, **133** (2), 337–338.

42 Hewitt, J. & Ormerod, A.D. (1992) Toxic epidermal necrolysis treated with cyclosporin. *Clinical and Experimental Dermatology*, **17** (4), 264–265.

43 Renfro, L., Grant-Kels, J.M. & Daman, L.A. (1989) Drug-induced toxic epidermal Necrolysis treated with cyclosporin. *International Journal of Dermatology*, **28** (7), 441–444.

44 Arevalo, J., Lorente, J., Gonzalez-Herrada, C. & Jiménez-Reyes, J. (2000) Treatment of toxic epidermal necrolysis with cyclosporin A. *Journal of Trauma*, **48**, 473–478.

45 Kreft, B., Wohlrab, J., Bramsiepe, I., Eismann, R., Winkler, M. & Marsch, W.C. (2010) Etoricoxib-induced toxic epidermal necrolysis: successful treatment with infliximab. *Journal of Dermatology*, **37** (10), 904–906.

46 Fischer, M., Fiedler, E., Marsch, W.C. & Wohlrab, J. (2002) Antitumour necrosis factor-a antibodies (infliximab) in the treatment of a patient with toxic epidermal necrolysis. *British Journal of Dermatology*, **146**, 707–709.

47 Al-Shouli, S., Abouchala, N., Bogusz, M.J., Al Tufail, M. & Thestrup-Pedersen, K. (2005) Toxic epidermal necrolysis associated with high intake of sildenafil and its response to infliximab. *Acta Dermato-Venereologica*, **85**, 534–535.

48 Wojtkiewicz, A., Wysocki, M., Fortuna, J., Chrupek, M., Matczuk, M. & Koltan, A. (2008) Beneficial and rapid effect of infliximab on the course of toxic epidermal necrolysis. *Acta Dermato-Venereologica*, **88**, 420–421.

49 Viard, L., Wehrli, P., Bullani, R. *et al.* (1998) Inhibition of toxic epidermal necrolysis by blockade of CD95 with human intravenous immunoglobulin. *Science*, **282**, 490–493.

50 Stella, M., Cassano, P., Bollero, D., Risso, D. & Dalmasso, P. (2001) Toxic epidermal necrolysis treated with intravenous high-dose immunoglobulins: our experience. *Dermatology (Basel, Switzerland)*, **203**, 45–49.

51 Metry, D.W., Jung, P. & Levy, M.L. (2003) Use of intravenous immunoglobulin in children with Stevens-Johnson syndrome and toxic epidermal necrolysis. *Pediatrics*, **112**, 1430–1436.

52 Morici, M.V., Galen, W.K., Shetty, A.K. *et al.* (2000) Intravenous immunoglobulin therapy for children with Stevens-Johnson syndrome. *Journal of Rheumatology*, **27**, 2494–2497.

53 Prins, C., Vittorio, C., Padilla, R.S. *et al.* (2003) Effect of high-dose intravenous immunoglobulin therapy in Stevens-Johnson syndrome: a retrospective, multicenter study. *Dermatology (Basel, Switzerland)*, **207**, 96–99.

54 Paquet, P., Jacob, E., Damas, P. & Piérard, G.E. (2001) Treatment of drug-induced toxic epidermal necrolysis (Lyell's syndrome) with intravenous human immunoglobulins. *Journal of the International Society for Burn Injuries*, **27**, 652–655.

55 Bachot, N., Revuz, J. & Roujeau, J.C. (2003) Intravenous immunoglobulin treatment for Stevens-Johnson syndrome and toxic epidermal necrolysis: a prospective noncomparative study showing no benefit on mortality or progression. *Archives of Dermatology*, **139**, 33–36.

56 Lee, C., Gianos, M. & Klaustermeyer, W.B. (2009) Diagnosis and management of hypersensitivity reactions related to common cancer chemotherapy agents. *Annals of Allergy, Asthma and Immunology*, **102**, 179–187.

57 Shepherd, G.M. (2003) Hypersensitivity reactions to chemotherapeutic drugs. *Clinical Reviews in Allergy and Immunology*, **24**, 253–262.

58 Sliesoraitis, S. & Chikhale, P.J. (2005) Carboplatin hypersensitivity. *International Journal of Gynecological Cancer*, **15**, 13–18.

59 Saif, M.W. (2006) Hypersensitivity reactions associated with oxaliplatin. *Expert Opinion on Drug Safety*, **5**, 687–694.

60 Oxaliplatin [package insert]. Available from: http://patient.cancerconsultants.com/druginserts/Oxaliplatin.pdf (accessed 13 May 2013).

61 Markman, M., Zanotti, K., Peterson, G., Kulp, B., Webster, K. & Belinson, J. (2003) Expanded experience with an intradermal skin test to predict for the presence or absence of carboplatin hypersensitivity. *Journal of Clinical Oncology*, **21**, 4611–4614.

62 Markman, M., Hsieh, F., Zanotti, K. *et al.* (2004) Initial experience with a novel desensitization strategy for carboplatin-associated hypersensitivity reactions: carboplatin-hypersensitivity reactions. *Journal of Cancer Research and Clinical Oncology*, **130**, 25–28.

63 Confino-Cohen, R., Fishman, A., Altaras, M. & Goldberg, A. (2005) Successful carboplatin desensitization in patients with proven carboplatin allergy. *Cancer*, **104**, 640–643.

64 Castells, M.C., Tennant, N.M., Sloane, D.E. *et al.* (2008) Hypersensitivity reactions to chemotherapy: outcomes and safety of rapid desensitizations in 413 cases. *Journal of Allergy and Clinical Immunology*, **122**, 574–580.

65 Meyer, L., Zuberbier, T., Worm, M., Oettle, H. & Riess, H. (2002) Hypersensitivity reactions to oxaliplatin: cross-reactivity to carboplatin and the introduction of a desensitization schedule. *Journal of Clinical Oncology*, **20**, 1146–1147.

66 Mis, L., Fernando, N.H., Hurwitz, H.I. & Morse, M.A. (2005) Successful desensitization to oxaliplatin. *Annals of Pharmacotherapy*, **39**, 966–969.

67 Gammon, D., Bhargava, P. & McCormick, M.J. (2004) Hypersensitivity reactions to oxaliplatin and the application of a desensitization protocol. *The Oncologist*, **9**, 546–549.

68 Rowinsky, E.K. & Donehower, R.C. (1995) Paclitaxel (Taxol). *New England Journal of Medicine*, **332**, 1004–1014.

69 Schrijvers, D., Wanders, J., Dirix, L. *et al.* (1993) Coping with toxicities of docetaxel (Taxotere). *Annals of Oncology*, **4**, 610–611.

70 Taxol (paclitaxel) injection [package insert]. Princeton, NJ: Bristol-Myers Squibb Company.

71 Gradishar, W.J., Tjulandin, S., Davidson, N. *et al.* (2005) Phase III trial of nanoparticle albumin-bound paclitaxel compared with polyethylated castor oil-based paclitaxel in women with breast cancer. *Journal of Clinical Oncology*, **23**, 7794.

72 Dizon, D.S., Schwartz, J., Rojan, A. *et al.* (2006) Cross-sensitivity between paclitaxel and docetaxel in a women's cancer program. *Gynecologic Oncology*, **100**, 149–151.

73 Semb, K.A., Aamdal, S. & Oian, P. (1998) Capillary protein leak syndrome appears to explain fluid retention in cancer patients who receive docetaxel treatment. *Journal of Clinical Oncology*, **16**, 3426–3432.

74 Piccart, M.J., Klijn, J., Paridaens, R. *et al.* (1997) Corticosteroids significantly delay the onset of docetaxel-induced fluid retention: final results of a randomized study of the European Organization for Reasearch and Treatment of Cancer Investigational Drug Branch for Breast Cancer. *Journal of Clinical Oncology*, **15**, 3149–3155.

75 Dellinger, C.T. & Miale, T.D. (1976) Comparison of anaphylactic reactions to asparaginase derived from *Escherichia coli* and from *Erwinia* cultures. *Cancer*, **38**, 1843–1846.

76 Evans, W.E., Tsiatis, A., Rivera, G. *et al.* (1982) Anaphylactoid reactions to Escherichia coli and Erwinia asparaginase in children with leukemia and lymphoma. *Cancer*, **49**, 1378–1383

77 Khan, A. & Hill, J.M. (1971) Atopic hypersensitivity to L-asparaginase: resistance to immunosuppression. *International Archives of Allergy and Applied Immunology*, **40**, 463–469.

78 Fabry, U., Korholz, D., Jurgens, H., Gobel, U. & Wahn, V. (1985) Anaphylaxis to L-asparaginase during treatment for acute lymphoblastic leukemia in children-evidence of a complement-mediated mechanism. *Pediatric Research*, **19**, 400–408.

79 Muller, H., Beier, R., Loning, L. *et al.* (2001) Pharmacokinetics of native *Escherichia coli* asparaginase (Asparaginase medac) and hypersensitivity reactions in ALL-BFM 95 reinduction treatment. *British Journal of Haematology*, **114**, 794–799.

80 Beard, M.E.J., Crowther, D., Galton, D.A. *et al.* (1970) L-asparaginase in treatment of acute leukaemia and lymphosarcoma. *British Medical Journal*, **1**, 191–195.

81 Larson, R.A., Fretzin, M.H., Dodge, R.K. & Schiffer, C.A. (1998) Hypersensitivity reactions to L-asparaginase do not impact on the remission duration of adults with acute lymphoblastic leukemia. *Leukemia*, **12**, 660–665.

82 Holle, L.M. (1997) Pegasparagase: an alternative. *Annals of Pharmacotherapy*, **31**, 616–624.

83 Soyer, O.U., Aytac, S., Tuncer, A., Cetin, M., Yetgin, S. & Sekerel, B.E. (2009) Alternative algorithm for L-asparaginase allergy in children with acute lymphoblastic leukemia. *Journal of Allergy and Clinical Immunology*, **123** (4), 895–899.

84 Weiss, R.B. (1992) Hypersensitivity reactions. *Seminars in Oncology*, **19**, 458–477.

85 Kellie, S.J., Crist, W.M., Pui, C.H. *et al.* (1991) Hypersensitivity reactions to epipodophyllotoxins in children with acute lymphoblastic leukemia. *Cancer*, **67**, 1070–1075.

86 Collier, K., Schink, C., Young, A.M., How, K., Seckl, M. & Savage, P. (2008) Successful treatment with etoposide phosphate in patients with previous etoposide hypersensitivity. *Journal of Oncology Pharmacy Practice*, **14** (1), 51–55.

87 O'Dwyer, P.J., King, S.A., Fortner, C.L. & Leyland-Jones, B. (1986) Hypersensitivity reactions to teniposide (VM-26): an analysis. *Journal of Clinical Oncology*, **4**, 1262–1269.

88 Zanotti, K.M. & Markman, M. (2001) Prevention and management of antineoplastic-induced hypersensitivity reactions. *Drug Safety*, **24**, 767–779.

89 Hoetelmans, R.M.W., Schornagel, J.H., Bokkeel Huinink, W.W. & Beijnen, J.H. (1996) Hypersensitivity reactions to etoposide. *Annals of Pharmacotherapy*, **30**, 367–371.

90 Lehmann, D.F., Hurteau, T.E., Newman, N. & Coyle, T.E. (1997) Anticonvulsant usage is associated with an increased risk of procarbazine hypersensitivity reactions in patients with brain tumors. *Clinical Pharmacology and Therapeutics*, **62**, 225–229.

91 Coyle, T., Bushunow, P., Winfield, J., Wright, J. & Graziano, S. (1992) Hypersensitivity reactions to procarbazine with mechlorethamine, vincristine, and procarbazine chemotherapy in the treatment of glioma. *Cancer*, **69**, 2532–2540.

92 Brooks, B.J., Hendler, N.B., Alvarez, S., Ancalmo, N. & Grinton, S.F. (1990) Delayed life-threatening pneumonitis secondary to procarbazine. *American Journal of Clinical Oncology*, **13**, 244–246.

93 Mahmood, T. & Mudad, R. (2002) Pulmonary toxicity secondary to procarbazine. *American Journal of Clinical Oncology*, **25**, 187–188.

94 Jones, R., Kirkup, M., Guglani, S. & Hopkins, K. (2006) Toxic epidermal necrolysis after PCV combination chemotherapy for relapsed B-cell lymphoma. *Clinical Oncology*, **18** (1), 90.

95 Giguere, J.K., Douglas, D.M., Lupton, G.P., Baker, J.R. & Weiss, R.B. (1988) Procarbazine hypersensitivity manifested as a fixed drug eruption. *Medical and Pediatric Oncology*, **16** (6), 378–380.

96 Millward, M.J., Cohney, S.J., Byrne, M.J. & Ryan, G.F. (1990) Pulmonary toxicity following MOPP chemotherapy. *Australian and New Zealand Journal of Medicine*, **20** (3), 245–248.

97 Saltzstein, S.L. & Ackerman, L.V. (1959) Lymphadenopathy induced by anticonvulsant drugs and mimicking clinically pathologically malignant lymphomas. *Cancer*, **12** (1), 164–182.

98 Bocquet, H., Bagot, M. & Roujeau, J.C. (1996) Drug-induced pseudolymphoma and drug hypersensitivity syndrome (Drug Rash with Eosinophilia and Systemic Symptoms: DRESS). *Seminars in Cutaneous Medicine and Surgery*, **15** (4), 250–257.

99 Hashimoto, K., Yasukawa, M. & Tohyama, M. (2003) Human herpesvirus 6 and drug allergy. *Current Opinion in Allergy and Clinical Immunology*, **3** (4), 255–260.

100 Shiohara, T., Iijima, M., Ikezawa, Z. & Hashimoto, K. (2007) The diagnosis of a DRESS syndrome has been sufficiently established on the basis of typical clinical features and viral reactivations. *British Journal of Dermatology*, **156** (5), 1083–1084.

101 Callot, V., Roujeau, J.C., Bagot, M. *et al.* (1996) Drug-induced pseudolymphoma and hypersensitivity syndrome: two different clinical entities. *Archives of Dermatology*, **132**, 1315–1321.

102 Rieder, M.J., Shear, N.H. & Kanee, A. (1991) Prominence of slow acetylator phenotype among patients with sulfonamide hypersensitivity reactions. *Clinical Pharmacology and Therapeutics*, **49**, 13–17.

103 Green, V.J., Pirmohamed, M., Kitteringham, N.R. *et al.* (1995) Genetic analysis of microsomal epoxide hydrolase in patients with carbamazepine hypersensitivity. *Biochemical Pharmacology*, **50**, 1353–1359.

104 Tohyama, M., Yahata, Y., Yasukawa, M. *et al.* (1998) Severe hypersensitivity syndrome due to sulfasalazine associated with reactivation of human herpesvirus 6. *Archives of Dermatology*, **134**, 1113–1117.

105 Descamps, V., Valence, A., Edlinger, C. *et al.* (2001) Association of human herpesvirus 6 infection with drug reaction with eosinophilia and systemic symptoms. *Archives of Dermatology*, **137**, 301–304.

106 Tohyama, M. & Hashimoto, K. (2002) Drug hypersensitivity syndrome and human herpesvirus 6 reactivation. *Archives of Dermatology*, **138**, 268–269.

107 Carrigan, D.R. & Knox, K. (2000) Human herpesvirus 6: diagnosis of active infection. *American Clinical Laboratory*, **19**, 12.

108 Suzuki, Y., Inagi, R., Aono, T., Yamanishi, K. & Shiohara, T. (1998) Human herpesvirus 6 infection as a risk factor for the development of severe drug-induced hypersensitivity syndrome. *Archives of Dermatology*, **134**, 1108–1112.

109 Peyrière, H., Dereure, O., Breton, H. *et al.* (2006) Network of the French Pharmacovigilance Centers. Variability in the clinical pattern of cutaneous side-effects of drugs with systemic symptoms: does a DRESS syndrome really exist? *British Journal of Dermatology*, **155** (2), 422–428.

110 Walsh, S.A. & Creamer, D. (2011) Drug reaction with eosinophilia and systemic symptoms (DRESS): a clinical update and review of current thinking. *Clinical and Experimental Dermatology*, **36**, 6–11.

111 Chen, Y.C., Chiu, H.C. & Chu, C.Y. (2010) Drug reaction with eosinophilia and systemic symptoms: a retrospective study of 60 cases. *Archives of Dermatology*, **146** (12), 1373–1379.

112 Shear, N.H. & Spielberg, S.P. (1988) Anticonvulsant hypersensitivity syndrome. In vitro assessment of risk. *Journal of Clinical Investigation*, **82**, 1826–1832.

113 Haruda, F. (1979) Phenytoin hypersensitivity: 38 cases. *Neurology*, **29**, 1480–1485.

114 Ganeva, M., Gancheva, T., Lazarova, R. *et al.* (2008) Carbamazepine-induced drug reaction with eosinophilia and systemic symptoms (DRESS) syndrome: report of four cases and brief review. *International Journal of Dermatology*, **47**, 853–860.

115 Jeung, Y.J., Lee, J.Y., Oh, M.J., Choi, D.C. & Lee, B.J. (2010) Comparison of the causes and clinical features of drug rash with eosinophilia and systemic symptoms and stevens-johnson syndrome. *Allergy Asthma Immunol Res.*, **2** (2), 123–126.

116 Tennis, P. & Stern, R.S. (1997) Risk of serious cutaneous disorders after initiation of use of phenytoin, carbamazepine, or sodium valproate: a record linkage study. *Neurology*, **49**, 542–546.

117 Cribb, A.E., Lee, B.L., Trepanier, L.A. & Spielberg, S.P. (1996) Adverse reactions to sulphonamide and sulphonamide-trimethoprim antimicrobials: clinical syndromes and pathogenesis. *Adverse Drug Reactions and Toxicological Reviews*, **15**, 9–50.

118 Hamanaka, H., Mizutani, H., Nouchi, N., Shimizu, Y. & Shimizu, M. (1998) Allopurinol hypersensitivity syndrome: hypersensitivity to oxypurinol but not allopurinol. *Clinical and Experimental Dermatology*, **23**, 32–34.

119 Sommers, L.M. & Schoene, R.B. (2002) Allopurinol hypersensitivity syndrome associated with pancreatic exocrine abnormalities and new-onset diabetes mellitus. *Archives of Internal Medicine*, **162**, 1190–1192.

120 Markel, A. (2005) Allopurinol-induced DRESS syndrome. *Israel Medical Association Journal*, **7** (10), 656–660.

121 Kardaun, S.H., Sidoroff, A., Valeyrie-Allanore, L. *et al.* (2007) Variability in the clinical pattern of cutaneous side-effects of drugs with systemic symptoms: does a DRESS syndrome really exist? *British Journal of Dermatology*, **156** (3), 609–611.

122 Kano, Y. & Shiohara, T. (2009) The variable clinical picture of drug-induced hypersensitivity syndrome/drug rash with eosinophilia and

systemic symptoms in relation to the eliciting drug. *Immunology and Allergy Clinics of North America*, **29** (3), 481–501.

123 Stalnikowicz, R., Mosseri, M. & Shalev, O. (1982) Phenytoin-induced arthritis. *Neurology*, **32**, 1317–1318.

124 Carfagna, P., Pistella, E., Paravati, V. & Serra, P. (2001) Arthritis as a rare side effect of phenytoin therapy. *European Journal of Internal Medicine*, **12**, 448–450.

125 Parker, W.A. & Shearer, C.A. (1979) Phenytoin hepatotoxicity: a case report and review. *Neurology*, **29**, 175–178.

126 Mahadeva, U., Al Mrayat, M., Steer, K. & Leen, E. (1999) Fatal phenytoin hypersensitivity syndrome. *Postgraduate Medical Journal*, **75**, 734–736.

127 Bonnetblanc, J.M. (1993) Drug hypersensitivity syndrome. *Dermatology (Basel, Switzerland)*, **187**, 84–85.

128 Yamakado, S., Yoshida, Y., Yamada, T., Kishida, T., Kobayashi, M. & Nomura, T. (1992) Pulmonary infiltration and eosinophilia associated with sulfasalazine therapy for ulcerative colitis: a case report and review of literature. *Internal Medicine (Tokyo, Japan)*, **31**, 108–113.

129 Syn, W.K., Naisbitt, D.J., Holt, A.P., Pirmohamed, M. & Mutimer, D.J. (2005) Carbamazepine-induced acute liver failure as part of the DRESS syndrome. *International Journal of Clinical Practice*, **59** (8), 988–991.

130 Hegarty, J., Picton, M., Agarwal, G., Pramanik, A. & Kalra, PA. (2002) Carbamazepine-induced acute granulomatous interstitial nephritis. *Clinical Nephrology*, **57**, 310–313.

131 Takahashi, N., Aizawa, H., Takata, S. *et al.* (1993) Acute interstitial pneumonitis induced by carbamazepine. *European Respiratory Journal*, **6**, 1409–1411.

132 Daniels, P.R., Berry, G.J., Tazelaar, H.D. & Cooper, L.T. (2000) Giant cell myocarditis as a manifestation of drug hypersensitivity. *Cardiovascular Pathology*, **9**, 287–291.

133 Lanzafame, M., Rovere, P., DeChecchi, G., Trevenzoli, M., Turazzini, M. & Parrinello, A. (2001) Hypersensitivity syndrome (DRESS) and meningoencephalitis associated with nevirapine therapy. *Scandinavian Journal of Infectious Diseases*, **33**, 475–476.

134 Gupta, A., Eggo, M.C., Uetrecht, J.P. *et al.* (1992) Drug-induced hypothyroidism: the thyroid as a target organ in hypersensitivity reactions to anticonvulsants and sulfonamides. *Clinical Pharmacology and Therapeutics*, **51**, 56–67.

135 Tas, S. & Simonart, T. (2003) Management of drug eruption with eosinophilia and systemic symptoms (DRESS syndrome): an update. *Dermatology (Basel, Switzerland)*, **206**, 353–356.

136 Chopra, S., Levell, N.J., Cowley, G. & Gilkes, J.J. (1996) Systemic corticosteroids in the phenytoin hypersensitivity syndrome. *British Journal of Dermatology*, **134**, 1109–1112.

137 Vittorio, C.C. & Muglia, J.J. (1995) Anticonvulsant hypersensitivity syndrome. *Archives of Internal Medicine*, **155**, 2285–2290.

138 Eshki, M., Allanore, L., Musette, P. *et al.* (2009) Twelve-year analysis of severe cases of drug reaction with eosinophilia and systemic symptoms: a cause of unpredictable multiorgan failure. *Archives of Dermatology*, **145** (1), 67–72.

139 Redondo, P., de Felipe, I., de la Pena, A., Aramendia, J.M. & Vanaclocha, V. (1997) Drug-induced hypersensitivity syndrome and toxic epidermal necrolyisis. Treatment with N-acetylcysteine. *British Journal of Dermatology*, **136**, 645–646.

31 Dermatologic Infections

Yevgeniy Balagula[1], Mario E. Lacouture[1] and James I. Ito[2]

[1]Dermatology Service, Memorial Sloan-Kettering Cancer Center, New York, NY, USA
[2]Division of Infectious Diseases, City of Hope Cancer Center, Duarte, CA, USA

Introduction

A wide spectrum of infections affecting the skin and its adnexae (i.e., hair and nails) are frequent in oncology (Figure 31.1). The increased susceptibility is multifactorial in nature and partially stems from the underlying disease with consequent alterations of the immune system such as neutropenia, lymphopenia, or hypogammaglobulinemia [1]. In addition, therapy with chemotherapy, radiation, or therapeutic hematopoietic cell transplantation (HCT) frequently result in myelosuppression, further predisposing patients to opportunistic infections. Anticancer treatments often disrupt skin structure and function, rendering patients susceptible to infections (Table 31.1). This chapter reviews the clinical spectrum of dermatologic bacterial, viral, fungal, and parasitic infections and their treatments in cancer patients.

Bacterial infections

Gram-positive organisms

Staphylococcus aureus

Staphylococcus aureus commonly colonizes skin, particularly anterior nares, axilla, and the intertriginous inguinal and perineal areas [2]. Carrier rates of 11–32% have been reported among healthy adults [3]. A relatively recent increase in the rate of community-acquired (CA) and healthcare acquired (HA) methicillin-resistant *S. aureus* (MRSA) infections has emerged, with many centers in the United States reporting rates exceeding 50% [4]. The predominant clinical manifestations of CA *S. aureus* are skin and soft tissue infections (SSTI), in approximately 85–95% of cases, manifested by abscesses, furuncles, carbuncles, folliculitis, and cellulitis [4]. Underlying diagnosis of cancer is a

risk factor for infections [5], and in patients with cancer SSTI can result in bacteremia, which is associated with increased morbidity and mortality [6]. In one series, *S. aureus* accounted for 23% of 142 identified cases of bacteremia, with skin and mucosal surfaces serving as a probable site of primary infection in 64% of cases [7]. Staphylococcal sepsis was a direct cause of death in 16% of these patients [7]. Similarly, a prospective analysis in non-neutropenic adults with malignancy demonstrated that surgical wound infections (17%), cellulitis (6%), furuncles (2%), decubitus ulcers (2%), and infections at nephrostomy sites (4%) were the primary foci of *S. aureus* bacteremia (SAB) [6]. Overall, MRSA and methicillin-susceptible strains (MSSA) accounted for 38% and 62% of cases, respectively. In addition to significant SAB-specific mortality (15%), secondary metastatic sequelae include infectious endocarditis, septic arthritis, paraspinal and brain abscesses, and osteomyelitis [6]. In another study of adult and pediatric patients undergoing allogenic HCT, SAB and late SAB (>50 days after HCT) were observed in 4.1% and 3.6% of patients, respectively. Among patients with late SAB, 11.5% presented with skin manifestations such as paronychia, superficial thrombophlebitis, and cutaneous septic emboli, and 15.3% with pocket or tunnel infections associated with an intravascular device [8]. Similarly, analysis of pediatric patients with leukemia, lymphoma, solid and brain tumors revealed that among patients infected with MRSA, 68% presented with cutaneous involvement [9]. These MRSA strains were resistant to ciprofloxacin (23%), clindamycin (18%), erythromycin (81%), and gentamicin (5%) [9].

Infections are common and the most common cause of mortality in patients with cutaneous T-cell lymphoma (CTCL). In this population, *S. aureus* is the most common cause of both skin infections and bacteremias [10,11], with beta-hemolytic streptococcus also commonly implicated (10%) [10]. Colonization by *S. aureus* in patients with mycosis fungoides (MF) and Sézary

Dermatologic Principles and Practice in Oncology: Conditions of the Skin, Hair, and Nails in Cancer Patients, First Edition. Edited by Mario E. Lacouture.
© 2014 John Wiley & Sons, Inc. Published 2014 by John Wiley & Sons, Inc.

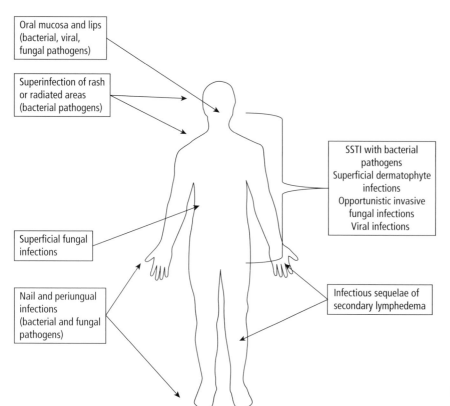

Oral mucosa and lips
(bacterial, viral,
fungal pathogens)

Superinfection of rash
or radiated areas
(bacterial pathogens)

SSTI with bacterial
pathogens
Superficial dermatophyte
infections
Opportunistic invasive
fungal infections
Viral infections

Superficial fungal
infections

Nail and periungual
infections
(bacterial and fungal
pathogens)

Infectious sequelae of
secondary lymphedema

Figure 31.1 Distribution of dermatologic infections in cancer patients. SSTI, skin and soft tissue infection.

syndrome (SS) has prognostic implications and is associated with disease progression and exacerbation of erythroderma and pruritus [11]. It was demonstrated that overall skin and nasal carriage rate was 31% in MF patients. Moreover, erythrodermic SS (erythroderma involving >80% of body surface area) patients had a higher rate of colonization than with patients without erythroderma (48% vs. 26%, $p < 0.0001$) [11]. In these patients, treatment with intranasal mupirocin and oral antibiotics (250 mg dicloxacillin qid or 1 g/day cephalexin for 4 weeks) eradicated bacteria in 91% of carriers and skin improvement in 57% of patients [11]. A regimen consisting of nasal mupirocin, oral rifampin, doxycycline, and chlorhexidine bathing resulted in successful MRSA decolonization for 74% at 3 months [12]. Patients with extensive skin involvement may benefit from baths with diluted sodium hypochlorite (1/4 cup of bleach in a bathtub of water), the frequency of which can range from once daily to once weekly [13]. However, there is significant controversy surrounding these decolonization or eradication strategies [93]. The majority of patients are recolonized within 6 months. MRSA decolonization has not always resulted in a reduction of infection rates. Finally, increased resistance to systemic antibiotics has also resulted. Thus, decolonization is not a recommended standard of care in most patient populations.

Staphylococcal scalded skin syndrome (SSSS) is mediated by an exfoliative exotoxin targeting desmoglein-1, and affects patients with cancer, immunosuppression, and renal failure, with mortality exceeding 50–60% [14]. It presents with localized blisters to widespread exfoliation with systemic symptoms.

Epidermal loss may lead to fluid and electrolyte imbalance and secondary infections [14].

Diagnosis of SSTI etiology may be difficult in the absence of a positive culture. Cultures from the site of a cellulitis or blood are rarely positive. Therapy of infection in the immunocompromised cancer patient is an immediate and empiric approach based upon epidemiologic and host factors. In the case of a suspected staphylococcal infection, the antibiotic chosen should be active against MRSA. Thus, the therapy recommended for SSTI where MRSA is a possible etiology (and vancomycin-resistant enterococcus (VRE), Gram negatives, and anaerobes are not), should be vancomycin, daptomycin, or linezolid (see Appendix 31.1). If there is a possibility of (or proven) vancomycin-resistant or tolerant *S. aureus* (VRSA), daptomycin or linezolid should be used. If an organism and its sensitivities are subsequently reported out from one of the cultures, the antibiotic regimen can be adjusted. It should be noted that if there is any suspicion that there may be a Gram-negative enteric, anaerobe, or VRE involved (e.g., SSTI in proximity to the gastrointestinal tract), other antibiotics (e.g., carbapenem, metronidazole, and linezolid or quinupristin/dalfopristin, respectively) should be added (see below). Finally, the mainstay and cornerstone of treatment of SSTI due to *S. aureus*, especially MRSA, is incision and drainage of the abscesses or necrotic skin lesions [15].

Other Gram-positive pathogens

Peptostreptococcus species were shown to be the predominant organisms isolated from wounds such as fasciitis, cellulitis,

Table 31.1 Selected pathogens and their clinical significance in cancer patients.

Pathogens	Clinical implications
Staphylococcus aureus	SSTI can serve as a site for systemic dissemination
	The most common cause of skin infections and bacteremias in patients with CTCL
	Exacerbation of cutaneous manifestations in patients with CTCL
	Cancer patients are at increased risk for staphylococcal scalded skin syndrome
	The most commonly isolated pathogen from areas of radiation-induced moist desquamation. Can produce superantigens that may potentially exacerbate skin dermatitis
	The most common pathogen in dermatologic infections at body sites affected by EGFRIs
Group A β-hemolytic Streptococci	The most common cause of erysipelas of upper extremities in breast cancer patients affected by lymphedema. Episodes of erysipelas tend to be recurrent
	Recurrent infection of the affected extremity, even subclinical, exacerbates and worsens lymphedema
Corynebacterium species	An emerging pathogen of SSTI in cancer patients
Stenotrophomonas maltophilia	An increasingly recognized emerging pathogen causing mucocutaneous and SSTI
Escherichia coli	An emergent pathogen that can cause pyomyositis, especially in patients with hematologic malignancies
Dermatophytes (microsporum, epidermophyton, and trichophyton)	May present with atypical manifestations affecting a larger body surface area
Aspergillus and *Fusarium* species	Onychomycosis due to these pathogens may lead to paronychia, invasive deep infection, and systemic dissemination, especially in patients with hematologic malignancies with profound and prolonged neutropenia
Aspergillus, Fusarium, Candida, Rhizopus, Mucor, Cryptococcal species	Cutaneous lesions may serve as initial and an indirect evidence of systemic disseminated infection with these organisms
	Cutaneous lesions can serve as a diagnostic source, especially in cases where blood cultures are of low yield
Rhizopus, Mucor, Aspergillus species	Cellulitis of the facial areas may indicate an underlying invasive fungal sinusitis, especially in patients with severe and profound neutropenia
Varicella zoster virus	High risk of reactivation in patients with leukemias, lymphomas, and those receiving HCT
	Increased risk of reactivation in CLL patients treated with alemtuzumab
	Significantly increased risk of reactivation in multiple myeloma patients treated with bortezomib
	Atypical clinical manifestation and more severe presentations
Cytomegalovirus	Increased risk of reactivation in patients treated with alemtuzumab
	Increased risk in patients undergoing HCT

CLL, chronic lymphocytic lymphoma; CTCL, cutaneous T-cell lymphoma; EGFRI, epidermal growth factor receptor inhibitor; HCT, hematopoietic cell transplantation; SSTI, skin and soft tissue infection.

decubitus ulcers, and post-surgical wounds [16]. VRE strains have become more prevalent, and many HCT programs now screen their patients routinely prior to transplantation.

Corynebacterium represent a diverse group of Gram-positive organisms, also known as diphtheroids (Figure 31.2) [17]. *C. diphtheriae* can initially present with a vesicle or a pustule that progresses to a nonhealing ulcer, with production of serosanguineous exudate [17]. Diphtheroids are common colonizers of human skin and mucosae. Only recently, they have been recognized as emerging organisms that can infect immunosuppressed patients [18,19]. A study demonstrated a spectrum of diphtheroids as a cause of cutaneous infections in cancer patients (adult and pediatric solid tumors and adult CNS tumors), of which *C. amycolatum* was the most common species isolated [19]. Among 16 pediatric oncology patients, 5 (31.3%) developed central venous catheter exit site or surgical wound site infections with *C. aquaticum, C. bovis,* or *C. jeikeium* species [18].

Gram-negative bacteria

Gram-negative infections in hospitalized patients with solid tumors and SSTI accounts for 64.5% of infections [20]. Organisms included *Klebsiella pneumoniae* (25.4%), *Escherichia coli* (22.2%),

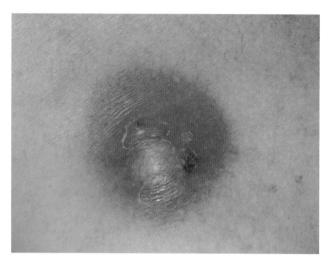

Figure 31.2 A cyst on the chest infected with *Diphtheroids* in a patient with cholangiocarcinoma.

and *Pseudomonas aeruginosa* (18.9%) [20]. In this study, isolates of *E. coli, Klebsiella, Enterobacter, Pseudomonas,* and *Acinetobacter* species were resistant to most antibiotics including non-beta-lactam antibiotics such as aminoglycosides and quinolones. *E. coli* were highly susceptible to imipenem, cefotetan, and amikacin; *Klebsiella* species were susceptible to imipenem and cefotetan, and meropenem was the most active antibiotic against *Pseudomonas* species [20]. Predominant Gram-negative anaerobic pathogens recovered from SSTI and wounds in cancer patients were *Prevotella* species and *Bacteroides* fragilis [16], whereas aerobic Gram-negatives from abscesses included *Proteus, Enterobacter* species, and other Enterobacteriaceae [16]. The emergence of extended spectrum beta-lactamase (ESBL) Gram-negative bacteria (e.g., *Klebsiella* species and *E. coli*) [21,22] and carbapenemase-producing organisms (e.g., *Klebsiella* species and *Pseudomonas aeruginosa*) [23] has been reported. The ESBL organisms are usually resistant to most antibiotics except for the carbapenems, while organisms producing *Klebsiella pneumoniae* carbapenemases (KPCs) are resistant to all beta-lactam antibiotics except for the polymyxins (polymyxin B or colistin) and tigecycline.

Stenotrophomonas maltophilia is an opportunistic aerobic Gram-negative organism that colonizes hospital nebulizers, dialysis machines, and intravenous fluids. In humans, respiratory tract, skin, and the gastrointestinal tract are some of the colonization sites. It is an increasingly recognized culprit of SSTI in immunosuppressed patients [24,25]. A recent review described 17 cases of patients with metastatic cellulitis (58%), primary cellulitis (23%), and ecthyma gangrenosum (17%). An underlying diagnosis of hematologic malignancy was present in 94% of chemotherapy-treated neutropenic patients, 84% received broad-spectrum antibiotics prior to the infection, and 17% had a central venous catheter, all considered risk factors [24]. Metastatic cellulitis presents as erythematous, nodular, and tender subcutaneous infiltrates, which can necrose and ulcerate [25,26]. Trimethoprim-sulfamethoxazole is recommended but increased

resistance to this agent (30–40%) has been reported [24,26]. Ticarcillin-clavulanate is an alternative drug, and can also be used in combination with trimethoprim-sulfamethoxazole for possible synergism. Other active drugs include tigecycline, moxifloxacin, and ceftazidime.

Pyomyositis, clinically presenting with fever and tenderness overlying the affected muscle area, is typically caused by *S. aureus* and other Gram-positive pathogens (>90%) of immunocompetent patients. *S. aureus* is also the most common cause (59% of cases) of pyomyositis in patients with hematologic malignancies [27]. *E. coli* has also been reported to cause pyomyositis in hematologic cancer patients [28] treated with chemotherapy and fluoroquinolone prophylaxis. Calf muscles were involved in five patients and three developed abscesses [28].

If a Gram-negative SSTI is suspected (e.g., proximity to the gastrointestinal or urinary tract), an empiric approach includes third generation cephalosporins (e.g., ceftazidime or cefepime). In cases of ESBL Gram-negative infections, imipenem or meropenem are advised. For KPC Gram-negative infections, polymyxins (polymyxin B or colistin) or tigecycline are indicated. Polymyxins are highly nephrotoxic. For an *S. maltophilia* infection, trimethoprim-sulfamethoxazole is indicated.

Prophylaxis against bacteremia is controversial and is usually reserved for cancer patients at highest risk (i.e., HCT recipients during the neutropenic pre-engraftment period) [29]. The antibacterial agent usually recommended is levofloxacin.

Fungal infections

Primary cutaneous infections or cutaneous sequelae of fungemia range from superficial dermatophyte or yeast to deeper and opportunistic mold infections [30]. The main risk factor for invasive and systemic infections is prolonged neutropenia (<500/mL for more than 1 week) in patients with hematologic malignancies undergoing high dose chemotherapy or HCT. In the post-engraftment period, major risk factors become graft versus host disease (GVHD) and immunosuppressive therapy. Other risk factors include intravascular and urinary catheters, disruption of gastrointestinal and oropharyngeal mucosa, total parenteral nutrition, broad-spectrum antibiotics, and immunosuppressive agents use [31].

Primary superficial dermatophyte and yeast infections
Superficial dermatophyte infections of the stratum corneum, hair shafts, and nails by *Microsporum, Epidermophyton,* and *Trichophyton* species are similar when compared with immunocompetent patients. Clinical manifestations include tinea pedis, tinea corporis (Figure 31.3), and onychomycosis. Invasion of the hair follicle may result in folliculitis, with discrete patches of alopecia with erythematous perifollicular papules and pustules, referred to as Majocchi granuloma, with lower legs being the most common sites [30]. Immunocompromised patients may have atypical presentations of tinea corporis, with annular or

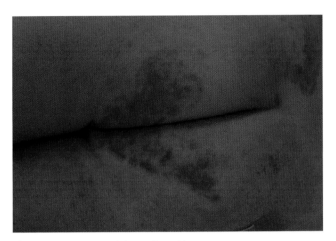

Figure 31.3 Tinea corporis in a patient with prostate cancer.

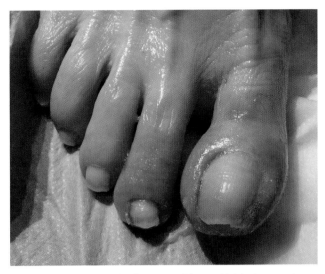

Figure 31.4 Acute paronychia from EGFR inhibitors with infection secondary to *Candida* species.

polycyclic lesions involving a large body surface area [30]. Clinical diagnosis is confirmed by microscopic examination of a potassium hydroxide (KOH) smear of skin scrapings, showing septate hyphae branching at various angles [30,31]. The risk of invasion and systemic dissemination of these superficial infections is negligible, even in immunocompromised patients [31].

Tinea corporis, cruris, or pedis can be treated topically with butenafine or terbinafine containing agents. Alternative treatments include oral terbinafine, ketoconazole, fluconazole, or griseofulvin. The drug of choice for tinea capitis is oral terbinafine. Alternatives are oral itraconazole, fluconazole, or griseofulvin. Perhaps the most difficult to treat is onychomycosis where the drug of choice is oral terbinafine which has a 76% success rate. Alternatives include oral itraconazole or fluconazole (see Appendix 31.1). The addition of topical ciclopirox or amorolfine to oral therapy may be synergistic and enhance its efficacy; when used alone, topical agents have a poor response.

Candida albicans is the most common culprit of these organisms, followed by *C. parapsilosis*, *C. krusei*, *C. pseudotropicalis*, *C. glabrata*, and *C. tropicalis* [31]. The emergence of *C. krusei* and *C. glabrata* is noteworthy because the former is innately resistant to fluconazole and the latter is becoming increasingly resistant to the azoles. The spectrum of infections includes intertrigo with satellite pustules, vulvovaginitis, balanitis, angular cheilitis, paronychia (Figure 31.4), and onychomycosis [32,33]. A pseudomembranous form is the most common manifestation of oral infection, and is characterized by friable white exudative plaques with pain and dysphagia [32]. Microscopic examination reveals either oval yeast-like cells, pseudohyphae, or hyphae, but different species cannot be distinguished based on histopathology [31]. For superficial cutaneous candidiasis, topical amphotericin B, clotrimazole, econazole, miconazole, or nystatin can be used. Alternatively, oral fluconazole or ketoconazole can be used. Stomatitis and esophagitis should be treated initially with oral fluconazole or itraconazole. However, if disease is refractory to these drugs, an echinocandin (caspofungin, micafungin, anidulafungin) should be used.

Malassezia furfur, yeast that is normally a part of adult skin flora, can lead to tinea versicolor or folliculitis, inflammation of the scrotum, and vaginitis with discharge [34]. The drug of choice is ketoconazole. Alternatives include fluconazole and itraconazole.

Primary opportunistic invasive nondermatophyte infections

Opportunistic dermatologic infections in cancer patients can be caused by *Aspergillus*, Zygomycetes, *Fusarium*, *Scedosporium*, *Candida*, and *Cryptococcus* species. Neutropenic patients with hematologic malignancies and HCT recipients are at highest risk [35,36]. Invasive *Aspergillus* or *Fusarium* infections occur in the setting of neutropenia, T-cell immunodeficiency, and immunosuppression [37]. Allogeneic HCT recipients develop these risk factors in stages:

1. Neutropenia during phase I, the pre-engraftment stage;
2. T-cell immunodeficiency and dysregulation associated with GVHD and corticosteroid therapy during phases II (engraftment to day +100) and III (after day +100), the post-engraftment acute GVHD and chronic GVHD stages, respectively.

The portal of entry for molds is the sinopulmonary tract from where they can disseminate. However, direct transdermal inoculation can occur and is facilitated by disrupted skin [30,35,36].

Primary *Aspergillus* and *Fusarium* infections limited to skin are uncommon (0.27%, n = 296) [35,38]. Most primary localized infections affect the hands, feet, or distal extremities [38], including paronychia, onychomycosis, black eschar formation, papulonodular lesions progressing to ulceronecrotic lesions, abscesses, superinfection of venous stasis ulcers, indurated areas of erythema at central venous catheter insertion sites, and hemorrhagic bullae [35,38,39].

Aspergillus, *Fusarium*, Zygomycetes, *Candida*, and *Cryptococcus* species can cause cellulitis, which may be difficult to distinguish from a bacterial etiology [30]. An underlying invasive fungal (i.e., *Aspergillus* and Zygomycetes) sinusitis may present as facial cellulitis [31].

Deep cutaneous *Candida* or *Cryptococcus* species infections in cancer patients may result in multiple erythematous papules, pustules, and ulcers with crusts [36,40–42]. Preceding cutaneous trauma and corticosteroid therapy are commonly reported risk factors [42]. Rarely, *Alternaria* species leads to localized skin infections, characterized by hemorrhagic, red to dark papules, and nodules or ulcers [40,43].

The presence of an eschar or purpura in the area of cellulitis may be suggestive of nondermatophytic fungal infection, resulting from angioinvasion [30]. A combination of cultures, histopathology, and molecular biology should be utilized for optimal diagnosis. Cultures should be interpreted with caution because these organisms are common environmental contaminants and may take weeks to grow. Hence, skin biopsies are useful in addition to immunohistochemistry and polymerase chain reaction (PCR) probes [31,32].

Primary dermatologic infection by molds and yeasts should be treated as if they represented an invasive systemic disease. If one does not have a specific fungal species diagnosis, empiric therapy with a lipid formulation of amphotericin B should be initiated to cover most possible fungal etiologies (see Appendix 31.1). In addition to antifungal therapy, an attempt must be made to eradicate all involved invaded and necrotic tissue:

1. Debridement of eschars;
2. Sinus drainage in sinusitis; and
3. Drainage of all abscesses.

Cutaneous manifestations of systemic disseminated disease

Aspergillus is rarely, if ever, found in the bloodstream, and skin involvement usually results from direct inoculation. *Fusarium*, on the other hand, commonly disseminates through the bloodstream and fusariosis almost always presents with cutaneous lesions [30].

Invasive yeast infections
Invasive candidiasis

Candidemia in cancer patients carries a 50% mortality risk. *C. albicans* is the most common cause, accounting for 33–64% of episodes [44]. In addition, *C. glabrata* and *C. krusei* were causative organisms in 11% and 15% of candidemia episodes in patients with hematologic malignancies, and 20% and 0.7% in patients with solid tumors, respectively [44]. Fluconazole resistance was evidenced in all cases of *C. krusei* and 68% of *C. glabrata* infections [44]. Major risk factors include hematologic malignancies, neutropenia, use of corticosteroids and cyclosporine, and chemotherapy and radiotherapy conditioning regimens [45].

Cutaneous involvement resulting from systemic candidiasis occurs in 13% of cases [45], with *C. tropicalis* being more prone to affect skin. In one series, *C. tropicalis*, *C. albicans*, and *C. glabrata* were responsible for skin infection in 63%, 26%, and 11% of patients, respectively [46]. The morphology of lesions can vary from multiple erythematous or purpuric maculopapules or nodules to plaques with central pustules [46]. The majority of patients present with a generalized rash, while others develop lower extremities lesions [46].

Blood cultures are negative in up to 75%, so skin biopsies are important, revealing dermal aggregates of pseudohyphae and spores with necrosis, vascular damage, and perivascular lymphocytic infiltrate [45]. The (1,3)-β-D-glucan assay may aid in diagnosis: (1,3)-β-D-glucan is produced by most fungi with the exception of Zygomycetes and *Cryptococcus* species. The treatment recommendations from the Infectious Diseases Society of America (IDSA) [47] suggest that in the non-neutropenic patient with invasive candidiasis, fluconazole can be considered. In the neutropenic patient, an echinocandin is recommended. Other factors that should be taken into consideration include the patient's hemodynamic stability, the local microbiologic epidemiology (i.e., Has your medical center observed azole or echinocandin resistant *Candida* infections?), and the recent history of antimicrobial therapy (Has the patient received azole or echinocandin prophylaxis or therapy recently?). With the rising incidence of azole and echinocandin resistant invasive candidiasis, it is advisable to consider initiating echinocandin or amphotericin B lipid formulation therapy until you receive microbiologic data that allows you to "step down" the therapy. Finally, if the patient has documented (positive blood cultures) candidemia, the central venous catheter should be removed.

Invasive cryptococcosis

Secondary involvement of skin as a sequela of disseminated cryptococcal infection can occur in patients with hematologic malignancies, underlying T-cell mediated immunity, and corticosteroid therapy [40]. In fact, the most common form of skin involvement is caused by systemic infection, acquired following lung inoculation, seen in 10–20% of cases [41]. The clinical presentation is nonspecific and varies from nodules and ulcerated plaques to umbilicated papules [30]. On histologic examination, spherical budding yeast with an accompanying polymorphous inflammatory infiltrate is observed [40]. An additional diagnostic test is the serum cryptococcal antigen assay. The treatment of choice for disseminated cryptococcosis in the immunocompromised host is liposomal (or conventional) amphotericin B plus flucytosine. An alternative therapy would be fluconazole with or without flucytosine.

Invasive mold infections
Invasive fusariosis

In contrast to systemic infections with *Candida* species, cutaneous involvement occurs much more frequently (75–90%) in patients with disseminated *Fusarium* infection [38]. Conversely, a primary cutaneous nidus of *Fusarium* infection can serve as a source for systemic dissemination in 33% of patients [38]. Among 16 patients with disseminated skin lesions, there was a preceding history of cellulitis adjacent to onychomycosis (11 patients), local trauma (3 patients), and insect bites (2 patients) [39].

Prolonged (>10 days) and profound (<100/mm^3) neutropenia are major risk factors, as seen in acute leukemia and HCT patients [37]. Patients with neutropenia are at much higher risk of developing disseminated *Fusarium* skin lesions than non-neutropenic counterparts (94% vs. 41%, *p* < 0.001) [39]. Multiple species may be implicated, including *F. solani, F. moniliforme, F. oxysporum,* or *F. proliferatum* [38]. The typical presentation is of rapidly developing, multiple, widespread erythematous papular or nodular painful lesions anywhere on the body with predilection for extremities. Lesions may mimic ecthyma gangrenosum. In 10% the lesions are targetoid, and lesions at different stages of evolution are commonly seen [37]. Of 148 patients with disseminated cutaneous *Fusarium* infection, 78 had negative blood cultures and skin lesions served as a diagnostic source in 76 [39]. Histopathologic examination reveals invasive hyaline acute-branching septate hyphae with extension into the blood vessels, with thrombosis and necrosis [39]. However, distinguishing *Fusarium* from *Aspergillus* species may not be possible and cultures, *in situ* hybridization and PCR-based methods should be performed [37,38]. Early diagnosis is critical, because the associated mortality is high, especially in patients with persistent neutropenia (100%) and with disseminated skin lesions (76%) [39].

Invasive aspergillosis

Cutaneous involvement with disseminated *Aspergillus* is uncommon and is seen in approximately 4% of acute leukemia patients with a documented infection [35]. Patients with hematologic malignancies, underlying neutropenia, HCT recipients with GVHD receiving corticosteroids are at greater risk [30]. Cutaneous lesions are characterized by erythematous macules that ulcerate and develop necrosis with a central black eschar [48]. In contrast to infection with *Fusarium*, these are usually larger (2–3 cm), and fewer in number [31]. *Aspergillus* species can rarely be cultured [38], highlighting the importance of biopsying skin. Microscopic appearance is characterized by septate hyphae branching at 45° angles with vessel wall destruction, necrosis, and hemorrhage [36]. In addition, serum *Aspergillus* galactomannan assays can assist with diagnosis [30], but if the patient is on an antimold agent, the assay is likely to be falsely negative. The serum test for (1,3)-β-D-glucan test can detect both *Aspergillus* and *Fusarium* infections, but a positive galactomannan essay would be highly suggestive of invasive aspergillosis [37].

Invasive zygomycosis

Disseminated zygomycosis (e.g., *Rhizopus, Mucor,* and *Cunninghamella* species), can be seen in approximately 5% of patients with hematologic malignancies and lymphopenia, with risk factors including disruption of mucocutaneous protective barrier, metabolic acidosis, and concurrent antibiotic therapy [31]. In the HCT setting it now accounts for more than 20% of mold infections [49] and is increasing in incidence [94]. Clinically, the lesions may resemble *Aspergillus* and *Fusarium* infections,

presenting with several 2–4 cm erythematous plaques with central purpura and formation of eschar [30]. Histopathologic examination often permits distinction between Zygomycetes and other molds. Zygomycetes appear as aseptate or pauciseptate hyphae with wide irregular branches oriented at 90° and are frequently twisted or collapsed [31].

Trichosporonosis

Trichosporon beigelii is a fungal organism that can lead to a potentially fatal disseminated infection in immunosuppressed neutropenic patients with hematologic malignancies, with lungs, gastrointestinal tract and skin as potential portals of entry [50]. Approximately 30% of patients present with purpuric papules and nodules which develop central necrosis and ulceration [50]. Histologic examination reveals pleomorphic yeast-like cells, septate hyphae, and arthroconidia, which may be difficult to distinguish from *Candida* species [31]. A culture of the infected tissue is positive in more than 90% of cases [50].

Diagnosis

Diagnosis of mold infections can be enhanced by serologic tests and histologic examination of (preferably) a deep skin biopsy. The *Aspergillus* galactomannan assay should be elevated in a patient with invasive aspergillosis, but a false-negative can result in a patient who is already on an antimold agent. The (1,3)-β-D-glucan assay may help, which is elevated in most yeast and mold infections except invasive zygomycosis and cryptococcosis. Also, false-positive results can occur in a patient receiving piperacillin-tazobactam. If there is evidence of a lung lesion, bronchoscopy (with bronchoalveolar lavage fluid) should be performed. If that is unrevealing, the patient should proceed to CT-guided needle biopsy/aspiration. If there is sinus involvement, sinusotomy with biopsy (or scraping) should be performed.

Approach

The initial approach to suspected invasive mold infection is an empiric one [51]. If zygomycosis cannot be ruled out, a Zygomycetes active antifungal agent should be initiated. This should be an amphotericin B lipid formulation such as amphotericin B lipid complex or liposomal amphotericin B. An alternative choice is posaconazole. If zygomycosis can be ruled out (e.g., the KOH fungal smears or cytologic stains demonstrate septate, acute branching hyphae), then voriconazole is the drug of choice. Amphotericin B lipid formulations, the echinocandins, and posaconazole are second-line choices. Combination therapy is controversial, but if a combination is to be used one of the following is suggested: (i) voriconazole + echinocandin; or (ii) amphotericin B lipid formulation + echinocandin. Therapy should also include the removal of any focus that is accessible and, preferably, singular. For example, a single lung nodule should be surgically removed. Also, an involved sinus should be accessed and drained. A single small peripheral brain lesion should also be considered for removal.

Prophylaxis

Antifungal prophylaxis is reserved for the highest risk groups: (i) HCT recipients; and (ii) acute myelogenous leukemia (AML) and myelodysplastic syndrome (MDS) patients with deep and prolonged neutropenia resulting from chemotherapy. There are many choices for antifungal prophylaxis in the HCT setting [29], but fluconazole remains the standard choice [52]. As fluconazole has no antimold activity [29,53], a prophylactic agent with antimold activity such as micafungin, voriconazole, or amphotericin B lipid formulation is recommended. The antifungal prophylaxis should be given from day 0 through at least day +75 in order to attain a survival benefit [52]. Prophylaxis should be continued beyond day +75 if the risk factors are present (GVHD and corticosteroid therapy). For the outpatient HCT recipient with GVHD and for neutropenic patients with AML and MDS, posaconazole is the recommended prophylaxis. Fluconazole and itraconazole are second-line choices. Finally, there are other measures that can be taken to prevent invasive mold infections in both the inpatient (HEPA-filtered rooms) and outpatient (N95 masks) settings.

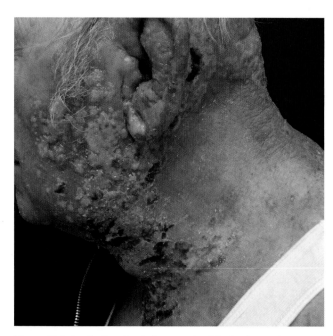

Figure 31.5 Reactivation of varicella zoster virus infection that can be associated with sequelae such as post-herpetic neuralgia.

Viral infections

Herpes simplex virus (HSV) and varicella zoster virus (VZV) are the primary viral pathogens in oncology. They share: (i) early acquisition (usually 90% acquisition before adulthood); (ii) latency until reactivation with immunosuppression; (iii) vesicular lesions; and (iv) ability to disseminate (both cutaneously and viscerally) in severely immunocompromised hosts. What differentiates these two viral infections is the timing of onset after HCT: HSV occurs from pre-day 0 (–7) up through the day of engraftment while VZV occurs after 3 months post-HCT. Although cytomegalovirus (CMV) is also a herpesvirus and was formerly the most devastating viral infection in HCT patients, it rarely manifests itself with cutaneous lesions.

Herpes simplex virus infections

Herpes simplex virus (HSV-1/HSV-2) can result in a primary infection or reactivation of a latent infection. Seropositive patients undergoing HCT have a risk ranging 37–62%, of developing mucocutaneous lesions. This is in contrast to less than 2% of those who develop a primary infection [54]. Up to 33% of acute leukemia patients being treated with conventional chemotherapy may develop reactivation of HSV [54]. Similarly, patients with chronic lymphocytic leukemia (CLL) are at increased risk for frequent and severe infections [55]. Immunosuppressed patients may have atypical presentations, including ulcerations developing over several years [56,57]. In cases in which diagnosis is not straightforward, direct fluorescent antibody test, culture, or a skin biopsy may be necessary [56].

Prophylaxis with oral acyclovir or valacyclovir in patients undergoing HCT results in significant reduction of lesions compared with no prophylaxis (0–7% vs. 85% and 2.7% vs. 45%, respectively). Treatment should begin with conditioning to at least 4 weeks after the transplant, or in patients with leukemia, particularly those treated with alemtuzumab and purine analogs [54].

The treatment approach to cutaneous HSV without evidence of visceral (e.g., lung, brain) involvement in a patient not on anti-HSV prophylaxis is 5 mg/kg acyclovir IV every 8 hours. However, if visceral involvement is suspected or cutaneous dissemination is evident, 10 mg/kg acyclovir IV every 8 hours should be given. If the patient is on acyclovir prophylaxis at the time of eruption of HSV, foscarnet should be administered [58].

Varicella zoster virus

Patients with leukemia, lymphoma, and HCT constitute a high-risk population for reactivation of VZV infection (Figure 31.5), with other risk factors including corticosteroid therapy, radiation, surgery, splenectomy, and immunosuppressive therapy [59]. It affects approximately 2% of chronic myelogenous leukemia patients treated with imatinib, 10–15% of CLL patients treated with fludarabine or alemtuzumab, and 25% of patients with Hodgkin lymphoma or autologous stem cell transplant [60]. A reactivation is a significant problem in allogeneic HCT patients without prophylaxis, with occurrence exceeding 30%, clinically manifesting mostly 3–12 months post-transplant [61]. The majority of patients develop localized dermatomal vesicular rash, which may disseminate in up to 30%, with mortality reaching 10% if left untreated [54]. Besides the acute pain, post-herpetic neuralgia, scarring, and bacterial superinfection occur in 25%,

19%, and 17% of patients, respectively [54]. In patients with CLL, infections tend to be more severe, recurrent, and disseminated, and may present atypically, such as edematous necrotic plaques mimicking embolic disease [56].

Certain anticancer agents can increase the rate of VZV infection. In patients with multiple myeloma, bortezomib is associated with an increased risk of VZV infection reactivation in contrast to those treated with high dose dexamethasone (13% vs. 5%) [62]. Prophylactic oral 400 mg/day acyclovir is the recommended prophylaxis in this population [63]. Rituximab has also been associated with VZV infection reactivation in 9.4% of lymphoma patients [64]. Temozolomide, which causes selective lymphopenia in 50% of patients, may increase the risk of disseminated VZV infection [65].

A randomized trial of 800 mg acyclovir bid 1 year following allogenic transplants, was shown to significantly reduce the risk of VZV disease within the first year (5% vs. 26%). There was also a reduction in disseminated disease (0% vs. 10.3%) [61]. However, there was no difference in the rates of VZV disease after discontinuation of acyclovir, with immunosuppression, unrelated and HLA-mismatched donor status being the most important risk factors. Thus, in the setting of HCT, acyclovir prophylaxis is recommended for the first year and longer if there are continuing risk factors (GVHD, immunosuppression) [66]. In leukemia patients who have not undergone HCT, acyclovir prophylaxis is not recommended [54]. Seronegative patients exposed to VZV should be treated with VZV immunoglobulin (if available), within 96 hours of exposure, or valacyclovir [54,66].

Treatment of an immunocompromised cancer patient with zoster not on acyclovir prophylaxis is 10 mg/kg acyclovir IV tid. If the patient was on acyclovir prophylaxis at the time of eruption, 60 mg/kg foscarnet IV tid should be considered. If the patient demonstrates evidence of visceral involvement, 12–15 mg/kg acyclovir IV tid is recommended.

Cytomegalovirus

CMV can cause disease in patients with hematologic malignancies and T-cell dysfunction, with an incidence of 5–75% without appropriate prophylaxis [60]. Serologic evidence of a latent CMV infection is found in 85% of the population. The risk of reactivation in patients with leukemia ranges from 5% in those treated with purine analogs to 15–66% in those receiving alemtuzumab [54]. In HCT patients, the risk of reactivation is higher and not seen until after engraftment, with a peak incidence between days 45 and 60 [54]. A viremia invariably precedes the disease by approximately 2 weeks, which may be asymptomatic to disseminated involvement of multiple organs, including the lungs, gastrointestinal tract, central nervous system, retina, liver, renal system, and bone marrow [60]. CMV pneumonitis is associated with a mortality of up to 100% [54]. In contrast, cutaneous manifestations of CMV infection are rare [67]. If present, they present as multiple ulcerations, erosions, or nodules affecting the anogenital region [67]. In the AIDS population,

lesions include vesicles, pruritic macules, verrucous lesions, erythematous and crusted papules, and digital infarcts [68]. The diagnosis can be established using a rapid culture, CMV antigen assays, and PCR-based molecular tests [60]. In the HCT setting, the standard of care for CMV infection is the "pre-emptive" approach [66], with monitoring (usually twice a week) for viremia beginning after engraftment. When CMV begins to rise, pre-emptive therapy (usually with ganciclovir or foscarnet) is initiated. If CMV disease arises while the patient is not receiving pre-emptive therapy, the drug of choice is ganciclovir. If the patient is neutropenic, foscarnet should be used. If either disease or CMV PCR does not respond to either ganciclovir or foscarnet, cidofovir should be considered.

Parasitic infections

In general, parasitic involvement of cutaneous structures is uncommon among cancer patients, but in an appropriate setting (e.g., recent immigration from or travel to an endemic area) should be considered as part of the differential diagnosis.

Disseminated toxoplasmosis is a potentially fatal infection, and in recipients of HCT most cases are diagnosed postmortem [69]. In general, among the HCT patients in the United States, the prevalence of toxoplasmosis is less than 0.5%, with skin involvement rare [69]. The prevalence in high risk cancer patients is low, likely because of the standard use of trimethoprim-sulfamethoxazole prophylaxis (for *Pneumocystis (carinii) jiroveci*). Reported clinical presentations vary, with purplish papules or nodules with mild hyperemia and indistinct borders affecting any body area [69–71]. Biopsy of affected skin can demonstrate multiple *Toxoplasma* bradyzoites within keratinocytes in the epidermis, skin appendages, dermal blood vessels, or tachyzoites (free parasites) in the dermis [69,70]. Distinction of *T. gondii* on histologic sections may not always be possible and the diagnosis should be confirmed with immunohistochemistry or PCR [70]. The primary therapy for toxoplasmosis is pyrimethamine/sulfadiazine and folinic acid or trimethoprim-sulfamethoxazole. Alternative therapy is pyrimethamine and folinic acid with one of the following: (i) clindamycin; (ii) clarithromycin; (iii) azithromycin; or (iv) atovaquone. If a seropositive patient (for *Toxoplasma*) cannot receive trimethoprim-sulfamethoxazole, PCRs may be used to follow levels and the patient treated as needed.

Cutaneous manifestations of disseminated *Strongyloides stercoralis* have been reported in a glioblastoma patient treated with temozolomide and corticosteroids, manifesting as a morbilliform rash affecting the abdomen and lower extremities [72]. Either ivermectin or albendazole can be used, but disseminated disease is potentially fatal and should be treated with a combination therapy [72].

Acanthamoeba infection can also be observed in HCT patients: papular and ulcerated lesions, involving the face, legs, and arms in a patient treated with tacrolimus, mycophenolate mofetil, and corticosteroids for chronic GVHD, have been reported [73]. Histopathologic examination of involved skin demonstrated amebic trophozoites and cyst forms. Similarly to *T. gondii*, diagnosis is challenging and in most patients is made postmortem [73]. Based on previous case reports and *in vitro* data, lipid amphotericin B, voriconazole, trimethoprim-sulfamethoxazole, and miltefosine have been used for treatment [73].

Infections attributable to specific anticancer treatment modalities or their sequelae

Novel targeted epidermal growth factor receptor inhibitors

The emergence of epidermal growth factor receptor inhibitors (EGFRIs) for a variety of solid malignancies has improved the outcome and made treatments more tolerable, reducing systemic toxicities such as myelosuppression [74]. The fundamental principle underlying the use of these agents is their ability to inhibit an epidermal growth factor receptor, which is commonly overexpressed in many epithelial tumors [75]. However, this receptor normally plays a critical part in the normal development and function of the integument, mediating formation of a protective layer of stratified squamous epithelium [76]. Thus, it is not unexpected that multiple dermatologic adverse events (AEs), including a papulopustular rash of the face and trunk (80%), nail toxicities (10–16%), xerosis (7–35%), pruritus (10–16%), and alopecia (5–6%) are observed [77]. These AEs render patients more susceptible to dermatologic infections; an analysis of 221 patients treated with EGFRIs revealed that 38% developed infection, which were polybacterial in 23.5% [77]. Bacterial infections were the most common type (29%), with *S. aureus* as the most common pathogen (22.6%, MRSA in 5.4% of patients; Figure 31.6). Among other pathogens, *Pseudomonas aeruginosa*, *Serratia marcescens*, *Enterobacter aerogenes*, and *Klebsiella pneumoniae* were encountered less commonly. The most common sites of bacterial infections were the seborrheic regions, commonly affected by the papulopustular rash. Other sites of infection

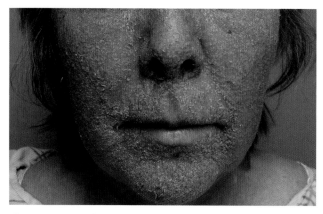

Figure 31.6 Superinfection of epidermal growth factor receptor inhibitor-induced rash with methicillin-resistant *Staphylococcus aureus*.

included periungual tissues, nails, trunk, and extremities. Fungal infections, of which candidal onychomycosis was the most common (13%), and viral infections, with HSV (3.2%) and VZV (1.8%), were also found. Leukopenia increased the risk for developing such infections [77]. Two cases of *Staphylococcus* bacteremia have been recently reported in patients with severe erlotinib-induced skin toxicities [78,79].

An empiric regimen should consist of antimicrobial agents that cover the most likely and most resistant organisms: (i) MRSA; (ii) ESBL Gram-negative bacteria; (iii) *Candida* species; and (iv) HSV and VZV. Thus, for systemic infections, an empiric regimen might consist of vancomycin, a carbapenem (imipenem or meropenem), fluconazole or an echinocandin, and acyclovir (high dose: i.e., 10 mg/kg intravenously every 8 hours). The regimen can be considerably narrowed as microbiologic reports are received.

It is the standard of practice at some cancer centers to initiate prophylactic therapy prior to initiating EGFRI therapy [77]. This usually consists of topical corticosteroid cream and a semisynthetic tetracycline antibiotic. The purpose of this regimen is to prevent moderate-to-severe EGFRI-induced rash, although it was also shown to decrease grade 3 pustular rash by approximately 70%.

Infectious sequelae of radiotherapy

Ionizing radiation has a suppressive effect on normal host defenses, and also leads to disruption of a normally protective layer of squamous epithelium, bacterial colonization, and superinfection [80]. Similarly, changes of chronic radiation dermatitis, characterized by skin fibrosis and atrophy, render patients susceptible to dermatologic infections [80]. Clinically, moist desquamation, a more severe form of acute radiation dermatitis characterized by edema, fibrinous exudates and pain, can be associated with a bacterial superinfection. However, even the growth of bacteria from the wound cultures may not always indicate an active superinfection, because colonization is common [81]. Among 146 patients with nasopharyngeal cancer that developed radiation-induced moist desquamation wounds, 123 (84%) had positive bacterial cultures without any overt clinical evidence of the wound infection. The most common isolated organisms were *S. aureus* (58.7%) and coagulase-negative *Staphylococcus* (25.7%) with >70% of wounds demonstrating a single species and >60% with heavy growth [81]. On the other hand, colonization with *Staphylococcus* and *Streptococcus* species that produce superantigens may result in prolonged and severe reaction because of activation of antigen-presenting cells and T cells, with subsequent upregulation of cytokines and inflammation [82]. Persistent nonhealing of the wound with increased or new onset of pain, excessive production of exudate, increased erythema, vesiculation, and presence of micropustules may be indicative of an infection (Figure 31.7) [81,82]. In the case of *S. aureus* infection, treatment with an appropriately chosen antibiotic in combination with topical and intranasal mupirocin is recommended [82].

Breast cancer patients treated with breast-conserving therapy appear to be at increased risk for developing breast cellulitis,

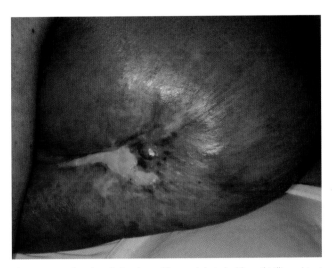

Figure 31.7 Chronic radiation dermatitis superinfected with methicillin-resistant *Staphylococcus aureus* and *Pseudomonas aeruginosa* of the right breast in a patient with breast cancer.

partially attributed to radiation-induced skin desquamation, endothelial injury, edema, and impaired lymphatic drainage, which are further compounded by surgery and axillary lymph node dissection [83]. The most common culprits are *S. aureus* and streptococcal species.

Superficial skin radiotherapy for MF has been reported to be associated with Kaposi varicelliform eruption, a rash characterized by vesicles localized to pre-existing lesions, most commonly caused by HSV, which may be related to cutaneous immunosuppression [84].

An interesting case of postmortem diagnosis of *Sarcoptes scabiei* infection in a patient with CTCL treated with radiation has been reported [85]. The infestation was limited to the upper chest, the area of previous irradiation, with histopathologic and immunohistochemical examination that revealed a reduced number of Langerhans cells, likely related to radiotherapy.

Infectious complications of lymphedema

Surgery and radiation cancer are the two most common causes of secondary lymphedema [86]. In breast cancer survivors, lymphedema has a 5-year cumulative incidence of approximately 42%, with 80% of cases developing within the first 2 years of diagnosis [87]. Recurrent infections requiring antibiotic treatment and potential hospitalizations are seen with increased frequency [88]. Increased susceptibility is multifactorial, with accumulated protein-rich fluid which serves as an ideal culture medium and disruption of the lymphatic system which results in impaired cell-mediated immunity [89]. Of 1877 women, those with lymphedema were twice as likely to develop cellulitis (15.9%) or lymphangitis (14.1%) [88]. Moreover, septicemia and thrombophlebitis were seen in 14% of patients compared with only 7.8% of patients without lymphedema [88]. Cellulitis or lymphangitis in the setting of lymphedema is usually caused by Gram-positive bacteria. Thus, the approach to empiric therapy is

to select the antimicrobial agent that is active against the most resistant possibility (i.e., MRSA) and yet cover the more likely etiologies (i.e., penicillin-sensitive streptococcal species). The choices would be vancomycin, daptomycin, or linezolid.

Erysipelas, a soft tissue infection of the dermis and dermal lymphatics, is most commonly caused by Group A β-hemolytic streptococci and tends to be recurrent [90,91]. In one series, there were more than 10 recurrences affecting 50% of breast cancer patients [91]. Clinically, erysipelas manifests with a raised erythematous tender well-demarcated area with raised borders. In patients with upper extremity lymphedema it can involve any part of the extremity, including the axilla, and is commonly accompanied by high fevers and chills [90]. A search for a potential portal of entry should be attempted as trauma, radiation burns, tinea pedis, paronychia, herpetic whitlow, and insect bites can facilitate the infection [90,92]. Intravenous penicillin G [90], with addition of clindamycin [92] are therapeutic options. In one series, intramuscular benzathine-penicillin G administered prophylactically in patients with three preceding episodes was able to prevent infection in 64% [91]. Although no standard approach exists to determine the onset and duration of prophylactic treatment, antibiotics may be administered for 6–12 months to patients at high risk of recurrence [91]. Even a mild recurrent infection, with erythema and induration, can over time result in significant lymphatic disruption and worsening of edema [89].

Conclusions

Oncology patients are highly susceptible to a wide spectrum of dermatologic infections, with bacterial, viral, fungal, and parasitic organisms being the topmost concerns. Individuals undergoing active treatments with chemotherapy, radiation, therapeutic transplantation, or a combination of these are particularly at risk, considering their relative immunosuppression. An impaired immune system may result in atypical or more severe manifestations and potentially lead to invasive and disseminated disease. Moreover, primary localized skin or adnexal infections may serve as a source for systemic dissemination. Thus, close vigilance and consideration of all potential infectious culprits as part of the differential diagnosis is critical in establishing an early and a correct diagnosis.

References

1 Polsky, B. & Armstrong, D. (1985) Infectious complications of neoplastic disease. *American Journal of Infection Control*, **13**, 199–209.

2 Kloos, W.E. & Bannerman, T.L. (1994) Update on clinical significance of coagulase-negative staphylococci. *Clinical Microbiology Reviews*, **7**, 117–140.

3 Maranan, M.C., Moreira, B., Boyle-Vavra, S. & Daum, R.S. (1997) Antimicrobial resistance in staphylococci: epidemiology, molecular mechanisms, and clinical relevance. *Infectious Disease Clinics of North America*, **11**, 813–849.

4 Miller, L.G. & Kaplan, S.L. (2009) *Staphylococcus aureus*: a community pathogen. *Infectious Disease Clinics of North America*, **23**, 35–52.

5 Trilla, A. & Miro, J.M. (1995) Identifying high risk patients for *Staphylococcus aureus* infections: skin and soft tissue infections. *Journal of Chemotherapy*, **7** (Suppl. 3), 37–43.

6 Gopal, A.K., Fowler, V.G. Jr, Shah, M. *et al.* (2000) Prospective analysis of Staphylococcus aureus bacteremia in nonneutropenic adults with malignancy. *Journal of Clinical Oncology*, **18**, 1110–1115.

7 Carney, D.N., Fossieck, B.E. Jr, Parker, R.H. & Minna, J.D. (1982) Bacteremia due to Staphylococcus aureus in patients with cancer: report on 45 cases in adults and review of the literature. *Reviews of Infectious Diseases*, **4**, 1–12.

8 Mihu, C.N., Schaub, J., Kesh, S. *et al.* (2008) Risk factors for late *Staphylococcus aureus* bacteremia after allogeneic hematopoietic stem cell transplantation: a single-institution, nested case-controlled study. *Journal of the American Society for Blood and Marrow Transplantation*, **14**, 1429–1433.

9 Srinivasan, A., Seifried, S., Zhu, L. *et al.* (2009) Panton-Valentine leukocidin-positive methicillin-resistant *Staphylococcus aureus* infections in children with cancer. *Pediatric Blood and Cancer*, **53**, 1216–1220.

10 Axelrod, P.I., Lorber, B. & Vonderheid, E.C. (1992) Infections complicating mycosis fungoides and Sézary syndrome. *Journal of the American Medical Association*, **267**, 1354–1358.

11 Talpur, R., Bassett, R. & Duvic, M. (2008) Prevalence and treatment of *Staphylococcus aureus* colonization in patients with mycosis fungoides and Sézary syndrome. *British Journal of Dermatology*, **159**, 105–112.

12 Simor, A.E., Phillips, E., McGeer, A. *et al.* (2007) Randomized controlled trial of chlorhexidine gluconate for washing, intranasal mupirocin, and rifampin and doxycycline versus no treatment for the eradication of methicillin-resistant *Staphlococcus aureus* colonization. *Clinical Infectious Diseases*, **44**, 178–185.

13 Nguyen, V., Huggins, R.H., Lertsburapa, T. *et al.* (2008) Cutaneous T-cell lymphoma and *Staphylococcus aureus* colonization. *Journal of the American Academy of Dermatology*, **59**, 949–952.

14 Scheinpflug, K., Schalk, E. & Mohren, M. (2008) Staphylococcal scalded skin syndrome in an adult patient with T-lymphoblastic non-Hodgkin's lymphoma. *Onkologie*, **31**, 616–619.

15 Daum, R.S. (2007) Skin and soft-tissue infections caused by methicillin-resistant *Staphlococcus aureus*. *New England Journal of Medicine*, **357**, 380–390.

16 Brook, I. & Frazier, E.H. (1998) Aerobic and anaerobic infection associated with malignancy. *Supportive Care in Cancer*, **6**, 125–131.

17 Frassetto, L. (2012) Corynebacterium infections. Available from: http://emedicine.medscape.com/article/215100-overview (accessed 19 April 2013).

18 Adderson, E.E., Boudreaux, J.W. & Hayden, R.T. (2008) Infections caused by coryneform bacteria in pediatric oncology patients. *Pediatric Infectious Disease Journal*, **27**, 136–141.

19 Martins, C., Faria, L., Souza, M. *et al.* (2009) Microbiological and host features associated with corynebacteriosis in cancer patients: a five-year study. *Memorias Do Instituto Oswaldo Cruz*, **104**, 905–913.

20 Ashour, H.M. & El-Sharif, A. (2009) Species distribution and antimicrobial susceptibility of gram-negative aerobic bacteria in hospitalized cancer patients. *Journal of Translational Medicine*, **7**, 14.

21 Johnson, M.P. & Ramphal, R. (1990) Beta-lactam-resistant Enterobacter bacteremia in febrile neutropenic patients receiving monotherapy. *Journal of Infectious Diseases*, **162**, 981–983.

22 Johnson, P.R., Liu Yin, J.A. & Tooth, J.A. (1992) A randomized trial of high-dose ciprofloxacin versus azlocillin and netilmicin in the empirical therapy of febrile neutropenic patients. *Journal of Antimicrobial Chemotherapy*, **30**, 203–214.

23 Aubron, C., Poirel, L., Fortineau, N., Nicolas, P., Collet, L. & Nordmann, P. (2005) Nosocomial spread of *Pseudomonas aeruginosa* isolates expressing the metallo-beta-lactamase VIM-2 in a hematology unit of a French hospital. *Microbial Drug Resistance*, **11**, 254–259.

24 Bin Abdulhak, A.A., Zimmerman, V., Al Beirouti, B.T., Baddour, L.M. & Tleyjeh, I.M. (2009) *Stenotrophomonas maltophilia* infections of intact skin: a systematic review of the literature. *Diagnostic Microbiology and Infectious Disease*, **63**, 330–333.

25 Safdar, A. & Rolston, K.V. (2007) *Stenotrophomonas maltophilia*: changing spectrum of a serious bacterial pathogen in patients with cancer. *Clinical Infectious Diseases*, **45**, 1602–1609.

26 Teo, W.Y., Chan, M.Y., Lam, C.M. & Chong, C.Y. (2006) Skin manifestation of *Stenotrophomonas maltophilia* infection: a case report and review article. *Annals of the Academy of Medicine, Singapore*, **35**, 897–900.

27 Falagas, M.E., Rafailidis, P.I., Kapaskelis, A. & Peppas, G. (2008) Pyomyositis associated with hematological malignancy: case report and review of the literature. *International Journal of Infectious Diseases*, **12**, 120–125.

28 Vigil, K.J., Johnson, J.R., Johnston, B.D. *et al.* (2010) *Escherichia coli* Pyomyositis: an emerging infectious disease among patients with hematologic malignancies. *Clinical Infectious Diseases*, **50**, 374–380.

29 National Comprehensive Cancer Network Prevention and Treatment of Cancer-Related Infection. v.1.2013. In: *NCCN Clinical Practice Guidelines in Oncology*. 2009.

30 Mays, S.R., Bogle, M.A. & Bodey, G.P. (2006) Cutaneous fungal infections in the oncology patient: recognition and management. *American Journal of Clinical Dermatology*, **7**, 31–43.

31 Quatresooz, P., Pierard-Franchimont, C., Arrese, J.E. & Pierard, G.E. (2008) Clinicopathologic presentations of dermatomycoses in cancer patients. *Journal of the European Academy of Dermatology and Venereology*, **22**, 907–917.

32 Venkatesan, P., Perfect, J.R. & Myers, S.A. (2005) Evaluation and management of fungal infections in immunocompromised patients. *Dermatologic Therapy*, **18**, 44–57.

33 Myskowski, P.L., White, M.H. & Ahkami, R. (1997) Fungal disease in the immunocompromised host. *Dermatologic Clinics*, **15**, 295–305.

34 Morrison, V.A. & Weisdorf, D.J. (2000) The spectrum of Malassezia infections in the bone marrow transplant population. *Bone Marrow Transplantation*, **26**, 645–648.

35 D'Antonio, D., Pagano, L., Girmenia, C. *et al.* (2000) Cutaneous aspergillosis in patients with haematological malignancies. *European Journal of Clinical Microbiology and Infectious Diseases*, **19**, 362–365.

36 Marcoux, D., Jafarian, F., Joncas, V., Buteau, C., Kokta, V. & Moghrabi, A. (2009) Deep cutaneous fungal infections in immunocompromised children. *Journal of the American Academy of Dermatology*, **61**, 857–864.

37 Nucci, M. & Anaissie, E. (2007) Fusarium infections in immunocompromised patients. *Clinical Microbiology Reviews*, **20**, 695–704.

38 Bodey, G.P., Boktour, M., Mays, S. *et al.* (2002) Skin lesions associated with Fusarium infection. *Journal of the American Academy of Dermatology*, **47**, 659–666.

39 Nucci, M. & Anaissie, E. (2002) Cutaneous infection by Fusarium species in healthy and immunocompromised hosts: implications for diagnosis and management. *Clinical Infectious Diseases*, **35**, 909–920.

40 Courville, P., Favennec, L., Viacroze, C. *et al.* (2002) Co-existent cutaneous cryptococcosis of the forearm and cutaneous alternariosis of the leg in patient with metastatic thymoma. *Journal of Cutaneous Pathology*, **29**, 55–58.

41 Devirgiliis, V., Panasiti, V., Borroni, R.G. *et al.* (2008) Cutaneous cryptococcosis in a patient affected by chronic lymphocytic leukaemia: a case report. *International Journal of Immunopathology and Pharmacology*, **21**, 463–466.

42 Christianson, J.C., Engber, W. & Andes, D. (2003) Primary cutaneous cryptococcosis in immunocompetent and immunocompromised hosts. *Medical Mycology*, **41**, 177–188.

43 Ben-Ami, R., Lewis, R.E., Raad, I.I. & Kontoyiannis, D.P. (2009) Phaeohyphomycosis in a tertiary care cancer center. *Clinical Infectious Diseases*, **48**, 1033–1041.

44 Slavin, M.A., Sorrell, T.C., Marriott, D. *et al.* (2010) Candidaemia in adult cancer patients: risks for fluconazole-resistant isolates and death. *Journal of Antimicrobial Chemotherapy*, **65**, 1042–1051.

45 Pedraz, J., Delgado-Jimenez, Y., Perez-Gala, S., Nam-Cha, S., Fernandez-Herrera, J. & Garcia-Diez, A. (2009) Cutaneous expression of systemic candidiasis. *Clinical and Experimental Dermatology*, **34**, 106–110.

46 Bae, G.Y., Lee, H.W., Chang, S.E. *et al.* (2005) Clinicopathologic review of 19 patients with systemic candidiasis with skin lesions. *International Journal of Dermatology*, **44**, 550–555.

47 Pappas, P.G., Kauffman, C.A., Andes, D. *et al.* (2009) Clinical practice guidelines for the management of candidiasis: 2009 update by the Infectious Diseases Society of America. *Clinical Infectious Diseases*, **48**, 503–535.

48 Khardori, N., Hayat, S., Rolston, K. & Bodey, G.P. (1989) Cutaneous *Rhizopus* and *Aspergillus* infections in five patients with cancer. *Archives of Dermatology*, **125**, 952–956.

49 Pappas, P.G. (2007) Prosective surveillance for invasive fungal infections in solid organ and stem cell transplant recipients. An overview of TRANSNET. In: Focus on Fugnal Infections 17. March 7–9. San Diego, CA.

50 Kim, J.C., Kim, Y.S., Park, C.S. *et al.* (2001) A case of disseminated *Trichosporon beigelii* infection in a patient with myelodysplastic syndrome after chemotherapy. *Journal of Korean Medical Science*, **16**, 505–508.

51 Ito, J.I., Kriengkauykiat, J., Dadwal, S.S., Arfons, L.M. & Lazarus, H.M. (2010) Approaches to the early treatment of invasive fungal infection. *Leukemia and Lymphoma*, **51**, 1623–1631.

52 Slavin, M.A., Osborne, B., Adams, R. *et al.* (1995) Efficacy and safety of fluconazole prophylaxis for fungal infections after marrow transplantation: a prospective, randomized, double-blind study. *Journal of Infectious Diseases*, **171**, 1545–1552.

53 Michallet, M. & Ito, J.I. (2009) Approaches to the management of invasive fungal infections in hematologic malignancy and hematopoietic cell transplantation. *Journal of Clinical Oncology*, **27**, 3398–3409.

54 Angarone, M. & Ison, M.G. (2008) Prevention and early treatment of opportunistic viral infections in patients with leukemia and allogeneic stem cell transplantation recipients. *Journal of the National Comprehensive Cancer Network*, **6**, 191–201.

55 Robak, E. & Robak, T. (2007) Skin lesions in chronic lymphocytic leukemia. *Leukemia and Lymphoma*, **48**, 855–865.

56 Khera, P., Haught, J.M., McSorley, J. & English, J.C. 3rd. (2009) Atypical presentations of herpesvirus infections in patients with chronic lymphocytic leukemia. *Journal of the American Academy of Dermatology*, **60**, 484–486.

57 Smith, E., Hallman, J.R., Pardasani, A. & McMichael, A. (2002) Multiple herpetic whitlow lesions in a patient with chronic lymphocytic leukemia. *American Journal of Hematology*, **69**, 285–288.

58 Ito, J.I. (2009) Herpes simplex virus infections. In: Applebaum, F.R., Forman, S.J., Negrin, R.S. & Blume, K.G. (eds), *Thomas' Hematopoietic Cell Transplantation*, 4th ed., pp. 1382–1387. Wiley-Blackwell, Oxford.

59 Mattiuzzi, G.N., Cortes, J.E., Talpaz, M. *et al.* (2003) Development of Varicella-Zoster virus infection in patients with chronic myelogenous leukemia treated with imatinib mesylate. *Clinical Cancer Research*, **9**, 976–980.

60 Wade, J.C. (2006) Viral infections in patients with hematological malignancies. *Hematology/the Education Program of the American Society of Hematology. American Society of Hematology. Education Program*, 368–374.

61 Boeckh, M., Kim, H.W., Flowers, M.E., Meyers, J.D. & Bowden, R.A. (2006) Long-term acyclovir for prevention of varicella zoster virus disease after allogeneic hematopoietic cell transplantation: a randomized double-blind placebo-controlled study. *Blood*, **107**, 1800–1805.

62 Chanan-Khan, A., Sonneveld, P., Schuster, M.W. *et al.* (2008) Analysis of herpes zoster events among bortezomib-treated patients in the phase III APEX study. *Journal of Clinical Oncology*, **26**, 4784–4790.

63 Vickrey, E., Allen, S., Mehta, J. & Singhal, S. (2009) Acyclovir to prevent reactivation of varicella zoster virus (herpes zoster) in multiple myeloma patients receiving bortezomib therapy. *Cancer*, **115**, 229–232.

64 Aksoy, S., Harputluoglu, H., Kilickap, S. *et al.* (2007) Rituximab-related viral infections in lymphoma patients. *Leukemia and Lymphoma*, **48**, 1307–1312.

65 Schwarzberg, A.B., Stover, E.H., Sengupta, T. *et al.* (2007) Selective lymphopenia and opportunistic infections in neuroendocrine tumor patients receiving temozolomide. *Cancer Investigation*, **25**, 249–255.

66 Tomblyn, M., Chiller, T., Einsele, H. *et al.* (2009) Guidelines for preventing infectious complications among hematopoietic cell transplantation recipients: a global perspective. *Biology of Blood and Marrow Transplantation*, **15**, 1143–1238.

67 Choi, Y.L., Kim, J.A., Jang, K.T. *et al.* (2006) Characteristics of cutaneous cytomegalovirus infection in non-acquired immune deficiency syndrome, immunocompromised patients. *British Journal of Dermatology*, **155**, 977–982.

68 Leal, L., Carrascosa, J.M., Boada, A. & Ferrandiz, C. (2009) Mucous membrane ulcers in an immunocompromised patient. Cutaneous cytomegalovirus infection. *Archives of Dermatology*, **145**, 931–936.

69 Lee, S.A., Diwan, A.H., Cohn, M., Champlin, R. & Safdar, A. (2005) Cutaneous toxoplasmosis: a case of confounding diagnosis. *Bone Marrow Transplantation*, **36**, 465–466.

70 Amir, G., Salant, H., Resnick, I.B. & Karplus, R. (2008) Cutaneous toxoplasmosis after bone marrow transplantation with molecular confirmation. *Journal of the American Academy of Dermatology*, **59**, 781–784.

71 Leyva, W.H. & Santa Cruz, D.J. (1986) Cutaneous toxoplasmosis. *Journal of the American Academy of Dermatology*, **14**, 600–605.

72 Aregawi, D., Lopez, D., Wick, M., Scheld, W.M. & Schiff, D. (2009) Disseminated strongyloidiasis complicating glioblastoma therapy: a case report. *Journal of Neuro-Oncology*, **94**, 439–443.

73 Kaul, D.R., Lowe, L., Visvesvara, G.S., Farmen, S., Khaled, Y.A. & Yanik, G.A. (2008) Acanthamoeba infection in a patient with chronic graft-versus-host disease occurring during treatment with voriconazole. *Transplant Infectious Disease*, **10**, 437–441.

74 Vokes, E.E. & Chu, E. (2006) Anti-EGFR therapies: clinical experience in colorectal, lung, and head and neck cancers. *Oncology (Williston Park, N.Y.)*, **20**, 15–25.

75 Li, T. & Perez-Soler, R. (2009) Skin toxicities associated with epidermal growth factor receptor inhibitors. *Targeted Oncology*, **4**, 107–119.

76 Jost, M., Kari, C. & Rodeck, U. (2000) The EGF receptor: an essential regulator of multiple epidermal functions. *European Journal of Dermatology*, **10**, 505–510.

77 Eilers, R.E. Jr, Gandhi, M., Patel, J.D. *et al.* (2010) Dermatologic infections in cancer patients treated with epidermal growth factor receptor inhibitor therapy. *Journal of the National Cancer Institute*, **102**, 47–53.

78 Li, J., Peccerillo, J., Kaley, K. & Saif, M.W. (2009) *Staphylococcus aureus* bacteremia related with erlotinib skin toxicity in a patient with pancreatic cancer. *Journal of the Pancreas*, **10**, 338–340.

79 Grenader, T., Gipps, M. & Goldberg, A. (2008) *Staphylococcus aureus* bacteremia secondary to severe erlotinib skin toxicity. *Clinical Lung Cancer*, **9**, 59–60.

80 Hymes, S.R., Strom, E.A. & Fife, C. (2006, 2006) Radiation dermatitis: clinical presentation, pathophysiology, and treatment. *Journal of the American Academy of Dermatology*, **54**, 28–46.

81 Mak, S.S., Yuen, M.L., Li, C. *et al.* (2006) Exploratory analysis of the bacteriological status of post-irradiation wounds and its relationship to healing. *Clinical Oncology (Royal College of Radiologists (Great Britain))*, **18**, 519–524.

82 Hill, A., Hanson, M., Bogle, M.A. & Duvic, M. (2004) Severe radiation dermatitis is related to *Staphylococcus aureus*. *American Journal of Clinical Oncology*, **27**, 361–363.

83 Hughes, L.L., Styblo, T.M., Thoms, W.W. *et al.* (1997) Cellulitis of the breast as a complication of breast-conserving surgery and irradiation. *American Journal of Clinical Oncology*, **20**, 338–341.

84 Smith, B.D., Son, C.B. & Wilson, L.D. (2003) Disseminated herpes simplex after total skin electron beam radiotherapy for mycosis fungoides. *Journal of the Royal Society of Medicine*, **96**, 500–501.

85 McGregor, D.H., Yang, Q., Fan, F., Talley, R.L. & Topalovski, M. (2001) Scabies associated with radiation therapy for cutaneous T-cell lymphoma. *Annals of Clinical and Laboratory Science*, **31**, 103–107.

86 Lacovara, J.E. & Yoder, L.H. (2006) Secondary lymphedema in the cancer patient. *Medsurg Nursing*, **15**, 302–306, quiz 307.

87 Norman, S.A., Localio, A.R., Potashnik, S.L. *et al.* (2009) Lymphedema in breast cancer survivors: incidence, degree, time course, treatment, and symptoms. *Journal of Clinical Oncology*, **27**, 390–397.

88 Shih, Y.C., Xu, Y., Cormier, J.N. *et al.* (2009) Incidence, treatment costs, and complications of lymphedema after breast cancer among women of working age: a 2-year follow-up study. *Journal of Clinical Oncology*, **27**, 2007–2014.

89 Sakorafas, G.H., Peros, G., Cataliotti, L. & Vlastos, G. (2006) Lymphedema following axillary lymph node dissection for breast cancer. *Surgical Oncology*, **15**, 153–165.

90 Masmoudi, A., Maaloul, I., Turki, H. *et al.* (2005) Erysipelas after breast cancer treatment (26 cases). *Dermatology Online Journal*, **11**, 12.

91 Vignes, S. & Dupuy, A. (2006) Recurrence of lymphoedema-associated cellulitis (erysipelas) under prophylactic antibiotherapy: a retrospective cohort study. *Journal of the European Academy of Dermatology and Venereology*, **20**, 818–822.

92 El Saghir, N.S., Otrock, Z.K., Bizri, A.R., Uwaydah, M.M. & Oghlakian, G.O. (2005) Erysipelas of the upper extremity following locoregional therapy for breast cancer. *Breast (Edinburgh, Scotland)*, **14**, 347–351.

93 Bradley, S.F. (2007) Eradication or decolonization of methicillin-resistant *Staphylococcus aureus* carriage: what are we doing and why are we doing it? *Clinical Infectious Diseases*, **44**, 186–189.

94 Park, B.J., Pappas, P.G., Wannemuehler, K.A. *et al.* (2011) Invasive non-Aspergillus mold infections in transplant recipients, United States, 2001–2006. *Emerging Infectious Diseases*, **17**, 1855–1864.

95 Slater, C.A., Sickel, J.Z., Visvesvara, G.S., Pabico, R.C., Gaspari, A.A. (1994) Brief report: successful treatment of disseminated acanthamoeba infection in an immunocompromised patient. *New England Journal of Medicine*, **331** (2), 85–87.

Appendix 31.1 Recommendations for treatment of specific microorganisms.

Microbial agent	Suggested regimens	
	Primary	Alternative
Bacteria		
Gram-positive bacteria		
Staphylococcus aureus		
MRSA	Vancomycin 1 g IV q 12 h	Daptomycin 4 mg/kg IV daily
		Linezolid 600 mg po/IV q 12 h
MSSA	Nafcillin or oxacillin 2 g IV q 6 h	Cefazolin 2 g IV q 8 h
		Vancomycin 1 g IV q 12 h
		Daptomycin 4 mg/kg IV daily
Decolonization:	Mupirocin calcium ointment 2% applied to nares 2×/day; diclox 250 mg po 4×/day × 1 mo (or cephalexin 1 g daily) for MSSA; for MRSA add chlorhexidine bathing daily and substitute rifampin 600 mg po daily + doxycycline 100 mg po q 12 h for diclox (and cephalexin); if MRSA doxycycline-resistant, substitute linezolid	
Enterococcus – VRE	Linezolid 600 mg po/IV q 12 h	Quinupristin/dalfopristin 7.5 mg/kg q 8 h
		Daptomycin 4 mg/kg IV daily
Clostridium species	Metronidazole 500 mg IV q 6 h	Clindamycin 900 mg IV q 8 h
Corynebacterium species	Vancomycin 1 g IV q 12 h	Daptomycin 4 mg/kg IV daily
Gram-negative bacteria		
Pseudomonas aeruginosa	Ceftazidime 2 g IV q 8 h or	
	Piperacillin-tazobactam 3.375 g IV q 6 h + aminoglycoside (e.g., amikacin 7.5 mg/kg q 12 h)	
ESBL	Imipenem 500 mg IV q 6 h or	
	Meropenem 1 g IV 8 h	
Carbapenemase	Colistin 2.5–5 mg/kg/day of base divided into 2–4 doses	Tigecycline 100 mg IV loading, then 50 mg IV q 12 h
Stenotrophomonas maltophilia	Trimethoprim-sulfamethoxazole 15 mg/kg/day in 4 divided doses	Ticarcillin-clavulanate 3.1 g IV q 4–6 h[a]
Anaerobes	Metronidazole 500 mg IV q 6 h	
Empiric therapy in febrile neutropenia		
(with cellulitis)	Vancomycin (or linezolid) + Piperacillin/tazobactam or Carbapenem or ceftazidime or cefepime	

(*Continued*)

Microbial agent	Suggested regimens	
	Primary	**Alternative**
Prophylaxis in HSCT		
	Levofloxacin 500 mg IV/po daily	
Fungi		
Yeasts		
Candida species[b]	Fluconazole 400 mg IV daily	Lipid form AmB 3 mg/kg IV daily
	Caspofungin 70 mg IV load, 50 mg IV daily	
	Micafungin 100 mg IV daily	
	Anidulafungin 200 mg IV load, 100 mg IV daily	
	Voriconazole 6 mg/kg IV q 12 h × 2, 4 mg/kg IV q 12 h	
Cryptococcus species (non-AIDS)	Fluconazole 400 mg IV/po daily × 8 weeks–6 months	Itraconazole 200–400 mg soln × 6–12 months
		AmB 0.3 mg/kg IV daily + 5FC 37.5 mg/kg po 4× daily × 6 wks
(severe disease)	AmB 0.5–0.8 mg/kg IV daily until response then change to fluconazole 400 mg po daily × 8–10 weeks	
(meningitis, non-AIDS)	AmB 0.5–0.8 mg/kg IV daily + 5FC 37.5 mg/kg	
(for less severely ill)	Fluconazole 400 mg po q 6 h until afebrile and cultures negative daily × 8–10 wks (approx. 6 wks) then fluconazole 200 mg po daily	
(HIV/AIDS cryptococcemia/ meningitis)	AmB 0.7 mg/kg IV daily + 5FC 25 mg/kg po q 6 h × 2 wks (or longer until CSF sterile) then consolidation rx fluconazole 400–800 mg po daily to complete 10-wk course, then suppression rx fluconazole 200 mg po daily	AmB 0.7 mg/kg IV daily or liposomal AmB 4 mg/kg IV daily alone or + fluconazole 400 mg po or IV daily
		Fluconazole 1200 mg po or IV + 5FC mg/kg po q 6 h
		All the above × 4–6 wks, then consolidation rx fluconazole 400–800 mg po daily to complete 10-wk course then suppression rx fluconazole 200 mg po daily
Molds		
Aspergillus species	Voriconazole 6 mg/kg IV q 12 h	Lipid form AmB 5 mg/kg IV daily
	Load, then 4 mg/kg IV q 12 h	Posaconazole 400 mg po q 12 h
		Itraconazole 200 mg soln po q 12 h
Zygomycetes	Lipid form AmB 5 mg/kg IV daily	Posaconazole 400 mg po q 12 h
Fusarium species	Lipid form AmB 5 mg/kg IV daily	Voriconazole 6 mg/kg IV q 12 h load, then 4 mg/kg IV q 12 h
Scedosporium species	Voriconazole 6 mg/kg IV q 12 h load then 4 mg/kg IV q 12 h	Itraconazole 400 mg soln po q 12 h (*S. apiospermum* only)

Microbial agent	Suggested regimens	
	Primary	**Alternative**
Molds		
Empiric therapy when mold unknown (i.e., cannot rule out Zygomycetes)	Lipid form AmB 5 mg/kg IV daily	Posaconazole 400 mg po q 12 h
Empiric therapy in febrile neutropenia		
(after 2–4 days of persistent fevers despite antibacterial therapy)	Caspofungin 70 mg load then 50 mg IV daily Liposomal AmB 3 mg/kg IV daily	Voriconazole 6 mg/kg IV q 12 h × 2 then 4 mg/kg IV q 12 h Posaconazole 400 mg po q 12 h Itraconazole 400 mg IV q 12 h Fluconazole 400 mg IV daily Micafungin 100 mg IV daily Anidulafungin 200 mg IV load 100 mg IV daily Lipid form AmB 3 mg/kg IV daily
Prophylaxis in HSCT		
Autologous Allogeneic	Fluconazole 400 mg IV/po daily	Micafungin 50 mg IV daily
Neutropenia (IV) to day +75 (po)	Fluconazole 400 mg IV/po daily	Itraconazole 400 mg po q 12 h Posaconazole 200 mg po q 8 h
Neutropenia (IV) to day +100 (po)	Voriconazole 200 mg IV/po q 12 h	Itraconazole 400 mg IV/po q 12 h Posaconazole 200 mg po q 8 h Fluconazole 400 mg IV/po daily
Neutropenia (IV) engraftment	Micafungin 50 mg IV daily	Lipid form AmB product 1 mg/kg IV daily Posaconazole 200 mg po q 8 h Fluconazole 400 mg IV daily
Post-engraftment, high risk	Posaconazole 200 mg po q 8 h	Voriconazole 200 mg po q 12 h Fluconazole 400 mg po daily Itraconazole 400 mg po q 12 h
Prophylaxis in neutropenic AML and MDS		
	Posaconazole 200 mg po q 8 h	Voriconazole 200 mg po q 12 h Itraconazole 400 mg po q 12 h Fluconazole 400 mg po daily

(Continued)

Microbial agent	Suggested regimens	
	Primary	**Alternative**
Viruses		
Herpes simplex virus (HSV)	Acyclovir 5 mg/kg IV q 8 h (if disseminated HSV: 10 mg/kg)	Valacyclovir 500 mg po q 12 h Famciclovir 500 mg po q 12 h Foscarnet 60 mg/kg IV q 8 h (if ACV-R)
Prophylaxis (HSCT)	Acyclovir 400–800 mg po q 12 h	Valacyclovir 500 mg po daily or q 12 h
Varicella zoster virus (VZV)	Acyclovir 10 mg/kg IV q 8 h (if visceral or disseminated VZV: 12–15 mg/kg IV q 8 h)	Valacyclovir 1 g po q 12 h Foscarnet 60 mg/kg q 8 h
Prophylaxis (HSCT)	Acyclovir 800 mg po twice daily	Valacyclovir 500 mg po twice daily
Cytomegalovirus		
Pre-emptive	Ganciclovir 5 mg/kg IV q 12 h induction × 2–3 wk, then daily maintenance	Foscarnet 60 mg/kg IV q 8 h Cidofovir 1 mg/kg q.o.d.
Treatment	Ganciclovir 5 mg/kg IV q 12 h + IVIG 500 mg/kg IV q.o.d. × 21 days	Foscarnet 60 mg/kg IV q 8 h + IVIG Cidofovir 1 mg/kg q.o.d. + IVIG
Parasites		
Toxoplasma gondii	Pyrimethamine 200 mg po load, then 75 mg po daily + sulfadiazine 1.5 g po 4× daily + folinic acid 20 mg po daily or trimethoprim-sulfamethoxazole 10/50 mg/kg IV or po daily in 2–4 divided doses	Pyrimethamine + folinic acid + one of the following: (1) clindamycin 600 mg po/IV q 6 h; (2) clarithromycin 1 g po q 12 h; (3) azithromycin 1.5 g po daily; or (4) atovaquone 750 mg po q 6 h
Strongyloides stercoralis	Ivermectin 200 μg/kg po daily	Albendazole 400 mg po twice daily
Acanthamoeba	No recommended standard of therapy[c]	
Empiric approach to dermatologic infections in setting of EGFRI		
Empiric treatment	Vancomycin 1 g IV q 12 h + carbapenem (imipenem 500 mg IV q 6 h or meropenem 1 g IV q 8 h) + echinocandin (caspofungin 70 mg IV load, 50 mg IV daily or micafungin 150 mg IV daily or anidulafungin 200 mg IV load, 100 mg IV daily) + (if herpetic infection suspected or proven) acyclovir 10 mg/kg IV q 8 h	Linezolid or daptomycin can be used instead of vancomycin
Prophylaxis	Doxycycline 100 mg po q 12 h + Hydrocortisone 1% cream	
Empiric approach to infection in setting of lymphedema		
Empiric treatment	Vancomycin 1 g IV q 12 h	Linezolid 600 mg po/IV q 12 h Daptomycin 4 mg/kg IV daily

AML, acute myelogenous leukemia; EGFRI, epithelial growth factor receptor inhibitor; ESBL, extended spectrum beta-lactamase; HSCT, hematopoietic stem cell transplantation; IVIG, intravenous immunoglobulin; MDS, myelodysplastic syndrome; MRSA, methicillin-resistant *Staphylococcus aureus*; MSSA, methicillin-susceptible strains; VRE, vancomycin-resistant enterococcus.

[a]Can be used in combination with trimethoprim-sulfamethoxazole in severe cases.
[b]Choice of antifungal agent should be based upon probability of an azole and/or echinocandin resistant *Candida* species (i.e., *C. krusei* or *C. glabrata*).
[c]A single successfully treated case of disseminated cutaneous infection was treated with pentamidine isethionate, topical chlorhexidine, and 2% ketoconazole cream followed by oral itraconazole [95]. Other cases of successful treatment (with trimethoprim-sulfamethoxazole, rifampin, and ketoconazole) of *Acanthamoeba* meningitis have been reported. *Acanthamoeba* isolates have been reported to be sensitive (*in vitro*) to pentamidine, ketoconazole, flucytosine, and amphotericin B.

5   Late Cutaneous Events from Cancer Treatment

32 Late Dermatologic Conditions

Jennifer Nam Choi

Yale University School of Medicine, New Haven, CT, USA

Introduction

With more than 12 500,000 cancer survivors in the United States alone, the late dermatologic adverse events from cancer and its treatment are being seen at an increasing rate. With improved survival, patients receiving cancer treatment are now living long enough to experience a range of late adverse events of cancer treatment. It is imperative for clinicians to continue long-term surveillance of cancer survivors and to educate them regarding possible cutaneous eruptions or lesions, as they can be a direct or indirect result of their underlying cancer or treatment. In some cases, they may herald rapidly progressive disease, so their recognition and prompt initiation of treatment can significantly affect clinical outcome. Described in this chapter are four main categories of late dermatologic conditions that can be seen in cancer patients: secondary neoplasms, cutaneous metastasis, radiation effects, and scars.

Secondary skin neoplasms

Secondary skin neoplasms occur in three main clinical settings:
1 In areas of prior radiation therapy;
2 In the setting of chronic immunosuppression; and
3 In association with particular therapeutic agents.

Radiation-induced cutaneous neoplasms

Radiation therapy has been well documented to induce both benign and malignant secondary cutaneous neoplasms (Table 32.1; Figure 32.1). One of the most concerning late effects of ionizing radiation is the induction of malignant diseases. Shortly after the discovery of X-rays by Roentgen, the first published report in 1902 documented the development of a squamous cell carcinoma (SCC) on the hand of an X-ray technician after accumulating large doses of radiation [1]. Since then, numerous reports have shown the association of ionizing radiation and development of skin cancer within the treatment sites, usually with a latency period of 20–30 years. In fact, the excess risk of skin cancer lasts for 45 years or more after treatment [2]. The onset of a radiation-induced SCC has been reported to be as long as 64 years after radiation exposure [3].

Nonmelanoma skin cancers (basal cell carcinoma and squamous cell carcinoma)

Cutaneous SCCs and basal cell carcinomas (BCCs) are among the most common secondary skin malignancies that develop within irradiated areas [4]. These tumors arising in irradiated areas may be quite aggressive and are associated with a higher risk of metastasis than those arising on nonirradiated skin [5]. In the head and neck region, the most common type of cancer following irradiation is BCC, often in multiple locations [6,7]. Over the years, many cases have been observed secondary to low-energy radiation that was used to treat a variety of benign dermatologic diseases, including tinea capitis, hypertrophic tonsillitis, acne vulgaris, atopic dermatitis, hirsutism, eczematous dermatitis, hemangioma, and hyperthyroidosis [6,8–13]. Frequently, this therapy was performed without regard for total accumulated dose. One study showed that in a group of 98 patients with 150 radio-induced cancers of the scalp following irradiation for tinea capitis, BCCs (125 cases) and SCCs (16 cases) were the most common [4]. In this series, there were also three cases of adnexal tumors, two malignant non-Hodgkin lymphomas, and four melanomas. The latent period for radiation-induced skin cancers was 36 (±14) years. In 62% of the patients the scalp appeared normal, while in 38% of patients there was coexistent radiodermatitis. A striking finding was that 82% of the patients had only one session of radiation. The average age at irradiation

Table 32.1 Classification of late dermatologic conditions in cancer patients and survivors.

Secondary neoplasms				
Malignant	Basal cell carcinomas			
	Squamous cell carcinomas			
	Angiosarcoma			
	Other sarcoma, including fibrosarcoma, dermatosarcoma, malignant fibrous histiocytoma			
	Melanoma			
Benign	Radiation keratoses (considered premalignant)			
	Benign lymphangiomatous papules (BLAP)			
	Verruca vulgaris			
	Eccrine poroma			
	Others			

Cutaneous metastases[a]	Men		Women	
	Primary site	**Percentage (total: n = 127)**	**Primary site**	**Percentage (total: n = 300)**
	Melanoma	32.3% (41)	Breast	70.7% (212)
	Head/neck	16.5% (21)	Melanoma	12.0% (36)
	Lung	11.8% (15)	Ovary	3.3% (10)
	Colon/rectum	11.0% (14)	Unknown	3.0% (9)
	Unknown	8.7% (11)	Head/neck	2.3% (7)
	Kidney	4.7% (6)	Lung	2.0% (6)
	Upper GI	3.9% (5)	Colon/rectum	1.3% (4)
	Breast	2.4% (3)	Endometrium	1.3% (4)
	Urinary bladder	2.4% (3)	Urinary bladder	1.3% (4)
	Esophagus	2.4% (3)	Uterine cervix	0.7% (2)
	Endocrine glands	1.7% (2)	Stomach	0.7% (2)
	Stomach	0.8% (1)	Bile ducts	0.7% (2)
	Pancreas	0.8% (1)	Pancreas	0.3% (1)
	Liver	0.8% (1)	Endocrine glands	0.3% (1)

Scars	Port and central venous lines
	Surgical

Radiation effects	Hypo/hyperpigmentation
	Telangiectasias
	Epidermal atrophy
	Xerosis, desquamation, sweat gland atrophy
	Alopecia
	Necrosis of soft tissue, cartilage, or bone
	Subdermal fibrosis (varying degrees)
	Morphea

[a]Adapted from Lookingbill *et al.* [107].

was 12 ($\pm$6) years. Patient age at diagnosis of malignancy varied from 20 to 83 years with an average of 47 years. In a report from the Childhood Cancer Survivor Study, radiation therapy was associated with a 6.3-fold increase in risk for nonmelanoma skin cancer (SCC and BCC). Of these cancers, 90% occurred within the radiation field [14].

Radiotherapy-induced SCC appears to develop after exposure to high doses of radiation, whereas radiation-induced BCC may occur subsequent to moderate or lower doses of radiation (e.g., 4–7 Gy [15–17]). The risk of radiogenic BCCs is suggested to increase with a lower age of exposure and by additive ultraviolet radiation [12,17]. Indeed, studies have shown increased incidence

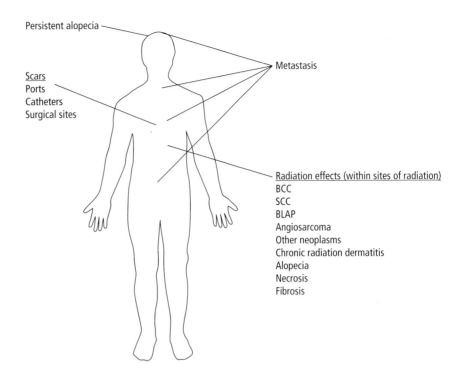

Persistent alopecia

Metastasis

Scars
Ports
Catheters
Surgical sites

Radiation effects (within sites of radiation)
BCC
SCC
BLAP
Angiosarcoma
Other neoplasms
Chronic radiation dermatitis
Alopecia
Necrosis
Fibrosis

Figure 32.1 Anatomic location of late dermatologic conditions in cancer patients and survivors.

in BCC development within irradiated areas among survivors of childhood and adolescent cancer [18]. Radiotherapy-induced BCCs tend to be multiple [6,8–13,19,20] (in approximately 40–46% of cases [12,16]), and may be present as conventional nodular BCC [9,10,13,20], superficial BCC [9–11,19,20], and, rarely, fibroepithelioma of Pinkus (FP, an indolent variant of BCC) [9]. In a retrospective analysis of 76 patients with chronic radiation dermatitis resulting from low-dose ionizing radiation (unspecified dose) for benign disease, approximately 5% of patients developed more than 50 skin cancers within the irradiated site [12]. The occurrence of multiple pigmented BCCs 38 years after radiotherapy for carcinoma of the cervix has been reported [21]. Even more rare are keloidal BCCs, which present as erythematous firm nodules that are hyperkeratotic with a crusted surface [22]. Histologically, keloidal BCCs show a dense collagenous stroma with bright eosinophilic thickened keloidal collagen bundles that contain irregular basaloid neoplastic cords and strands. The cutaneous carcinomas may occur on skin showing concurrent chronic radiation dermatitis or on skin with normal appearance but often with histopathologic changes suggestive of radiation dermatitis.

The frequent and often multiple occurrence of FP in chronic radiation-damaged skin is a known phenomenon. FP was first described as an entity in 1953 [23], the classification of which has been a matter of debate. It is most widely accepted that FP is a type of BCC with a very low malignant behavior. Interestingly, Hartschuh & Schulz [24] showed that hyperplasia of Merkel cells is demonstrated in chronic radiation-damaged skin (similar to that seen in chronically sun-damaged skin and actinic keratoses), as well as in FPs. As Merkel cells have a regulative function on the growth of follicular epithelium, Merkel cell hyperplasia suggests

a causal role in the development of FPs. The hyperplasia of Merkel cells in chronic radiation dermatitis may explain the frequent occurrence of FP due to radiation exposure.

SCC in radiation fields or scars are often ill-defined and exhibit aggressive behavior and metastases [25]. In one study, the incidence of recurrent disease for SCC arising in irradiated skin was found to be 70%. The site of initial recurrence of radiation-induced SCC was local skin in 30% of cases, regional lymph nodes in 35%, and distant metastasis in 5% [26]. When distant metastases occurred, the most common site was bone, followed by lung and distant skin. SCC arising in irradiated skin was associated with a 5-year survival of only 50%, in contrast to the 90% 5-year survival observed in patients with sunlight-induced SCC [26].

The long latency period between development of SCC and BCC after radiation may be due to promotion by ultraviolet radiation. Previous studies showed a trend for higher numbers of skin cancers in patients with sun-reactive skin type I compared with those of types II and III (10% of patients with sun-reactive skin type I had more than 10 skin cancers versus 4% and 5% of patients with sun-reactive skin types II and III, respectively) [12]. Patients with types I and II skin also had a shorter latency period than patients with type III (average of 28 years versus 34 years) [12]. Therefore, patients who have undergone radiation treatment should be counseled regarding avoidance of future excessive sunlight.

The molecular mechanisms underlying ionizing radiation-induced carcinogenesis of the skin is not clear. The most frequently mutated gene in a wide variety of human cancers is p53 [27]. p53 encodes a nuclear phosphoprotein that functions as a transacting transcriptional regulator, controlling the expression of genes involved in cell-cycle regulation. Cells exposed to ionizing

Table 32.2 Treatment options for management of radiation-induced keratoses.

Agent	Mechanism of action	Treatment regimen
Imiquimod cream (5% and 3.75% available)	Activates immune cells via TLR-7 and TLR-8, leading to production of monocyte–macrophage-derived proinflammatory cytokines and chemokines; proapoptotic and direct antitumoral effects	2–5 times a week for 2–16 weeks (best if individualized). Discontinue when severe inflammation occurs. Suggest a test spot within the radiation site for the first week to determine tolerance of individual's skin as severe skin reactions can occur. Associated with influenza-like symptoms in 1–3% of patients
Cryotherapy	Liquid nitrogen provides local destruction of lesion	Liquid nitrogen is applied to individual lesions for 10–15 seconds each. Associated with temporary burning sensation. May result in vesicles or bullae at the site of treatment. Treated lesions will form crust and heal within 2 weeks. Does not address diffuse ill-defined keratoses
5-fluorouracil cream (5% and 0.5% available)	Antineoplastic antimetabolite that interferes with the synthesis of DNA and RNA	Once a night for 14 days. Consider intermittent 'pulse' courses to reduce adverse events. Associated with severe inflammation, pruritus, pain, erosions, possible ulcerations
Diclofenac 3% gel	COX-2 inhibitor; inhibits enzymes involved in arachidonic acid metabolism	2 times a day for up to 90 days (best if individualized). Discontinue if severe inflammation occurs
PDT	Topical MAL or ALA acts as photosensitizer of rapidly dividing cells, and is photoactivated by red or blue light illumination, respectively	Topical MAL or ALA is applied to lesions with an incubation period of 1 or more hours; red or blue light is illuminated for a predetermined number of minutes. Associated with pain and burning sensations during and after treatment. Lesions typically crust and heal over within 7–14 days

ALA, aminolevulinic acid; COX-2, cyclooxygenase 2; MAL, methylaminolevulinic acid; PDT, photodynamic therapy; TLR, toll-like receptor.

radiation accumulate high levels of p53 protein and may be induced into G1 arrest of the cell cycle [28]. DNA damage-induced p53 accumulation may either inhibit cell growth, allowing DNA repair processes, or, in the case of severe damage, initiate apoptosis [29]. It has been shown that irradiation induces significant p53 alterations in the skin, which may be relevant in the modification of epithelial maturation processes and may be responsible for the high risk for development of carcinomas in radiodermatitis [30]. It has indeed been shown that p53 is expressed by neoplastic cells in cutaneous BCCs and SCCs arising in radiodermatitis [30].

Because SCC and BCC arising in scars and radiation fields may exhibit more aggressive behavior and may present with ill-defined margins, surgical excision is the preferred modality of treatment. Microscopically monitored surgery with margin control, otherwise known as Mohs surgery, is an excellent option, which has a high 5-year cure rate of 99% for BCC [31] and 97% for SCC [32] and can be performed under local anesthesia in an office setting. Mohs micrographic surgery has been shown to be effective for high-risk cutaneous SCC, with one study showing a 1.2% local recurrence rate, 4.6% rate of perineural invasion, and 2.3% rate of metastasis [33]. Patients with positive lymph nodes, positive margins after surgery, extensive nerve involvement, and those who are not surgical candidates should be treated with radiation therapy [34].

As a potential precursor to SCC, radiation-induced keratoses occur not infrequently within radiation sites as well. Clinically, these appear identical to actinic keratoses induced by chronic ultraviolet radiation exposure. They are most often pink gritty macules and papules that can coalesce into ill-defined patches and plaques. At times, they can become hyperkeratotic with a thick crust or cutaneous horn. Due to their premalignant potential, radiation-induced keratoses are frequently treated rather than left alone. Among actinic keratoses induced by chronic ultraviolet irradiation, the potential risk for progression to malignancy is approximately 0.025–16% per year [35]. There are no studies specifically addressing therapy of keratoses in irradiated skin, but in practice these keratoses are treated like actinically induced lesions because of the potential risk for progressive to invasive SCC. There are several treatment options for radiation-induced keratoses, particularly when they present as widespread lesions within the radiation site, often referred to as field cancerization (Table 32.2). Cryotherapy is one of the most common means of treating localized lesions, which results in a clinical clearance rate of approximately 68% and histologic clearance rate of 32% [36]. Recurrence rate with cryotherapy tends to be high, with a 12-month sustained clearance rate of 28% [36]. With diffuse ill-defined keratoses, other measures that can target larger areas are used. Options include chemical peels, dermabrasion, laser, or photodynamic therapy (PDT). Methylaminolevulinic acid (MAL) PDT has been shown to clear 50–70% of actinic keratoses clinically, with a histologic clearance of 42% [37].

Specific topical therapies have also proven beneficial. The topical therapies include 5-fluorouracil, diclofenac, and imiquimod. Fluorouracil acts as an antineoplastic antimetabolite agent that interferes with the synthesis of DNA and RNA, thus preventing the proliferation of damaged cells [38]. The short-term average clearance rates of actinic keratoses can reach 96% with a 67% histologic clearance rate, but the recurrence rate is high. The 12-month sustained clearance of initially cleared individual lesions is 54%, while sustained clearance of total treatment field is 33% [36]. Diclofenac is a cyclooxygenase 2 (COX-2) inhibitor, which inhibits the enzymes involved in arachadonic acid metabolism. This inhibition is important as arachadonic acid metabolites have been shown to promote epithelial tumor growth by stimulating angiogenesis, inhibiting apoptosis, and increasing invasiveness of tumor cells [39,40]. Topical 3% diclofenac in a hyaluronic acid-based gel that is applied topically twice daily for 90 days can achieve clinical clearance in approximately 50% of patients [41]. Another promising therapy for widespread keratoses is topical imiquimod [41]. Imiquimod is an immune response modifier of the imidazoquinoline group that binds to toll-like receptor 7 [42], affecting both the innate and acquired immune responses. An increase of mRNA expression of cytokines, including interferon α, tumor necrosis factor α (TNF-α), and interleukin 12 (IL-12), promotes a helper T-cell type 1-mediated immune response, which induces apoptosis of atypical cells [43]. Imiquimod 5% cream has been used successfully in treating chronic radiation dermatitis associated with multiple keratoses, SCCs, and BCCs [44]. Imiquimod 5% cream can produce an initial clearance rate of 85%, histologic clearance rate of 73%, and a 12-month sustained clearance rate of 73% [36]. Patients treated with topical imiquimod have also been found to have better cosmetic outcomes than those treated with cryotherapy or topical 5-fluorouracil.

Angiosarcoma

The definition of a radiation-associated sarcoma includes:

1 Site of origin must be within the field of previous irradiation;

2 Patients should have received a significant amount of radiation therapy (25–80 Gy);

3 An interval of at least 3–5 years must elapse between the time of irradiation and the development of the sarcoma; and

4 The secondary sarcoma should be histologically different from the primary neoplasm [45,46].

The occurrence of angiosarcoma (AS) in cutaneous areas previously treated with radiation therapy is rare. Post-radiation sites is one of the characteristic clinical settings, the other two being on the head and neck in elderly subjects, and on the limbs associated with chronic lymphedema. In women with breast carcinoma treated with radiotherapy, the incidence of AS is estimated to be around 0.4% [47]. The patient's age at the time of diagnosis of mammary AS ranges between 45 and 83 years with a latency period of 29–178 months [48]. In addition to the breast, AS may arise in any cutaneous region subjected to radiotherapy. It has been described in the setting of post-radiation for cervical carcinoma [49], congenital hemangioma [50], on the abdominal wall following radiation for endometrial carcinoma [51], in an angiomatous nevus following irradiation in childhood [52], and in the vagina and bladder [53], among others. In such cases, the

latency period is longer, 48–600 months, with an average of approximately 207 months [48]. It has been reported that the average latency period in the setting of breast cancer patients is 5–6 years following an average dose of radiation of 40–60 Gy in contrast to patients in other clinical settings who develop post-radiation cutaneous angiosarcomas with an average latency period of 30 years [54]. Overall, the latency period between the radiotherapy and the appearance of angiosarcoma appears inversely related to the total dose and strength of the radiation applied, with an average of 23.3 years (range 4–40 years) in medium to low radiation, and of 12.3 years (range 3–25 years) in high dosage [55].

Angiosarcomas often present as numerous erythematoviolaceous macules and papules with a tendency to merge into plaques. AS developing in radiation sites, however, should be considered in any of the following clinical settings: late skin thickening, induration, edema, or dyspigmentation [56]. In some cases there will be evidence of adjacent or preceding radiation dermatitis [48,57].

Histopathology will reveal a proliferation of irregular anastomosing vascular channels lined by a single layer of atypical and pleomorphic endothelial cells in the whole thickness of the dermis. In the deep dermis, the vascular structures may infiltrate the connective tissue with a characteristic dissecting pattern. In the stroma, there may be foci of hemorrhage and an inflammatory infiltrate. Rarely, angiosarcomas exhibit pure spindle cell phenotype [58]. Immunohistochemical studies may reveal positivity for factor VIII and CD31, highlighting the endothelial nature of the neoplastic elements.

The majority of patients (approximately 75%) who develop post-irradiation AS have undergone conservative surgery (partial mastectomy or quandrantectomy). Also in the majority of patients (86%), the removal of the breast carcinoma was accompanied by ipsilateral axillary lymph node dissection. While the majority had undergone axillary lymphadenectomy, chronic lymphedema occurs in only a minority of cases [48]. Because chronic lymphedema is not present in a large majority of post-irradiation AS cases, the role of lymphedema is questionable in their pathogenesis. In contrast, the role of chronic lymphedema in the development of AS arising in the upper limbs of women who have undergone lymph node dissection and mastectomy, known as Stewart–Treves syndrome, is presumed [59]. Additionally, it is presumed to be part of the pathogenesis in the setting of AS arising on lower limbs [60]. The carcinogenic effect of lymphedema may be correlated to the biochemical and immunologic changes in the tissue, resulting in immunologic suppression [59,60].

The best method of treatment for AS is wide surgical excision [61]. However, even surgical excision with negative margins is associated with very high rates of disease recurrence (up to 73% after a minimum of 1 year follow-up) [62]. Given the high recurrence rates, hyperfractionated radiotherapy can be applied before and after primary surgical treatment, as it seems to successfully prevent local disease recurrences in a limited number of cases [63,64]. Not infrequently, wide excision may not be possible because of the width of the involved area. Adoptive immunotherapeutic trials for IL-2-actived killer (IAK or LAK) cells and IL-2 have been introduced for angiosarcomas [65]. The reported overall median survival time for patients with post-irradiation AS is 12 months, in contrast to 20 months for those with nonradiation-associated AS [61]. The overall survival is quoted from 72% after 2 years to 10–35% survival rate after 5 years [66,67].

The differential diagnosis of rapidly growing skin lesions in the mammary region of a patient affected by mammary carcinoma and subjected to radiation therapy should include cutaneous metastasis of the original malignancy, Kaposi sarcoma, and radiotherapy-induced atypical vascular proliferation (AVP). AVP in the setting of post-irradiated skin usually presents as single or multiple papular or nodular violaceous lesions that remain stable over time. There is relative circumscription, empty vascular spaces, and wisp-like projections of stroma in the lumens. Features that are often observed in foci of an AS, including infiltration into the subcutis, prominent dissection of collagen, hemorrhage, tufting and papillary proliferation of severely atypical endothelial cells, are absent [48]. In one study, 83% of benign-behaving vascular proliferations of the skin after radiation therapy for breast cancer stained positively with D2.40, which is an O-linked sialoglycoprotein that targets an oncofetal antigen, M2A [68]. D2.40 is a marker of normal and neoplastic lymphatic endothelial cells. Because positive D2.40 staining has been reported in a subset of angiosarcomas [54], this antibody cannot be used reliably to distinguish between benign and malignant radiation-associated vascular lesions.

Other sarcomas

Radiotherapy is known to rarely cause other sarcomas. Post-radiation sarcomas account for 0.5–5.5% of all sarcomas [69–71]. Most post-radiation sarcomas are now related to radiation for soft tissue neoplasms, including breast cancer [72], lymphoma [73], and genitourinary cancer [74]. A history of radiation for head and neck cancer is also common [75]. The most common histopathologies include osteosarcoma, extraskeletal osteosarcoma, fibrosarcoma, and malignant fibrous histiocytoma [76]. Osteosarcomas account for 17–63% of cases, extraskeletal osteosarcomas can account for 10–40% of cases, malignant fibrous histiocytomas can account for 22–56% of cases, while fibrosarcoma can account for 3–41% of cases.

The mean latency periods for post-radiation soft tissue sarcomas range from 6 to 17 years (range 3–45 years). It has been suggested that a shorter latency period is related to a larger radiation dose. The reported mean and median radiation doses associated with the development of post-radiation sarcomas is 36–49 Gy (range 25–124 Gy) for all post-radiation sarcomas. The latency period may also be affected by the age at the time of radiotherapy. Post-radiation sarcomas have been documented in patients aged 5–86 years.

The edge of the radiation field is at particular risk for the development of a secondary malignancy. It is indeed within or at the edge of the radiotherapy field that post-radiation sarcomas typically occur [77]. Due to lack of homogeneity of dose at the periphery of the radiation field, this area receives a low to intermediate dose range, which is less radiation than the putative tumor dose. This lower radiation dose may be insufficient to kill all viable cells, while causing cell damage and genetic mutations [75]. Tumor development may be initiated as a consequence of a disorganized reparative proliferation. It is therefore the low to intermediate dose range that is particularly important for second cancer risk [78].

Clinically, sarcomas on the skin can present as dome-shaped nodules or tumors that are soft and smooth-surfaced, or can be subcutaneous masses. They may be tender or nontender, and at times can be fluctuant or ulcerated [79,80].

The diagnosis of skin tumors with a sarcoma-like histology requires in-depth immunohistochemical investigations using a panel of antibodies including vimentin, cytokeratin, S-100, desmin, and CD34 [81]. The prognosis for post-radiation sarcomas is generally poor, with a median or mean survival of 0.66–2.4 years [75].

Melanoma and pigmented lesions

The occurrence of malignant melanoma in skin areas exposed to ionizing radiation has been reported, but is exceedingly rare [82–85]. Cutaneous melanoma may account for as many as 7% of malignant neoplasms in survivors of retinoblastoma, although a minority arise within the radiation field [86]. Reports of melanoma occurring within the radiation field have documented intervals ranging from simultaneous with the radiation up to 45 years later. The role of ionizing radiation in producing carcinogenic effects on melanocytes is not known. One study has shown that the ultrastructural effect of Grenz rays on melanocytes was similar to those caused by ultraviolet A: an increase in the number of premature and mature melanosomes, elongation and protrusion of cytoplasm, indented nuclei, and development of multilamella of basal lamina [87]. The prognosis of cutaneous melanoma occurring within a radiation field is unknown because case reports rarely give long-term follow-up. While secondary melanomas resulting from radiation are very uncommon, the diagnosis must be considered when evaluating any pigmented lesion that arises in a site of prior radiation.

Apart from melanoma, melanocytic nevi with atypia are also known to occur within radiation sites. Due to coexistent atrophy and fibrosis in these sites, pigmented lesions can develop features that make them highly suspicious for malignant melanoma. Such lesions have been called "pseudomelanoma" through the disorganization of the normal cutaneous structure caused by fibrosis and atrophy [88]. In such cases, complete excisional biopsies are usually recommended in order to rule out malignancy and clinicopathologic correlation is crucial.

Radiation-induced benign neoplasms

Radiation therapy can induce a variety of secondary neoplasms that are benign in histology and behavior. Among these is an entity that has been termed benign lymphangiomatous papules

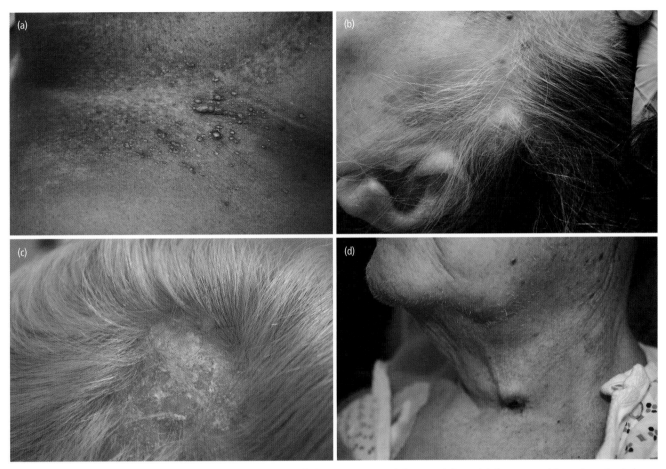

Figure 32.2 (a) Benign lymphagiomatous papules within the radiation site for breast cancer. Several discrete and clustered 1–5 mm tan to pink papules and vesicular papules. Histology confirmed benign lymphangiomas. (b) Skin-colored, slightly erythematous firm nodule on the temple of a patient with metastatic breast cancer. (c) Alopecia neoplastica showing a patch of hair loss with erythema and scale in a patient with metastatic breast cancer. Histology confirmed underlying breast metastasis. (d) Erythematous firm nodules on the left mandibular area and left neck on a patient with metastatic lung adenocarcinoma. Histology confirmed lung metastases.

(BLAP) after radiotherapy. In the past 20 years, various terminologies have been used to describe the same entity, including acquired lymphangiectasis, acquired (progressive) lymphangioma, lymphangioma circumscriptum, and benign lymphangioendothelioma. BLAP typically occurs in females who have undergone radiotherapy, most frequently for breast cancer. Patients present with solitary or few papules or vesicles, usually each less than 5 mm in size, which can be skin-colored or erythematous (Figure 32.2a) [89,90]. Because of their vesicular nature, the papules can also appear translucent or hemorrhagic and be associated with clear fluid exudate when traumatized. Histology reveals a wedge-shaped lesion with dilated vascular spaces in the upper dermis. There is relative circumscription, monomorphous nuclei of endothelial cells with small or no nucleoli, and absence of mitotic features [89]. These features help to distinguish BLAP from angiosarcoma, which is the main differential diagnosis. BLAP do not progress into malignant lesions, but therapy may be pursued through excision or electrodessication if they become problematic because of traumatization or growth.

The occurrence of other benign lesions, such as numerous grouped verruca vulgaris, appearing as 1–7 mm verrucous papules strictly in the radiotherapy fields of the chest wall and axilla 6 months after breast cancer radiation therapy, has been described [91]. Additionally, the development of eccrine poromas, which typically present as well-circumscribed skin-colored firm nodules within a radiation field, has been reported [92].

Association with chronic immunosuppression

It is well-recognized that chronic immunosuppression is a risk factor for cutaneous SCC. Organ transplant patients are greater than 100 times more likely to develop SCC during their lifetime than the general population [93]. Similarly, patients with chronic lymphocytic leukemia (CLL) have been found to have an 8- to 10-fold increased risk for developing skin cancer, particularly SCCs [94]. Due to their lack of both cell-mediated and humoral immunity, patients with CLL are susceptible to tumor recurrence and metastasis of aggressive SCCs and BCCs. It has been demonstrated that after Mohs micrographic surgical excisions, the rate of recurrence in patients with CLL is 7 times higher for

SCC and 14 times higher for BCC than in similar patients without CLL [95,96]. Studies of cutaneous secondary skin cancers from CLL patients have found a significantly increased rate of human papilloma virus (HPV) presence by polymerase chain reaction (PCR) when compared with skin cancers from a control population without CLL (62.5% versus 0%, $p = 0.003$) [97], indicating that HPV may have a pathogenic role in immunosuppressed cancer patients.

Among patients with mycosis fungoides (MF) and Sézary syndrome, the rate of secondary malignancy is also elevated, reported as being 2.4 times that of a control population, with a relative frequency of 15.6% [98]. Among these secondary malignancies, cutaneous SCCs and BCCs are the most common. The SCCs that occur in MF patients tend to be more aggressive, more likely to metastasize, and more likely to occur on non-sun-exposed areas, compared with SCCs in the general population. It is possible that the treatment modalities for MF may compound the risk, as many of them have carcinogenic potential. Increased rates of nonmelanoma skin cancer have been reported in association with use of topical nitrogen mustard, photo-chemotherapy (e.g., PUVA), and radiotherapy (e.g., total skin electron beam). The latency period can be 2–21 years [99]. The risk of developing a second malignancy in MF appears to be greater in patients who have more advanced disease or have been treated with multiple modalities. Many of these nonmelanoma skin cancers occur in sun-exposed areas, suggesting that sun exposure or prior actinic damage may have a role. However, the fact that these skin cancers also occur in non-sun-exposed areas and in patients with no history of increased sun exposure or prior carcinogenic therapies implies that innate T-cell immunity defects in MF are also likely to have a role [99].

Regular skin cancer screening is important for cancer patients, particularly in certain diseases such as CLL and MF. Because of the aggressive behavior of secondary malignancies in these patients, rapid detection and treatment is imperative to minimize risk of a fatal outcome.

Association with therapeutic agents

There have been few associations of development of skin cancer with certain therapeutic agents. Keratoacanthomas, as well as actinic keratoses progressing to SCCs, have been reported in patients being treated with sorafenib, which is a multikinase inhibitor that suppresses the actions of Raf kinase and vascular endothelial growth factor receptor [100]. In these cases, patients rapidly develop SCCs after initiation of sorafenib, and do not develop new tumors after discontinuation. It has been hypothesized that the effects on protein signaling of sorafenib through the Ras/Raf/mitogen-activated protein kinase/ERK kinase (MEK)/extracellular signal-regulated kinase [14] signaling circuit, which has been implicated in cutaneous squamous cell carcinogenesis, play a key role [100].

Voriconazole has been increasingly identified as a medication that causes significant photosensitivity. Patients treated with long-term voriconazole (years) show signs of accelerated photodamage, including actinic keratoses, and lentigo formation. There have been numerous reports of development of aggressive or multifocal SCCs in association with prolonged voriconazole therapy [101,102], and more recently the development of melanoma in association with long-term voriconazole therapy has been implicated in a report of five melanoma *in situ* lesions developing in two patients in the setting of extreme photosensitivity [103]. The mechanism of voriconazole-induced photosensitivity is not known. Based on the growing body of evidence of its association with development of skin cancer as a result of its phototoxic and/or photosensitivity feature, surveillance for skin cancer formation in all patients requiring long-term voriconazole treatment is advised.

Cutaneous metastases

Metastasis is defined as a neoplastic lesion arising from another neoplasm with which it is no longer in contiguity or in close proximity within the same tissue [104]. Cutaneous metastases (CM) of internal malignancies can occur in up to 10.4% of patients [105–108]. They account for 0.7–9.0% of all metastases [109]. It is important for clinicians to keep a high level of awareness to detect metastatic skin disease, as prompt recognition can lead to appropriate treatment. The delay or failure in diagnosis may impact the patient's morbidity and quality of life, and recognition of a cutaneous metastasis can certainly lead to restaging of disease and a more accurate prognosis.

In a large majority of cases, CM develop as an evolution of the primary tumor. Approximately 5% of visceral malignancies (excluding cases of malignant melanoma, leukemia, and lymphoma) eventually become cutaneous metastases [108]. When CM occur, the large majority of patients (approximately 75% [110]) have concomitant visceral metastases (usually involving bone, lung, or liver), at the time of cutaneous presentation or during the course of disease. In few cases, they may represent the first sign of an undiscovered unknown internal malignancy (in less than 1% of cases [111] but up to 13.5% in one series [110]) or a sign of recurrence of a supposedly adequately treated tumoral disease. CM can occur in the setting of widely disseminated disease or as the only sign of metastatic involvement.

Tumor invasion of the skin can occur by several different routes: hematogenous, lymphatic, direct contiguous tissue invasion, and iatrogenic implantation [112]. Metastasis is a complex process, in which malignant cells need to detach from the primary tumor, invade and intravasate into a blood or lymphatic vessel, pass through the blood or lymphatic circulatory system, extravasate through a vessel wall, invade the recipient tissue bed, and proliferate within the tissue [112].

The mean age at diagnosis of CM is approximately 60 years, but can range from 22 to 88 years [110]. The time interval between initial diagnosis of a primary tumor and associated cutaneous metastases averages 2–3 years, although metastases arising as late as 22 years after its primary tumor have been described [113].

While the time to appearance may be independent of tumor type, newer data suggest that the time intervals vary depending on the primary tumor type. Hu *et al.* [110] found that cutaneous metastases from cancers of the lung and gastrointestinal tract (colorectal and gastric cancers) occurred earlier (mean of 15.7–19.8 months), whereas metastases from the breast present several years after primary tumor diagnosis (mean of 47.2 months). CM rarely occur in children, mainly because carcinoma rarely occurs in this group. Of the CM that do occur in children, the most common sources are neuroblastoma and leukemia [114].

CM have a range of clinical presentations. Hu *et al.* [110] found that among 141 CM, the most common clinical presentations were multiple nodules in 46.4% of cases, single nodule in 37.7%, plaques or erythematous patches in 9.4%, and ulcers in 6.5%. CM can be mobile or fixed, hard or flexible, pruritic, painful or painless, with colors ranging from skin-colored to pink, red or violaceous. They can have minimal to no overlying skin changes or be associated with bleeding, erosion, or ulceration [113]. Because CM frequently present as asymptomatic and painless, a high index of suspicion must be used when considering the diagnosis of such lesions, or else a CM may be mistaken for a benign epidermoid cyst or other benign neoplasm. CM may be mistaken for other benign entities as well, including hemangioma, pyogenic granuloma, cellulitis, dermatitis, facial lymphedema, or herpes zoster [110,115,116]. Renal cell carcinoma has presented as a cutaneous horn [117]. Gastric adenocarcinoma has presented as an isolated painless swelling of the superior and inferior eyelid [118].

When CM occur, they are generally considered a grave prognostic sign. While the overall prognosis depends on the pathology and biologic behavior of the primary neoplasm and its response to treatment, the cumulative overall survival tends to be less than 12 months [119,120]. Half of patients with CM may die within the first 6 months after the diagnosis [120]. One study found cumulative overall survival rates at 1, 3, 5, and 10 years to be 36%, 23%, 18%, and 3%, respectively [110]. There does appear to be some discrepancy in median survival based on primary neoplasm. Breast cancer patients with CM appear to have a better survival rate than other cancer types (e.g., median survival of 42 months versus 6 months for non-breast cancer) [110]. Patients with CM of lung carcinoma, on the other hand, have particularly poor prognosis, with a median survival of 2.9 months [120]. There is also a better survival for patients with CM only versus those with CM and visceral metastases. In one study, 19 patients with breast cancer with only skin metastasis had 1, 3, 5, and 10-year cumulative overall survival rates of 79%, 51%, 37%, and 11%, respectively. The median survival was 42.15 months, and the mean survival was 57.43 months. In contrast to this group, 32 patients with breast cancer with skin and visceral metastasis had 1, 3, and 5-year cumulative survival rates of 43%, 27%, and 22%, respectively. The median survival was 12.08 months, and the mean survival was 25.22 months (*p* = 0.012) [110]. Overall, CM portends a poor prognosis particularly for patients with cancers of the lung, ovary, upper respiratory tract, or upper digestive tract [107].

Histology

Skin biopsy for histologic examination combined with immunohistochemical staining remains the gold standard for diagnosis. The majority of CM are confined to the dermis and/or subcutaneous fatty tissue. Tumor cells can grow either in a nodular or star-like pattern, within or around dilated lymphatic and blood vessels, or in small groups in a linear arrangement dissecting collagen bundles referred to as "Indian filing" [113]. The histologic appearance of the CM may be identical to the primary malignancy, but, more commonly, the metastasis is dedifferentiated. Particularly in cases when the CM is phenotypically dedifferentiated, a panel of immunohistochemical stains can help in determining the organ of origin. For example, CK-7 and CK-20 staining can distinguish pulmonary and colorectal adenocarcinomas in up to 95% of cases, with the majority of colonic cancers showing a CD7−/CD20+ profile and most pulmonary adenocarcinomas showing the reverse staining pattern [105]. When the histologic findings are ambiguous, there may also be clues to suggest the primary site. For example, signet ring cells may suggest origin from adenocarcinomas of the gastrointestinal tract, while lobules of clear-staining cells containing glycogen in a highly vascular stroma may indicate origin from renal cell carcinoma.

Anatomic distribution

Cutaneous metastases frequently occur in anatomic areas in close proximity to the primary tumor (Table 32.3) [105,107]. The most likely reason is the spread of carcinoma cells through the lymphatic route to areas having common lymphatic drainage as that of the primary site. Breast and lung cancers frequently metastasize to the chest wall, while cancers of the bowel, ovary, and bladder often metastasize to the abdomen [107]. The most common locations of metastases overall are the chest, abdomen, and scalp. Reviews of CM, including a meta-analysis of 1103 lesions, have identified locations on the chest in 28–30% of cases, abdomen in 20%, scalp in 7–12%, extremities in 7–12%, neck in 11%, pelvis in 6%, and face in 5% [108,110]. Multiple sites of CM involving two or more anatomic regions can be seen in up 19% of patients [110]. Distant metastases are not rare, with melanoma, lung, and breast cancers accounting for the most metastases remote from the primary site. CM to the scalp are disproportionately higher in patients with renal cell carcinoma, with up to 50% of CM at this site [107,121,122]. The high degree of vascularity, immobility, and warmth of this region may explain the high predilection for this site.

CM may also develop in scars at a surgical incision site [123]. Examples include CM in the tracheostomy site for laryngeal cancer, a nephrectomy incisional site for a renal cell cancer, and a thoracotomy site for lung cancer [107].

Metastases from solid organ malignancies

In women, the most common cancer that metastasizes to the skin is breast cancer, which accounts for up to 70% of all cases (Table 32.1) [107,121]. In men, the most common CM comes from

Table 32.3 Cutaneous metastases originating from different internal malignancies and their common locations and descriptions.

Internal malignancy	Location of cutaneous metastasis	Physical description
Breast cancer	Chest, abdomen > scalp, neck, upper extremities, back	Distinct clinicopathologic types (see text)
Melanoma	Chest, back, lower extremities	Skin-colored, pink, or dark blue–black papules, nodules, or tumors
Colorectal cancer	Abdomen, pelvis	Dome-shaped, whitish or red nodules; soft plaques; ulcerations; subcutaneous tumors
Lung cancer	Chest wall, back, scalp	Skin-colored, pink, brown, or blue–black; firm nodules, plaques, erysipelas-like, vascular; within thoracotomy incisional sites
Ovarian cancer	Abdomen, back	Firm, dermal and/or subcutaneous papules or nodules; inflammatory, zosteriform, sclerodermoid, within laparoscopy port sites
Head/neck cancer (mainly SCC)	Head, neck > scalp, abdomen, chest, back, extremities	Red nodules, masses; tender, ulcerate; within tracheostomy sites
Renal cell carcinoma	Chest, abdomen, scalp, extremities	Lobulated tumors, fragile, ulcerated or bleeding; involvement of deeper skin layers
Esophageal cancer	Scalp, back, axilla, fingers	Isolated or widespread cutaneous or subcutaneous nodules
Gastric carcinoma	Chest, abdomen, extremities, scalp, face, neck	Firm, red nodules and plaques; erysipeloid-like; within abdominal excision scars
Liver, gallbladder, pancreatic carcinoma	Scalp, chest, legs; peri-umbilical region for pancreas	Inflammatory nodules; eroded or ulcerated tumors; within laparoscopy or catheter sites
Prostate, urinary bladder, uterine cancer	Suprapubic region > abdomen, head/neck, chest, extremities, back	Hard nodules, associated edema or lymphedema, nonspecific macules or papules

SCC, squamous cell carcinoma.

melanoma, comprising 32% of cases [107]. Other common primary malignancies that metastasize to the skin include lung, colorectal, renal, ovarian, and bladder, all with rates between 3.4 and 4.0% for CM [108]. Metastases from head and neck and oral cavity cancers also have a predilection for the skin [105,107]. In contrast, it is rare to see CM from the prostate, pancreas, and liver.

The relative frequencies of CM from different internal organs do not necessarily parallel the overall incidence of the various primary malignancies. In a study of CM among patients in Taiwan, Hu *et al.* [110] found that hepatocellular carcinoma, which has a higher incidence than breast or lung cancer in Taiwan, rarely gives rise to cutaneous metastasis. Similarly, carcinoma of the bladder and ureter, nasopharyngeal carcinoma, and cervical cancer are not frequently associated with CM. These results indicate that the risk of CM depends largely on the characteristics of tumor cells, which is similar among different ethnic groups.

Melanoma

Melanoma is a primary skin cancer; however, it frequently metastasizes to other parts of the skin. In a large analysis of 4020 patients with metastatic disease, Lookingbill *et al.* [107] found that melanoma was the tumor with the highest overall frequency of CM (44.8% of patients with metastatic melanoma had CM). CM in melanoma can occur as in-transit metastases, in which tumor spreads through the lymphatic vessels between the primary

tumor and draining lymph node basin and seeds into the skin. These CM occur in close proximity to the original tumor. Melanoma CM can also occur as distant metastases through hematogenous spread, in which CM can appear anywhere on the skin surface. Clinically, melanoma CM can be skin-colored, pink, or dark blue to black in color, and can appear as papules, nodules, or large tumors [124]. They can appear as singular, clustered, or multiple scattered lesions. Any new nodule in the setting of history of melanoma should be monitored carefully and considered for skin biopsy. In a study of 200 cases of cutaneous metastases, 31 patients with melanoma had a median survival of 13.5 months after diagnosis of CM [120].

Breast cancer

Breast cancer accounts for the most common source of CM in women, partly because of its high prevalence overall. It is the most common cancer in women, and the second greatest cause of cancer mortality in women [125]. At the time of diagnosis, 33% of cases have spread to regional lymph nodes or directly beyond the primary site, while 5% are metastatic [126]. Thirty percent of patients with breast cancer that is already metastatic will have cutaneous manifestations [107]. The average interval between diagnosis of breast cancer and CM is 47–60 months [110,127].

Of all the types of CM, those from breast cancer have the most well-described clinicopathologic types [128]. While these patterns are not restricted to breast cancer, they are encountered more often in this patient population because of the high frequency of this type of malignancy [124]. A study of 164 cases of CM from breast carcinoma showed that 80% of cases presented as papules and/or nodules, 11.2% as telangiectatic carcinoma, 3% as erysipeloid carcinoma, 3% as carcinoma en cuirasse, 2% as alopecia neoplastica, and 0.8% as a zosteriform pattern [129]. In comparison with patients with other forms of visceral malignancy, breast cancer patients and CM tend to have a better prognosis. One-third of breast cancer patients who present with CM may have no evidence of visceral metastases, representing a subset of patients with significantly better prognosis when compared with breast cancer patients with metastasis not confined to the skin [110]. Described briefly below are the common well-described clinicopathologic types.

Clinicopathologic types of breast cancer metastasis

Nodules are the most common clinical presentation of breast CM. They are usually firm and located in the dermis or subcutaneous tissue, ranging in size from 1 to 3 cm. The nodules can be solitary or multiple, and can appear skin-colored, pink, or red–brown (Figure 32.2b) [130]. Carcinoma en cuirasse consists of swelling with pitting edema, with scattered firm papules and nodules overlying an erythematous or red–blue smooth surface. As time progresses, the affected area becomes thickened into a sclerodermoid plaque with minimal inflammatory changes [124]. Clinically, it can resemble morphea. Carcinoma erysipelatoides, also known as inflammatory metastatic carcinoma, is most frequently associated with intraductal breast cancer [131,132]. Clinically, it presents as erythematous warm tender patches or plaques with well-defined, actively spreading borders, resembling erysipelas or cellulitis [133]. If the neoplastic infiltrate causes lymphatic blockage leading to lymphedema, the clinical presentation can change over several weeks into a fibrotic plaque, overlapping with carcinoma en cuirasse. Telangiectatic carcinoma is characterized by pinpoint telangiectasias caused by dilated capillaries [134]. However, telangiectatic CM can also present as purpuric papules, nodules, or plaques on the chest wall, resembling vasculitis [135], sometimes on a background resembling inflammatory metastatic carcinoma. Alopecia neoplastica is characterized by hair loss in association with a cutaneous metastatic lesion to the scalp [136]. Breast cancer is the primary malignancy in 84% of patients with alopecia neoplastica [137]. Clinically, alopecia neoplastica presents as circular patches or plaques of hair loss in a single or multiple areas (Figure 32.2c). They are painless, nonpruritic, and well-demarcated, often with a smooth surface and overlying pink–red color [138]. The consistency is usually firm and the surface may become uneven over time as a result of progression of the underlying metastasis. Eyelid metastases are rare, representing less than 1% of malignant eyelid lesions [139]. Breast cancer accounts for more than 50% of all eyelid metastases [130]. Clinically, they present as painless

eyelid swelling with induration, nodules, or ulcerations, frequently with surrounding erythema. They can involve both the upper and lower eyelids, usually unilaterally, but has been described to involve all four eyelids giving a mask-like appearance [140,141].

Paget disease of the breast nipple and areola complex represents cutaneous infiltration by primary breast cancer, usually in the setting of an intraductal carcinoma reaching the epidermis through a lactiferous duct [109]. Metastatic breast carcinoma can assume the appearance of Paget disease, as a sharply demarcated erythematous scaly plaque or patch on the nipple or areola. It can be unilateral or bilateral [124], and can at times be pigmented [142]. Other, even rarer, clinical presentations of breast CM have been described: zosteriform unilateral vesicular eruption [143], targetoid [144], clown nose (reddish nodule on tip of the nose) [145], nodule in intradermal nevus [146], subungual mimicking acute paronychia [147], pyogenic granuloma-like [115], Sister Mary Joseph nodule [148], and dermatitis-like [149].

Histologically, the metastatic lesions will reveal tumor cells, often associated with fibrosis, and sometimes within blood vessels (such as in telangiectatic carcinoma) or within lymphatic vessels (such as in carcinoma erysipelatoides).

Other solid organ malignancies

Lung CM most commonly present on the chest wall and back, but have also been reported on the scalp, face, abdomen, extremities, and genitalia. They commonly present as single or multiple firm nodules that can vary in color from skin-colored to brown or blue–black (Figure 32.2d). They have also been reported to occur as plaques, ulcerated nodules, erysipelas-like, vascular-appearing, in a zosteriform pattern, and arising in thoracotomy incisional sites and within a burn scar [107,123,150–152]. The incidence of lung cancer metastasizing to the skin in men has been reported to be 24–29%, and 4% in women [105,121]. Colorectal CM appear on the abdomen and perineal regions, but have been documented on the scalp, face, chest, back, and genitalia. Several have been documented to occur within the abdominal incision site [107]. They have been described as nodular, pedunculated, inflammatory, vascular, and cyst-like [109,111,131]. The incidence of colorectal cancer metastasizing to the skin has been reported to be 11–19% in men, and 9% in women [107,121]. SCC of the pharynx/larynx are the most common source of CM associated with head and neck cancers. Other tumor types of the pharynx/larynx associated with CM include epidermoid carcinoma, neuroendocrine carcinoma, and adenocarcinoma [113]. Lesions can appear as multiple nodules, frequently red to red–lilac in color, which may be tender, ulcerate, and grow to large masses [109,113]. CM can involve the abdomen, chest, back, extremities, neck, and scalp, as well as tracheostomy sites [107].

Renal cell carcinomas metastasize to the skin in 4–6% of cases [107,108]. The most common sites of metastasis include the torso (40%), the scalp (25.3%), and the extremities (10.7%) [113,122,153]. Renal cell carcinomas often metastasize to distant sites through hematogenous spread because of its highly vascular nature. Renal cancer CM tend to present as lobulated nodules or masses that ulcerate or bleed easily and involve the deeper layers of the skin [113]. They can be erythematous or violaceous, and can be brown to black in color. Clinically, these vascular nodules can resemble Kaposi sarcoma, hemangiomas, or pyogenic granulomas [124]. Ovarian cancer accounts for 4–10% of all CM in females [154,155]. The most common location is the overlying abdominal wall and contiguous perineal skin, but CM can also occur on the extremities and axillae [156]. They have been described most commonly as discrete, firm, dermal and/or subcutaneous papules or nodules [109,157]. CM from esophageal cancer is rare, accounting for only 2.1% of all CM in men and women [110]. However, among those with metastatic esophageal cancer, up to 8.6% will have skin involvement [107]. They can appear as isolated subcutaneous nodules or as widespread cutaneous nodules, on the scalp, back, axilla, or fingers [124,158]. The most common histologic types are adenocarcinoma and SCC, followed by mucoepidermoid carcinoma and small cell carcinoma [107,159].

Gastric cancer presents as CM as the first clinical manifestation of cancer in 6.4–7.8% of cases [105,107]. CM occur preferentially in males (7 : 3), and usually present as multiple lesions on the chest and face or as single lesions on the chest or abdomen [160]. Clinically, they can be red, violet, or hyperpigmented nodules. Survival time after diagnosis of CM is less than 12 months [160]. Histologically, gastric adenocarcinomas represent approximately 95% of gastric tumors and are further classified as papillary adenocarcinomas, tubular adenocarcinomas, mucinous adenocarcinomas, or signet ring cell carcinomas [160]. Metastatic gastric adenocarcinoma has also been known to present as umbilical nodules, referred to as Sister Mary Joseph nodules. They present as irregular firm nodules ranging in size from 1 to 1.5 cm, with occasional cases as large as 10 cm [161]. The most common origins are gastrointestinal (52%), gynecologic (28%), stomach (23%), and ovarian (16%) cancer [162]. In 14–33% of cases, the presence of a Sister Mary Joseph nodule leads to the diagnosis of a previously occult neoplasm [163]. Survival can range from 2.3 to 17.6 months [162]. CM from carcinoma of the genitourinary system is rare, with an incidence of 0.36% for prostate cancer [153], 0.84% for the urinary bladder [153], and 0.8% for the uterine corpus [164]. Most commonly, they present as firm nodules with a predisposition for the inguinal and umbilical regions [165].

Treatment

When CM are detected, the main treatment options include excision or radiation. There have been few reports of excision of CM leading to increased survival [166,167], and radiation or pulsed brachytherapy leading to durable palliation of metastases [168,169]. Local tumor destruction can also be achieved with electrocoagulation, electroporation, and electrovaporization. Investigational measures for cutaneous metastasis control have included topical 6% miltefosine solution for breast cancer metastases [170], intratumoral injections with a recombinant single-chain antibody-toxin targeted to ErbB2/HER2 [171],

intralesional immunotherapies with interferon-α or IL-2 [172,173], and bleomycin-based electrochemotherapy [174]. Investigations on the control of melanoma CM have included use of isolated limb perfusion [175], topical imiquimod [176,177], intralesional BCG (bacille Calmette–Guérin) [178], intralesional interferon-α and IL-2 [179–181], intralesional interferon-β [182–184], intralesional Rose Bengal [185,186], and bleomycin-based electrochemotherapy [187,188]. Topical metronidazole has also been found to reduce malodor in fungating wounds [189]. Beyond local control, treatment is systemic therapy according to the histopathologic type of tumor disease.

Surveillance

Because of the potential for CM, all cancer patients should receive thorough skin examinations on a regular basis including the scalp, face, eyelids, ears, neck, extremities, chest, abdomen, back, umbilicus, genital and anal areas, in addition to oral mucosa, hair, and nails. Skin biopsies of any new or persistent skin lesions should always be considered in this patient population. In patients with known disease, detection of CM may help in restaging, determining accurate prognosis, and directing optimal treatment strategies. Early recognition of CM will also aid in avoiding complications of the metastases themselves such as ulceration, bleeding, pain, pruritus, infection, and malodor, which could negatively impact the quality of life of these patients.

Metastases from hematologic malignancies

Hematologic malignancies, such as leukemia and lymphoma, can also result in CM. The cutaneous manifestations can arise at any time during the course of the disease and their appearance has a wide range of variation, making it difficult to distinguish them from other lesions. Clinically, they can present as macules, papules, plaques, and nodules that can be pink, red, blue, brown, or purple. The nodules and plaques can ulcerate or form bullae, and the lesions are characteristically painless [124,190].

Leukemia cutis

Leukemia cutis is defined as cutaneous infiltration by neoplastic leukocytes, resulting in clinically identifiable cutaneous lesions [191]. Leukemia cutis has been described in patients with acute myeloid leukemia, acute myelomonocytic leukemia, acute monocytic leukemia, chronic myeloproliferative disease, including chronic myelogenous leukemia, and myelodysplastic/lymphoproliferative diseases [192]. The incidence can range from 1% of patients (such as in precursor B or T-cell lymphoblastic leukemia) to 50% (such as in acute melomonocytic and monocytic leukemia types) [192]. Leukemia cutis can present as single or multiple lesions. They are usually described as erythematous, violaceous, red–brown, or hemorrhagic papules, nodules, and plaques of varying sizes. Legs, followed by arms, back, chest, scalp, and face, are the most common locations [192,193]. Skin infiltration by congenital leukemia is one of the underlying causes of the "blueberry muffin" appearance with widely disseminated erythematous and violaceous papules and nodules [194]. Most cases present after a diagnosis of systemic leukemia has been established and portend a poor prognosis. Studies have shown that patients with leukemia cutis with acute myeloid leukemia or chronic myelogenous leukemia tend to have an aggressive disease course with short survival [195]. Up to 88% of patients with leukemia cutis die within 1 year of diagnosis [196]. In less than 10% of cases, skin infiltration can occur before bone marrow or peripheral blood involvement, and even in the absence of systemic symptoms [196]. This phenomenon has been referred to as aleukemic leukemia cutis, and frequently presents as widespread papulonodular lesions [197]. Diagnosis is confirmed by biopsy, which typically shows dense dermal collections of neoplastic and benign inflammatory cells dissecting collagen bundles and surrounding adnexal structures [193]. Treatment usually consists of chemotherapy targeted to the specific underlying leukemia, though localized electron beam therapy or bone marrow transplant can be considered.

Lymphoma cutis

Skin involvement of lymphomas occur more frequently with histiocytic and lymphocytic lymphomas [124]. It can occur in up to 9.1% of patients with non-Hodgkin lymphoma [109]. The incidence rate is lower in Hodgkin disease, ranging 0.5–3.4% [124,198]. The trunk is the most common site of involvement [199]. Lymphoma cutis may present as widely disseminated papulonodules and plaques, or as single or multiple nodules with no apparent site predilection. They can be erythematous, violaceous, or ulcerated. Histologically, the cutaneous lesions resemble the primary disease. The predominant cell infiltrate is atypical lymphocytes with occasional eosinophils and plasma cells. Depending on the histologic subtype, lacunar and Reed–Sternberg cells can be seen [124].

Chronic radiation dermatitis and other cutaneous radiation effects

The late cutaneous adverse effects (AEs) from radiotherapy often appear months to years after completion of treatment, and are a result of normal tissue injury after cancer therapy. The late skin AEs can be divided into "consequential" late effects, which are late reactions directly deriving from severe acute reactions, and "chronic" or "true late" effects. These late radiotherapy reactions range from the more common manifestations of chronic radiation dermatitis and fibrosis to the less common effects of post-radiation morphea or necrosis (Table 32.1). It is important for the clinician to be aware of the range of different post-radiation skin manifestations in order to prepare their patients for these possible effects, as well as to recognize these entities even if they occur years after radiotherapy has been completed.

Factors influencing skin reactions

Radiogenic skin reactions usually occur in the regions of the radiation beam entry and exit. The cutaneous effects of radiation differ in nature and intensity depending on different parameters, including technique, target, total dose, volume, and individual variations [200]. The effect of single and total radiotherapy doses and the duration of the radiotherapy course upon acute and late skin reactions is known as the fractionation effect. It appears that late skin reactions, as opposed to acute, are influenced more by the fractionation schemes, including fraction size and dose/fraction schedules [201,202]. For example, among over 400 patients treated with radiotherapy for BCC and SCC, 92% had a good or excellent cosmetic result [203]. However, there was an increasing proportion of poor cosmesis (up to 20–24%) associated with increasing total radiotherapy dose (>60 Gy even when given in ≤2 Gy fractions). The surface of the irradiated skin is also important for the development of early and late skin reactions, known as the volume effect. If a total skin dose of 70 Gy is delivered to 100 cm^2, 50% of the treated patients will have skin necrosis within 5 years [204]. If the field dose is reduced to 10 cm^2, the same radiotherapy dose will lead to skin necrosis in only 5% of patients within 5 years. So far, no threshold dose has been found at which cutaneous AEs can be avoided [201]. Overall, the late cutaneous effects tend to occur if there has been continued unprotected sun exposure after radiotherapy, when a large dose per fraction (>3–4 Gy) was delivered, if the total dose of radiotherapy was more than 40 Gy [201], and when large fields were irradiated [205]. While smaller treatment fields, such as 2–3 cm, tolerate hypofractionation better than do larger areas, larger fractions should be avoided if cosmesis is an important consideration [205].

Individual factors, such as age, comorbidities, poor nutritional status, smoking [206], obesity [207], and underlying skin conditions such as actinic damage and problems with skin integrity, may also influence the observed skin changes. Additionally, the use of concomitant medications, such as chemotherapy or radiosensitizers [208], can also affect the cutaneous AEs of radiotherapy.

Chronic radiation dermatitis

The most common manifestations of chronic radiation dermatitis include desquamation, skin atrophy, telangiectasias, and irregular dyspigmentation. The term poikiloderma is often used, referring to the combination of epidermal atrophy, telangiectasias, and hypopigmentation or hyperpigmentation. These clinical features usually occur within the field of the previously irradiated skin, and may present months to years after radiation exposure (Figure 32.3a). In one study of 245 women with breast cancer treated with whole-breast irradiation delivered in the prone position, 27.8% of patients developed grade 1 chronic cutaneous radiation changes, while 2.8% and 1.6% of patients developed grade 2 and 3 chronic cutaneous changes, respectively [209].

The histopathologic features of chronic radiodermatitis include predominant epidermal atrophy with focal areas of acanthosis and hyperkeratosis. Dyskeratotic keratinocytes can be observed throughout the epidermis. Melanin can be seen in the basal layer with melanin deposits in the upper part of the dermis. Dermal

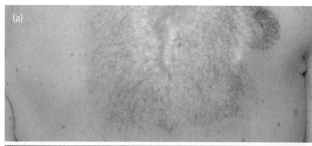

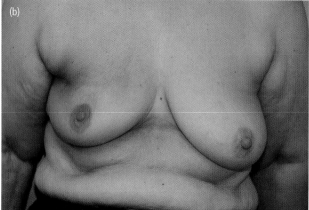

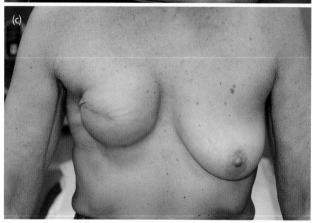

Figure 32.3 (a) Chronic radiation dermatitis with dyschromia, atrophy, and telangiectasias. (Photo courtesy of Dr Mario. E. Lacouture.) (b) Right breast 6 months after radiation therapy for breast cancer. Slight fibrosis with minimal retraction of breast tissue. Overlying skin shows hyperpigmentation and xerosis. (c) Right breast 2 years after radiation therapy for breast cancer. Marked fibrosis with significant retraction of breast tissue.

changes include hyalinization of collagen, dilation of blood vessels, and presence of atypical dermal fibroblasts [30].

Hypopigmentation and hyperpigmentation

Post-inflammatory hypopigmentation and hyperpigmentation occur as one component of chronic radiation changes. One study found that breast cancer patients treated with conventional wedge-based radiotherapy developed chronic grade ≥2 hyperpigmentation in 17% of cases [210]. When intensity-modulated

radiotherapy (IMRT) was used, resulting in a more homogeneous dose distribution, only 7% of patients developed chronic grade ≥2 hyperpigmentation ($p = 0.06$) [210].

Post-inflammatory hypopigmentation and hyperpigmentation may persist or slowly normalize, depending on the severity of the initial reaction and skin type of the patient. In darker skinned individuals, post-inflammatory dyspigmentation persists more frequently than in lighter skinned individuals. Apart from cosmetic concerns, the dyspigmentation itself does not pose medical risks. Treatment of dyspigmentation is limited both in options and efficacy. Options include topical bleaching agents such as hydroquinone, topical retinoids such as tretinoin, and chemical peels. The successful use of a 755-nm long-pulse alexandrite laser to remove hyperpigmentation within chronic radiodermatitis has recently been reported [211]. In general, any potential treatments should be approached with caution to prevent damage to atrophied skin, which is a frequent component of chronic radiation dermatitis. Cosmetic camouflage is the safest, albeit not permanent, option for cosmetic concerns. Exposure to ultraviolet irradiation should be avoided during both the acute healing phase of radiation dermatitis, as well as thereafter, as ultraviolet irradiation can significantly worsen post-inflammatory hyperpigmentation. Patients should be counseled on regular daily use of broad-spectrum sunscreens on sun-exposed and treated areas, the use of sun protective hats and clothing, and seeking shade when outdoors.

Telangiectasias

Persistent telangiectasias occur within the radiation field more commonly after boost dosing, acute grade 3 injury, and moist desquamation [212,213]. While the underlying pathogenesis of the development of telangiectasias is unknown, it may be due in part to the inflammatory microvascular damage that occurs during the acute injury [25]. Damaged endothelial cells or macrophages are stimulated to produce platelet derived growth factor (PDGF) and fibroblast growth factor (FGF) [214]. The number of papillary vessels decreases with increasing radiotherapy dose, while the remaining vessels enlarge further in diameter and become visible [201]. Genetic polymorphisms may also have a role. In a study of over 400 breast cancer patients who received radiotherapy after breast-conserving surgery, patients with variant TP53 genotypes either for the Arg72Pro or the PIN3 polymorphism were at significantly increased risk of telangiectasias [215]. Telangiectasias become clinically evident at total doses of 50–60 Gy, and usually at 6 months to years later [201]. The presence of telangiectasias is not of medical concern. However, they may become a matter of cosmesis, particularly if they are in a readily visible area. Pulsed-dye laser treatment has been beneficial in clearing such radiation-induced telangiectasias [216].

Skin atrophy

Over time, radiated skin becomes thinner in the epidermis and/or dermis, leading to cutaneous atrophy. With increasing radiotherapy dose, the number of papillary vessels decreases and becomes shallower until they disappear, resulting in decreased perfusion of the epidermis and increasing malnutrition [201]. This vascular degeneration leads to basal cell death, and thus secondary skin atrophy. Leukocyte infiltration, mediated in part by cell adhesion molecules, is also commonly seen in irradiated skin and is likely to lend to parenchymal atrophy [217]. Additionally, there is decreased population of dermal fibroblasts and the reabsorption of collagen [218]. Atrophy becomes clinically evident at total doses of 50–60 Gy. Atrophic skin often appears white and shiny, at times with a cigarette-paper-like quality on the surface. These changes are frequently associated with the concomitant appearance of underlying telangiectasias. If atrophy is associated with underlying fibrosis, the skin will appear shiny and bound-down. Due to the thinning of the epidermis and/or dermis, atrophic skin is also associated with fragility, lending to easy tearing or bruising of the skin and predisposing to erosions and ulcerations.

Xerosis and desquamation

Weeks to months after radiation therapy, it is common to see xerosis and dry desquamation of the previously treated field. Xerosis is due in part to the atrophy or loss of sebaceous glands by the radiation treatment. Textural changes, such as hyperkeratosis, can also be seen. These changes are usually minor and minimally, if at all, symptomatic. Occasionally, the xerosis can be associated with pruritus. The majority of patients will benefit from bland petrolatum-based emollients. In general, creams and ointments are better tolerated than lotions in dry skin as they have a lower concentration of water which eventually evaporates. Patients should be counseled to avoid use of alcohol-containing topical products, as this can lead to increased dryness and irritation of the skin. It should be noted that approximately 10% of patients have allergic-type reactions with topical agents [219], particularly to fragrances or preservatives. Some moisturizers, such as Aquaphor®, contain lanolin (wool) alcohol, which can lead to contact dermatitis in approximately 1.3% of the population [220]. Therefore, if irritation of the skin is exacerbated or xerosis of the skin becomes edematous, erythematous, and/or more pruritic, an allergic contact dermatitis to a topical product should be considered.

Sweat gland atrophy can lend not only to xerosis, but also to decreased or absent sweating. This consequence is especially significant when large surface areas are treated, such as when treating MF with electron beam therapy [25]. The main danger of generalized hypohidrosis or anhidrosis is the potential for hyperthermia, which can lead to heat exhaustion, heat stroke, coma, or death. While this would be a very rare consequence of radiation therapy, it must be considered in an applicable setting.

Alopecia

Hair loss secondary to radiation therapy can be an emotionally difficult component of cancer treatment, particularly if most or all of the scalp hair is lost. Hair loss occurs after 3–5 Gy single doses and at a total of 4–8 Gy when given as fractionations of 2 Gy as single dose [201]. Hair loss may be temporary after treatment, and new hair regrowth may occur for up to a year [221].

When radiation is given at a higher dose, radiotherapy-induced alopecia can become permanent. A tolerance dose for complete and permanent hair loss has not been established. However, in an animal model of pig skin, single doses of 7–8 Gy lead to a measurable thinning of the hair, doses above 14.4 Gy lead to obvious hair loss, and doses above 17.4 Gy lead to complete and irreversible hair loss [221]. In humans, fractionated radiotherapy using 2 Gy single doses and total radiotherapy doses of 14–20 Gy induce measurable hair changes. Doses greater than 40–50 Gy lead to complete and irreversible hair loss [202]. This type of permanent destruction of hair follicles and resultant alopecia is usually associated with high-dose radiotherapy for treating intracranial malignancies. Typically, there is clinical scarring of the skin as well. The histologic findings include a decreased number of follicular units with streams of fibrosis or hyalinization of surrounding collagen [222]. Occasionally, scarring alopecia can occur due to radiotherapy without the associated dermal fibrosis. In such cases, hair transplantation can be considered as a treatment option [222].

There is no cure for permanent radiotherapy-induced alopecia. As hair loss secondary to cancer treatment can significantly impact quality of life and self-image in a negative way [223], counseling regarding use of wigs, scarves, and other cosmetic cover-ups is beneficial. In addition, particularly for scalp alopecia, because chronic ultraviolet irradiation subsequent to radiation therapy may be a risk factor for secondary cutaneous malignancies, it is imperative for clinicians to counsel patients to protect their alopecic skin from the sun with use of sunscreens and sun-protective clothing and hats.

Necrosis of soft tissue, cartilage, or bone

When acute radiation changes of persistent tender or edematous erythema progresses to epidermal necrosis, the formation of ulcers, hemorrhage, and further necrosis can ensue. When acute changes do not resolve, they can result in chronic skin ulceration, fibrosis, or necrosis of underlying structures, including soft tissue, cartilage, or bone. Such changes are considered the "consequential" late effects. Pathologically, radiation therapy can lead to proliferation of the myointima within small arteries and arterioles, which may progress to thrombosis or obstruction, increasing the predisposition for ulcers and skin breakdown [224]. These erosions and ulcerations may be painful, slow to heal, and predisposed to infection. They rarely heal spontaneously and can further progress over decades [202,225]. Radiation necrosis in particular is associated with high-dose radiotherapy, failure to heal, acute dermatitis, and dermal ischemia [226]. Radiation necrosis is particularly difficult to manage because these affected tissues are relatively avascular, leading to impaired healing and superinfection. Underlying issues including peripheral vascular disease, hypertension, diabetes, and connective tissue disease exacerbate the problem [25].

The mainstay of wound care, which is not specific to irradiated skin but rather derived from generic wound care experience, includes managing wound secretions, protecting the skin from superinfection, promoting re-epithelialization, and pain control. Wound dressings can be very useful to achieve these goals. It is possible to tailor dressing decisions according to the particular characteristics of each individual wound to optimize the healing [227]. Hydrogel dressings can be used in conjunction with hydrophilic and lipophilic creams and ointments in order to promote a moist environment and enhance barrier function. The moist environment also helps lysis of necrotic tissue and phagocytosis of necrotic debris and bacteria [224]. They can be used on granular and necrotic wounds of all depths. Hydrogel dressings are not self-adherent, and therefore must be kept in place. They can be cleaned and reapplied if the wounds are not exudative. Hydrocolloid dressings are also often used, indicated for partial-thickness wounds and shallow full-thickness wounds with clean or necrotic bases. They are effective particularly to hydrate the wound in the setting of minimal exudate. They are self-adherent and are frequently left in place for several days at a time [228]. When wounds are highly exudative, more appropriate wound dressings include burn pads or alginate or foam dressings, as they are highly absorptive [25].

Persistent eschars on ulcerations will generally impede wound healing as they prevent re-epithelialization. Therefore, it is recommended that they be gently removed under local anesthesia or treated with enzymatic debridement or autolytic dressings. Biosynthetic dressings or artificial or bioengineered skin can also be useful for persistent ulcerations. Novel therapies have also been described in the treatment of chronic nonhealing skin ulcers after radiotherapy. Low-intensity helium-neon laser has been successfully used to treat chronic radiation ulcers in patients with breast cancer [229]. Targeted biologic therapy consisting of a recombinant PDGF and hydrophilic copolymer membrane dressing has also been used to successfully treat chronic radiation ulcers [230]. In some cases, hyperbaric oxygen therapy has been a successful therapeutic option for radiation-induced ulcers [231,232].

The role of topical or oral antibiotics is crucial, particularly for chronic wounds that are already infected or are at high risk for infection. If a patient has evidence for Gram-positive bacterial infections, including methicillin-resistant *Staphylococcus aureus*, topical mupirocin 2% cream or ointment can be applied on the wound. If the wound has evidence of Gram-negative bacterial growth, topical gentamicin ointment can be beneficial. More nonspecific antibacterial agents that have been effective include silver-based dressings. It should be noted that if used during radiotherapy treatment, caution should be used with any metal-based dressing as they can potentially increase skin dose.

Subdermal fibrosis

Subcutaneous fibrosis of the skin is a common late manifestation of radiation-induced injury. Post-irradiation fibrosis occurs in up to 23% of patients receiving breast radiation therapy [233]. It can be of varying degrees, ranging from mild (with no clinical evidence of fibrosis) to severe. As degree of fibrosis increases, the clinical changes become more apparent, with the affected area becoming more firm and bound-down and associated with retraction (Figure 32.3b,c). In general, radiation-induced fibrosis tends to affect the deep subcutaneous tissues such as fascia and muscle, largely sparing the dermis and epidermis with little to no overlying skin changes [234,235]. The overlying skin of fibrotic areas is usually skin-colored, but occasionally will present with post-inflammatory hyperpigmentation. Notably, there is lack of inflammation or erythema. These fibrotic changes can occur as early as 10 weeks after irradiation and slowly progress within the radiation port [236]. The severity of the ensuing fibrosis tends to correlate with the radiation dose [234]. Additionally, the latency period between radiation treatment and development of fibrosis positively correlates with the grade of damage. Grade ≥1 fibrosis occurs in 91% of patients with a latency period of less than 2 years, grade ≥2 fibrosis occurs in 58% with a latency period of 3.2 years, and grade 3 fibrosis occurs in 22% with a latency period of 4.4 years [234]. This trend for longer latency periods for higher grade damage has been demonstrated in patients treated with very high doses (80–110 Gy) who continued to develop very severe fibrosis and skin necrosis up to 10 years after irradiation [237]. It is rare for patients to develop severe fibrosis if treated with less than 80 Gy.

Subcutaneous fibrosis, when left untreated, can remain focal or become widespread. Over time, the ongoing process will induce an increasing loss of elasticity and hardening of the skin, which can lead to further functional deficits. If around joints, the fibrosis can lead to joint restriction and immobility. Additionally, fluid retention within the dermis and subcutis may cause a painful lymphedema of the arm, such as in breast cancer patients after lymphadenectomy, or submental and neck regions, such as in patients with head and neck tumors after resection [201].

Once believed to be irreversible dead scar tissue, fibrosis can better be described as a "wound that does not heal" [238]. While the pathogenesis of fibrosis is not entirely elucidated, it has been postulated that a complex network of interacting cytokines and growth factors have a central role in the chronic activation of myofibroblasts within the treated areas. Transforming growth factor-β1 (TGF-β1) is considered the master switch for the fibrotic program [238]. Continuous production of TGF-β1 has been demonstrated in irradiated tissues [238]. Other factors that have a role include PDGF, IL-1, insulin-like growth factor-1 (IGF-1), and TNF-α [238,239]. There is also increasing evidence that chronic normal tissue hypoxia develops after exposure to radiation therapy, which may have a role in the development of late normal tissue injury [240]. Hypoxia has been shown to promote the production of profibrotic cytokines and stimulate collagen deposition through TGF-β1 [241].

With growing insight into the pathogenesis of radiation-induced fibrosis, new possible targets for therapeutic agents with potential antifibrotic effects have been discovered. Approaches have been taken to prevent the binding of TGF-β1 to its receptor, including the use of anti-TGF-β1 antibodies, small molecule receptor tyrosine kinase inhibitors, and gene therapy to induce production of a soluble TGF-β1 type II receptor [240]. Other approaches have targeted TGF-β1 indirectly, such as by reducing the stimulus for TGF-β1 activation. As reactive oxygen species are produced as a result of radiation exposure, administration of liposomal copper/zinc (Cu/Zn) superoxide dismutase (SOD) was shown to effectively reduce long-standing radiation fibrosis [242]. A clinical trial of topical applications of Cu/Zn-SOD in a concentration of 3600 units/mg was applied as ointment to affected areas of radiation fibrosis twice daily for 90 days, in a total dose of 40 mg [243]. Cu/Zn SOD effectively reduced fibrosis by lowering pain score in 36/39 patients and by decreasing the size of the fibrotic area in half of the patients. Additionally, mammography density showed decreased fibrosis in one-third of patients and subcutaneous temperature by infrared thermography was significantly decreased in 36 of 44 patients [243]. *In vivo* experiments of reconstituted fibrotic skin have also indeed shown that SOD enters the cells and reduced TGF-β1 and tissue inhibitor metalloproteinase gene expression [238]. Other therapeutic intervention trials have included colchicines, interferon-γ, interferon-α, α-tocopherol (vitamin E), pentoxifylline, direct TNF-α antagonists, and antibodies to integrins. In animal studies, amifostine has been shown to reduce the development of fibrosis [244], but there are no correlative convincing studies in humans. For now, corticosteroids are still the first-line therapeutics, though they are effective mainly against symptoms associated with inflammatory reactions [239].

Diseases induced by radiation therapy

Apart from the common radiation-induced late cutaneous reactions described above, there are several other dermatologic conditions that can be induced by radiation therapy that are seen less commonly. These conditions include diseases that occur confined to sites of radiation, which include acne, folliculitis, bullous pemphigoid, erythema multiforme, graft versus host disease, lichen planus, lichen sclerosus, morphea (localized scleroderma), and pseudosclerodermatous panniculitis [217]. Diseases induced by radiation therapy but not confined to the sites of radiation have included erythema multiforme, bullous pemphigoid, pemphigus foliaceus, pemphigus vulgaris, Brunsting–Perry cicatricial pemphigoid, paraneoplastic pemphigus, and herpes zoster [217].

Post-irradiation morphea

Post-irradiation morphea is rare, with less than 50 cases reported in the literature since 1989. The vast majority of cases occur in breast cancer patients, among whom the incidence has been estimated at 0.2% [245]. The onset of post-irradiation morphea is anywhere from a few weeks to 32 years after irradiation therapy, but the majority occur within 1 year after radiation exposure [246]. While the majority of cases remain confined to the area of radiation, up to 20% of the reported cases spread beyond the irradiated areas [247]. Clinically, morphea presents as an acute-onset eruption consisting mainly of erythema and induration. During this stage, it is frequently mistaken for infectious cellulitis. As time progresses, the affected area becomes hard, sclerotic, and bound-down. The sclerotic surface may appear shiny and whitish with an inflammatory lilac ring indicating still active inflammation [248]. If the breast is affected, the overall size of the affected breast typically shrinks due to the progressive sclerosis. Over time, the affected area may then turn hyperpigmented.

The proposed factors involved in pathogenesis of morphea are similar to those of radiation-induced fibrosis, including injury to cellular components, such as fibroblasts and endothelial cells, and dysregulation of collagen production. In morphea, as opposed to fibrosis, it may be possible that an exposure to an unknown environmental stimulus initiates immunologic phenomena to occur, leading B and/or T-cell lymphocytes to produce a local inflammatory response [247]. Resultant cytokines and growth factors may then stimulate fibroblasts to overproduce collagen, even beyond the radiation port.

Recognition of post-irradiation morphea is important for clinicians in order to distinguish it from clinical mimickers, including infectious cellulitis, Lyme disease, recurrent carcinoma, metastatic carcinoma, or second primary carcinoma [247]. In such a scenario, lack of fever, normal peripheral leukocyte count, and poor response to antibiotic therapy will help to distinguish morphea from cellulitis. In order to confirm the diagnosis, a biopsy that contains the entire thickness of the affected skin is recommended. On histology, there will typically be a moderate to severe mixed dermal inflammatory infiltrate, frequently with lymphocytes and plasma cells. The reticular dermis typically shows fibrosis with thickened hyalinized collagen bundles and absence of adnexal structures. There can be vascular ectasia and rare atypical fibroblasts [247,248].

Treatment options for morphea are limited. In the acute inflammatory stage, immunosuppressive medications, including topical steroids, calcineurin inhibitors, and low doses of systemic immunosuppressants (including steroids, methotrexate, and cyclosporine), have been used. Oral antibiotics have also been used as anti-inflammatory agents. Topical therapies, including heparin, hyaluronidase, UVA1 irradiation, and PUVA (psoralen + UVA) irradiation may produce topical softening of the tissue [248].

Grading

The Common Terminology Criteria for Adverse Events (CTCAE), developed by the National Cancer Institute (NCI), is one of the most commonly used grading systems to document adverse events to cancer therapy. The most recent version 4.03 for the common late AEs from radiation therapy was released in June 2010.

Treatment

The prevention and treatment of radiation-induced skin injury is best provided in a multidisciplinary format, involving dermatology, radiation oncology, and wound care specialists. Identifying patients at risk for significant cutaneous AEs is useful in order to provide heightened awareness and careful surveillance for the first signs of injury during and after radiation treatment. Ongoing technologic advances in radiation delivery may also help to reduce the frequency or severity of skin AEs. For example, conformal radiotherapy targets the tumor while minimizing exposure of normal tissue. IMRT focuses multiple beams on the intended target, resulting in a smaller high-dose target. A study of 172 patients with breast cancer treated with lumpectomy followed by whole breast irradiation compared the incidence of cutaneous toxicities in patients treated with IMRT with those treated with conventional wedge-based radiotherapy [210]. A significant reduction in acute grade 2 or worse dermatitis, edema, and hyperpigmentation was seen with IMRT compared with wedges. Additionally, there was a significant reduction in the development of chronic grade 2 or worse breast edema with IMRT compared with conventional wedges.

The linear accelerator and in-room computed tomography provide increased precision. In addition, the combination of positron emission tomographic scans and computed tomography helps to further define treatment targets. The utilization of photons may potentially treat targets while avoiding the skin altogether [25]. Certainly, ongoing research and clinical trials are warranted in order to identify future potentially effective ways to prevent and treat the late AEs of cancer treatment, of which we will likely see at an increasing rate because of the prolonged survival of patients.

Scars

Surgical procedures are a mainstay of cancer therapy, for diagnostic biopsies, tumor removal, and placement of devices for the administration of therapy. The appearance of scars can be very disturbing to patients, both physically and psychologically, and can be challenging to treat for physicians. Adverse events of surgical intervention in 22 childhood cancer survivors included scars, partial urinary and fecal incontinence, intestinal obstruction, nerve injury, and thorax deformity, with scars resulting in psychological problems being the most common (n = 12) [249]. Scars have been associated with anxiety, social avoidance, and depression [250]. Scar formation can become a major clinical problem also due to loss of function, particularly if over joints, and hindrance of growth in children [251].

The stages of wound healing are inflammation, proliferation, matrix remodeling, and scar formation. As only the epidermis is truly regenerative, any injury that extends into the dermis will heal with a scar. If aberrant wound healing occurs, hypertrophic scars or keloids can form, which appear as raised nodules or plaques that are initially pink to purple, and can be painful, pruritic, or both. Hypertrophic scars remain in the area of original injury, while keloids spread into adjacent areas with active borders.

Several therapies for scar prevention and reduction have been described. Proper surgical techniques that ensure minimal tension and inflammation, in addition to avoiding incisions over the midchest and joints when possible, can lead to better cosmetic results [251]. Occlusive therapy can be effective by reducing proinflammatory and profibrotic cytokine levels, and by increasing temperature which has been found to upregulate collagenase expression [252]. Occlusive therapy includes silicone gels and sheets, nonsilicone occlusive sheets, flurandrenolide tape, as well as other topical medications containing silicone. Silicone gel sheets placed over keloids from median sternotomy surgery in nine patients, maintained over the keloids 24 hours a day and replaced every 4 weeks for a duration of 24 weeks, showed improvement in protuberance and redness [253]. In nine additional patients who underwent a median sternotomy, application of silicone gel sheets 24 hours a day that were changed every 4 weeks for 24 weeks resulted in all patients being free of a keloid scar at the end of 24 weeks [254]. Interestingly, other studies have indicated that occlusive therapy with both silicone and nonsilicone-based therapies appears to be of equal value [255], suggesting that wound hydration may be the primary beneficial mechanism.

Topical application of hyaluronic acid or saponins, which upregulate hyaluronic acid, may lead to an antiscarring effect [256]. Additionally, onion extract gel has been shown to significantly improve scar softness, redness, texture, and overall appearance at the excision site [257]. Topical application of imiquimod and vitamin E, a TGF-β inhibitor, have not been demonstrated to be effective in scar prevention or reduction [258,259]. It should be noted that while several agents claim to accelerate healing time, there is no evidence that faster healing time is associated with decreased scar formation [260].

Several other therapies exist for scar reduction, including intralesional and topical steroids, surgery, cryosurgery, radiotherapy, intralesional interferon, and intralesional 5-fluorouracil. Additionally, laser therapy has emerged as a treatment of choice for many types of scars. The 585-nm pulsed-dye laser represents an excellent safe choice for hypertrophic and keloid scars [261]. Pulsed-dye laser primarily reduces erythema, but also reduces scar volume and improves scar surface texture [262]. It is possible that pulsed-dye laser results in photothermolysis, in which thermal injury to scar microvasculature leads to ischemia and reduced collagen within the scar [261]. Atrophic scars can be effectively treated with ablative lasers, including carbon dioxide (CO_2) and erbium-doped yttrium-aluminum-garnet (Er:YAG), which are used for skin resurfacing. Recently, the use of ablative lasers based on the fractional approach has become a new strategy for the treatment of scars, as this method can enable the use of higher pulse energy and lead to decreased complications by leaving an intact epidermal architecture surrounding each coagulated microtreatment area [263]. The ablative 10600-nm CO_2 fractional laser system has been shown to significantly improve the appearance of scarring in 23 women with thyroidectomy scars after a single session of treatment [264].

Ongoing research is being conducted on novel therapies for scar reduction, such as agents targeting TGF-β1 and TGF-β2, connexin 43, which mediates TGF-β signaling, and Smad3, which is implicated in TGF-β-induced fibrosis [251].

References

1 Getzrow, P.L. (1966) Histological architecture of basal cell epitheliomas ectodermal-mesodermal interaction. *Archives of Dermatology*, **94**, 44–49.

2 Shore, R.E. (2001) Radiation-induced skin cancer in humans. *Medical and Pediatric Oncology*, **36**, 549–554.

3 Sugita, K., Yamamoto, O. & Suenaga, Y. (2000) [Seven cases of radiation-induced cutaneous squamous cell carcinoma]. *Journal of UOEH*, **22**, 259–267.

4 Maalej, M., Frikha, H., Kochbati, L. *et al.* (2004) Radio-induced malignancies of the scalp about 98 patients with 150 lesions and literature review. *Cancer Radiotherapie*, **8**, 81–87.

5 Goldschmidt, H. & Sherwin, W.K. (1980) Reactions to ionizing radiation. *Journal of the American Academy of Dermatology*, **3**, 551–579.

6 Martin, H., Strong, E. & Spiro, R.H. (1970) Radiation-induced skin cancer of the head and neck. *Cancer*, **25**, 61–71.

7 Karagas, M.R., McDonald, J.A., Greenberg, E.R. *et al.* (1996) Risk of basal cell and squamous cell skin cancers after ionizing radiation therapy. For The Skin Cancer Prevention Study Group. *Journal of the National Cancer Institute*, **88**, 1848–1853.

8 Lazar, P. & Cullen, S.I. (1963) Basal cell epithelioma and chronic radiodermatitis. *Archives of Dermatology*, **88**, 172–175.

9 Stone, N.H. & Montiel, M.M. (1970) Multiple basal cell carcinomas arising in radiated burn scars. Case report. *Plastic and Reconstructive Surgery*, **46**, 506–509.

10 van Dijk, T.J. & Mali, W.J. (1979) Multiple basal cell carcinoma 58 years after X-ray therapy. *Archives of Dermatology*, **115**, 1287.

11 Allison, J.R. Jr. (1984) Radiation-induced basal-cell carcinoma. *Journal of Dermatologic Surgery and Oncology*, **10**, 200–203.

12 Davis, M.M., Hanke, C.W., Zollinger, T.W., Montebello, J.F., Hornback, N.B. & Norins, A.L. (1989) Skin cancer in patients with chronic radiation dermatitis. *Journal of the American Academy of Dermatology*, **20**, 608–616.

13 Ekmekci, P., Bostanci, S., Anadolu, R., Erdem, C. & Gurgey, E. (2001) Multiple basal cell carcinomas developed after radiation therapy for tinea capitis: a case report. *Dermatologic Surgery*, **27**, 667–669.

14 Perkins, J.L., Liu, Y., Mitby, P.A. *et al.* (2005) Nonmelanoma skin cancer in survivors of childhood and adolescent cancer: a report from the childhood cancer survivor study. *Journal of Clinical Oncology*, **23**, 3733–3741.

15 Shore, R.E., Albert, R.E., Reed, M., Harley, N. & Pasternack, B.S. (1984) Skin cancer incidence among children irradiated for ringworm of the scalp. *Radiation Research*, **100**, 192–204.

16 Shore, R.E., Moseson, M., Xue, X., Tse, Y., Harley, N. & Pasternack, B.S. (2002) Skin cancer after X-ray treatment for scalp ringworm. *Radiation Research*, **157**, 410–418.

17 Ron, E., Modan, B., Preston, D., Alfandary, E., Stovall, M. & Boice, J.D. Jr. (1991) Radiation-induced skin carcinomas of the head and neck. *Radiation Research*, **125**, 318–325.

18 Levi, F., Moeckli, R., Randimbison, L., Te, V.C., Maspoli, M. & La Vecchia, C. (2006) Skin cancer in survivors of childhood and adolescent cancer. *European Journal of Cancer*, **42**, 656–659.

19 Wollenberg, A., Peter, R.U. & Przybilla, B. (1995) Multiple superficial basal cell carcinomas (basalomatosis) following cobalt irradiation. *British Journal of Dermatology*, **133**, 644–646.

20 Iwamoto, I., Endo, M., Kakinuma, H. & Suzuki, H. (1998) Multiple basal cell carcinoma developing two years after 60Co irradiation. *European Journal of Dermatology*, **8**, 180–182.

21 Handa, Y., Miwa, S., Yamada, M., Ono, H., Suzuki, T. & Tomita, Y. (2003) Multiple pigmented basal cell carcinomas arising in the normal-appearing skin after radiotherapy for carcinoma of the cervix. *Dermatologic Surgery*, **29**, 1233–1235.

22 Misago, N., Ogusu, Y. & Narisawa, Y. (2004) Keloidal basal cell carcinoma after radiation therapy. *European Journal of Dermatology*, **14**, 182–185.

23 Pinkus, H. (1953) Premalignant fibroepithelial tumors of skin. *Archives of Dermatology and Syphilology*, **67**, 598–615.

24 Hartschuh, W. & Schulz, T. (1997) Merkel cell hyperplasia in chronic radiation-damaged skin: its possible relationship to fibroepithelioma of Pinkus. *Journal of Cutaneous Pathology*, **24**, 477–483.

25 Hymes, S.R., Strom, E.A. & Fife, C. (2006) Radiation dermatitis: clinical presentation, pathophysiology, and treatment 2006. *Journal of the American Academy of Dermatology*, **54**, 28–46.

26 Edwards, M.J., Hirsch, R.M., Broadwater, J.R., Netscher, D.T. & Ames, F.C. (1989) Squamous cell carcinoma arising in previously burned or irradiated skin. *Archives of Surgery*, **124**, 115–117.

27 Fei, P. & El-Deiry, W.S. (2003) P53 and radiation responses. *Oncogene*, **22**, 5774–5783.

28 Harris, C.C. (1993) p53: at the crossroads of molecular carcinogenesis and risk assessment. *Science*, **262**, 1980–1981.

29 Fritsche, M., Haessler, C. & Brandner, G. (1993) Induction of nuclear accumulation of the tumor-suppressor protein p53 by DNA-damaging agents. *Oncogene*, **8**, 307–318.

30 Franchi, A., Massi, D., Gallo, O., Santucci, M. & Porfirio, B. (2006) Radiation-induced cutaneous carcinoma of the head and neck: is there an early role for p53 mutations? *Clinical and Experimental Dermatology*, **31**, 793–798.

31 Rowe, D.E., Carroll, R.J. & Day, C.L. Jr. (1989) Long-term recurrence rates in previously untreated (primary) basal cell carcinoma: implications for patient follow-up. *Journal of Dermatologic Surgery and Oncology*, **15**, 315–328.

32 Rowe, D.E., Carroll, R.J. & Day, C.L. Jr. (1992) Prognostic factors for local recurrence, metastasis, and survival rates in squamous cell carcinoma of the skin, ear, and lip. Implications for treatment modality selection. *Journal of the American Academy of Dermatology*, **26**, 976–990.

33 Pugliano-Mauro, M. & Goldman, G. (2010) Mohs surgery is effective for high-risk cutaneous squamous cell carcinoma. *Dermatologic Surgery*, **36**, 1544–1553.

34 Ozgediz, D., Smith, E.B., Zheng, J., Otero, J., Tabatabai, Z.L. & Corvera, C.U. (2008) Basal cell carcinoma does metastasize. *Dermatology Online Journal*, **14**, 5.

35 Glogau, R.G. (2000) The risk of progression to invasive disease. *Journal of the American Academy of Dermatology*, **42**, 23–24.

36 Krawtchenko, N., Roewert-Huber, J., Ulrich, M., Mann, I., Sterry, W. & Stockfleth, E. (2007) A randomised study of topical 5% imiquimod vs. topical 5-fluorouracil vs. cryosurgery in immunocompetent patients with actinic keratoses: a comparison of clinical and histological outcomes including 1-year follow-up. *British Journal of Dermatology*, **157** (Suppl. 2), 34–40.

37 Kim, H.S., Yoo, J.Y., Cho, K.H., Kwon, O.S. & Moon, S.E. (2005) Topical photodynamic therapy using intense pulsed light for treatment of actinic keratosis: clinical and histopathologic evaluation. *Dermatologic Surgery*, **31**, 33–36, discussion 6–7.

38 Ceilley, R.I. (2010) Mechanisms of action of topical 5-fluorouracil: Review and implications for the treatment of dermatological disorders. *Journal of Dermatological Treatment*.

39 Masferrer, J.L., Leahy, K.M., Koki, A.T. *et al.* (2000) Antiangiogenic and antitumor activities of cyclooxygenase-2 inhibitors. *Cancer Research*, **60**, 1306–1311.

40 Wolf, J.E. Jr., Taylor, J.R., Tschen, E. & Kang, S. (2001) Topical 3.0% diclofenac in 2.5% hyaluronan gel in the treatment of actinic keratoses. *International Journal of Dermatology*, **40**, 709–713.

41 Pierard, G.E., Pierard-Franchimont, C., Paquet, P. & Quatresooz, P. (2009) Emerging therapies for ionizing radiation-associated skin field carcinogenesis. *Expert Opinion on Pharmacotherapy*, **10**, 813–821.

42 Stockfleth, E., Trefzer, U., Garcia-Bartels, C., Wegner, T., Schmook, T. & Sterry, W. (2003) The use of Toll-like receptor-7 agonist in the treatment of basal cell carcinoma: an overview. *British Journal of Dermatology*, **149** (Suppl. 66), 53–56.

43 Stanley, M.A. (2002) Imiquimod and the imidazoquinolones: mechanism of action and therapeutic potential. *Clinical and Experimental Dermatology*, **27**, 571–577.

44 Sachse, M.M., Zimmermann, J. & Bahmer, F.A. (2006) Efficiency of topical imiquimod 5% cream in the management of chronic radiation dermatitis with multiple neoplasias. *European Journal of Dermatology*, **16**, 56–58.

45 Amendola, B.E., Amendola, M.A., McClatchey, K.D. & Miller, C.H. Jr. (1989) Radiation-associated sarcoma: a review of 23 patients with postradiation sarcoma over a 50-year period. *American Journal of Clinical Oncology*, **12**, 411–415.

46 Laskin, W.B., Silverman, T.A. & Enzinger, F.M. (1988) Postradiation soft tissue sarcomas. An analysis of 53 cases. *Cancer*, **62**, 2330–2340.

47 Cafiero, F., Gipponi, M., Peressini, A. *et al.* (1996) Radiation-associated angiosarcoma: diagnostic and therapeutic implications: two case reports and a review of the literature. *Cancer*, **77**, 2496–2502.

48 Tomasini, C., Grassi, M. & Pippione, M. (2004) Cutaneous angiosarcoma arising in an irradiated breast: case report and review of the literature. *Dermatology (Basel, Switzerland)*, **209**, 208–214.

49 Krasagakis, K., Hettmannsperger, U., Tebbe, B. & Garbe, C. (1995) Cutaneous metastatic angiosarcoma with a lethal outcome, following radiotherapy for a cervical carcinoma. *British Journal of Dermatology*, **133**, 610–614.

50 Caldwell, J.B., Ryan, M.T., Benson, P.M. & James, W.D. (1995) Cutaneous angiosarcoma arising in the radiation site of a congenital hemangioma. *Journal of the American Academy of Dermatology*, **33**, 865–870.

51 Paik, H.H. & Komorowski, R. (1976) Hemangiosarcoma of the abdominal wall following irradiation therapy of endometrial carcinoma. *American Journal of Clinical Pathology*, **66**, 810–814.

52 Handfield-Jones, S.E., Kennedy, C.T. & Bradfield, J.B. (1988) Angiosarcoma arising in an angiomatous naevus following irradiation in childhood. *British Journal of Dermatology*, **118**, 109–112.

53 Morgan, M.A., Moutos, D.M., Pippitt, C.H. Jr., Suda, R.R., Smith, J.J. & Thurnau, G.R. (1989) Vaginal and bladder angiosarcoma after therapeutic irradiation. *Southern Medical Journal*, **82**, 1434–1436.

54 Brenn, T. & Fletcher, C.D. (2005) Radiation-associated cutaneous atypical vascular lesions and angiosarcoma: clinicopathologic analysis of 42 cases. *American Journal of Surgical Pathology*, **29**, 983–996.

55 Requena, L. & Sangueza, O.P. (1998) Cutaneous vascular proliferations. Part III. Malignant neoplasms, other cutaneous neoplasms with significant vascular component, and disorders erroneously considered as vascular neoplasms. *Journal of the American Academy of Dermatology*, **38**, 143–175, quiz 76–8.

56 Rao, J., Dekoven, J.G., Beatty, J.D. & Jones, G. (2003) Cutaneous angiosarcoma as a delayed complication of radiation therapy for carcinoma of the breast. *Journal of the American Academy of Dermatology*, **49**, 532–538.

57 Funaki, M., Koike, S., Dekio, S., Jidoi, J. & Ohno, H. (1997) Angiosarcoma which developed on the abdominal wall: report of a case. *Journal of Dermatology*, **24**, 342–344.

58 Kiyohara, T., Kumakiri, M., Kobayashl, H. *et al.* (2002) Spindle cell angiosarcoma following irradiation therapy for cervical carcinoma. *Journal of Cutaneous Pathology*, **29**, 96–100.

59 Stewart, F.W. & Treves, N. (1948) Lymphangiosarcoma in postmastectomy lymphedema; a report of six cases in elephantiasis chirurgica. *Cancer*, **1**, 64–81.

60 Alessi, E., Sala, F. & Berti, E. (1986) Angiosarcomas in lymphedematous limbs. *American Journal of Dermatopathology*, **8**, 371–378.

61 Nanus, D.M., Kelsen, D. & Clark, D.G. (1987) Radiation-induced angiosarcoma. *Cancer*, **60**, 777–779.

62 Kunkel, T., Mylonas, I., Mayr, D., Friese, K. & Sommer, H.L. (2008) Recurrence of secondary angiosarcoma in a patient with post-radiated breast for breast cancer. *Archives of Gynecology and Obstetrics*, **278**, 497–501.

63 Monroe, A.T., Feigenberg, S.J. & Mendenhall, N.P. (2003) Angiosarcoma after breast-conserving therapy. *Cancer*, **97**, 1832–1840.

64 Feigenberg, S.J., Mendenhall, N.P., Reith, J.D., Ward, J.R. & Copeland, E.M. 3rd. (2002) Angiosarcoma after breast-conserving therapy: experience with hyperfractionated radiotherapy. *International Journal of Radiation Oncology, Biology, Physics*, **52**, 620–626.

65 Furue, M., Yamada, N., Takahashi, T. *et al.* (1994) Immunotherapy for Stewart–Treves syndrome: usefulness of intrapleural administration of tumor-infiltrating lymphocytes against massive pleural effusion caused by metastatic angiosarcoma. *Journal of the American Academy of Dermatology*, **30**, 899–903.

66 Strobbe, L.J., Peterse, H.L., van Tinteren, H., Wijnmaalen, A. & Rutgers, E.J. (1998) Angiosarcoma of the breast after conservation therapy for invasive cancer, the incidence and outcome: an unforseen sequela. *Breast Cancer Research and Treatment*, **47**, 101–109.

67 Kuten, A., Sapir, D., Cohen, Y., Haim, N., Borovik, R. & Robinson, E. (1985) Postirradiation soft tissue sarcoma occurring in breast cancer patients: report of seven cases and results of combination chemotherapy. *Journal of Surgical Oncology*, **28**, 168–171.

68 Gengler, C., Coindre, J.M., Leroux, A. *et al.* (2007) Vascular proliferations of the skin after radiation therapy for breast cancer:

clinicopathologic analysis of a series in favor of a benign process: a study from the French Sarcoma Group. *Cancer*, **109**, 1584–1598.

69 Wiklund, T.A., Blomqvist, C.P., Raty, J., Elomaa, I., Rissanen, P. & Miettinen, M. (1991) Postirradiation sarcoma. Analysis of a nationwide cancer registry material. *Cancer*, **68**, 524–531.

70 Davidson, T., Westbury, G. & Harmer, C.L. (1986) Radiation-induced soft-tissue sarcoma. *British Journal of Surgery*, **73**, 308–309.

71 Huvos, A.G., Woodard, H.Q., Cahan, W.G. *et al.* (1985) Postradiation osteogenic sarcoma of bone and soft tissues: a clinicopathologic study of 66 patients. *Cancer*, **55**, 1244–1255.

72 Pendlebury, S.C., Bilous, M. & Langlands, A.O. (1995) Sarcomas following radiation therapy for breast cancer: a report of three cases and a review of the literature. *International Journal of Radiation Oncology, Biology, Physics*, **31**, 405–410.

73 Gunko, R.I., Bardychev, M.S., Fomin, S.D., Fedjaev, E.B. & Belichenko, L.V. (1990) Radiation-induced sarcomas of the clavicle following treatment of Hodgkin's disease. Report of two cases. *European Journal of Surgical Oncology*, **16**, 512–516.

74 Mark, R.J., Poen, J., Tran, L.M., Fu, Y.S., Heaps, J. & Parker, R.G. (1996) Postirradiation sarcoma of the gynecologic tract. A report of 13 cases and a discussion of the risk of radiation-induced gynecologic malignancies. *American Journal of Clinical Oncology*, **19**, 59–64.

75 Sheppard, D.G. & Libshitz, H.I. (2001) Post-radiation sarcomas: a review of the clinical and imaging features in 63 cases. *Clinical Radiology*, **56**, 22–29.

76 Fang, Z., Matsumoto, S., Ae, K. *et al.* (2004) Postradiation soft tissue sarcoma: a multiinstitutional analysis of 14 cases in Japan. *Journal of Orthopaedic Science*, **9**, 242–246.

77 Tucker, M.A., D'Angio, G.J., Boice, J.D. Jr. *et al.* (1987) Bone sarcomas linked to radiotherapy and chemotherapy in children. *New England Journal of Medicine*, **317**, 588–593.

78 Kim, J.H., Chu, F.C., Woodward, H.Q. & Huvos, A. (1983) Radiation induced sarcomas of bone following therapeutic radiation. *International Journal of Radiation Oncology, Biology, Physics*, **9**, 107–110.

79 Yamamoto, Y., Arata, J. & Yonezawa, S. (1985) Angiomatoid malignant fibrous histiocytoma associated with marked bleeding arising in chronic radiodermatitis. *Archives of Dermatology*, **121**, 275–276.

80 Biswas, S. & Badiuddin, F. (2008) Radiation induced malignant histiocytoma of the contralateral breast following treatment of breast cancer: a case report and review of the literature. *Cases Journal*, **1**, 313.

81 Samitz, M.H. (1967) Pseudosarcoma. Pseudomalignant neoplasm as a consequence of radiodermatitis. *Archives of Dermatology*, **96**, 283–285.

82 Margo, C.E., Duncan, W.C., Rich, A., Garcia, E. & Stricker, J. (2004) Periocular cutaneous melanoma arising in a radiotherapy field. *Ophthalmic Plastic and Reconstructive Surgery*, **20**, 319–320.

83 de Giorgi, V., Santi, R., Grazzini, M. *et al.* (2010) Synchronous angiosarcoma, melanoma and morphea of the breast skin 14 years after radiotherapy for mammary carcinoma. *Acta Dermato-Venereologica*, **90**, 283–286.

84 Conley, J. (1970) Irradiation as an etiologic factor in the development of melanoma. *Archives of Otolaryngology*, **92**, 627–631.

85 Trefzer, U., Voit, C., Milling, A., Audring, H. & Sterry, W. (2003) Malignant melanoma arising in a radiotherapy field: report of two cases and review of the literature. *Dermatology (Basel, Switzerland)*, **206**, 265–268.

86 Traboulsi, E.I., Zimmerman, L.E. & Manz, H.J. (1988) Cutaneous malignant melanoma in survivors of heritable retinoblastoma. *Archives of Ophthalmology*, **106**, 1059–1061.

87 Nakatani, T. & Beitner, H. (1995) A qualitative ultrastructural study of melanocytes after grenz-ray and UVA irradiation. *Okajimas Folia Anatomica Japonica*, **72**, 59–68.

88 Arpaia, N., Cassano, N. & Vena, G.A. (2006) Melanocytic nevus with atypical dermoscopic features at the site of radiodermatitis. *Dermatologic Surgery*, **32**, 100–102.

89 Brunasso, A.M., Delfino, C., Ketabchi, S., Difonzo, E.M. & Massone, C. (2009) Papules arising after radiotherapy for rhabdomyosarcoma. *Acta Dermatovenerologica Alpina, Panonica, et Adriatica*, **18**, 24–27.

90 Diaz-Cascajo, C., Borghi, S., Weyers, W., Retzlaff, H., Requena, L. & Metze, D. (1999) Benign lymphangiomatous papules of the skin following radiotherapy: a report of five new cases and review of the literature. *Histopathology*, **35**, 319–327.

91 Genc, M., Yavuz, M., Cimsit, G., Cobanoglu, O. & Yavuz, A. (2006) Radiation port wart: a distinct cutaneous lesion after radiotherapy. *Journal of the National Medical Association*, **98**, 1193–1196.

92 Ullah, K., Pichler, E. & Fritsch, P. (1989) Multiple eccrine poromas arising in chronic radiation dermatitis. *Acta Dermato-Venereologica*, **69**, 70–73.

93 Weinberg, A.S., Ogle, C.A. & Shim, E.K. (2007) Metastatic cutaneous squamous cell carcinoma: an update. *Dermatologic Surgery*, **33**, 885–899.

94 Manusow, D. & Weinerman, B.H. (1975) Subsequent neoplasia in chronic lymphocytic leukemia. *Journal of the American Medical Association*, **232**, 267–269.

95 Mehrany, K., Weenig, R.H., Pittelkow, M.R., Roenigk, R.K. & Otley, C.C. (2005) High recurrence rates of squamous cell carcinoma after Mohs' surgery in patients with chronic lymphocytic leukemia. *Dermatologic Surgery*, **31**, 38–42, discussion.

96 Mehrany, K., Weenig, R.H., Pittelkow, M.R., Roenigk, R.K. & Otley, C.C. (2004) High recurrence rates of Basal cell carcinoma after mohs surgery in patients with chronic lymphocytic leukemia. *Archives of Dermatology*, **140**, 985–988.

97 Flynn, J.M., Andritsos, L., Lucas, D. & Byrd, J.C. (2010) Second malignancies in B-cell chronic lymphocytic leukaemia: possible association with human papilloma virus. *British Journal of Haematology*, **149**, 388–390.

98 Olsen, E.A., Delzell, E. & Jegasothy, B.V. (1984) Second malignancies in cutaneous T cell lymphoma. *Journal of the American Academy of Dermatology*, **10**, 197–204.

99 Le, K., Lim, A., Samaraweera, U., Morrow, C. & See, A. (2005) Multiple squamous cell carcinomas in a patient with mycosis fungoides. *Australasian Journal of Dermatology*, **46**, 270–273.

100 Hong, D.S., Reddy, S.B., Prieto, V.G. *et al.* (2008) Multiple squamous cell carcinomas of the skin after therapy with sorafenib combined with tipifarnib. *Archives of Dermatology*, **144**, 779–782.

101 McCarthy, K.L., Playford, E.G., Looke, D.F. & Whitby, M. (2007) Severe photosensitivity causing multifocal squamous cell carcinomas secondary to prolonged voriconazole therapy. *Clinical Infectious Diseases*, **44**, e55–e56.

102 Cowen, E.W., Nguyen, J.C., Miller, D.D. *et al.* (2010) Chronic phototoxicity and aggressive squamous cell carcinoma of the skin in children and adults during treatment with voriconazole. *Journal of the American Academy of Dermatology*, **62**, 31–37.

103 Miller, D.D., Cowen, E.W., Nguyen, J.C., McCalmont, T.H. & Fox, L.P. (2010) Melanoma associated with long-term voriconazole

therapy: a new manifestation of chronic photosensitivity. *Archives of Dermatology*, **146**, 300–304.

104 Lambert, W.C. & Schwartz, R.A. (1992) Metastasis. *Journal of the American Academy of Dermatology*, **27**, 131–133.

105 Saeed, S., Keehn, C.A. & Morgan, M.B. (2004) Cutaneous metastasis: a clinical, pathological, and immunohistochemical appraisal. *Journal of Cutaneous Pathology*, **31**, 419–430.

106 Kleyn, C.E., Lai-Cheong, J.E. & Bell, H.K. (2006) Cutaneous manifestations of internal malignancy: diagnosis and management. *American Journal of Clinical Dermatology*, **7**, 71–84.

107 Lookingbill, D.P., Spangler, N. & Helm, K.F. (1993) Cutaneous metastases in patients with metastatic carcinoma: a retrospective study of 4020 patients. *Journal of the American Academy of Dermatology*, **29**, 228–236.

108 Krathen, R.A., Orengo, I.F. & Rosen, T. (2003) Cutaneous metastasis: a meta-analysis of data. *Southern Medical Journal*, **96**, 164–167.

109 Schwartz, R.A. (1995) Cutaneous metastatic disease. *Journal of the American Academy of Dermatology*, **33**, 161–182, quiz 83–6.

110 Hu, S.C., Chen, G.S., Wu, C.S., Chai, C.Y., Chen, W.T. & Lan, C.C. (2009) Rates of cutaneous metastases from different internal malignancies: experience from a Taiwanese medical center. *Journal of the American Academy of Dermatology*, **60**, 379–387.

111 Lookingbill, D.P., Spangler, N. & Sexton, F.M. (1990) Skin involvement as the presenting sign of internal carcinoma. A retrospective study of 7316 cancer patients. *Journal of the American Academy of Dermatology*, **22**, 19–26.

112 Brodland, D.G. & Zitelli, J.A. (1992) Mechanisms of metastasis. *Journal of the American Academy of Dermatology*, **27**, 1–8.

113 Nashan, D., Meiss, F., Braun-Falco, M. & Reichenberger, S. (2010) Cutaneous metastases from internal malignancies. *Dermatologic Therapy*, **23**, 567–580.

114 Maher-Wiese, V.L., Wenner, N.P. & Grant-Kels, J.M. (1992) Metastatic cutaneous lesions in children and adolescents with a case report of metastatic neuroblastoma. *Journal of the American Academy of Dermatology*, **26**, 620–628.

115 Hager, C.M. & Cohen, P.R. (1999) Cutaneous lesions of metastatic visceral malignancy mimicking pyogenic granuloma. *Cancer Investigation*, **17**, 385–390.

116 Jang, K.A., Choi, J.H., Sung, K.J., Moon, K.C. & Koh, J.K. (1998) Cutaneous metastasis presenting as facial lymphedema. *Journal of the American Academy of Dermatology*, **39**, 637–638.

117 Peterson, J.L. & McMarlin, S.L. (1983) Metastatic renal-cell carcinoma presenting as a cutaneous horn. *Journal of Dermatologic Surgery and Oncology*, **9**, 815–818.

118 Rodriguez-Garcia, C., Gonzalez-Hernandez, S., Perez-Robayna, N., Martin-Herrera, A., Sanchez, R. & Guimera, F. (2010) Eyelid metastasis as an initial presentation of a gastric adenocarcinoma. *Journal of the American Academy of Dermatology*, **63**, e49–e50.

119 Braverman, I.M. (2002) Skin manifestations of internal malignancy. *Clinics in Geriatric Medicine*, **18**, 1–19, v.

120 Schoenlaub, P., Sarraux, A., Grosshans, E., Heid, E. & Cribier, B. (2001) [Survival after cutaneous metastasis: a study of 200 cases]. *Annales de Dermatologie et de Venereologie*, **128**, 1310–1315.

121 Brownstein, M.H. & Helwig, E.B. (1972) Patterns of cutaneous metastasis. *Archives of Dermatology*, **105**, 862–868.

122 Dorairajan, L.N., Hemal, A.K., Aron, M. *et al.* (1999) Cutaneous metastases in renal cell carcinoma. *Urologia Internationalis*, **63**, 164–167.

123 Brownstein, M.H. & Helwig, E.B. (1973) Spread of tumors to the skin. *Archives of Dermatology*, **107**, 80–86.

124 Rolz-Cruz, G. & Kim, C.C. (2008) Tumor invasion of the skin. *Dermatologic Clinics*, **26**, 89–102, viii.

125 Jemal, A., Siegel, R., Xu, J. & Ward, E. (2010) Cancer statistics, 2010. *CA: A Cancer Journal for Clinicians*, **60**, 277–300.

126 Altekruse, S.F., Kosary, C.L., Krapcho, M. *et al.* (eds) (2010) *SEER Cancer Statistics Review, 1975–2007*, National Cancer Institute., Bethesda, MD. Available from: http://seer.cancer.gov/csr/1975_2007/ (accessed 13 May 2013) based on November 2009 SEER data submission, posted to the SEER website.

127 Marcoval, J., Moreno, A. & Peyri, J. (2007) Cutaneous infiltration by cancer. *Journal of the American Academy of Dermatology*, **57**, 577–580.

128 Calonje, E., Brenn, T. & Lazar, A. (2005) Cutaneous metastases and Paget's disease of the skin. In: E. Calonje, T. Brenn, A. Lazar & P.H. McKee (eds), McKee's *Pathology of the Skin with Clinical Correlations*, 4th edn, pp. 1421–1444. Elsevier: Saunders, UK.

129 Perisic, D., Jancic, S., Kalinovic, D. & Cekerevac, M. (2007) Metastasis of lobular breast carcinoma to the cervix. *Journal of Obstetrics and Gynaecology Research*, **33**, 578–580.

130 De Giorgi, V., Grazzini, M., Alfaioli, B. *et al.* (2010) Cutaneous manifestations of breast carcinoma. *Dermatologic Therapy*, **23**, 581–589.

131 Cox, S.E. & Cruz, P.D. Jr. (1994) A spectrum of inflammatory metastasis to skin via lymphatics: three cases of carcinoma erysipeloides. *Journal of the American Academy of Dermatology*, **30**, 304–307.

132 Tschen, E.H. & Apisarnthanarax, P. (1981) Inflammatory metastatic carcinoma of the breast. *Archives of Dermatology*, **117**, 120–121.

133 Rudolph, P., MacGrogan, G., Bonichon, F. *et al.* (1999) Prognostic significance of Ki-67 and topoisomerase IIalpha expression in infiltrating ductal carcinoma of the breast: a multivariate analysis of 863 cases. *Breast Cancer Research and Treatment*, **55**, 61–71.

134 Newcomb, G.M., Seymour, G.J. & Adkins, K.F. (1982) An unusual form of chronic gingivitis: an ultrastructural, histochemical, and immunologic investigation. *Oral Surgery, Oral Medicine, and Oral Pathology*, **53**, 488–495.

135 Whitaker-Worth, D.L., Carlone, V., Susser, W.S., Phelan, N. & Grant-Kels, J.M. (2000) Dermatologic diseases of the breast and nipple. *Journal of the American Academy of Dermatology*, **43**, 733–751, quiz 52–4.

136 Mallon, E. & Dawber, R.P. (1994) Alopecia neoplastica without alopecia: a unique presentation of breast carcinoma scalp metastasis. *Journal of the American Academy of Dermatology*, **31**, 319–321.

137 Conner, K.B. & Cohen, P.R. (2009) Cutaneous metastasis of breast carcinoma presenting as alopecia neoplastica. *Southern Medical Journal*, **102**, 385–389.

138 Cohen, I., Levy, E. & Schreiber, H. (1961) Alopecia neoplastica due to breast carcinoma. *Archives of Dermatology*, **84**, 490–492.

139 Fonseca, N.L. Jr., Lucci, L.M., Cha, S.B., Rossetti, C. & Rehder, J.R. (2009) Metastatic eyelid disease associated with primary breast carcinoma: case report. *Arquivos Brasileiros de Oftalmologia*, **72**, 390–393.

140 Martorell-Calatayud, A., Requena, C., Diaz-Recuero, J.L. *et al.* (2010) Mask-like metastasis: report of 2 cases of 4 eyelid metastases and review of the literature. *American Journal of Dermatopathology*, **32**, 9–14.

141 Douglas, R.S., Goldstein, S.M., Einhorn, E., Ibarra, M.S. & Gausas, R.E. (2002) Metastatic breast cancer to 4 eyelids: a clinicopathologic report. *Cutisr*, **70**, 291–293.

142 Bourlond, A. (1994) Pigmented epidermotropic metastasis of a breast carcinoma. *Dermatology (Basel, Switzerland)*, **189** (Suppl. 2), 46–49.

143 Savoia, P., Fava, P., Deboli, T., Quaglino, P. & Bernengo, M.G. (2009) Zosteriform cutaneous metastases: a literature meta-analysis and a clinical report of three melanoma cases. *Dermatologic Surgery*, **35**, 1355–1363.

144 Singh, G., Mohan, M., Srinivas, C. & Valentine, P. (2002) Targetoid cutaneous metastasis from breast carcinoma. *Indian Journal of Dermatology, Venereology and Leprology*, **68**, 51–52.

145 Soyer, H.P., Cerroni, L., Smolle, J. & Kerl, H. (1990) ["Clown nose"–skin metastasis of breast cancer]. *Zeitschrift fur Hautkrankheiten*, **65**, 929–931.

146 Hayes, A.G. & Chesney, T.M. (1993) Metastatic adenocarcinoma of the breast located within a benign intradermal nevus. *American Journal of Dermatopathology*, **15**, 280–282.

147 Cohen, P.R. & Buzdar, A.U. (1993) Metastatic breast carcinoma mimicking an acute paronychia of the great toe: case report and review of subungual metastases. *American Journal of Clinical Oncology*, **16**, 86–91.

148 Brunelli, M., Manfrin, E., Miller, K. *et al.* (2009) Her-2/neu evaluation in Sister Mary Joseph's nodule from breast carcinoma: a case report and review of the literature. *Journal of Cutaneous Pathology*, **36**, 702–705.

149 Ai-Ping, F., Yue, Q. & Yan, W. (2007) A case report of remote cutaneous metastasis from male breast carcinoma. *International Journal of Dermatology*, **46**, 738–739.

150 Matarasso, S.L. & Rosen, T. (1988) Zosteriform metastasis: case presentation and review of the literature. *Journal of Dermatologic Surgery and Oncology*, **14**, 774–778.

151 Rubinstein, R.Y., Baredes, S., Caputo, J., Galati, L. & Schwartz, R.A. (2000) Cutaneous metastatic lung cancer: literature review and report of a tumor on the nose from a large cell undifferentiated carcinoma. *Ear, Nose, and Throat Journal*, **79**, 96–97, 100–101.

152 Beachkofsky, T.M., Wisco, O.J., Osswald, S.S., Osswald, M.B. & Hodson, D.S. (2009) Pulmonary cutaneous metastasis: a case report and review of common cutaneous metastases. *Cutis*, **84**, 315–322.

153 Mueller, T.J., Wu, H., Greenberg, R.E. *et al.* (2004) Cutaneous metastases from genitourinary malignancies. *Urology*, **63**, 1021–1026.

154 Brownstein, M.H. & Helwig, E.B. (1972) Metastatic tumors of the skin. *Cancer*, **29**, 1298–1307.

155 Sariya, D., Ruth, K., Adams-McDonnell, R. *et al.* (2007) Clinicopathologic correlation of cutaneous metastases: experience from a cancer center. *Archives of Dermatology*, **143**, 613–620.

156 Lalich, D., Tawfik, O., Chapman, J. & Fraga, G. (2010) Cutaneous metastasis of ovarian carcinoma with shadow cells mimicking a primary pilomatrical neoplasm. *American Journal of Dermatopathology*, **32**, 500–504.

157 Abbas, O., Salem, Z., Haddad, F. & Kibbi, A.G. (2010) Perforating cutaneous metastasis from an ovarian adenocarcinoma. *Journal of Cutaneous Pathology*, **37**, e53–e56.

158 Hedeshian, M.H., Wang, X., Xu, B., Fontaine, J.P. & Podbielski, F.J. (2006) Subcutaneous metastasis from esophageal cancer. *Asian Cardiovascular and Thoracic Annals*, **14**, 520–521.

159 Schwartz, R.A. (1995) Histopathologic aspects of cutaneous metastatic disease. *Journal of the American Academy of Dermatology*, **33**, 649–657.

160 Aneiros-Fernandez, J., Husein-ElAhmed, H., Arias-Santiago, S. *et al.* (2010) Cutaneous metastasis as first clinical manifestation of signet ring cell gastric carcinoma. *Dermatology Online Journal*, **16**, 9.

161 Barrow, M.V. (1966) Metastatic tumors of the umbilicus. *Journal of Chronic Diseases*, **19**, 1113–1117.

162 Galvan, V.G. (1998) Sister Mary Joseph's nodule. *Annals of Internal Medicine*, **128**, 410.

163 Majmudar, B., Wiskind, A.K., Croft, B.N. & Dudley, A.G. (1991) The Sister (Mary) Joseph nodule: its significance in gynecology. *Gynecologic Oncology*, **40**, 152–159.

164 Damewood, M.D., Rosenshein, N.B., Grumbine, F.C. & Parmley, T.H. (1980) Cutaneous metastasis of endometrial carcinoma. *Cancer*, **46**, 1471–1475.

165 Wang, S.Q., Mecca, P.S., Myskowski, P.L. & Slovin, S.F. (2008) Scrotal and penile papules and plaques as the initial manifestation of a cutaneous metastasis of adenocarcinoma of the prostate: case report and review of the literature. *Journal of Cutaneous Pathology*, **35**, 681–684.

166 Fruh, M., Ruhstaller, T., Neuweiler, J. & Cerny, T. (2005) Resection of skin metastases from gastric carcinoma with long-term follow-up: an unusual clinical presentation. *Onkologie*, **28**, 38–40.

167 Ambrogi, V., Tonini, G. & Mineo, T.C. (2001) Prolonged survival after extracranial metastasectomy from synchronous resectable lung cancer. *Annals of Surgical Oncology*, **8**, 663–666.

168 Gay, H.A., Cavalieri, R., Allison, R.R., Finley, J. & Quan, W.D. Jr. (2007) Complete response in a cutaneous facial metastatic nodule from renal cell carcinoma after hypofractionated radiotherapy. *Dermatology Online Journal*, **13**, 6.

169 Fritz, P., Hensley, F.W., Berns, C., Harms, W. & Wannenmacher, M. (2000) Long-term results of pulsed irradiation of skin metastases from breast cancer. Effectiveness and sequelae. *Strahlentherapie und Onkologie*, **176**, 368–376.

170 Leonard, R., Hardy, J., van Tienhoven, G. *et al.* (2001) Randomized, double-blind, placebo-controlled, multicenter trial of 6% miltefosine solution, a topical chemotherapy in cutaneous metastases from breast cancer. *Journal of Clinical Oncology*, **19**, 4150–4159.

171 Azemar, M., Djahansouzi, S., Jager, E. *et al.* (2003) Regression of cutaneous tumor lesions in patients intratumorally injected with a recombinant single-chain antibody-toxin targeted to ErbB2/HER2. *Breast Cancer Research and Treatment*, **82**, 155–164.

172 Lifshitz, O.H., Berlin, J.M., Taylor, J.S. & Bergfeld, W.F. (2005) Metastatic gastric adenocarcinoma presenting as an enlarging plaque on the scalp. *Cutis*, **76**, 194–196.

173 Tjalma, W.A. & Watty, K. (2003) Skin metastases from vulvar cancer: a fatal event. *Gynecologic Oncology*, **89**, 185–188.

174 Campana, L.G., Mocellin, S., Basso, M. *et al.* (2009) Bleomycin-based electrochemotherapy: clinical outcome from a single institution's experience with 52 patients. *Annals of Surgical Oncology*, **16**, 191–199.

175 Deroose, J.P., Eggermont, A.M., van Geel, A.N. & Verhoef, C. (2010) Isolated limb perfusion for melanoma in-transit metastases: developments in recent years and the role of tumor necrosis factor alpha. *Current Opinion in Oncology*.

176 Wolf, I.H., Smolle, J., Binder, B., Cerroni, L., Richtig, E. & Kerl, H. (2003) Topical imiquimod in the treatment of metastatic melanoma to skin. *Archives of Dermatology*, **139**, 273–276.

177 Turza, K., Dengel, L.T., Harris, R.C. *et al.* (2010) Effectiveness of imiquimod limited to dermal melanoma metastases, with simultaneous resistance of subcutaneous metastasis. *Journal of Cutaneous Pathology*, **37**, 94–98.

178 Good, L.M., Miller, M.D. & High, W.A. (2010) Intralesional agents in the management of cutaneous malignancy: A review. *Journal of the American Academy of Dermatology*.

179 Ikic, D., Spaventi, S., Padovan, I. *et al.* (1995) Local interferon therapy for melanoma patients. *International Journal of Dermatology*, **34**, 872–874.

180 Weide, B., Derhovanessian, E., Pflugfelder, A. *et al.* (2010) High response rate after intratumoral treatment with interleukin-2: results from a phase 2 study in 51 patients with metastasized melanoma. *Cancer*, **116**, 4139–4146.

181 Radny, P., Caroli, U.M., Bauer, J. *et al.* (2003) Phase II trial of intralesional therapy with interleukin-2 in soft-tissue melanoma metastases. *British Journal of Cancer*, **89**, 1620–1626.

182 Kubo, H., Ashida, A., Matsumoto, K., Kageshita, T., Yamamoto, A. & Saida, T. (2008) Interferon-beta therapy for malignant melanoma: the dose is crucial for inhibition of proliferation and induction of apoptosis of melanoma cells. *Archives of Dermatological Research*, **300**, 297–301.

183 Fujimura, T., Okuyama, R., Ohtani, T. *et al.* (2009) Perilesional treatment of metastatic melanoma with interferon-beta. *Clinical and Experimental Dermatology*, **34**, 793–799.

184 Rapprich, H. & Hagedorn, M. (2006) Intralesional therapy of metastatic spreading melanoma with beta-interferon. *Journal der Deutschen Dermatologischen Gesellschaft*, **4**, 743–746.

185 Foote, M.C., Burmeister, B.H., Thomas, J. & Mark Smithers, B. (2010) A novel treatment for metastatic melanoma with intralesional rose bengal and radiotherapy: a case series. *Melanoma Research*, **20**, 48–51.

186 Thompson, J.F., Hersey, P. & Wachter, E. (2008) Chemoablation of metastatic melanoma using intralesional Rose Bengal. *Melanoma Research*, **18**, 405–411.

187 Heller, R., Jaroszeski, M.J., Reintgen, D.S. *et al.* (1998) Treatment of cutaneous and subcutaneous tumors with electrochemotherapy using intralesional bleomycin. *Cancer*, **83**, 148–157.

188 Gaudy, C., Richard, M.A., Folchetti, G., Bonerandi, J.J. & Grob, J.J. (2006) Randomized controlled study of electrochemotherapy in the local treatment of skin metastases of melanoma. *Journal of Cutaneous Medicine and Surgery*, **10**, 115–121.

189 Adderley, U. & Smith, R. (2007) Topical agents and dressings for fungating wounds. *Cochrane Database of Systematic Reviews*, 2, CD003948.

190 Sabir, S., James, W.D. & Schuchter, L.M. (1999) Cutaneous manifestations of cancer. *Current Opinion in Oncology*, **11**, 139–144.

191 Weedon, D. (1977) Bullous skin diseases: a selective review. *Australasian Journal of Dermatology*, **18**, 99–105.

192 Cho-Vega, J.H., Medeiros, L.J., Prieto, V.G. & Vega, F. (2008) Leukemia cutis. *American Journal of Clinical Pathology*, **129**, 130–142.

193 Paydas, S. & Zorludemir, S. (2000) Leukaemia cutis and leukaemic vasculitis. *British Journal of Dermatology*, **143**, 773–779.

194 Resnik, K.S. & Brod, B.B. (1993) Leukemia cutis in congenital leukemia. Analysis and review of the world literature with report of an additional case. *Archives of Dermatology*, **129**, 1301–1306.

195 Kaddu, S., Zenahlik, P., Beham-Schmid, C., Kerl, H. & Cerroni, L. (1999) Specific cutaneous infiltrates in patients with myelogenous leukemia: a clinicopathologic study of 26 patients with assessment of diagnostic criteria. *Journal of the American Academy of Dermatology*, **40**, 966–978.

196 Su, W.P. (1994) Clinical, histopathologic, and immunohistochemical correlations in leukemia cutis. *Seminars in Dermatology*, **13**, 223–230.

197 Tomasini, C., Quaglino, P., Novelli, M. & Fierro, M.T. (1998) "Aleukemic" granulomatous leukemia cutis. *American Journal of Dermatopathology*, **20**, 417–421.

198 Smith, J.L. Jr. & Butler, J.J. (1980) Skin involvement in Hodgkin's disease. *Cancer*, **45**, 354–361.

199 Smoller, B.R. & Warnke, R.A. (1998) Cutaneous infiltrate of chronic lymphocytic leukemia and relationship to primary cutaneous epithelial neoplasms. *Journal of Cutaneous Pathology*, **25**, 160–164.

200 Sun, W., Metz, J.M., Gallagher, M. *et al.* (2010) Two phase I studies of concurrent radiation therapy with continuous-infusion 5-fluorouracil plus epirubicin, and either cisplatin or irinotecan for locally advanced upper gastrointestinal adenocarcinomas. *Cancer Chemotherapy and Pharmacology*.

201 Seegenschmiedt, H. (2006) Management of skin and related reactions to radiotherapy. *Frontiers of Radiation Therapy and Oncology*, **39**, 102–119.

202 Turesson, I. & Thames, H.D. (1989) Repair capacity and kinetics of human skin during fractionated radiotherapy: erythema, desquamation, and telangiectasia after 3 and 5 year's follow-up. *Radiotherapy and Oncology*, **15**, 169–188.

203 Locke, J., Karimpour, S., Young, G., Lockett, M.A. & Perez, C.A. (2001) Radiotherapy for epithelial skin cancer. *International Journal of Radiation Oncology, Biology, Physics*, **51**, 748–755.

204 Emami, B., Lyman, J., Brown, A. *et al.* (1991) Tolerance of normal tissue to therapeutic irradiation. *International Journal of Radiation Oncology, Biology, Physics*, **21**, 109–122.

205 Veness, M. & Richards, S. (2003) Role of modern radiotherapy in treating skin cancer. *Australasian Journal of Dermatology*, **44**, 159–166, quiz 67–8.

206 Porock, D., Kristjanson, L., Nikoletti, S., Cameron, F. & Pedler, P. (1998) Predicting the severity of radiation skin reactions in women with breast cancer. *Oncology Nursing Forum*, **25**, 1019–1029.

207 Twardella, D., Popanda, O., Helmbold, I. *et al.* (2003) Personal characteristics, therapy modalities and individual DNA repair capacity as predictive factors of acute skin toxicity in an unselected cohort of breast cancer patients receiving radiotherapy. *Radiotherapy and Oncology*, **69**, 145–153.

208 Azria, D., Gourgou, S., Sozzi, W.J. *et al.* (2004) Concomitant use of tamoxifen with radiotherapy enhances subcutaneous breast fibrosis in hypersensitive patients. *British Journal of Cancer*, **91**, 1251–1260.

209 Stegman, L.D., Beal, K.P., Hunt, M.A., Fornier, M.N. & McCormick, B. (2007) Long-term clinical outcomes of whole-breast irradiation delivered in the prone position. *International Journal of Radiation Oncology, Biology, Physics*, **68**, 73–81.

210 Harsolia, A., Kestin, L., Grills, I. *et al.* (2007) Intensity-modulated radiotherapy results in significant decrease in clinical toxicities compared with conventional wedge-based breast radiotherapy. *International Journal of Radiation Oncology, Biology, Physics*, **68**, 1375–1380.

211 Santos-Juanes, J., Coto-Segura, P., Galache Osuna, C., Sanchez Del Rio, J. & Soto de Delas, J. (2009) Treatment of hyperpigmentation component in chronic radiodermatitis with alexandrite epilation laser. *British Journal of Dermatology*, **160**, 210–211.

212 Turesson, I., Nyman, J., Holmberg, E. & Oden, A. (1996) Prognostic factors for acute and late skin reactions in radiotherapy patients. *International Journal of Radiation Oncology, Biology, Physics*, **36**, 1065–1075.

213 Bentzen, S.M. & Overgaard, J. (1994) Patient-to-patient variability in the expression of radiation-induced normal tissue injury. *Seminars in Radiation Oncology*, **4**, 68–80.

214 Denham, J.W. & Hauer-Jensen, M. (2002) The radiotherapeutic injury – a complex 'wound'. *Radiotherapy and Oncology*, **63**, 129–145.

215 Chang-Claude, J., Ambrosone, C.B., Lilla, C. *et al.* (2009) Genetic polymorphisms in DNA repair and damage response genes and late normal tissue complications of radiotherapy for breast cancer. *British Journal of Cancer*, **100**, 1680–1686.

216 Lanigan, S.W. & Joannides, T. (2003) Pulsed dye laser treatment of telangiectasia after radiotherapy for carcinoma of the breast. *British Journal of Dermatology*, **148**, 77–79.

217 Quarmby, S., Kumar, P. & Kumar, S. (1999) Radiation-induced normal tissue injury: role of adhesion molecules in leukocyte-endothelial cell interactions. *International Journal of Cancer*, **82**, 385–395.

218 Harper, J.L., Franklin, L.E., Jenrette, J.M. & Aguero, E.G. (2004) Skin toxicity during breast irradiation: pathophysiology and management. *Southern Medical Journal*, **97**, 989–993.

219 Lokkevik, E., Skovlund, E., Reitan, J.B., Hannisdal, E. & Tanum, G. (1996) Skin treatment with bepanthen cream versus no cream during radiotherapy – a randomized controlled trial. *Acta Oncologica*, **35**, 1021–1026.

220 Nguyen, J.C., Chesnut, G., James, W.D. & Saruk, M. (2010) Allergic contact dermatitis caused by lanolin (wool) alcohol contained in an emollient in three postsurgical patients. *Journal of the American Academy of Dermatology*, **62**, 1064–1065.

221 Malkinson, F.D. & Keane, J.T. (1981) Radiobiology of the skin: review of some effects on epidermis and hair. *Journal of Investigative Dermatology*, **77**, 133–138.

222 Severs, G.A., Griffin, T. & Werner-Wasik, M. (2008) Cicatricial alopecia secondary to radiation therapy: case report and review of the literature. *Cutis*, **81**, 147–153.

223 Snobohm, C., Friedrichsen, M. & Heiwe, S. (2010) Experiencing one's body after a diagnosis of cancer – a phenomenological study of young adults. *Psycho-Oncology*, **19**, 863–869.

224 Mendelsohn, F.A., Divino, C.M., Reis, E.D. & Kerstein, M.D. (2002) Wound care after radiation therapy. *Advances in Skin and Wound Care*, **15**, 216–224.

225 Thames, H.D., Bentzen, S.M., Turesson, I., Overgaard, M. & Van den Bogaert, W. (1990) Time-dose factors in radiotherapy: a review of the human data. *Radiotherapy and Oncology*, **19**, 219–235.

226 Hopewell, J.W. (1990) The skin: its structure and response to ionizing radiation. *International Journal of Radiation Biology*, **57**, 751–773.

227 Hom, D.B., Adams, G., Koreis, M. & Maisel, R. (1999) Choosing the optimal wound dressing for irradiated soft tissue wounds. *Otolaryngology and Head and Neck Surgery*, **121**, 591–598.

228 Margolin, S.G., Breneman, J.C., Denman, D.L., LaChapelle, P., Weckbach, L. & Aron, B.S. (1990) Management of radiation-induced moist skin desquamation using hydrocolloid dressing. *Cancer Nursing*, **13**, 71–80.

229 Schindl, A., Schindl, M., Pernerstorfer-Schon, H., Mossbacher, U. & Schindl, L. (2000) Low intensity laser irradiation in the treatment of recalcitrant radiation ulcers in patients with breast cancer–long-term results of 3 cases. *Photodermatology, Photoimmunology and Photomedicine*, **16**, 34–37.

230 Wollina, U., Liebold, K. & Konrad, H. (2001) Treatment of chronic radiation ulcers with recombinant platelet-derived growth factor and a hydrophilic copolymer membrane. *Journal of the European Academy of Dermatology and Venereology*, **15**, 455–457.

231 Borg, M., Wilkinson, D., Humeniuk, V. & Norman, J. (2001) Successful treatment of radiation induced breast ulcer with hyperbaric oxygen. *Breast (Edinburgh, Scotland)*, **10**, 336–341.

232 Dall'Era, M.A., Hampson, N.B., Hsi, R.A., Madsen, B. & Corman, J.M. (2006) Hyperbaric oxygen therapy for radiation induced proctopathy in men treated for prostate cancer. *Journal of Urology*, **176**, 87–90.

233 Clarke, D., Martinez, A. & Cox, R.S. (1983) Analysis of cosmetic results and complications in patients with stage I and II breast cancer treated by biopsy and irradiation. *International Journal of Radiation Oncology, Biology, Physics*, **9**, 1807–1813.

234 Bentzen, S.M., Thames, H.D. & Overgaard, M. (1989) Latent-time estimation for late cutaneous and subcutaneous radiation reactions in a single-follow-up clinical study. *Radiotherapy and Oncology*, **15**, 267–274.

235 Archambeau, J.O., Pezner, R. & Wasserman, T. (1995) Pathophysiology of irradiated skin and breast. *International Journal of Radiation Oncology, Biology, Physics*, **31**, 1171–1185.

236 James, W.D. & Odom, R.B. (1980) Late subcutaneous fibrosis following megavoltage radiotherapy. *Journal of the American Academy of Dermatology*, **3**, 616–618.

237 Spanos, W.J. Jr., Montague, E.D. & Fletcher, G.H. (1980) Late complications of radiation only for advanced breast cancer. *International Journal of Radiation Oncology, Biology, Physics*, **6**, 1473–1476.

238 Martin, M., Lefaix, J. & Delanian, S. (2000) TGF-beta1 and radiation fibrosis: a master switch and a specific therapeutic target? *International Journal of Radiation Oncology, Biology, Physics*, **47**, 277–290.

239 Liu, W., Ding, I., Chen, K. *et al.* (2006) Interleukin 1beta (IL1B) signaling is a critical component of radiation-induced skin fibrosis. *Radiation Research*, **165**, 181–191.

240 Anscher, M.S. (2010) Targeting the TGF-beta1 pathway to prevent normal tissue injury after cancer therapy. *The Oncologist*, **15**, 350–359.

241 Falanga, V., Zhou, L. & Yufit, T. (2002) Low oxygen tension stimulates collagen synthesis and COL1A1 transcription through the action of TGF-beta1. *Journal of Cellular Physiology*, **191**, 42–50.

242 Delanian, S., Baillet, F., Huart, J., Lefaix, J.L., Maulard, C. & Housset, M. (1994) Successful treatment of radiation-induced fibrosis using liposomal Cu/Zn superoxide dismutase: clinical trial. *Radiotherapy and Oncology*, **32**, 12–20.

243 Campana, F., Zervoudis, S., Perdereau, B. *et al.* (2004) Topical superoxide dismutase reduces post-irradiation breast cancer fibrosis. *Journal of Cellular and Molecular Medicine*, **8**, 109–116.

244 Rojas, A., Stewart, F.A., Soranson, J.A., Smith, K.A. & Denekamp, J. (1986) Fractionation studies with WR-2721: normal tissues and tumour. *Radiotherapy and Oncology*, **6**, 51–60.

245 Bleasel, N.R., Stapleton, K.M., Commens, C. & Ahern, V.A. (1999) Radiation-induced localized scleroderma in breast cancer patients. *Australasian Journal of Dermatology*, **40**, 99–102.

246 Morganroth, P.A., Dehoratius, D., Curry, H. & Elenitsas, R. (2010) Postirradiation morphea: a case report with a review of the literature

and summary of the clinicopathologic differential diagnosis. *American Journal of Dermatopathology*.

247 Schaffer, J.V., Carroll, C., Dvoretsky, I., Huether, M.J. & Girardi, M. (2000) Postirradiation morphea of the breast presentation of two cases and review of the literature. *Dermatology (Basel, Switzerland)*, **200**, 67–71.

248 Herrmann, T., Gunther, C. & Csere, P. (2009) Localized morphea: a rare but significant secondary complication following breast cancer radiotherapy. Case report and review of the literature on radiation reaction among patients with scleroderma/morphea. *Strahlenther Onkol*, **185**, 603–607.

249 Pinter, A.B., Hock, A., Kajtar, P. & Dober, I. (2003) Long-term follow-up of cancer in neonates and infants: a national survey of 142 patients. *Pediatric Surgery International*, **19**, 233–239.

250 Rumsey, N., Clarke, A. & White, P. (2003) Exploring the psychosocial concerns of outpatients with disfiguring conditions. *Journal of Wound Care*, **12**, 247–252.

251 Namazi, M.R., Fallahzadeh, M.K. & Schwartz, R.A. (2011) Strategies for prevention of scars: what can we learn from fetal skin? *International Journal of Dermatology*, **50**, 85–93.

252 Berman, B., Perez, O.A., Konda, S. *et al.* (2007) A review of the biologic effects, clinical efficacy, and safety of silicone elastomer sheeting for hypertrophic and keloid scar treatment and management. *Dermatologic Surgery*, **33**, 1291–1302, discussion 302–3.

253 Sakuraba, M., Takahashi, N., Akahoshi, T., Miyasaka, Y. & Suzuki, K. (2010) Experience of silicone gel sheets for patients with keloid scars after median sternotomy. *General Thoracic and Cardiovascular Surgery*, **58**, 467–470.

254 Sakuraba, M., Takahashi, N., Akahoshi, T., Miyasaka, Y. & Suzuki, K. (2011) Use of silicone gel sheets for prevention of keloid scars after median sternotomy. *Surgery Today*, **41**, 496–499.

255 Wolfram, D., Tzankov, A., Pulzl, P. & Piza-Katzer, H. (2009) Hypertrophic scars and keloids – a review of their pathophysiology,

risk factors, and therapeutic management. *Dermatologic Surgery*, **35**, 171–181.

256 Mast, B.A., Flood, L.C., Haynes, J.H. *et al.* (1991) Hyaluronic acid is a major component of the matrix of fetal rabbit skin and wounds: implications for healing by regeneration. *Matrix (Stuttgart, Germany)*, **11**, 63–68.

257 Draelos, Z.D. (2008) The ability of onion extract gel to improve the cosmetic appearance of postsurgical scars. *Journal of Cosmetic Dermatology*, **7**, 101–104.

258 Berman, B., Frankel, S., Villa, A.M., Ramirez, C.C., Poochareon, V. & Nouri, K. (2005) Double-blind, randomized, placebo-controlled, prospective study evaluating the tolerability and effectiveness of imiquimod applied to postsurgical excisions on scar cosmesis. *Dermatologic Surgery*, **31**, 1399–1403.

259 Baumann, L.S. & Spencer, J. (1999) The effects of topical vitamin E on the cosmetic appearance of scars. *Dermatologic Surgery*, **25**, 311–315.

260 Cohen, J.L., Jorizzo, J.L. & Kircik, L.H. (2007) Use of a topical emulsion for wound healing. *Journal of Supportive Oncology*, **5**, 1–9.

261 Elsaie, M.L. & Choudhary, S. (2010) Lasers for scars: a review and evidence-based appraisal. *Journal of Drugs in Dermatology*, **9**, 1355–1362.

262 Alster, T.S. (1994) Improvement of erythematous and hypertrophic scars by the 585-nm flashlamp-pumped pulsed dye laser. *Annals of Plastic Surgery*, **32**, 186–190.

263 Manstein, D., Herron, G.S., Sink, R.K., Tanner, H. & Anderson, R.R. (2004) Fractional photothermolysis: a new concept for cutaneous remodeling using microscopic patterns of thermal injury. *Lasers in Surgery and Medicine*, **34**, 426–438.

264 Jung, J.Y., Jeong, J.J., Roh, H.J. *et al.* (2011) Early postoperative treatment of thyroidectomy scars using a fractional carbon dioxide laser. *Dermatologic Surgery*, **37**, 217–223.

6 Dermatologic Practice in Oncology

33 Management Algorithms for Dermatologic Adverse Events

Alyx Rosen[1], Iris Amitay-Laish[2] and Mario E. Lacouture[1]

[1]Dermatology Service, Memorial Sloan-Kettering Cancer Center, New York, NY, USA
[2]Department of Dermatology, Rabin Medical Center, Beilinson Hospital, Petah Tikva, Israel

Regardless of the anticancer therapy involved, skin adverse events (AEs) can cause discomfort and diminish quality of life. Not only can AEs necessitate dose modifications that may adversely affect treatment outcomes, but they can also restrict activities of daily living. Thus, it is important to educate patients and provide effective treatments. This chapter is meant to serve as a quick reference for physicians involved in the treatment and care of patients on anticancer therapies who develop skin toxicities. Detailed preventive and treatment algorithms are set forth below in Figures 33.1–33.22 and represent expert opinions from experienced dermatologists. Table 33.1 provides a summary of various topical and systemic treatment groups that are referenced throughout the treatment algorithms. Although the recommendations set forth in this section represent the best approaches to treatment of patients with dermatologic AEs, there is still a need for improved management strategies.

- Overview [1–17] Figure 33.1
- Acneiform (papulopustular) rash [11,15,18–29] Figures 33.2, 33.3, 33.4
- Hand-foot syndrome/hand-foot skin reaction [30–35] Figures 33.5, 33.6, 33.7
- Radiation dermatitis [36–44] Figure 33.9
- Maculopapular rash [45] Figure 33.8
- Intertriginous rash [46] Figure 33.10
- Infusion site extravasation reaction and antidotes [47–49] Figure 33.11
- Injection site reaction Figure 33.12
- Xerosis, pruritus, fissures [5,14,28,43,50–64] Figure 33.13, 33.14, 3.15
- Hyperpigmentation [43,46] Figure 33.16
- Paronychia [7,8,16,65–69] Figure 33.17
- Oral mucositis and anal mucositis/proctitis [70–75] Figures 33.18, 33.19, 33.20
- Hair changes [76–81] Figures 33.21, 33.22.

Table 33.1 Topical and systemic treatment options.

Examples of topical steroids	
Topical steroids low/moderate potency (increasing potency) (face)	Hydrocortisone 2.5% cream (Hytone); Alclometasone 0.05% cream (Aclovate); Fluocortolone Caproate 0.25% cream (Ultralan); Triamcinolone Acetonide 0.1% cream (Kenalog, Aristocort A)
Topical steroids high-potency (increasing potency) (body)	Mometasone Furoate 0.1% cream (Elocon); Clobetasol Propionate 0.05% cream (Temovate or Dermovate); Betamethasone Dipropionate 0.25% cream (Diprolene)
Combined topical steroid and topical antibiotics ± anti-fungal agent	Threolone ointment (Chloramphenicol 3% and Prednisolone 0.5%); Tevacutan cream (Clotrimazole 1%, Dexamethasone Acetate 0.044%, and Neomycin Sulfate 0.645%); Lotrisone cream(Betamethasone 0.05% and Clotrimazole 1%)
Topical steroids for scalp application	Shampoo: Clobetasol Propionate 0.05% (Clobex)
	Foam (decreasing potency):Clobetasol propionate 0.05% (Olux/Olux E); Betamethasone Valerate 0.12% (Luxiq); Desonide 0.05%, (Verdeso)
	Solution: Betamethasone Valerate 0.1% (Betacorten Scalp Application); Fluocinonide 0.05% (Lidex)
Topical steroids recommended for oral application	Dexamethasone Elixir: 0.5 mg/5 mL (swish and spit with 5 mL qid); no eating/drinking 30 minutes after use
Examples of topical retinoids	
Tretinoin 0.025% cream; Tazarotene 0.05% cream; Tretinoin 0.1% lotion	
Examples of topical antibiotics	
Mupirocin 1% cream (Bactroban); Clindamycin 1–2% cream or gel (Cleocin T); Erythromycin 1–2% gel (Erygel) or ointment (Akne-mycin); Metronidazole 1% cream or gel (MetroGel); Polysporin 1% ointment; Fusidic Acid cream 20 mg/g (Fucidin); Gentamicin 0.1% cream; Silver Sulfadiazine 1% cream (Silvadene)	
Topical antibiotics recommended for Radiation Dermatitis: Mupirocin 1% (Bactroban); Silver sulfadiazine 1% cream (Silvadene)	
Topical antibiotics recommended for Intertriginous Rash: Polysporin 1% ointment; Silver sulfadiazine 1% cream (Silvadene)	
Examples of topical antipruritics	
Pramoxine 1% (cream, lotion, foam, gel , or spray); Doxepin 5% cream (Zonalon)	
Examples of moisturizers/keratolytics for Hand-Foot Skin Reaction to Multikinase Inhibitors	
Urea 20–40% cream; Salicylic Acid of up to 30% (6%–30%)	
Do not apply in between fingers and on deep fissures	
Examples of sunscreens and ingredients (Broad-spectrum with SPF>15 applied every 2 hours and before going outside)	
Zinc Oxide; Titanium Dioxide; Ecamsule; Helioplex (contains Avobenzone and Oxybenzone)	
Oral steroids: Dexamethasone for Hand-Foot Syndrome to Doxorubicin (Doxil) or Taxanes	
8 mg bid for 5 days beginning the day before infusion, followed by 4 mg bid for 1 day, then 4 mg once daily for 1 day	
Oral antibiotics with *anti-Staphylococcus aureus* and Gram + coverage	
Cephalexin (Keflex) 500 mg q6h for 2 weeks ; Doxycycline (Doxy) or Minocycline (Minocin) 100 mg bid or Oxytetracycline 500 mg bid for 2 weeks; Trimethoprim/sulfamethoxazole DS (double strength) (Bactrim DS) 1 tab bid for 2 weeks. Definite treatment should be given according the appropriate **antibiogram**.	
Examples of oral antipruritics and dosing	
Antihistamines	Diphenhydramine 25–50 mg tid; (Benadryl) Hydroxyzine 10–25 mg tid (Vistaril); Fexofenadine 60 mg tid (Allegra), Cetirizine 10 mg daily (Zyrtec); Loratadine 10 mg bid (Claritin)
GABA agonists (adjust if renal impairment)	Gabapentin 300 mg q8 hours; Pregabalin 50–75 mg q8 hours
Antihistamine/Tricyclic antidepressant	Doxepin 25–50 mg q8 hours

Box 33.1 Levels of evidence for recommended guidelines

Level I evidence is reserved for meta-analyses of randomized controlled trials or randomized trials with high power.

Level II evidence includes randomized trials with low power.

Level III evidence includes nonrandomized trials, such as cohort or case-controlled series.

Level IV evidence includes descriptive and case studies.

Level V evidence includes case reports and clinical examples.

Note: Levels of evidence and recommendation grades are used by the American Society of Clinical Oncology. Statements and algorithms without are considered standard clinical practice based on expert opinion.

Box 33.2 Grade of recommendation for recommended guidelines

Grade A is reserved for level I evidence of consistent findings from multiple studies of levels II, III, or IV evidence.

Grade B is for levels II, III, or IV evidence with generally consistent findings.

Grade C is similar to grade B but with inconsistencies.

Grade D implies little or no evidence.

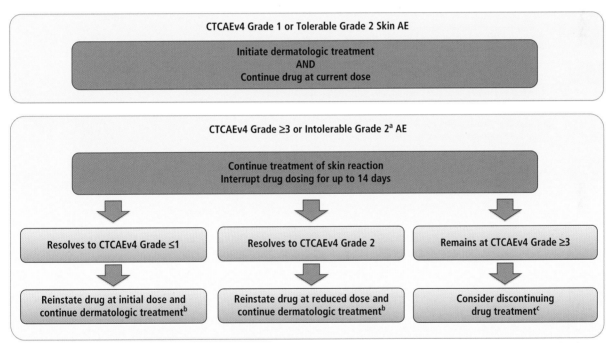

CTCAEv4 Grade 1 or Tolerable Grade 2 Skin AE

Initiate dermatologic treatment
AND
Continue drug at current dose

CTCAEv4 Grade ≥3 or Intolerable Grade 2[a] AE

Continue treatment of skin reaction
Interrupt drug dosing for up to 14 days

Resolves to CTCAEv4 Grade ≤1 → Reinstate drug at initial dose and continue dermatologic treatment[b]

Resolves to CTCAEv4 Grade 2 → Reinstate drug at reduced dose and continue dermatologic treatment[b]

Remains at CTCAEv4 Grade ≥3 → Consider discontinuing drug treatment[c]

[a] Intolerable grade 2 is defined as a grade 2 adverse event (AE) that does not decrease to grade ≤1 after 2 weeks of therapy OR that is considered intolerable as per patient.

[b] If a patient was previously started on oral corticosteroids, they should be continued for at least one week after resumption of reduced dose of drug.

[c] You can request additional advice from the company or dermatologist if a patient has not responded to intervention and permanent discontinuation of causal drug is being considered.

Figure 33.1 Recommended dose modifications for dermatologic adverse events based on Common Terminology Criteria for Adverse Events (CTCAE) grade.

Severity (CTCAE v.4)	Intervention	Level of Evidence	Recommendation Grade
Grade 0	Begin EGFR inhibitor at standard dose (Prophylactic treatment during weeks 1–6 and 8 of EGFR inhibitors initiation); Skin evaluation at initial visit and treat any underlying skin conditions		
	Oral antibiotics for 6 weeks at start of therapy (doxycycline 100 mg bid OR minocycline 100 mg bid OR oxytetracycline 500 mg bid) **AND**	II	A
	Alcohol-free OTC moisturizing creams or ointment bid	II	C
	Sunscreen SPF≥15 applied to exposed areas of body and every 2 hours when outside	II	C
	Topical low/moderate potency steroid to face and chest bid	II	C

OTC: Over the counter

Figure 33.2 Skin adverse event management for epidermal growth factor receptor (EGFR) inhibitors: prophylactic treatment for acneiform (papulopustular) rash.

Severity (CTCAE v.4)	Intervention	Level of Evidence	Recommendation Grade
Grade 0	See: Skin Toxicity Management for EGFR Inhibitors: Prophylactic Treatment		
Grade 1	Continue drug at current dose and monitor for change in severity		
	Topical low/moderate potency steroid daily AND Topical antibiotic bid OR Combined topical steroid and antibiotic	IV	C
	Reassess after 2 weeks (either by healthcare professional or patient self-report); if reactions worsen or do not improve proceed to next step		
Grade 2	Continue drug at current dose and monitor for change in severity		
	Stop topical antibiotic if being used Oral antibiotic for 6 weeks (doxycycline 100 mg bid OR minocycline 100 mg bid OR oxytetracycline 500 mg bid) AND	IV	C
	Topical low/moderate potency steroid	IV	C
	Reassess after 2 weeks (either by healthcare professional or patient self-report); if reactions worsen or do not improve proceed to next step		
Grade ≥3 Or intolerable grade 2	Dose modify as per protocol; obtain bacterial/viral/fungal cultures if infection is suspected; continue treatment of skin reaction with the following:		
	Oral antibiotic for 6 weeks (doxycycline 100 mg bid OR minocycline 100 mg bid OR oxytetracycline 500 mg bid) AND Topical low/moderate potency steroid ±	IV	C
	Isotretinoin at low doses (20–30 mg/day)	IV	C
	Reassess after 2 weeks; if reactions worsen or do not improve, dose interruption or discontinuation per protocol may be necessary		

Figure 33.3 Treatment algorithm for acneiform (papulopustular) rash to EGFR, multikinase, and mTOR inhibitors.

Severity (CTCAE v.4)	Intervention
Grade 0	Sunscreen SPF ≥ 15; OTC Moisturizing creams; Gentle skin care instructions given
Grade 1	Continue corticosteroids at current dose and monitor for change in severity
	Topical antibiotic daily ± Topical retinoid
	Reassess after 2 weeks (either by healthcare professional or patient self-report); if reactions worsen or do not improve proceed to next step
Grade 2	Continue corticosteroids at current dose and monitor for change in severity
	Oral antibiotics for 6 weeks (doxycycline 100 mg bid OR minocycline 100 mg bid OR oxytetracycline 500 mg bid) AND Stop topical antibiotics if being used ± Topical retinoid
	Reassess after 2 weeks (either by healthcare professional or patient self-report); if reactions worsen or do not improve proceed to next step
Grade ≥3 Or intolerable grade 2	Dose modify as per protocol; obtain bacterial/viral/fungal cultures if infection is suspected; and continue treatment of skin reaction with the following:
	Oral antibiotics for 6 weeks (doxycycline 100 mg bid OR minocycline 100 mg bid OR oxytetracycline 500 mg bid) AND Benzoyl peroxide 8% wash daily ± topical retinoid
	Reassess after 2 weeks; if reactions worsen or do not improve, dose interruption or discontinuation per protocol may be necessary

OTC: Over the counter

Figure 33.4 Treatment algorithm for acneiform (papulopustular) rash to corticosteroids (steroid acne).

Severity (CTCAE v.4)	Intervention
Grade 0	Gentle skin care instructions given; Avoid irritation to the hands and feet; Urea 10% tid
Grade 1	Continue drug at current dose and monitor for change in severity
	Topical high-potency steroid bid AND urea 10% tid
	Reassess after 2 weeks (either by healthcare professional or patient self-report); if reactions worsen or do not improve proceed to next step
Grade 2	Continue drug at current dose and monitor for change in severity
	Topical high-potency steroid bid (may be combined concomitantly with topical moisturizer/keratolytic with occlusion) AND Pain control with NSAIDs/GABA agonists/Narcotics
	Reassess after 2 weeks (either by healthcare professional or patient self-report); if reactions worsen or do not improve proceed to next step
Grade ≥3 Or intolerable grade 2	Interrupt treatment until severity decreases to grade 0–1; and continue treatment of skin reaction with the following:
	Topical high-potency steroid bid (may combine concomitantly with topical moisturizer/keratolytic with occlusion) AND Pain control with NSAIDs/GABA agonists/Narcotics
	Reassess after 2 weeks; if reactions worsen or do not improve, dose interruption or discontinuation per protocol may be necessary

Figure 33.5 Treatment algorithm for hand-foot skin reaction to multikinase inhibitors. GABA, gamma-aminobutyric acid; NSAID, nonsteroidal anti-inflammatory drug.

Severity (CTCAE v.4)	Intervention	Level of Evidence	Recommendation Grade
Grade 0	Gentle skin care instructions given; Avoid irritation to the hands and feet; Celecoxib 200 mg/m² bid		
		I	A
Grade 1	Continue drug at current dose and monitor for change in severity		
	Celecoxib 200 mg/m² bid AND Topical high-potency steroid bid	I	A
	Reassess after 2 weeks (either by healthcare professional or patient self-report); if reactions worsen or do not improve proceed to next step		
Grade 2	Continue drug at current dose and monitor for change in severity		
	Celecoxib 200 mg/m² bid AND Topical high-potency steroid bid AND Pain control with NSAIDs/GABA agonists/Narcotics	I	A
	Reassess after 2 weeks (either by healthcare professional or patient self-report); if reactions worsen or do not improve proceed to next step		
Grade ≥3 Or intolerable grade 2	Interrupt treatment until severity decreases to grade 0–1; and continue treatment of skin reaction with the following:		
	Celecoxib 200 mg/m² bid AND Topical high-potency steroid bid AND Pain control with NSAIDs/GABA agonists/Narcotics	I	A
	Reassess after 2 weeks; if reactions worsen or do not improve, dose interruption or discontinuation per protocol may be necessary		

Figure 33.6 Treatment algorithm for hand-foot syndrome to capecitabine.

Severity (CTCAE v.4)	Intervention
Grade 0	Gentle skin care instructions given; Avoid irritation to the hands and feet
Grade 1	Continue drug at current dose and monitor for change in severity
	Topical high-potency steroid bid
	Reassess after 2 weeks (either by healthcare professional or patient self-report); if reactions worsen or do not improve proceed to next step
Grade 2	Continue drug at current dose and monitor for change in severity
	Topical high-potency steroid bid AND Pain control with NSAIDs/GABA agonists/Narcotics AND Oral dexamethasone (8 mg twice daily for 5 days beginning the day before infusion followed by 4 mg twice daily for 1 day, then 4 mg once daily for 1 day)
	Reassess after 2 weeks (either by healthcare professional or patient self-report); if reactions worsen or do not improve proceed to next step
Grade ≥3 Or intolerable grade 2	Interrupt treatment until severity decreases to grade 0–1; and continue treatment of skin reaction with the following:
	Topical high-potency steroid bid AND Pain control with NSAIDs/GABA agonists/Narcotics AND Oral dexamethasone (see above)
	Reassess after 2 weeks; if reactions worsen or do not improve, dose interruption or discontinuation per protocol may be necessary

Figure 33.7 Treatment algorithm for hand-foot syndrome to doxorubicin (or PEGylated doxorubicin) and taxanes.

Severity (CTCAE v.4)	Intervention
Grade 0	OTC Moisturizing creams; Gentle skin care instructions given
Grade 1	Continue drug at current dose and monitor for change in severity
	Topical steroid bid AND Oral antihistamines
	Reassess after 2 weeks (either by healthcare professional or patient self-report); if reactions worsen or do not improve proceed to next step
Grade 2	Continue drug at current dose and monitor for change in severity
	Topical steroid bid AND Oral antihistamines AND Oral steroids (Prednisone 0.5 mg/kg or equivalent)
	Reassess after 2 weeks (either by healthcare professional or patient self-report); if reactions worsen or do not improve proceed to next step
Grade ≥3 Or intolerable grade 2	Dose modify as per protocol; obtain bacterial/viral/fungal cultures if infection is suspected; and continue treatment of skin reaction with the following:
	Topical steroid bid AND Oral antihistamines AND Oral steroids (Prednisone 0.5 mg/kg or equivalent)
	Reassess after 2 weeks; if reactions worsen or do not improve, dose interruption or discontinuation per protocol may be necessary

OTC: Over the counter

Figure 33.8 Treatment algorithm for maculopapular rash.

Severity (CTCAE v.4)	Intervention	Level of Evidence	Recommendation Grade
Grade 0	Maintain hygiene, gently clean and dry skin in radiation field shortly before each radiation treatment AND **no topicals within 4 hrs of radiation therapy;**	IV	A
	Topical high-potency steroid daily for the duration of radiation;	I	A
	If concurrent EGFR inhibitor therapy, oral antibiotics for 6 weeks (doxycycline 100 mg bid OR minocycline 100 mg bid OR oxytetracycline 500 mg bid)	II	A
Grade 1	Continue drug at current dose and monitor for change in severity		
	Maintain hygiene, gently clean and dry skin in radiation field shortly before each radiation treatment AND	IV	A
	Topical high-potency steroid daily	I	A
	Reassess after 2 weeks (either by healthcare professional or patient self-report); if reactions worsen or do not improve proceed to next step		
Grade 2	Continue drug at current dose and monitor for change in severity		
	Topical high-potency steroid daily AND	I	A
	Topical antibiotic* to moist desquamative areas bid	IV	B
	Reassess after 2 weeks (either by healthcare professional or patient self-report); if reactions worsen or do not improve proceed to next step		
Grade ≥3 Or intolerable grade 2	Continue radiation at current dose; obtain bacterial/viral/fungal cultures if infection is suspected; and continue treatment of skin reaction with the following:		
	Topical high-potency steroid daily AND	I	A
	Topical antibiotic daily* to moist desquamative areas bid AND	IV	B
	Pain control with NSAIDs/GABA agonists/Narcotics AND		
	If infection suspected, begin oral antibiotics with anti-*Staphylococcus aureus* and Gram + coverage; obtain bacterial skin culture	II	B
	Reassess after 2 weeks; if reactions worsen or do not improve, dose interruption or discontinuation per protocol may be necessary		

* See Table 1 for topical antibiotics recommended for radiation dermatitis

Figure 33.9 Treatment algorithm for acute radiation dermatitis.

Severity (CTCAE v.4)	Intervention
Grade 0	Gentle skin care instructions given
Grade 1	Continue drug at current dose and monitor for change in severity
	Topical antibiotics AND Topical low/moderate potency steroid to affected areas bid AND If candida is suspected, apply combined topical steroid and antibiotic + anti-fungal agent and Agispor shampoo[a]
	Reassess after 2 weeks (either by healthcare professional or patient self-report); if reactions worsen or do not improve proceed to next step
Grade 2	Continue drug at current dose and monitor for change in severity; obtain bacterial/viral/fungal cultures if infection is suspected; continue treatment of skin reaction with the following:
	Topical antibiotics AND Topical moderate potency steroid to affected areas bid AND If candida is suspected, apply combined topical steroid and antibiotic + anti-fungal agent and Agispor shampoo[a]
	Reassess after 2 weeks (either by healthcare professional or patient self-report); if reactions worsen or do not improve proceed to next step
Grade ≥3 Or intolerable grade 2	Interrupt treatment until severity decreases to grade 0–1; obtain bacterial/viral/fungal cultures if infection is suspected; and continue treatment of skin reaction with the following:
	Topical antibiotics AND Topical moderate potency steroid to affected areas bid AND If candida is suspected, apply combined topical steroid and antibiotic + anti-fungal agent and Agispor shampoo[a]
	Reassess after 2 weeks; if reactions worsen or do not improve, dose interruption or discontinuation per protocol may be necessary

[a]Agispor shampoo contains bifonazole 1%

Figure 33.10 Treatment algorithm for intertriginous rash from doxorubicin or liposomal doxorubicin.

(a)

Severity (CTCAE v4.0)	Intervention
Grade 0	Use strong viable veins for infusions; Monitor patients closely for early signs of extravasation (especially patients treated with highly vesicant potential drugs); Use proper infusion technique and proper infusion cannula

No CTCAE v4.0 Grade 1 for Infusion Site Extravasation

Severity (CTCAE v4.0)	Intervention
Grade 2	Stop infusion immediately. For vesicant compounds: Disconnect IV tubing from IV device but DO NOT remove the IV device or needle. Attempt to aspirate residual vesicant from the IV device using a small (1–3 cc) syringe. Instill appropriate amount of antidote through existing IV, then remove the peripheral IV device or needle. Elevate the affected limb and clearly mark the affected area.
	Non-vesicant compounds[a]: Intermittent cooling and observation; Vesicant compounds[a]: Administer antidote when available[b]; If infection suspected, begin oral (or IV) antibiotics
	Reassess patient frequently by healthcare professional; if reactions worsen (evidence of ulceration or necrosis) or do not improve, surgical intervention may be necessary.

Severity (CTCAE v4.0)	Intervention
Grade ≥3	Stop infusion immediately, disconnect IV tubing from IV device. Attempt to aspirate residual vesicant from the IV device using a small (1–3 cc) syringe. Instill appropriate amount of antidote through existing IV, then remove the peripheral IV device or needle. Elevate the affected limb and clearly mark the affected area.
	Administer antidote when available[b]; Surgical intervention with wide local excisions and skin grafting may be indicated; If infection suspected, begin oral (or IV) antibiotics
	Reassess patient frequently by healthcare professional

Grade 3 reactions: Caused by vesicant compounds only, which can cause tissue necrosis/blistering.
[a]See section 3.09: Extravasation Reactions, for a complete list of vesicant and non-vesicant compounds.
[b]See section 3.09: Extravasation Reactions and Figure 11B, for detailed compound-specific acute antidotes.

(b)

Drug Classification and Name	Immediate Topical Therapy	Antidote or Treatment
DNA-binding Vesicant Drugs		
Alkylating agents: Mechlorethamine	Apply ice for 6–12 hours following antidote injection	Sodium thiosulfate[a]
Anthracyclines: Doxorubicin, Daunorubicin, Epirubicin, Idarubicin	Apply ice pack and remove at least 15 minutes prior to treatment	Dexrazoxane IV[a] (Totect[TM], Savene[TM])
Non-Anthracycline Antitumor Antibiotics: Mitomycin, Dactinomycin	Apply ice pack for 15–20 minutes qid for the first 24 hours	DMSO 99%[a]
Non-DNA-binding Vesicant Drugs		
Vinca alkaloids: Vinblastine, Vincristine, Vinorelbine, Vindesine	1–3mL subcutaneous normal saline immediately at extravasation site; Apply warm pack for 15–20 minutes qid for the first 24–48 hours	Hyaluronidase[a]
Taxanes (mild vesicants/irritants): Paclitaxel, Docetaxel	Apply ice pack for 15–20 minutes qid for the first 24 hours	Hyaluronidase[a]

[a]Formulations for antidotes	
Sodium thiosulfate	4 mL of 10% sodium thiosulfate is mixed with 6 mL of sterile water producing a 1/6 molar solution which is injected SC. A dose example is 2 mL for each milligram of extravasated mechlorethamine
Dexrazoxane	Treatment is started within 6 hours of the extravasation. Intravenous infusion of 1,000 mg/m^2 on days 1 and 2, and 500 mg/m^2 on day 3 of the prepared solution.
DMSO	A solution of 50–100% is applied topically q2–8 hrs for up to 14 days. (DMSO 99% is ideal but DMSO 50% can be used temporarily)
Hyaluronidase	1–6 mL of a 150 Units/mL solution is injected SC into the area of extravasation. Often 1 mL of solution is used for each mL of extravasated drug

Guidelines adapted from the Oncology Nursing Society and from the European Oncology Nursing Society.
SC: Subcutaneous, IV: Intravenous.
Refer to section 3.09: Extravasation Reactions, for further information.

Figure 33.11 (a) Treatment algorithm for infusion site extravasation reactions. (b) Infusion site extravasation reaction antidotes.

Severity (CTCAE v.4)	Intervention
Grade 0	Observe for correct placement and infusion rate
Grade 1	Continue drug at current dose and monitor for change in severity
	Topical corticosteroids AND Daily warm compresses
	Reassess after 2 weeks (either by healthcare professional or patient self-report); if reactions worsen or do not improve proceed to next step
Grade 2	Continue drug at current dose using alternate access and monitor for change in severity;
	Topical corticosteroids AND Daily warm compresses
	Reassess after 2 weeks (either by healthcare professional or patient self-report); if reactions worsen or do not improve proceed to next step
Grade ≥3 Or intolerable grade 2	Continue drug at current dose using alternate access and monitor for change in severity; and continue treatment of skin reaction with the following:
	Plastic surgery/wound care team consultation AND Oral antibiotics if infection suspected
	Reassess after 2 weeks; if reactions worsen or do not improve, dose interruption or discontinuation per protocol may be necessary

Figure 33.12 Treatment algorithm for injection site reactions.

Severity (CTCAE v.4)	Intervention	Level of Evidence	Recommendation Grade
Grade 0	Gentle skin care instructions given; Sunscreen SPF≥15; OTC Moisturizing creams; Avoid extreme temperatures; Use tepid water when showering/bathing or washing dishes	III	B
Grade 1	Continue drug at current dose and monitor for change in severity		
	OTC Moisturizing cream or ointment to face bid AND	III	B
	Ammonium lactate 12% cream to body bid	III	B
	Reassess after 2 weeks (either by healthcare professional or patient self-report); if reactions worsen or do not improve proceed to next step		
Grade 2	Continue drug at current dose and monitor for change in severity		
	OTC Moisturizing cream or ointment to face bid AND	III	B
	Ammonium lactate 12% cream OR salicylic acid 6% cream to body bid	III	B
	Reassess after 2 weeks (either by healthcare professional or patient self-report); if reactions worsen or do not improve proceed to next step		
Grade ≥3 Or intolerable grade 2	Dose modify as per protocol; obtain bacterial/viral/fungal cultures if infection is suspected; and continue treatment of skin reaction with the following:		
	OTC Moisturizing cream or ointment to face bid AND	III	B
	Ammonium lactate 12% cream OR salicylic acid 6% cream to body bid AND	III	B
	Topical moderate/high-potency steroid to eczematous areas bid	III	B
	Reassess after 2 weeks; if reactions worsen or do not improve, dose interruption or discontinuation per protocol may be necessary		

OTC: Over the counter

Figure 33.13 Treatment algorithm for xerosis.

	Intervention	Level of Evidence	Recommendation Grade
Prevention	Skin fissures form due to significant xerosis and are a late adverse effects of EGFR inhibitor therapy; treating xerosis is the best way to prevent fissures		
	Wear protective footwear and cover fingertips to avoid friction with fingers, toes, and heels	III	B
Treatment	Thick ointments or zinc oxide (13–40%) creams; *Silverol OR combined topical steroid and antibiotic; Liquid glues of cyanoacrylate to seal cracks; Occlusion during sleep with cotton gloves/socks	III	B

*Silverol contains silver sulfadiazine 1%

Figure 33.14 Treatment algorithm for palmoplantar fissures.

Severity (CTCAE v.4)	Intervention	Level of Evidence	Recommendation Grade
Grade 0	Gentle skin care instructions given	IV	D
Grade 1	Continue drug at current dose and monitor for change in severity		
	Topical moderate/high-potency steroid OR	III	B
	Topical antipruritics with menthol applied bid	V	D
	Reassess after 2 weeks (either by healthcare professional or patient self-report); if reactions worsen or do not improve proceed to next step		
Grade 2	Continue drug at current dose and monitor for change in severity		
	Topical moderate/high-potency steroid OR	III	B
	Topical antipruritics with menthol applied bid AND	V	D
	Oral antipruritics	I	A
	Reassess after 2 weeks (either by healthcare professional or patient self-report); if reactions worsen or do not improve proceed to next step		
Grade ≥3 Or intolerable grade 2	Dose modify as per protocol; and continue treatment of skin reaction with the following:		
	Oral antipruritics AND Oral corticosteroids (Prednisone 0.5–1 mg/kg or equivalent for 5 days)	I	A
	Oral gabapentin or pregabalin* ± Phototherapy (narrowband ultraviolet B) at dermatologist office	V	D
	Reassess after 2 weeks; if reactions worsen or do not improve, dose interruption or discontinuation per protocol may be necessary		

* Recommended as second-line only if oral antipruritics fail

Figure 33.15 Treatment algorithm for pruritus.

Severity (CTCAE v.4)	Intervention
Grade 0	Prophylaxis with sunscreen SPF ≥15 to face, ears, neck, arms and hands when exposed to sun and reapply every 2 hours; Use hats and protective clothing
Grade 1	Continue drug at current dose and monitor for change in severity
	Hydroquinone 4% cream to affected areas bid ± Tretinoin 0.05–0.1% OR Azelaic Acid 20% Strict sun protection
	Reassess after 2 weeks (either by healthcare professional or patient self-report); if reactions worsen or do not improve proceed to next step
Grade 2	Do not interrupt drug treatment; continue treatment of skin reaction with the following:
	Hydroquinone 4% cream to affected areas bid ±Tretinoin 0.05–0.1% OR Azelaic Acid 20% Strict sun protection
	Reassess after 2 weeks (either by healthcare professional or patient self-report); if reactions worsen or do not improve, counsel patient and encourage continuation of anticancer treatment

Figure 33.16 Treatment algorithm for hyperpigmentation.

Severity (CTCAE v.4)	Intervention	Level of Evidence	Recommendation Grade
Grade 0	Gentle skin care instructions given	II	A
	Recommend wearing comfortable shoes, wearing gloves while cleaning, and avoiding biting nails or cutting nails too short;	II	A
	Biotin to improve nail strength	III	B
Grade 1	Continue drug at current dose and monitor for change in severity		
	Topical high-potency steroid AND Vinegar soaks*; Topical iodine** OR Combined topical steroid and antibiotic + anti-fungal agent	II	A
	Reassess after 2 weeks (either by healthcare professional or patient self-report); if reactions worsen or do not improve proceed to next step		
Grade 2	Continue drug at current dose and monitor for change in severity; obtain bacterial/viral/fungal cultures if infection is suspected		
	Topical high-potency steroid AND Vinegar soaks*; Topical iodine** OR Combined topical steroid and antibiotic + anti-fungal agent	II	A
	If infection suspected, begin oral antibiotics with anti-*Staphylococcus aureus* and Gram + coverage	II	A
	Reassess after 2 weeks (either by healthcare professional or patient self-report); if reactions worsen or do not improve proceed to next step		
Grade ≥3 Or intolerable grade 2	Dose modify as per protocol; obtain bacterial/viral/fungal cultures if infection is suspected; and continue treatment of skin reaction with the following:		
	Topical high-potency steroid AND Vinegar soaks*; Topical iodine** OR Combined topical steroid and antibiotic + anti-fungal agent	II	A
	If infection suspected, begin oral antibiotics with anti-*Staphylococcus aureus* and Gram + coverage AND	II	A
	Silver nitrate weekly ± consider nail avulsion by a dermatologist/surgeon	IV	D
	Reassess after 2 weeks; if reactions worsen or do not improve, dose interruption or discontinuation per protocol may be necessary		

*Vinegar soaks consist of soaking fingers or toes in a solution of white vinegar in water (1:1) for 15 minutes every day
** Recommend topical povidone iodine ointment

Figure 33.17 Treatment algorithm for paronychia.

Intervention	Level of Evidence	Recommendation Grade
Oral Mucositis from Radiotherapy (RT) for Head and Neck Cancer		
Basic oral care and oral care protocols[a]; Baseline dental examination;	III	B
Midline radiation blocks AND	II	B
Benzydamine oral rinse (15 mL, 0.15%) for 2 minutes up to 5 times a day for the duration of RT (available internationally but not in the US)	I	A
Elixir (dexamethasone 0.5 mg/5 mL); swish and spit 2 tsp qid; no eating/drinking 30 minutes after use	II	C
Oral Mucositis from Standard and High-dose Chemotherapy		
Basic oral care and oral care protocols[a]; Baseline dental examination ±	III	B
Topical steroids[b]	III	B
30 minutes of oral cryotherapy (ice chips) during bolus 5-fluorouracil (5-FU) chemotherapy or bolus doses of edatrexate	I	A
Oral Mucositis from High-dose Chemotherapy ± Total Body Irradiation Plus Hematopoietic Stem Cell Transplantation (HSCT)		
Basic oral care and oral care protocols[a]; Baseline dental examination ±	III	B
Topical steroids[b]	III	B
Palifermin 60 µg/kg/day for 3 days prior to conditioning treatment **and** 3 days post-transplant for patients with hematologic malignancies;	I	A
Cryotherapy (ice chips) in patients receiving high-dose melphalan;	I	A
Low-level laser therapy (LLLT) for patients receiving high-dose chemotherapy or chemoradiotherapy **prior to HSCT**	II	B

[a]Basic oral care includes using a soft-bristle toothbrush, bland rinses, and flossing daily. Oral care protocols provide comprehensive patient education about mucositis and oral care with an emphasis on feasibility and adherence.
[b]See Table 1 for topical steroids recommended for oral application.

Figure 33.18 Management algorithm for prevention of oral mucositis.

Intervention	Level of Evidence	Recommendation Grade
Oral Mucositis from Radiotherapy (RT) for Head and Neck Cancer		
Basic oral care and oral care protocols[a] AND	III	B
Benzydamine oral rinse (15 mL, 0.15%) for 2 minutes up to 5 times a day for the duration of RT (available internationally but not in the US) AND	I	A
Pain control with NSAIDs/GABA agonists/Narcotics or PCA with morphine AND	II	B
Elixir (dexamethasone 5 mg/5 mL); swish and spit 2 tsp qid; no eating/drinking 30 minutes after use	II	C
Oral Mucositis from Standard and High-dose Chemotherapy		
Basic oral care and oral care protocols[a] AND	III	B
30 minutes of oral cryotherapy (ice chips) during bolus 5-fluorouracil (5-FU) chemotherapy or bolus doses of edatrexate AND	I	A
Pain control with NSAIDs/GABA agonists/Narcotics or PCA with morphine	II	B
Oral Mucositis from High-dose Chemotherapy ± Total Body Irradiation Plus Hematopoietic Stem Cell Transplantation (HSCT)		
Basic oral care and oral care protocols[a] ±Topical steroids AND	III	B
Pain control with NSAIDs/GABA agonists/Narcotics or PCA with morphine	II	B
Palifermin 60 µg/kg/day for 3 days prior to conditioning treatment **and** 3 days post-transplant for patients with hematologic malignancies;	I	A
Cryotherapy (ice chips) in patients receiving high-dose melphalan;	I	A
Low-level laser therapy (LLLT) for patients receiving high-dose chemotherapy or chemoradiotherapy **prior to HSCT**	II	B

[a]Basic oral care includes using a soft-bristle toothbrush, bland rinses, and flossing daily. Oral care protocols provide comprehensive patient education about mucositis and oral care with an emphasis on feasibility and adherence.
PCA: Patient-controlled analgesia.
Grade 1 oral mucositis: Continue RT/drug therapy and monitor for change in severity; recommend dental evaluation. Reassess patient after 2 weeks (either by healthcare professional or patient self-report).
Grades ≥ 3 oral mucositis: Interrupt RT/drug therapy until severity decreases to grade 0–1; assess/manage pain; recommend dental evaluation; continue treatment of therapy specific mucositis. Reassess after 2 weeks; if reactions worsen or do not improve, RT/drug therapy interruption or discontinuation per protocol may be necessary.

Figure 33.19 Management algorithm for treatment of oral mucositis.

Severity (CTCAE v.4)	Intervention	Level of Evidence	Recommendation Grade
Grade 0[a]	Intrarectal Amifostine ≥ 340 mg/m^2 for radiation proctitis in patients receiving standard-dose radiotherapy; Silver leaf dressing	III	B
	Reassess after 2 weeks (either by healthcare professional or patient self-report); if reactions worsen or do not improve proceed to next step		
Grade 1	Continue drug at current dose and monitor for change in severity		
	Silver sulfadiazine 1% AND Hydrocortisone 2.5% AND Lidocaine 4% (for pain control); Silver leaf dressing		
	Reassess after 2 weeks (either by healthcare professional or patient self-report); if reactions worsen, or do not improve, proceed to next step		
Grade 2	Continue drug at current dose; assess/manage pain; and continue treatment of skin reaction with the following:		
	Silver sulfadiazine 1% AND Hydrocortisone 2.5% AND Lidocaine 4% AND Pain control with NSAIDs/GABA agonists/Narcotics		
	Reassess after 2 weeks (either by healthcare professional or patient self-report); if reactions worsen or do not improve proceed to next step		
Grade ≥3 Or intolerable grade 2	Interrupt treatment until severity decreases to grade 0–1; assess/manage pain; and continue treatment of skin reaction with the following:		
	Silver sulfadiazine 1% AND Hydrocortisone 2.5% AND Lidocaine 4% AND Pain control with NSAIDs/GABA agonists/Narcotics Sucralfate enema for chronic radiation-induced proctitis in patients with rectal bleeding	III	B
	Reassess after 2 weeks; if reactions worsen or do not improve, dose interruption or discontinuation per protocol may be necessary		

[a]Encourage limiting self care ADLs

Figure 33.20 Treatment algorithm for anal mucositis and proctitis.

Severity (CTCAE v.4)	Intervention	Level of Evidence	Recommendation Grade
Grade 0	None recommended for non-scarring alopecia; Follow rash recommendations for scarring alopecia	V	D
Grade 1	Continue drug at current dose and monitor for change in severity; Check TSH, Vitamin D, Zinc, and Ferritin serum levels (Fe ≥ 70 ng/mL)		
	Minoxidil 2%, 5% bid during chemotherapy; Biotin[a] AND Orthosilicic acid 10mg qd[b] after chemotherapy is completed; Eyelash hair loss: Bimatoprost ophthalmic solution 0.03% (Latisse)	I	B
	Reassess after 2 weeks (either by healthcare professional or patient self-report); if reactions worsen, or do not improve, proceed to next step		
Grade 2	Continue drug at current dose and monitor for change in severity; Check TSH, Vitamin D, Zinc, and Ferritin serum levels (Fe ≥ 70 ng/mL)		
	Minoxidil 2%, 5% bid during chemotherapy; Biotin[a] AND Orthosilicic acid 10mg qd[b] after chemotherapy is completed; Eyelash hair loss: Bimatoprost ophthalmic solution 0.03% (Latisse)	I	B
	Reassess after 2 weeks (either by healthcare professional or patient self-report); if reactions worsen, or do not improve, counsel patient about use of hats, scarves, or wigs		

[a]Biotin: Appearex 2.5 mg or 2500 mcg qd
[b]Orthosilicic acid 10 mg qd: Biosil, 1 capsule bid

Figure 33.21 Management algorithm for hair loss (alopecia).

Severity (CTCAE v.4)	Intervention	Level of Evidence	Recommendation Grade
Grade 0	Proper patient education and support	IV	B
Grade 1	Continue anticancer agent at current dose and monitor for change in severity; Provide treatment options if concerning to the patient		
	Facial hypertrichosis: Eflornithine; Lasers; Threading	IV	B
	Eyelash trichomegaly: Regularly trim eyelashes to avoid corneal abrasions AND Ophthalmologic evaluation	IV	B
	Reassess after 2 weeks (either by healthcare professional or patient self-report); if reactions worsen or do not improve proceed to next step		
Grade 2	Continue drug at current dose and monitor for change in severity		
	Facial hypertrichosis: Eflornithine; Lasers; Threading	IV	B
	Eyelash trichomegaly: Regularly trim eyelashes to avoid corneal abrasions AND Ophthalmologic evaluation	IV	B
	Reassess after 2 weeks (either by healthcare professional or patient self-report); if reactions worsen or do not improve counsel patient and encourage continuation of anticancer treatment		

Figure 33.22 Management algorithm for hair growth (hypertrichosis).

References

1 Agero, A.L., Dusza, S.W., Benvenuto-Andrade, C., Busam, K.J., Myskowski, P. & Halpern, A.C. (2006) Dermatologic side effects associated with the epidermal growth factor receptor inhibitors. *Journal of the American Academy of Dermatology*, **55** (4), 657–670.

2 Balagula, E. & Lacouture, M.E. (2011) Dermatologic toxicities. In: Olver, I.N. (ed), *The MASCC Textbook of Cancer Supportive Care and Survivorship*, pp. 361–380. Springer.

3 Balagula, Y., Garbe, C., Myskowski, P.L. *et al.* (2011) Clinical presentation and management of dermatological toxicities of epidermal growth factor receptor inhibitors. *International Journal of Dermatology*, **50** (2), 129–146.

4 Balagula, Y., Lacouture, M.E. & Cotliar, J.A. (2010) Dermatologic toxicities of targeted anticancer therapies. *Journal of Supportive Oncology*, **8** (4), 149–161.

5 Burtness, B., Anadkat, M., Basti, S. *et al.* (2009) NCCN Task Force Report: management of dermatologic and other toxicities associated with EGFR inhibition in patients with cancer. *Journal of the National Comprehensive Cancer Network*, **7** (Suppl. 1), S5–S21, quiz S22–24.

6 Busam, K.J., Capodieci, P., Motzer, R., Kiehn, T., Phelan, D. & Halpern, A.C. (2001) Cutaneous side-effects in cancer patients treated with the antiepidermal growth factor receptor antibody C225. *British Journal of Dermatology*, **144** (6), 1169–1176.

7 Eames, T., Grabein, B., Kroth, J. & Wollenberg, A. (2010) Microbiological analysis of epidermal growth factor receptor inhibitor therapy-associated paronychia. *Journal of the European Academy of Dermatology and Venereology*, **24** (8), 958–960.

8 Fox, L.P. (2007) Nail toxicity associated with epidermal growth factor receptor inhibitor therapy. *Journal of the American Academy of Dermatology*, **56** (3), 460–465.

9 Han, S.S., Lee, M., Park, G.H. *et al.* (2010) Investigation of papulopustular eruptions caused by cetuximab treatment shows altered differentiation markers and increases in inflammatory cytokines. *British Journal of Dermatology*, **162** (2), 371–379.

10 Lacouture, M.E. (2006) Mechanisms of cutaneous toxicities to EGFR inhibitors. *Nature Reviews. Cancer*, **6** (10), 803–812.

11 Lacouture, M.E., Basti, S., Patel, J. & Benson, A. 3rd. (2006) The SERIES clinic: an interdisciplinary approach to the management of toxicities of EGFR inhibitors. *Journal of Supportive Oncology*, **4** (5), 236–238.

12 Lacouture, M.E., Mitchell, E.P., Piperdi, B. *et al.* (2010) Skin toxicity evaluation protocol with panitumumab (STEPP), a phase II, open-label, randomized trial evaluating the impact of a pre-emptive skin treatment regimen on skin toxicities and quality of life in patients with metastatic colorectal cancer. *Journal of Clinical Oncology*, **28** (8), 1351–1357.

13 Lacouture, M.E., Reilly, L.M., Gerami, P. & Guitart, J. (2008) Hand foot skin reaction in cancer patients treated with the multikinase inhibitors sorafenib and sunitinib. *Annals of Oncology*, **19** (11), 1955–1961.

14 Roé, E., García Muret, M.P., Marcuello, E., Capdevila, J., Pallarésm C. & Alomar, A. (2006) Description and management of cutaneous side effects during cetuximab or erlotinib treatments: a prospective study of 30 patients. *Journal of the American Academy of Dermatology*, **55** (3), 429–437.

15 Scope, A., Agero, A.L., Dusza, S.W. *et al.* (2007) Randomized double-blind trial of prophylactic oral minocycline and topical tazarotene for cetuximab-associated acne-like eruption. *Journal of Clinical Oncology*, **25** (34), 5390–5396.

16 Tosti, A., Piraccini, B.M., Ghetti, E. & Colombo, M.D. (2002) Topical steroids versus systemic antifungals in the treatment of chronic paronychia: an open, randomized double-blind and double dummy study. *Journal of the American Academy of Dermatology*, **47** (1), 73–76.

17 Joshi, S.S., Ortiz, S., Witherspoon, J.N. *et al.* (2010) Effects of epidermal growth factor receptor inhibitor-induced dermatologic toxicities on quality of life. *Cancer*, **116** (16), 3916–3923.

18 Alexandrescu, D.T., Vaillant, J.G. & Dasanu, C.A. (2007) Effect of treatment with a colloidal oatmeal lotion on the acneform eruption induced by epidermal growth factor receptor and multiple tyrosine-kinase inhibitors. *Clinical and Experimental Dermatology*, **32** (1), 71–74.

19 Bidoli, P., Cortinovis, D.L., Colombo, I. *et al.* (2010) Isotretinoin plus clindamycin seem highly effective against severe erlotinib-induced skin rash in advanced non-small cell lung cancer. *Journal of Thoracic Oncology*, 5 (10), 1662–1663.

20 Gutzmer, R., Werfel, T., Mao, R., Kapp, A. & Elsner, J. (2005) Successful treatment with oral isotretinoin of acneiform skin lesions associated with cetuximab therapy. *British Journal of Dermatology*, 153 (4), 849–851.

21 Jatoi, A. (2007) Sunshine and rash: testing the role of sunscreen to prevent epidermal growth factor receptor inhibitor-induced rash. *Supportive Cancer Therapy*, 4 (4), 198–202.

22 Jatoi, A., Dakhil, S.R., Sloan, J.A. *et al.* (2011) Prophylactic tetracycline does not diminish the severity of epidermal growth factor receptor (EGFR) inhibitor-induced rash: results from the North Central Cancer Treatment Group (Supplementary N03CB). *Supportive Care in Cancer*, 19 (10), 1601–1607.

23 Jatoi, A., Rowland, K., Sloan, J.A. *et al.* (2008) Tetracycline to prevent epidermal growth factor receptor inhibitor-induced skin rashes: results of a placebo-controlled trial from the North Central Cancer Treatment Group (N03CB). *Cancer*, 113 (4), 847–853.

24 Jatoi, A., Thrower, A., Sloan, J.A. *et al.* (2010) Does sunscreen prevent epidermal growth factor receptor (EGFR) inhibitor-induced rash? Results of a placebo-controlled trial from the North Central Cancer Treatment Group (N05C4). *The Oncologist*, 15 (9), 1016–1022.

25 Lynch, T.J. Jr, Kim, E.S., Eaby, B., Garey, J., West, D.P. & Lacouture, M.E. (2007) Epidermal growth factor receptor inhibitor-associated cutaneous toxicities: an evolving paradigm in clinical management. *The Oncologist*, 12 (5), 610–621.

26 Melosky, B., Burkes, R., Rayson, D., Alcindor, T., Shear, N. & Lacouture, M. (2009) Management of skin rash during EGFR-targeted monoclonal antibody treatment for gastrointestinal malignancies: Canadian recommendations. *Current Oncology*, 16 (1), 16–26.

27 Pomerantz, R.G., Chirinos, R.E. & Falo, L.D. Jr & Geskin, L.J. (2008) Acitretin for treatment of EGFR inhibitor-induced cutaneous toxic effects. *Archives of Dermatology*, 144 (7), 949–950.

28 Shah, N.T., Kris, M.G., Pao, W. *et al.* (2005) Practical management of patients with non-small-cell lung cancer treated with gefitinib. *Journal of Clinical Oncology*, 23 (1), 165–174.

29 Vezzoli, P., Marzano, A.V., Onida, F. *et al.* (2008) Cetuximab-induced acneiform eruption and the response to isotretinoin. *Acta Dermato-Venereologica*, 88 (1), 84–86.

30 Brown, J., Burck, K., Black, D. & Collins, C. (1991) Treatment of cytarabine acral erythema with corticosteroids. *Journal of the American Academy of Dermatology*, 24 (6 Pt 1), 1023–1025.

31 Chu, D., Lacouture, M.E., Fillos, T. & Wu, S. (2008) Risk of hand-foot skin reaction with sorafenib: a systematic review and meta-analysis. *Acta Oncologica (Stockholm, Sweden)*, 47 (2), 176–186.

32 Lacouture, M.E., Wu, S., Robert, C. *et al.* (2008) Evolving strategies for the management of hand-foot skin reaction associated with the multitargeted kinase inhibitors sorafenib and sunitinib. *The Oncologist*, 13 (9), 1001–1011.

33 von Moos, R., Thuerlimann, B.J., Aapro, M. *et al.* (2008) Pegylated liposomal doxorubicin-associated hand-foot syndrome: recommendations of an international panel of experts. *European Journal of Cancer*, 44 (6), 781–790.

34 Zhang, R.-X., Wu, X.J., Lu, S.X., Pan, Z.Z., Wan, D.S. & Chen, G. (2011) The effect of COX-2 inhibitor on capecitabine-induced hand–foot syndrome in patients with stage II/III colorectal cancer: a phase

II randomized prospective study. *Journal of Cancer Research and Clinical Oncology*, 137 (6), 953–957.

35 Zhang, R.X., Wu, X.J., Wan, D.S. *et al.* (2011) Celecoxib can prevent capecitabine-related hand-foot syndrome in stage II and III colorectal cancer patients: result of a single-center, prospective randomized phase III trial. *Annals of Oncology*.

36 Bernier, J., Bonner, J., Vermorken, J.B. *et al.* (2008) Consensus guidelines for the management of radiation dermatitis and coexisting acne-like rash in patients receiving radiotherapy plus EGFR inhibitors for the treatment of squamous cell carcinoma of the head and neck. *Annals of Oncology*, 19 (1), 142–149.

37 Boström, A., Lindman, H., Swartling, C., Berne, B. & Bergh, J. (2001) Potent corticosteroid cream (mometasone furoate) significantly reduces acute radiation dermatitis: results from a double-blind, randomized study. *Journal of the European Society for Therapeutic Radiology and Oncology*, 59 (3), 257–265.

38 Campbell, I.R. & Illingworth, M.H. (1992) Can patients wash during radiotherapy to the breast or chest wall? A randomized controlled trial. *Clinical Oncology (Royal College of Radiologists (Great Britain))*, 4 (2), 78–82.

39 Roy, I., Fortin, A. & Larochelle, M. (2001) The impact of skin washing with water and soap during breast irradiation: a randomized study. *Journal of the European Society for Therapeutic Radiology and Oncology*, 58 (3), 333–339.

40 Salvo, N., Barnes, E., van Draanen, J. *et al.* (2010) Prophylaxis and management of acute radiation-induced skin reactions: a systematic review of the literature. *Current Oncology*, 17 (4), 94–112.

41 Schmuth, M., Wimmer, M.A., Hofer, S. *et al.* (2002) Topical corticosteroid therapy for acute radiation dermatitis: a prospective, randomized, double-blind study. *British Journal of Dermatology*, 146 (6), 983–991.

42 Segaert, S., Tabernero, J., Chosidow, O. *et al.* (2005) The management of skin reactions in cancer patients receiving epidermal growth factor receptor targeted therapies. *Journal der Deutschen Dermatologischen Gesellschaft*, 3 (8), 599–606.

43 Segaert, S. & Van Cutsem, E. (2005) Clinical signs, pathophysiology and management of skin toxicity during therapy with epidermal growth factor receptor inhibitors. *Annals of Oncology*, 16 (9), 1425–1433.

44 Tejwani, A., Wu, S., Jia, Y., Agulnik, M., Millender, L. & Lacouture, M.E. (2009) Increased risk of high-grade dermatologic toxicities with radiation plus epidermal growth factor receptor inhibitor therapy. *Cancer*, 115 (6), 1286–1299.

45 Agha, R., Agha, R., Kinahan, K., Bennett, C.L. & Lacouture, M.E. (2007) Dermatologic challenges in cancer patients and survivors. *Oncology (Williston Park)*, 21 (12), 1462–1472, discussion 1473, 1476, 1481 passim.

46 Wyatt, A.J., Leonard, G.D. & Sachs, D.L. (2006) Cutaneous reactions to chemotherapy and their management. *American Journal of Clinical Dermatology*, 7 (1), 45–63.

47 Wengstrom, Y. & Margulies, A. (2008) European Oncology Nursing Society extravasation guidelines. *European Journal of Oncology Nursing*, 12 (4), 357–361.

48 Polovich, M., Whitford, J.M. & Olsen, M. (eds) (2009) Immediate complications of cytotoxic therapy. In: *Chemotherapy and Biotherapy Guidelines and Recommendations for Practice*, 3rd edn, pp. 105–116. Oncology Nursing Society, Pittsburg, PA.

49 Goolsby, T.V. & Lombardo, F.A. (2006) Extravasation of chemotherapeutic agents: prevention and treatment. *Seminars in Oncology*, 33 (1), 139–143.

50 Aygenc, E., Celikkanat, S., Kaymakci, M., Aksaray, F. & Ozdem, C. (2004) Prophylactic effect of pentoxifylline on radiotherapy complications: a clinical study. *Otolaryngology and Head and Neck Surgery*, **130** (3), 351–356.

51 Bromm, B., Scharein, E., Darsow, U. & Ring, J. (1995) Effects of menthol and cold on histamine-induced itch and skin reactions in man. *Neuroscience Letters*, **187** (3), 157–160.

52 Drake, L.A. & Millikan, L.E. (1995) The antipruritic effect of 5% doxepin cream in patients with eczematous dermatitis. Doxepin Study Group. *Archives of Dermatology*, **131** (12), 1403–1408.

53 Eschler, D.C. & Klein, P.A. (2010) An evidence-based review of the efficacy of topical antihistamines in the relief of pruritus. *Journal of Drugs in Dermatology*, **9** (8), 992–997.

54 Goutos, I., Eldardiri, M., Khan, A.A., Dziewulski, P. & Richardson, P.M. (2010) Comparative evaluation of antipruritic protocols in acute burns. The emerging value of gabapentin in the treatment of burns pruritus. *Journal of Burn Care and Research*, **31** (1), 57–63.

55 Gunal, A.I., Ozalp, G., Yoldas, T.K., Gunal, S.Y., Kirciman, E. & Celiker, H. (2004) Gabapentin therapy for pruritus in haemodialysis patients: a randomized, placebo-controlled, double-blind trial. *Nephrology, Dialysis, Transplantation*, **19** (12), 3137–3139.

56 Hu, J.C., Sadeghi, P., Pinter-Brown, L.C., Yashar, S. & Chiu, M.W. (2007) Cutaneous side effects of epidermal growth factor receptor inhibitors: clinical presentation, pathogenesis, and management. *Journal of the American Academy of Dermatology*, **56** (2), 317–326.

57 Jennings, M.B., Alfieri, D., Ward, K. & Lesczczynski, C. (1998) Comparison of salicylic acid and urea versus ammonium lactate for the treatment of foot xerosis: a randomized, double-blind, clinical study. *Journal of the American Podiatric Medical Association*, **88** (7), 332–336.

58 Porzio, G., Aielli, F., Verna, L. *et al.* (2006) Efficacy of pregabalin in the management of cetuximab-related itch. *Journal of Pain and Symptom Management*, **32** (5), 397–398.

59 Racca, P., Fanchini, L., Caliendo, V. *et al.* (2008) Efficacy and skin toxicity management with cetuximab in metastatic colorectal cancer: outcomes from an oncologic/dermatologic cooperation. *Clinical Colorectal Cancer*, **7** (1), 48–54.

60 Saif, M.W., Kaley, K., Lamb, L. *et al.* (2010) Management of skin toxicities of anti-EGFR agents in patients with pancreatic cancer and other GI tumors by using electronic communication: effective and convenient. *JOP: Journal of the Pancreas*, **11** (2), 176–182.

61 Shohrati, M., Tajik, A., Harandi, A.A., Davoodi, S.M. & Akmasi, M. (2007) Comparison of hydroxyzine and doxepin in treatment of pruritus due to sulfur mustard. *Skinmed*, **6** (2), 70–72.

62 Vincenzi, B., Tonini, G. & Santini, D. (2010) Aprepitant for erlotinib-induced pruritus. *New England Journal of Medicine*, **363** (4), 397–398.

63 Wollenberg, A., Kroth, J., Hauschild, A. & Dirschka, T. (2010) Cutaneous side effects of EGFR inhibitors: appearance and management. *Deutsche Medizinische Wochenschrift (1946)*, **135** (4), 149–154.

64 Wollenberg, A., Staehler, M. & Eames, T. (2010) [Cutaneous side effects of the multikinase inhibitors sorafenib and sunitinib]. *Der Hautarzt; Zeitschrift fur Dermatologie, Venerologie, Und Verwandte Gebiete*, **61** (8), 662–667.

65 Hochman, L.G., Scher, R.K. & Meyerson, M.S. (1993) Brittle nails: response to daily biotin supplementation. *Cutis; Cutaneous Medicine for the Practitioner*, **51** (4), 303–305.

66 Robert, C., Soria, J.C., Spatz, A. *et al.* (2005) Cutaneous side-effects of kinase inhibitors and blocking antibodies. *Lancet Oncology*, **6** (7), 491–500.

67 Sassone, L.M., Fidel, R.A., Murad, C.F., Fidel, S.R. & Hirata, R. Jr. (2008) Antimicrobial activity of sodium hypochlorite and chlorhexidine by two different tests. *Australian Endodontic Journal*, **34** (1), 19–24.

68 Scotte, F., Tourani, J.M., Banu, E. *et al.* (2005) Multicenter study of a frozen glove to prevent docetaxel-induced onycholysis and cutaneous toxicity of the hand. *Journal of Clinical Oncology*, **23** (19), 4424–4429.

69 Suh, K.Y., Kindler, H.L., Medenica, M. & Lacouture, M. (2006) Doxycycline for the treatment of paronychia induced by the epidermal growth factor receptor inhibitor cetuximab. *British Journal of Dermatology*, **154** (1), 191–192.

70 Epstein, J.B., Elad, S., Eliav, E., Jurevic, R. & Benoliel, R. (2007) Orofacial pain in cancer: part II: clinical perspectives and management. *Journal of Dental Research*, **86** (6), 506–518.

71 Keefe, D.M., Schubert, M.M., Elting, L.S. *et al.* (2007) Updated clinical practice guidelines for the prevention and treatment of mucositis. *Cancer*, **109** (5), 820–831.

72 Rubenstein, E.B., Peterson, D.E., Schubert, M. *et al.* (2004) Clinical practice guidelines for the prevention and treatment of cancer therapy-induced oral and gastrointestinal mucositis. *Cancer*, **100** (9 Suppl.), 2026–2046.

73 Rothwell, B.R. & Spektor, W.S. (1990) Palliation of radiation-related mucositis. *Special Care in Dentistry*, **10** (1), 21–25.

74 Peterson, D.E., Bensadoun, R.J., Roila, F.; ESMO Guidelines Working Group (2011) Management of oral and gastrointestinal mucositis: ESMO Clinical Practice Guidelines. *Annals of Oncology*, **22** (Suppl. 6), vi78–vi84.

75 Kazemian, A., Kamian, S., Aghili, M., Hashemi, F.A. & Haddad, P. (2009) Benzydamine for prophylaxis of radiation-induced oral mucositis in head and neck cancers: a double-blind placebo-controlled randomized clinical trial. *European Journal of Cancer Care*, **18** (2), 174–178.

76 Amin, S.P. & Goldberg, D.J. (2006) Clinical comparison of four hair removal lasers and light sources. *Journal of Cosmetic and Laser Therapy*, **8** (2), 65–68.

77 Duvic, M., Lemak, N.A., Valero, V. *et al.* (1996) A randomized trial of minoxidil in chemotherapy-induced alopecia. *Journal of the American Academy of Dermatology*, **35** (1), 74–78.

78 Hamzavi, I., Tan, E., Shapiro, J. & Lui, H. (2007) A randomized bilateral vehicle-controlled study of eflornithine cream combined with laser treatment versus laser treatment alone for facial hirsutism in women. *Journal of the American Academy of Dermatology*, **57** (1), 54–59.

79 Olsen, E.A., Dunlap, F.E., Funicella, T. *et al.* (2002) A randomized clinical trial of 5% topical minoxidil versus 2% topical minoxidil and placebo in the treatment of androgenetic alopecia in men. *Journal of the American Academy of Dermatology*, **47** (3), 377–385.

80 Olsen, E.A., Whiting, D., Bergfeld, W. *et al.* (2007) A multicenter, randomized, placebo-controlled, double-blind clinical trial of a novel formulation of 5% minoxidil topical foam versus placebo in the treatment of androgenetic alopecia in men. *Journal of the American Academy of Dermatology*, **57** (5), 767–774.

81 Smith, S.R., Piacquadio, D.J., Beger, B. & Littler, C. (2006) Eflornithine cream combined with laser therapy in the management of unwanted facial hair growth in women: a randomized trial. *Dermatologic Surgery*, **32** (10), 1237–1243.

34 Dermatologic Therapeutics and Formulations

Judy H. Borovicka[1], Jennifer R.S. Gordon[1], Ann Cameron Haley[1], Nicole E. Larsen[1,2] and Dennis P. West[1,2]

[1]Department of Dermatology, Northwestern University, Chicago, IL, USA
[2]Robert H. Lurie Comprehensive Cancer Center, Feinberg School of Medicine, Chicago, IL, USA

Introduction

In this chapter we discuss the most common dermatologic therapeutic agents and their uses. When appropriate, management strategies for oncology-related dermatologic adverse events (AEs) or immunocompromised patients are highlighted (Table 34.1).

Moisturizing therapy

Emollients are a mainstay in dermatology both for damaged and undamaged skin as prophylaxis and therapy. Vehicles used in moisturizers include creams, lotions, and ointments. Creams are emulsions (two-phase systems) containing oil and water, and are the most common type of delivery system used for moisturizers. Lotions are usually emulsions with a lower content of oils than creams. Ointments contain oleaginous solids and are a single-phase system usually composed of a lipophilic drug in a base such as petrolatum, organic alcohols, mineral oil, or waxes [1]. Ointments spread easily on the skin (although not as easily as creams) and are completely water-insoluble with maximal water-retaining occlusive properties. They usually form a greasy film on the skin and can cause excessive heat retention, which may cause discomfort to the patient. Common fats in moisturizers are mono-, di-, and triglycerides, waxes, long-chain esters, fatty acids, lanolin (wool) alcohol, and mineral oils [1].

Foams deliver active drug at an increased rate compared with other vehicles by enhancing penetration and altering barrier properties of the outer stratum corneum. This is in contrast to other topical delivery vehicles that first require hydration of an intercellular space in the stratum corneum. Foam vehicles consist of oil, water, and an organic solvent, and may be a liquid pressurized in an aluminum container with hydrocarbon propellant [2].

- Moisturization for dryness associated with anticancer therapies typically involves application of emollients to face, hands, feet, neck, and back at least daily [3]
- Incidence of grade 2 or higher skin toxicities was shown to be reduced by more than 50% in the pre-emptive topical emollient group compared with the group receiving emollient treatment upon reaction [4]

Types of moisturizers

Types of moisturizers include occlusives, humectants, and hydrophilic matrices. The additives found in moisturizers include exfoliants, antioxidants, humectants, emollients, and bioactive ingredients [5].

Occlusive moisturizers

Occlusive moisturizers form a barrier that retains water by preventing transepidermal water loss (TEWL). A complete barrier is not desirable because of impeded barrier recovery. Of the various types of occlusive moisturizers, one of the most effective is petrolatum. Because petrolatum permeates through the stratum corneum interstices, it accelerates recovery of barrier function while promoting hydration [5]. Occlusives can feel greasy or heavy and are not as cosmetically appealing as the alternative moisturizers.

Humectant moisturizers

Humectants are hygroscopic agents that can draw moisture to the skin from deeper tissues but minimally from surrounding air. TEWL maybe increased in low humidity by drawing water from the skin. The majority of humectants used in moisturizers are

Dermatologic Principles and Practice in Oncology: Conditions of the Skin, Hair, and Nails in Cancer Patients, First Edition. Edited by Mario E. Lacouture.

Table 34.1 Characteristics of commonly used delivery vehicles.

Vehicle	Ease of application	Irritancy potential	Moisturizing ability	Cosmetic acceptance
Lotion	Excellent	Moderate	Fair	Excellent
Cream	Good	Minimal	Good	Good
Ointment	Fair	Minimal	Excellent	Fair
Gel	Good	Moderate	Fair	Good
Foam	Good	Moderate	Fair	Good, especially in hair-bearing areas
Solution	Good	Moderate	Fair	Good
Orabase (Kenalog®)	Good for oral mucosa	Minimal	Not Applicable	Good for oral mucosa

hydrophilic with low molecular weight substances. Glycerol, propylene glycol, and butylene glycol are the most commonly used humectants. Alpha hydroxyl acids (AHAs), including lactic, glycolic, and tartaric acids, are another common group of humectants [1].

Hydrophilic matrices

The standard hydrophilic matrix is colloidal oatmeal, which is used in bath, lotion, and cream formulations. Hyaluronic acid, a mucopolysaccharide found in the dermis, is a hydrophilic matrix substance that functions as both a humectant and a penetration enhancer [6].

Recommendations

Moisturizers are commonly recommended for the treatment of xerosis and dermatitis.

Xerosis

The right vehicle choice is vital to alleviate skin dryness associated with anticancer therapies. When the first signs of dryness appear on the face, chest, or back, alcoholic lotions or gels should be discontinued and switched to oil-in-water creams or ointments. Greasy (water-in-oil) creams or even ointments can be used for moderate to severe xerosis of the limbs. The right balance of oil and water should always be kept because occlusive ointments may facilitate the development of folliculitis lesions [7].

Radiation dermatitis

Plain nonscented lanolin-free hydrophilic cream is recommended for patients experiencing radiation skin reactions. These creams attract and trap moisture at the skin surface to increase the skin's moisture and maintain skin pliability. The cream should be discontinued when skin breakdown occurs [8]. It should be noted that topical moisturizers, gels, emulsions, and dressings should not be applied immediately before radiation treatment as they can artificially increase the radiation dose to the epidermis as a bolus effect [8].

AEs of moisturizers

Moisturizers are rarely associated with AEs. The most common AEs to moisturizers are sensory reactions immediately after application, including burning and stinging sensations [9]. Fragrances and preservatives are the major sensitizers in topical formulations, because over 100 fragrance ingredients have been identified as allergens [10]. Lanolin (wool) alcohol (an example of a lanolin-containing agent is Aquaphor®) is an allergen for approximately 1.3% of the [11] population. Skin irritation from topical preparations is commonly encountered, particularly in atopics, because of impaired barrier function [1]. Humectants, emulsifiers, and oils rarely cause contact allergy [12]. Some products such as Chinese herbal creams have been found to be contaminated with corticosteroids, which can cause serious AEs [1].

General dispensing recommendations for topical therapy

Recommendations for applying emollients are typically nonspecific and require covering the affected areas. However, for prescription preparations it is important to know how much product is sufficient for a specific treatment area and the duration of treatment required. Table 34.2 is a general guideline using "fingertip" units to help calculate an appropriate tube size when prescribing topical medication.

- Various topical formulations (vehicles) provide different benefits and are important to consider when prescribing or recommending therapy
- The effectiveness of topical medications are dependent on medication concentration, vehicle, frequency, and compliance of applications, as well as integrity of the stratum corneum
- Active ingredient(s) *or* vehicle components can cause local toxicity
- Topical medications can have systemic absorption, especially when applied to large body surface areas

Keratolytic therapy

The mechanism of action of keratolytics is somewhat unknown but is thought to be related to proteolysis and keratinolysis [14]. These agents cause peeling of the epidermis. At low concentrations, most keratolytics act as humectants, or moisturizing agents.

Table 34.2 Amount of topical medication required to treat affected body area [13].

Affected body area	Amount of topical medication needed per 1 application		Amount to dispense for coverage of area for 7 days bid (grams)
	FTU	grams	
Head	4	2	30
Face and neck	2.5	1.25	20
Trunk (either front or back)	7	3.5	50
One arm	3	1.5	25
One hand (either palmar or dorsal)	0.5	0.25	5
One leg	6	3	50
One foot	2	1	20

bid, twice daily; FTU, fingertip unit (the amount of ointment or cream expressed from a tube with a 5-mm diameter nozzle) applied from the distal skin crease to the tip of the finger.

Keratolytics are most commonly used for hyperkeratotic diseases including psoriasis and ichthyosis, as well as photoaging and hand-foot syndrome [15].

Common keratolytics
Salicylic acid
Salicylic acid dissolves the intercellular matrix and softens hyperkeratotic areas by enhancing the shedding of skin [16]. For keratolysis, ≤6% creams are typically used (see also Salicylic acid in the section on topical antiviral therapy).

Urea
Urea moisturizes the skin and acts as a mild keratolytic by promoting skin penetration. Urea dissolves the intercellular matrix, resulting in the loosening of the horny layer and shedding of scaly skin. Thus, hyperkeratotic areas are softened by reducing epidermal thickness and proliferation [14]. Hydrocortisone penetration is enhanced when combined with urea [17].

AEs of keratolytics
Salicylic acid preparations to extensive areas of skin should be used cautiously as they may induce systemic toxicity [16]. Urea cream is acidic (pH 3) and may sting when applied to the skin. Formulations containing urea must keep an acid pH to prevent degradation of urea to ammonia.

Table 34.3 Common sunscreen components.

UVB blockers	Padimate O Octyl methoxycinnamate (Octinoxate) Octyl salicylate (Octisalate) Octocrylene Phenylbenzimidazole sulfonic acid
UVA blockers	Oxybenzone Methyl anthranilate Avobenzone (Parsol 1789)
UVA-UVB blockers (physical)	Titanium dioxide Zinc oxide
UVA-UVB blockers (chemical)	Methoxyphenyltriazene Ecamsule (Mexoryl™SX)

For grade 1 and higher hand-foot syndrome and dry skin, keratolytics such as urea 20–40% or salicylic acid 6% may be useful.

Sunscreens

Sunscreens and sun blocks
Sunscreens and sun blocks are useful in the prevention of dry skin caused by photodamage and are widely available in moisturizing formulations for the treatment of photodamaged dry skin. Sunscreens minimize radiation damage to cells by either physically blocking UV rays (physical blockers) or by absorbing and converting UV rays to heat energy (chemical blockers). Sunscreens are only part of a complete program for sun protection that includes use of protective clothing, shade, and sun avoidance [18].

Sun protection products can be classified as UVB blockers, UVA blockers, or physical blockers (Table 34.3). A broad-spectrum sunscreen protects against both UVA and UVB light. UVA blockers are active in the range 320–400 nm while UVB blockers are active in the range 290–320 nm [19]. Sunscreens such as oxybenzone and octocrylene have UVA activity in the 320–340 nm range. Avobenzone, benzopheonomes, and dicamphor sulfonic acid are effective in most of the UVA range [19]. Most currently available sunscreen formulations aim for coverage of both UVA and UVB spectra. Methoxyphenyltriazine is a recently introduced sunscreen in Europe with a broad-spectrum filter that stabilizes avobenzone-containing sunscreens and offers broad-spectrum protection [19]. Physical blockers, including titanium dioxide and zinc oxide, are effective in both the UVA and UVB ranges [20].

Sun-protective clothing is often recommended as an alternative to sunscreen use. The Skin Cancer Foundation has recommended Rit Sun Guard™, a photoprotective laundry additive with TINOSORB™FD as the active ingredient. The additive washes into the clothing fibers and absorbs broadband UV. A single treatment sustains a sun protection factor (SPF) of 30 for approximately 20 launderings [21].

Sun protection factor

The term SPF refers to the effectiveness of a sunscreen to reduce UVB radiation to skin. If the product label contains the words "broad spectrum" it also protects against UVA radiation in accordance with FDA labeling guidelines (www.fda.gov/ForConsumers/ConsumerUpdates/ucm258416.htm). An SPF of 15 indicates that the length of time spent in the sun without erythema is increased by a factor of 15. A fair-skinned person who normally sunburns after 20 minutes is theoretically able to tolerate 300 minutes after applying a sunscreen with an SPF of 15. The efficiency of sunscreen is related to the spectrum of wavelengths absorbed, amount of product applied (2 mg/cm^2 recommended), time sunscreen dries before UV exposure (15 minutes recommended), and the resistance to washing off during swimming or sweating [19,22]. The US Food and Drug Administration (FDA) labeling guidelines specify that sunscreen labeled "Broad Spectrum" and "SPF 15" (or higher) protects against sunburn and can help prevent skin cancer. Sunscreen that has an SPF between 2 and 14 or sunscreen that is not labeled "Broad Spectrum" only assists in the prevention of sunburn (www.fda.gov/ForConsumers/ConsumerUpdates/ucm258416.htm).

Recommendations

In general, most dermatologists recommend daily sunscreen of SPF 30 or higher, especially for sun-exposed areas, 15 minutes prior to sun exposure and every 2 hours thereafter. Special populations that are at higher risk for sun-induced toxicities and neoplasms are advised to avoid sun exposure by using para-aminobenzoic acid (PABA) free UVA and UVB protection as well as sun-protective clothing [4,7,23].

The recommended amount of sunscreen needed for one application to an adult is 2 mg/cm^2, or about 35 g (www.fda.gov/downloads/Drugs/GuidanceComplianceRegulatoryInformation/Guidances/UCM330696) [24]. Only about 20–60% of the recommended amount of sunscreen is applied by most consumers [23]. A simplified method of recommending an amount to patients is the teaspoon rule: more than half a teaspoon each on the head and neck area, right arm, and left arm; more than one teaspoon each on the anterior torso, posterior torso, right leg, left leg [25]. Practitioners will often recommend a higher SPF value than is necessary in order to compensate for skimpy application [26].

AEs of sunscreens

AEs reportedly caused by sunscreens include stinging, burning, pruritus, contact urticaria, irritant contact dermatitis, allergic contact dermatitis, photosensitivity, and worsening or causing acne [27]. Some AEs are caused by vehicle ingredients. A common complaint is stinging or burning in the eye area, which is an irritant reaction. Care should be taken to avoid the immediate eye area and, if facial sweating occurs, choose a vehicle that will not wash into the eye area, such as a dry lotion or gel. Acne problems usually can be managed by selection of oil-free or gel-based product.

PABA is no longer used in sunscreen products in the United States because of the relatively high incidence of allergic contact dermatitis. Though photoallergic reactions are not common, the leading agents causing these reactions are sunscreens. Oxybenzone is now the most common of the sunscreen agents to cause photoallergic contact dermatitis [28]. If photoallergy is present, the physical sunscreens, zinc oxide and titanium oxide, can be used because they have not been reported to cause photoallergy reaction [28].

Insect repellants

Insect repellants are applied to the skin or clothing and produce a vapor layer that has an offensive smell or taste to insects [29]. Insects are repelled only when they reach the repellent barrier, which extends to less than 4 cm from the skin surface [30]. More frequent reapplication is required when external factors such as abrasion by clothing, sweating, washing with water, and wind are present [31].

DEET (*N,N*-diethyl-3-methylbenzamide)

DEET (*N,N*-diethyl-3-methylbenzamide) is considered to be a broad-spectrum insect repellent and has been used since the 1950s [32]. It is available in concentrations from 5% to 100% and comes in many formulations including lotions, sprays, and cloth-impregnating laundry emulsions [33]. Under most conditions, products with 10–35% DEET provide adequate protection [32]. Repellents may be applied directly to the skin, or they may be applied to clothing and other items such as tents and sleeping bags. DEET should be used cautiously as cases of systemic toxicity have been reported after topical use. Case reports of potential DEET toxicity include the central nervous system (CNS, including cases of encephalopathy), cardiovascular system, cutaneous system, and/or allergic reactions [32].

DEET has been used as an insect repellent for almost 60 years and remains the gold standard. According to the US Environmental Protection Agency, approximately 30% of the US population is expected to use this product annually.

IR3535 (ethyl-butylacetylaminopropionate)

IR3535 (ethyl-butylacetylaminopropionate) is classified as a biopesticide in the United States. It is effective against mosquitoes, ticks, and flies. In general, IR3535 provides longer lasting repellency than the botanical citronella-based repellents, but does not match the overall efficacy of DEET [34,35].

Picaridin

Picaridin, commonly used in Europe and Australia, is becoming increasingly popular in the United States. Picardin offers low toxicity and comparable efficacy. Further, it does not feel sticky or greasy, is less irritating to skin, and does not damage plastics and fabrics [32]. Although picaridin seems to have similar efficacy to DEET, there are few supporting data [36].

Citronella
Citronella was originally extracted from the grass plant *Cymbopogon nardus*. Although generally less effective than other insect repellants, citronella is rarely noted to cause systemic toxicity or allergic contact sensitization [28].

Local anesthetic and analgesic therapy

Local anesthetic therapy
Lidocaine
Lidocaine is available topically in 3% cream and 5% ointment. It causes sensory and motor blockade by inhibiting axonal sodium channels. Injectable lidocaine is often combined with epinephrine, which causes vasoconstriction, for use in laceration repair. Topical preparations (LET and EMLA) are typically used before lidocaine injection to prevent pain, but can also be used alone. Any compound with epinephrine should not be used on end-arterial locations including fingers, toes, nose, and penis [37]. Liposomal lidocaine (LMX) is a lidocaine preparation that is encapsulated in liposomes. These liposomes facilitate drug absorption and protect against rapid metabolism [38]. It is available over-the-counter. The recommended duration to keep on the skin is 30 minutes. Topical lidocaine-based products should also be avoided on mucous membranes and should not exceed 5 g per dose. A 2% viscous solution also exists for oral ulcers or other mouth pain. This is used as a swish-and-spit formulation up to eight times daily.

> Topical lidocaine gel and cream may be used for painful rashes, especially hand-foot skin syndrome or perianal dermatitis secondary to radiation or sunitinib therapy. The viscous solution is also used for the painful oral ulcers that occur with many antineoplastic therapies.

Local analgesic therapy
Capsaicin
Capsaicin is a natural alkaloid derived from the Solanaceae family, and is what gives chili peppers their heat. Capsaicin cream activates vanilloid receptors in the skin and sensory neurons, leading to release of substance P which produces a burning or itching sensation. Continual application will desensitize neurons and eventually deplete substance P [39]. Limiting AEs include pain and burning sensation at the site of application. Capsaicin is approved for post-herpetic neuralgia and diabetic neuropathy, but is used off-label for many other conditions, including pruritus. It is available in cream, dermal patches, and a nasal preparation. Initial applications result in stinging; however, after repeated application (>4 times a day) the area becomes less sensitive to pain or itch.

Topical antibacterial therapy
In addition to oral antibiotics [40,41], topical antibacterials are used for targeted therapy-induced rashes and include clindamycin, erythromycin, metronidazole, and benzoyl peroxide [7]. Topical antibiotics appear to be effective and, because many rashes are often associated with xerosis and increased skin fragility, there may be an increased risk of secondary infection with *Staphylococcus aureus* and thus the benefit of antibacterial agents [42]. A moisturizing effect is provided by creams while solutions or alcohol-containing gels may be too drying and irritating [43].

Clindamycin
Clindamycin is a broad-spectrum antibiotic that inhibits bacterial protein synthesis [44]. It is available as a 1% solution, lotion, and gel for topical application [42]. The gel formulation is recommended for a grade 1–3 rash [45] to epidermal growth factor receptor (EGFR) inhibitors and scalp rash to taxanes. In rash grade <2, topical clindamycin is used in conjunction with topical corticosteroids. Mild local reactions can occur and include burning, itching, dryness, erythema, oily skin, and peeling [46]. Very rarely, cases of pseudomembraneous colitis have been reported with topical treatment [47].

Erythromycin
Erythromycin is a macrolide antibiotic which also inhibits bacterial protein synthesis [48]. It is available as a 2% topical solution and gel. Topical erythromycin is used as a single agent for mild (grade 1) rashes, steroid acne, and folliculitis [7,42]. AEs such as burning, itching, dryness, erythema, oily skin, and peeling have been reported.

Metronidazole
Metronidazone is classified as both an antibacterial and an antiprotozoal agent and has anti-inflammatory effects [49]. It is available as a 0.75% gel, lotion, or cream and 1% gel. The main use for topical metronidazole is the treatment of rosacea but it is also used for malignant malodorous wounds [7,50]. Burning and stinging are the most frequently reported AEs followed by erythema, skin irritation, and pruritus.

Benzoyl peroxide
Benzoyl peroxide is an antibacterial agent whose activity appears secondary to the release of oxygen [51]. It is available in cleansers, lotions, creams, and gels in varying concentrations. Benzoyl peroxide cream or gel is used for folliculitis [7]. The main AEs of topical therapy include allergic contact dermatitis and dryness [52]. If dryness occurs, the dose can be decreased by using a lower concentration, changing to a less irritating vehicle, or using alternate-day dosing [7]. Patients should be informed that benzoyl peroxide can bleach or discolor fabric, hair, and other colored materials.

> Topical antibacterial agents are recommended for grade 1 rash and folliculitis and, in conjunction with an oral agent, for grade 2–3 skin rash.

- Topical antibacterials are used for prophylaxis and treatment of local skin and wound infections. These are available in different combinations to broaden the spectrum of activity
- Mupirocin twice daily is useful for nasal colonization by *S. aureus*

Bacitracin

Bacitracin is bactericidal via inhibition of bacterial cell wall synthesis and is active against Gram-positive and some Gram-negative organisms [53]. When combined with polymyxin B or neomycin, a wider spectrum of bacterial coverage exists. Bacitracin is available in a variety of topical ointments and creams and is used for the prophylaxis and treatment of local skin and wound infections. Bacitracin should not be used in treating chronic wounds and ulcers because of the increased risk of sensitization [54]. There is some risk of allergic reaction and cases of systemic anaphylaxis have been reported with topical bacitracin [56].

Polymyxin B

Polymyxin B disrupts bacterial cell membranes via a surfactant-like mechanism and is bactericidal against some Gram-negative bacteria [53]. It is commonly combined with other topical antibiotics to broaden the spectrum of activity. Polysporin ointment consists of bacitracin and polymyxin B. Polymyxin B is also used for prophylaxis and treatment of local skin and wound infections.

Neomycin

Neomycin is an aminoglycoside antibiotic that inhibits bacterial protein synthesis [53]. This antibiotic is bactericidal against most Gram-negative bacteria (not *Pseudomonas aueruginosa*), some Gram-positive bacteria (not streptococci), but does not cover aenarobes [54]. Neosporin ointment consists of bacitracin, polymyxin B, and neomycin [55]. Deafness has been reported with use of this antibiotic in the irrigation of a large wound [57]. The incidence of allergy in the US population is 11% [58,59]. In general, neomycin is not used because of its high rate of sensitization.

Mupirocin

Mupirocin is derived from a fermentation process by *Pseudomonas fluorescens* and inhibits bacterial protein synthesis [53]. It is active against a wide range of Gram-positive bacteria including methicillin-resistant *Staphylococcus aureus* (MRSA) and some Gram-negatives [60]. As mupirocin has a unique mechanism of action, it does not cross-react with other topical antibiotics. A 2% ointment is available and can be used for topical treatment of impetigo caused by *Staphylococcus aureus* and *Streptococcus pyogenes*. Mupirocin nasal is a paraffin-based formulation that is available for use intranasally. Adverse reactions such as burning, stinging, pain, pruritus, erythema, xerosis, and contact dermatitis have been reported. It is very useful for nasal dryness, crusting, and epistaxis associated with *S. aureus* colonization.

Systemic antibiotic therapy

Tetracyclines

Tetracyclines as a class inhibit bacterial protein synthesis and have a similar spectrum of activity against bacteria, including Gram-positive and Gram-negative coverage [61]. This class of antibiotics should not be used for streptococcal infections unless susceptibility is confirmed. Tetracyclines are not the drug of choice when treatment of staphylococcal infection is required. Care must be taken when treating patients with renal impairment, as excessive accumulation and liver toxicity may ensue [62]. Common AEs include nausea, vomiting, epigastric burning, and abdominal discomfort. Tetracyclines can also cause photosensitivity (more common with doxycycline and demeclocycline), oral and skin hyperpigmentation (especially minocycline), and, rarely, pseudotumor cerebri [63]. Minocycline may cause light-headedness, dizziness, and vertigo and has been noted to cause a lupus-like syndrome [40,41]. These antibiotics are also recommended because of their immunomodulating and anti-inflammatory effects and can be used in conjunction with other topical medications [7,40,41,64]. These treatments are typically given for 4–6 weeks and may be extended into maintenance therapy at a dose of 50–100 mg orally twice daily, or may be restarted in the case of recurrence [45].

Clindamycin

Clindamycin inhibits bacterial protein synthesis and is bacteriostatic against Gram-positive aerobes and anaerobes as well as Gram-negative anaerobes [46]. It is used for treating serious infections including skin and soft tissue infections. Colitis associated with *Clostridium difficile* toxin has been reported from use of this antibiotic in 0.1–10% of treated patients [65]. The most common AEs include nausea, vomiting, and diarrhea.

> Oral antibiotics are recommended for grade 2–3 skin rash, secondarily infected paronychia, and other skin and soft tissue infections.

Antiviral therapy

Topical antiviral therapy

Acyclovir

Topical acyclovir is available as a 5% cream or ointment [66]. The benefit of using topical acyclovir for recurrent herpes labialis in adolescents and adults is negligible. The ointment formulation can be useful for management of initial genital herpes infection and in limited mucocutaneous herpes simplex virus (HSV) infection in immunocompromised patients [67]. Oral acyclovir is preferable to topical therapy.

Penciclovir
Penciclovir is available in a 1% cream for the treatment of recurrent herpes labialis in adults [68]. Treatment should begin when lesions or prodrome symptoms (tingling) first appear and be applied every 2 hours while awake for 4 days.

Topical therapy for cutaneous warts
Cutaneous warts are the clinical manifestation of epithelial infection with human papillomavirus. Therapy is not directly aimed at the virus and the majority of treatments focus on destruction of the affected skin. This often takes multiple office visits and/or rigorous home care. Location and morphology (flat, filiform, mosaic) are also important to take into account when choosing a therapy, as well as patient compliance and immune status. In general, paring of dead skin is essential for successful resolution of warts. This can be accomplished at home with pumice stones, nail files, or cuticle trimmers; or in the office with scalpel blades or currettes. Spontaneous regression does occur and observation is an option in most patients. The majority of patients desire treatment before enlargement or spreading occurs. Despite a few controlled trials, there is not enough evidence to compare treatment efficacy [69]. The most common treatment options are described below.

Liquid nitrogen cryotherapy
Liquid nitrogen cryotherapy is a destructive therapy that is applied to the wart and 2 mm of surrounding skin via spray, probe, or cotton-tip applicator to provide a thaw cycle of 10–60 seconds. One to two cycles per treatment are recommended to cause a response ranging from erythema to hemorrhagic vesicles. Lesions may take multiple or adjunctive treatments to resolve. Patients often need to be seen every 2–3 weeks until resolution, but cure rates can be as high as 70% [70]. Difficulties associated with this therapy include pain and scarring.

Salicylic acid
Salicylic acid is a beta-hydroxy acid that causes desquamation of the epithelium. It is a useful agent for most warts, especially in a patient who is willing to do home treatments. Preparations range from lower strength liquid (17%, Compound W®, Wart-off®, Duofilm®, Duoplant®, and Occlusal HP®) to patches (15%, Trans Ver Sal® and 21%, Trans Plantar®), and finally to plasters (40%, Mediplast® or Duofilm®). With appropriate application, cure rates can be as high as 75% [70]. Most formulations are a combination with lactic acid, an α-hydroxy acid, which is also a keratolytic. Treatment duration is variable, but should continue 2–3 weeks after clinical resolution to prevent recurrence.

Bichloroacetic acid and trichloroacetic acid
Bichloroacetic acid and trichloroacetic acid (80% solution) cause destruction via protein coagulation [70]. Typically, the solution is applied to warts weekly in a physician's office, taking note to avoid the surrounding normal skin. The lesion is then covered for 5 days and the cycle is repeated every week. Resolution can take many weeks and AEs are generally mild localized irritation.

Fluorouracil
5-Fluorouracil (Efudex® and others) is a topical preparation of a commonly used chemotherapeutic antimetabolite agent. Recommendations include application once to twice daily for 6 weeks (for warts), but is variable for other skin lesions. Topical formulations include 2% and 5% solution as well as 5% cream. AEs are local irritation, with measurable systemic absorption rarely seen [71].

Imiquimod
Imiquimod (Aldara®) is a non-nucleoside heterocyclic amine that acts as an immunomodulator via activation of toll-like receptor 7 to induce cytokines. It also enhances the skin's immune system by the production of intracellular interferon α (INFα), interleukin 12 (IL-12), tumour necrosis factor α (TNFα) and TNFγ [72]. It is FDA approved for external genital and perianal warts in patients 12 years of age and older, as well as superficial basal cell carcinomas and actinic keratosis in immunocompetent patients (www.accessdata.fda.gov/drugsatfda_docs/label/2010/020723s022lbl). Off-label uses have included cutaneous warts, molluscum contagiosum, Bowen's disease, lentigo maligna, and herpes simplex virus [73]. Erythema and irritation are the most common AEs but may also be considered by some as a response to treatment. Reported recommendations include application to affected areas up to five times a week before bed (to allow 6–10 hours before washing off) as tolerated until resolution of the lesions or up to 16 weeks.

Podophyllotoxin
Podophyllotoxin (podofilox) is a standardized solution or gel containing podophyllin which is a plant resin that causes tissue necrosis by arresting mitosis [70]. It is FDA-approved for at-home application by patients and is preferred over podophyllin because the dose is standardized and overall systemic AEs are reduced. Application recommendation is twice daily for 3 days followed by 4 days without therapy for up to 6 weeks. The treatment area should be restricted to <10 cm^2, with a daily maximum dose of 0.5 mL to reduce systemic AEs. Local AEs can be minimal but clearance rates are variable.

Silver nitrate
Sliver nitrate is available in solution (0.5%, 10%, 25%, 50%) and topical applicators (75%, Lunar Caustic®). Contact with skin causes a chemical reaction that coagulates bacterial proteins and destroys tissue [74]. Topical applicators are commonly used for small lesions such as warts or hemostasis by first dipping into water and then pressing on the lesion for cauterization. AEs are typically local irritation and brown discoloration at the site, which resolves within 1–2 weeks.

Silver nitrate sticks can be used for warts or paronychia caused by EGFR or mTOR inhibitors, typically at weekly intervals.

Systemic antiviral therapy

Table 34.4 illustrates three of the oral antiviral agents along with their indications and appropriate dosing.

Acyclovir

Acyclovir is used for treatment of HSV-1 and HSV-2 as well as varicella zoster virus (VZV) [75]. Continuous suppressive therapy reduces recurrence of genital herpes by 80–90% and reduces asymptomatic viral shedding of HSV-2 by 95% [76]. Acute herpes zoster dosing has been shown to reduce the mean duration of the

Table 34.4 Dosing of select systemic antivirals. Information adapted from package inserts for acyclovir, valacyclovir, and famciclovir.

Drug	Uses	Dosage
Acyclovir	Herpes zoster (acute)	800 mg orally every 4 hours, 5 times daily × 7–10 days
	Genital herpes (initial infection)	200 mg orally every 4 hours, 5 times daily × 10 days
	Genital herpes (chronic suppressive therapy)	400 mg orally twice daily, for up to 12 months
	Genital herpes (intermittent therapy)	200 mg orally every 4 hours, 5 times daily × 5 days
	Varicella zoster (adults and children >40 kg)	800 mg orally four times daily × 5 days
Valacyclovir	Herpes zoster	1 g three times daily × 7 days
	Herpes labialis	2 g orally twice daily × 1 day
	Genital herpes (initial infection)	1 g orally twice daily × 10 days
	Genital herpes (recurrence)	500 mg orally twice daily × 3 days
	Genital herpes (chronic suppressive therapy)	1 g orally once daily or if ≤9 recurrences per year, 500 mg orally once daily
Famciclovir	Herpes zoster	500 mg orally three times daily × 7 days
	Herpes labialis (recurrent)	1.5 g orally × 1 dose
	First episode of genital herpes	250 mg orally three times daily for 10 days
	Genital herpes (recurrence)	1 g orally twice daily × 1 day
	Genital herpes (chronic suppressive therapy)	250 mg orally twice daily, for up to 12 months

acute pain of post-herpetic neuralgia from 62 days for patients treated with placebo to 20 days for patients treated with acyclovir [77]. Adjustment in dosing regimen is recommended for patients with impaired renal function. In immunocompromised patients, thrombotic thrombocytopenic purpura/hemolytic uremic syndrome (TTP/HUS) has been reported.

Valacyclovir

Valacyclovir is an oral prodrug of acyclovir. In treating herpes labialis and recurrent genital herpes, valacyclovir should be initiated at the earliest onset of symptoms (tingling, burning, or itching). For initial genital herpes and herpes zoster, treatment is most effective when initiated within 48 hours from the onset of signs and symptoms [78]. Similar to acyclovir, dosing should be adjusted in patients with renal impairment.

Famciclovir

Famciclovir is an oral prodrug of penciclovir and has a greater bioavailability than oral acyclovir and valacyclovir [79,80]. Again, dose reduction is recommended in patients with reduced renal function [78].

Antifungal therapy

Four main classes exist for antifungal therapy: polyenes, azoles, allylamines, and echinocandins. In general, topical and systemic therapies are available and treatment recommendation is dependent upon extent and location of infection, suspected microbe, and immune status of patient.

Polyene

Polyene agents are nystatin and its derivatives and amphotericin B. Nystatin is an antibiotic produced by *Streptomyces noursei* and *S. albidus*. It elicits both fungistatic and fungicidal activity by binding to membrane sterols of susceptible *Candida* species, but is not effective against dermatophyte infections [81]. Nystatin is available topically in cream, ointment, and powder formulations and is typically used twice daily. In cases of oral thrush a solution is available for use four to five times a day. AEs are rarely reported but include local irritation and hypersensitivity.

Amphotericin B

Amphotericin B is a polyene antifungal derived from *Streptomyces nodosus*. It acts similarly to nystatin by binding membrane sterols and causing instability of the organism. It can be fungistatic or fungicidal, depending on concentration. It is used only for life-threatening fungal infections, including aspergillosis, cryptococcosis, blastomycosis, histoplasmosis, zygomycosis (including *Mucor* and *Rhizopus*), sporotrichosis, and systemic candidiasis [82,83]. Amphotericin B is only available in IV form and is typically dosed initially at 0.25 mg/kg/day and gradually increased to 0.3–1.0 mg/kg/day. It is usually limited by its toxic AEs. Acutely these reactions include fevers, shaking chills, nausea, vomiting, and tachypnea. Overdose has been associated with fatal cardiac and cardiopulmonary events. Other AEs include hypotention, hypokalemia, arrhythmias, nephrotoxicity, and it should be used with caution in renal patients. Newer lipid preparations are still under investigation in the United States but are designed to have an improved AE profile [84].

Azoles

Azoles are the most commonly used antifungal drug class because of their effectiveness against *Candida* and dermatophytes. Their mechanism of action is inhibition of 14-alpha-demethylase, blocking the synthesis of ergosterol, a primary component in the fungal cell membrane [85]. There are two groups of azoles: the imidazoles (ketoconazole, miconazole, clotrimazole, and econazole) and the triazoles (fluconazole, itraconazole, voriconazole, and posaconazole). They are available in systemic and topical preparations, and some are available IV for severe infections. Overall they are well-tolerated; however, all azoles inhibit CYP3A4 to different extents and the majority are also metabolized via the CYP450 enzyme system, so drug–drug interactions need to be taken into account [86]. Table 34.5 and Table 34.6 describe the utilization of the most common azoles including uses, dosing, and specific limitations.

Echinocandins

Echinocandins (caspofungin, anidulafungin, and micafungin) are noncompetitive inhibitors of the synthesis of 1,3-beta-D-glucan, which is a main component of the fungal cell wall. They are used for *Candida* and *Aspergillus* infections, and micafungin is used for azole-resistant *C. albicans*, *C. glabrata*, and *C. krusei* [85]. It is also used for prevention of *Candida* infections in hematopoietic stem cell transplant patients. Caspofungin is as effective as amphotericin B for invasive candidiasis and empiric antifungal treatment in neutropenic patients [87]. All echinocandins are only available in IV form. Dosing is as follows: caspofungin is started at 70 mg IV on the first day, followed by 50 mg/day; micafungin is given daily at 100 mg IV; and anidulafungin is started at 200 mg IV on the first day followed by 100 mg/day. AEs are minimal and include headache, fever, and elevated aminotransferases.

Hydroxypyridones

Ciclopirox is a topical antifungal agent used for dermatophyte infections, onychomycosis, candidiasis, as well as seborrheic dermatitis [88]. It is available in a cream (0.77%), gel (0.77%), shampoo (1%), and solution (nail lacquer, 8% and solution, 0.77%). Cicopirox is structurally unlike other antifungals and acts by inhibiting cellular uptake via metal-dependent enzymes [89]. It is a good alternative to systemic agents for onychomycosis and dermatophyte infections, showing good efficacy and minimal AEs. For dermatophyte infections, preparations are typically applied once to twice daily for 4 weeks. Nail lacquer is used every day to the nail and surrounding skin. A new coat is put over the previous day's application and every 7 days is removed with alcohol to restart the cycle.

Table 34.5 Dosages for triazole systemic antifugal therapies.

Drug	Uses/dosage
Fluconazole Oral (capsule, solution), IV	Oropharyngeal candidiasis: 200 mg loading then 100–200 mg/day for 7–14 days
	Esophageal candidiasis: 400 mg loading then 200–400 mg/day for 7–14 days
	Vaginal candidiasis: 150 mg once
	Candidemia: 800 mg loading dose, then 400 mg/day
Itraconazole Oral (capsule, solution)	Oropharyngeal or esophageal candidiasis, histoplasmosis, blastomycosis: 200 mg/day to bid if needed
	Coccidiodomycosis: 400–600 mg/day in divided doses
	Onychomycosis: 200 mg bid for 1 week (fingernails); and 200 mg/day for 12 weeks (toenails)
Voriconazole Oral (capsule, solution), IV	Invasive apergillosis, severe fungal infections or candidemia: load with 6 mg/kg q 12 h for two doses, then 4 mg/kg IV q 12 h
	Candidiasis: load with 400 mg q 12 h for two doses, then 200 mg PO q 12 h
Posaconazole Oral (solution)	Prophylaxis: 200 mg tid
	Candidiasis: 100 mg bid for 1 day then 100 mg/day × 13 days
	Candidiasis resistant to fluconazole/itraconazole: 400 mg bid

Table 34.6 Dosages for imidazole topical antifugal therapies.

Drug	Uses/dosage
Ketoconazole (Nizoral) 2% cream	Daily
Clotrimazole (Lotrimin) 1% cream, 1% lotion, 1% solution, 10 mg troches	bid Troches qid (for oral candidiasis)
Econazole (Spectazole) 1% cream	Daily to bid
Miconazole (Monistat) 2% cream, suppositories	Vaginal candidiasis: 1200 mg supp × 1; 200 mg supp qHS × 3 days, 100 mg supp qHS × 7 days or 2% cream qHS × 7 days
	Topical: bid

bid, twice daily; qHS, at night; qid, four times daily.

Table 34.7 Benzylamines for common dermatophyte infections.

Drug	Uses/dosage
Terbinafine (Lamisil) Oral, 1% cream, 1% gel, 1% solution	Onychomycosis: 250 mg PO daily for 6 weeks (fingernails) or 12 weeks (toenails) Tinea pedis: topical application bid for 7 days Tinea corporis/cruris: topical application daily for 7 days
Naftifine (Naftil) 1% cream, 1% gel	Tinea pedis/corporis/cruris: twice daily (cream) or daily (gel) until resolution
Butenafine (Lotrimin Ultra, Mentax) 1% cream	Tinea versicolor: Mentax daily for 2 weeks Tinea pedis: Lotrimin Ultra twice daily for 1 week Tinea corporis/cruris: Lotrimin Ultra daily for 2 weeks

bid, twice daily.

Allylamines and benzylamines

Allylamines and benzylamines (terbinafine, naftifine, butenafine) are broad-spectrum antifungal agents with both fungistatic and fungicidal activity. They act by preventing ergosterol synthesis via inhibition of squalene epoxidase, which leads to membrane instability. They are P-450 independent, but terbinafine is metabolized by multiple CYP enzymes. Terbinafine is used systemically for onychomycosis, tinea corporis/cruris, interdigital and chronic tinea pedis, tinea versicolor, and cutaneous candidiasis [90]. Naftifine and butenafine are also available as topical preparations for common dermatophytes [90]. For common usage information see Table 34.7. AEs for all benzylamines are rare and include irritation and hypersensitivity.

- Topical antifungal classes include polyenes, azoles, echinocandins, and benzylamines
- Topical antifungal treatments are preferred for superficial fungal infections
- Systemic agents are preferred for large surface areas, terminal hair or nail involvement, and in those with resistance

Steroid therapy

Topical corticosteroids

Topical corticosteroids (TCs) are a mainstay in dermatology practice and are used in a variety of inflammatory disorders. TCs decrease inflammation in the same manner as systemic glucocorticoids (see below). In addition to anti-inflammatory properties, TCs have immunosuppressive, vasoconstrictive, and antiproliferative properties [91]. The effectiveness of TCs vary greatly depending on strength, vehicle, and adjuncts. Hydration of the stratum corneum can enhance absorption up to fivefold [92] and occlusion can enhance it up to 10-fold [93]. TCs are also absorbed more efficiently on inflamed, desquamated, or thin skin. Application site and area of involvement must therefore be taken into account when choosing a treatment regimen. Frequency and duration of treatment is also variable, but 2–4 weeks of twice-daily application is often recommended [91]. Tachyphylaxis and rebound after drug cessation are potential obstacles of TC treatment, and using pulse therapy and medication taper, respectively, can sometimes help avoid these complications.

Common AEs of TCs include atrophy, telangiectasias, striae, purpura, hypertrichosis, and pigmentation changes, and are commonly seen on areas of thin skin or with high potency and prolonged use. Allergic contact dermatitis is seen with TC use and should be considered with worsening or no resolution of the condition. Steroid acne and perioral dermatitis can also be seen with facial application. In adults, systemic suppression of the hypothalamic–pituitary axis, Cushing syndrome and hyperglycemia have been reported, although these are rare [91]. TCs are divided into classes based on potency: super potent (class I), potent (classes II and III), intermediate (classes IV and V), and mild (classes VI and VII).

- Topical corticosteroids are the most commonly prescribed of all dermatologic drug products.
- They are used for symptomatic treatment of inflammation, but do not usually treat the underlying disease
- Vehicle and potency are important considerations when prescribing these medications, ointments being more potent than creams or solutions
- Foams, shampoos, and solutions are preferable for rashes or pruritus on the scalp
- Orabase® is an ideal vehicle to deliver triamcinolone to mucositis or stomatitis
- Topical corticosteroids are typically used in hand-foot skin syndrome grades 2 and 3. Generally, a class I or II ointment or cream is used twice daily until resolution or discontinuation of anticancer therapy

Systemic corticosteroids

Corticosteroids are involved in many physiologic systems but are used in dermatology mainly for their anti-inflammatory effects [94]. Systemic corticosteroids are typically reserved for acute severe reactions or refractory conditions and are available in oral, intramuscular, and intravenous form. Oral therapy is typically begun at 40–60 mg prednisone every morning, but can be alternated with methylprednisolone to reduce mineralocorticoid effects. If therapy is needed for longer than 2–3 weeks, a taper is required to prevent withdrawal symptoms. Intramuscular

Table 34.8 Characteristics of common systemic corticosteroids.

Class	Name	Relative glucocorticoid potency	Relative mineralocorticoid potency	Biologic half-life (hours)
Short acting	Cortisone	0.8	Moderate	8–12
	Hydrocortisone	1	Moderate	8–12
Intermediate acting	Prednisone	4	Mild	24–36
	Prednisolone	4	Mild	24–36
	Methylprednisolone	5	Minimal	24–36
	Triamcinolone	5	Minimal	24–36
Long acting	Dexamethasone	20–30	Minimal	36–54
	Betamethasone	20–30	Minimal	36–54

administration can be used for acute control of dermatoses with betamethasone and dexamethasone. Intralesional injection can also be used for chronic localized cutaneous lesions with triamcinolone, which should be limited to a maximum of six doses per year. Intravenous corticosteroids are used in life-threatening dermatologic conditions. Systemic corticosteroids have significant AEs that need to be taken into account when determining dose and duration of therapy. The most common include suppression of hypothalamic–pituitary axis, hyperglycemia, cushingoid changes, hyperlipidemia, osteoporosis, and cataracts [95]. Table 34.8 lists the most common systemic glucocorticoids, relative glucocorticoid and mineralocorticoid potency, and effective biologic (tissue) half-life [94,96].

- Systemic glucocorticoids are anti-inflammatory and potent immunosuppressive agents that are used for severe dermatologic diseases
- Oral, intralesional, intramuscular, and intravenous administrations are available
- Complications are commonly associated with higher doses and longer duration of therapy; therefore careful monitoring and/or prophylaxis should be performed

Antipruritic therapy

There are many causes of pruritus spanning from skin disorders and infections to systemic disorders such as blood and metabolic disorders and malignancies. In general, treatment of the underlying disorder (if known) is the mainstay of therapy. Appropriate skin care and avoidance behaviors for scratching are also paramount [97]. Adjunctive therapies may be beneficial when the underlying disorder is unknown or refractory, as well as in primary skin disorders.

Topical antipruritic therapy
Diphenhydramine
Diphenhydramine (a first generation H1-antihistamine) is available in a 2% cream which can be used 3–4 times daily. Topical diphenhydramine can be used for mild pruritus or pain, but data are limited on its efficacy with dermatologic toxicity-associated conditions. Topical diphenhydramine is not typically used in dermatology because of a high incidence of allergic contact dermatitis [98].

Menthol
Menthol elicits the sensation of cooling via the TRPM8 receptor in sensory neurons which can lead to relief of itch, especially in patients who have pruritus that responds to cooling [99]. Although data are limited and the mechanism is poorly understood, menthol has been used for decades and concentrations of 1–3% are safe for topical use.

Topical corticosteroids
Topical corticosteroids are commonly not used for pruritus unless the underlying cause is inflammatory.

Topical calcineurin inhibitors
Tacrolimus and pimecrolimus are topical calcineurin inhibitors that share similar structures and properties. Tacrolimus is a macrolide produced by *Streptomyces tsukubaensis*, and pimecrolimus is a derivative of a macrolactam that was isolated from *Streptomyces hygroscopicus*. Their main mechanisms of action prevents transcription of IL-2 via calcineurin complex binding. This blocks T-cell activation and proliferation and prevents release of T-cell-derived cytokines [100,101]. The reported antipruritic effect of calcineurin inhibitors is thought to result from this reduction of inflammation.

Tacrolimus and pimecrolimus are FDA approved for atopic dermatitis, though are often used off-label for other conditions. They are not only effective and have a rapid rate of onset, but can be used safely up to 12 months and in conjunction with topical steroids as "steroid sparing agents." [102] Tacrolimus is available in a 0.03% or 0.1% ointment and pimecrolimus as a 1% cream, to be applied twice daily. AEs are typically mild and include headache, local irritation, and skin infection. Topical calcineurin inhibitors are not commonly used for pruritus unless the underlying cause is inflammatory. Caution must be taken with their use, based on preclinical data and anecdotal reports of secondary malignancies (cutaneous squamous cell cancer and lymphomas), which led to the FDA issuing a boxed warning for "possible cancer risk" for these drugs. However, the American Academy of Dermatology has issued a statement in response to the FDA warning, disagreeing with the warning and stating that current research does not prove that these drugs are dangerous when used properly. Despite these conflicts, in the oncology setting it may be difficult to assuage patients that these drugs are safe.

Systemic antipruritic therapy
Antihistamines

Antihistamines target the histamine receptor proteins which are categorized into four subtypes: H1–H4. H1 and H2 antihistamines are considered inverse agonists of histamine receptor proteins because of their effect of downregulating the constitutively activated state of the receptor [103]. H1 receptors are involved most extensively in pruritus, erythema, edema, and axon reflex flare of disorders such as chronic urticaria. Along with H1 receptors, H2 receptors have also been found on epithelial and endothelial cells, and may contribute to vascular permeability, inflammatory mediator release, cellular recruitment, and antigen presentation. H2 receptors are usually associated with gastric acid secretion; however, they also mediate downregulation of T-lymphocyte activation, which supports their role in treating mucocutaneous candidiasis and human papillomavirus infections. H2 antihistamines have been shown to have efficacy with concurrent H1 antihistamines in chronic urticaria [104]. H3 receptors are presynaptic and do not seem to have a role in pruritus [105]. The recently described H4 receptor has been reported to have some anti-inflammatory and antipruritic effects [106,107].

H1 antihistamines

H1 antihistamines are commonly used to treat pruritus independent of cause. They are categorized into first and second generation drugs. The first generation drugs include diphenhydramine, cyproheptadine, promethazine, and hydroxyzine. This generation is very lipophilic and readily crosses the blood–brain barrier, which causes the sedating and anticholinergic AEs that often limit their use [105]. Second generation H1 antihistamines include fexofenadine, cetirizine, loratadine, and desloratadine. These drugs are less lipophilic and therefore have less sedating and anticholinergic effects [105]. Second generation H1 antihistamines are typically first-line treatment for pruritus, but first generation drugs are sometimes substituted for nighttime relief. Dosing varies per medication but most are available in oral, intramuscular, or intravenous formulations.

> Toxicities that have pruritic symptoms, such as xerosis and rash can be treated with second generation H1 antihistamines during the day and first generation H1 antihistamines before bedtime, although data on the efficacy with regards to dermatologic AE are limited.

H2 antihistamines

H2 antihistamines include cimetidine, famotidine, and ranitidine. Although H2 antihistamines are typically used for gastric ulcer disease, evidence has shown that cimetidine may provide an antipruritic activity and may enhance cell-mediated immunity [108]. There is some evidence that combination H1 and H2 antihistamines may be of benefit for pruritus, and at high doses they have been found to act as immunomodulators [104]. Dermatologic uses for H2 blockers include acute allergy, chronic urticaria, pruritus associated with other diseases, and urticaria pigmentosa. Dosing regiments are the same as for gastroesophageal reflux disease.

Doxepin

Doxepin is a tricyclic antidepressant that has H1 and H2 antihistamine effects, making it effective for pruritus. It has both oral and topical preparations but should be used with caution in patients with liver or cardiac disease, should not be abruptly withdrawn, or used with CYP3A4 inhibitors (macrolides, azoles, grapefruit juice) [109]. Dosing should start at 25–75 mg PO at bedtime and escalate to no more than 300 mg/day. A 5% cream is available for topical application every 4 hours for no more than 8 days, which has shown efficacy for pruritus in clinical trials [110].

Opiate antagonists and agonists

Opiate antagonists and agonists such as naloxone, naltrexone, nalmefene, and nalfurafine have been used in multiple pruritic dermatoses but are most often used for pruritus of cholestasis [110].

> - H1 antihistamines are first-line treatment for urticarias and histamine-related pruritus
> - H2 antihistamines may be a useful adjunct to H1 antihistamines

Retinoid therapy

Topical retinoids

Topical retinoids (TRs) are vitamin A derivatives that alter gene transcription in cellular differentiation and proliferation. The comedolytic effect of TRs is secondary to the targeting of abnormal follicular epithelial proliferation, resulting in a reduction in follicular plugging [111]. In immunosuppressed individuals, nonmelanoma skin cancers, along with warts, premalignant keratoses, and keratoacanthomas occur more frequently and aggressively [112]. TRs have been shown to be an effective treatment in such individuals; however, systemic retinoids have shown better efficacy [112]. TRs are typically applied once daily at night as tolerated and AEs include local

Table 34.9 Formulations and uses for common topical retinoids.

Drug	Uses and available formulations
Tretinoin (Retin-A, Renova, Atralin)	Acne: cream (02025%, 0.05%, 0.1%), gel (0.05%, 0.1%), solution (0.05%)
	Photoaging: cream (0.05%, 0.02%)
Tazarotene (Avage, Tazorac)	Photoaging: cream 0.1%
	Acne: gel (0.05%, 0.1%), lotion (0.05%, 0.1%)
	Psoriasis: gel (0.05%, 0.1%), lotion (0.05%, 0.1%)
Adapalene (Differin)	Acne: gel (0.1%), lotion (0.1%)

Source: Kang [113].

irritation, dryness, and erythema. The most common agent is tretinoin (all-*trans* retinoic acid), which is used for acne vulgaris as well as rhytides, hyperpigmentation, and resurfacing of facial skin. Adapalene_is another common agent also used for acne. Tazarotene is used in both acne and psoriasis. Table 34.9 describes the formulations of the most common TRs. Alitretinoin is used most often for Kaposi sarcoma and bexarotene is used in cutaneous T-cell lymphoma stage 1A and 1B. Tretinoin and adapalene are pregnancy category C, whereas alitretinoin is category D and tazarotene and bexarotene are category X.

Topical retinoids have been considered by some as useful in the treatment of actinic purpura on the dorsal arms induced by photoaging and corticosteroids, in order to stimulate collagen formation by the dermis and to minimize the development of purpuric lesions.

Systemic retinoids

Systemic retinoids (SRs) are vitamin A derivatives that alter nuclear transcription by binding to the families of retinoic acid receptors or retinoid X receptors. Retinoids have large effects on cell differentiation and may have a role in chemoprevention [111]. The three major generations of drugs are described below.

Isotretinoin

Isotretinoin is a first generation retinoid FDA approved for use in nodulocystic acne, but is also commonly used for other acne-related disorders, rosacea, hidradenitis suppurativa, and disorders of keratinization. Dosing strategy is based on a total cumulative dose of 120–150 mg/kg. Patients typically take 0.5–1.0 mg/kg/day until goal cumulative dose is achieved. Clearance rates average

70% without relapse for acne. It should be noted that if relapse occurs, patients typically respond well to conventional therapy, even if they failed it previously. A second course of isotretinoin may be used for recalcitrant cases, and clearance rates (without relapse) are similar to the first course. Oral isotretinoin at low doses (20 mg/day) has reported anecdotal benefit in the treatment of EGFR inhibitor rash that has not responded to oral antibiotic therapy (M.E. Lacouture, personal communication, 8 March 2011).

Acitretin

Acitretin is a second generation active form of etretinate, which is no longer available in the United States because of its narrow therapeutic index and long half-life of approximately 120 days. Acitretin is FDA approved for psoriasis and is especially efficacious for generalized pustular psoriasis. It is also used in chemoprevention of malignancies (transplant and xeroderma pigmentosum patients) such as nonmelanoma skin cancers, along with prevention of keratotic and premalignant lesions [112,114,115]. Treatment efficacy of Kaposi sarcoma, graft versus host disease and human papillomavirus has also been reported [111]. Typical dosing starts at 25 mg/day and can be escalated up to 75 mg/day as tolerated to achieve desired results. Maintenance therapy as low as 10 mg every other day has been shown to be effective. Ethanol ingestion can convert acitretin to etretinate, and because of this, women should not ingest alcohol while taking this medication and should not become pregnant within 3 years of stopping this medication. Oral acitretin at low doses (10 mg/day) has reported benefit in the treatment of EGFR inhibitor rash that has not responded to oral antibiotic [116] therapy.

Bexarotene

Bexarotene is a selective third generation retinoid X receptor modulator which is FDA approved for patients with cutaneous T-cell lymphoma who were refractory to at least one other oral antineoplastic therapy. The optimal dosage is 300 mg/m^2/day [117].

AEs

The risk of teratogenicity is an extremely important factor to consider when prescribing systemic retinoids [118]. Pregnancy is an absolute contraindication and women should not become pregnant for at least 1 month after the drug has been discontinued. Any patient taking isotretinoin must be registered in the iPledge system, which was designed to help prevent women from becoming pregnant while taking the medication. Other notable AEs include mucocutaneous complaints such as photosensitivity, xerosis, dry mucous membranes, dry and abnormal hair texture, along with nail softness and fragility. Patients on any SRs should also be followed with monthly CBCs, serum lipids, and liver function tests for the first 3–6 months, followed by every 3 months.

- Retinoids bind and activate the retinoic acid receptor to modulate gene transcription and cellular proliferation
- Topical and systemic retinoids are useful for steroid acne, psoriasis, and photoaging but are used off-label for many other conditions
- Systemic retinoids are used in acne, psoriasis, cutaneous T-cell lymphoma and other disorders of keratinization, and for EGFR inhibitor rash that has not responded to antibiotics or topical steroids. On the other hand, topical retinoids have not shown benefit for EGFR inhibitor rash
- Systemic retinoids are considered to be universally teratogenic (major and minor malformations), as well as embryotoxic, and contraindications include pregnancy, breastfeeding, and noncompliance with contraception

References

1 Loden, M. (2005) The clinical benefit of moisturizers. *Journal of the European Academy of Dermatology and Venereology*, **19**, 672–688, quiz 686–7.

2 Huang, X., Tanojo, H., Lenn, J. Deng, C.H &, Krochmal, L. (2005) A novel foam vehicle for delivery of topical corticosteroids. *Journal of the American Academy of Dermatology*, **53**, S26–S38.

3 Haley, A.C., Calahan, C., Gandhi, M., West, D.P., Rademaker, A. & Lacouture, M.E. (2010) Skin care management in cancer patients: an evaluation of quality of life and tolerability. *Supportive Care in Cancer*.

4 Lacouture, M.E., Mitchell, E.P., Piperdi, B. *et al.* (2010) Skin toxicity evaluation protocol with panitumumab (STEPP), a phase II, open-label, randomized trial evaluating the impact of a pre-Emptive Skin treatment regimen on skin toxicities and quality of life in patients with metastatic colorectal cancer. *Journal of Clinical Oncology*, **28**, 1351–1357.

5 Ghadially, R., Halkier-Sorensen, L. & Elias, P.M. (1992) Effects of petrolatum on stratum corneum structure and function. *Journal of the American Academy of Dermatology*, **26**, 387–396.

6 Draelos, Z.D. (1996) *Cosmetics in Dermatology*, 2nd ed., Churchill-Livingstone, New York.

7 Segaert, S. & Van Cutsem, E. (2005) Clinical signs, pathophysiology and management of skin toxicity during therapy with epidermal growth factor receptor inhibitors. *Annals of Oncology*, **16**, 1425–1433.

8 Bolderston, A., Lloyd, N.S., Wong, R.K., Holden, L., Robb-Blenderman, L.; Supportive Care Guidelines Group of Cancer Care Ontario Program in Evidence-Based Care. (2006) The prevention and management of acute skin reactions related to radiation therapy: a systematic review and practice guideline. *Supportive Care in Cancer*, **14**, 802–817.

9 Zirwas, M.J., Stechschulte, S.A. (2008) Moisturizer Allergy Diagnosis and Management. *The Journal of Clinical and Aesthetic Dermatology*, **1**, 38-44.

10 Lodén, M. & Maibach, H.I. (1999) *Dry Skin and Moisturizers: Chemistry and Function*, CRC Press, Boca Raton.

11 Nguyen, J.C., Chesnut, G., James, W.D., Saruk, M. (2010) Allergic contact dermatitis caused by lanolin (wool) alcohol contained in an emollient in three postsurgical patients. *Journal of the American Academy Dermatology*. **62**, 1064-5.

12 Ernst, E. (2000) Adverse effects of herbal drugs in dermatology. *British Journal of Dermatology*, **143**, 923–929.

13 Long, C.C. & Finlay, A.Y. (1991) The finger-tip unit: a new practical measure. *Clinical and Experimental Dermatology*, **16**, 444–447.

14 Hagemann, I. & Proksch, E. (1996) Topical treatment by urea reduces epidermal hyperproliferation and induces differentiation in psoriasis. *Acta Dermato-Venereologica*, **76**, 353–356.

15 Lacouture, M.E., Wu, S., Robert, C., Atkins, M.B., Kong, H.H., Guitart, J. *et al.* (2008) Evolving strategies for the management of hand-foot skin reaction associated with the multitargeted kinase inhibitors sorafenib and sunitinib. *The Oncologist*, **13**, 1001–1011.

16 Loden, M., Bostrom, P. & Kneczke M. (1995) Distribution and keratolytic effect of salicylic acid and urea in human skin. *Skin Pharmacology*, **8**, 173–178.

17 Polano, M.K. & Ponec, M. (1980) *Percutaneous Absorption of Steroids*, Academic Press, New York.

18 El Sayed, F., Ammoury, A., Nakhle, F., Dhaybi, R. & Marguery, M.C. (2006) Photoprotection in teenagers. *Photodermatology, Photoimmunology and Photomedicine*, **22**, 18–21.

19 MacNeal, R.J. & Dinulos, J.G. (2007) Update on sun protection and tanning in children. *Current Opinion in Pediatrics*, **19**, 425–429.

20 Mitchnick, M.A., Fairhurst, D. & Pinnell, S.R. (1999) Microfine zinc oxide (Z-cote) as a photostable UVA/UVB sunblock agent. *Journal of the American Academy of Dermatology*, **40**, 85–90.

21 Edlich, R.F., Cox, M.J., Becker, D.G., Horowitz, J.H., Nichter, L.S., Britt, L.D. *et al.* (2004) Revolutionary advances in sun-protective clothing: an essential step in eliminating skin cancer in our world. *Journal of Long-Term Effects of Medical Implants*, **14**, 95–106.

22 Kim, S.M., Oh, B.H., Lee, Y.W., Choe, Y.B. & Ahn, K.J. (2010) The relation between the amount of sunscreen applied and the sun protection factor in Asian skin. *Journal of the American Academy of Dermatology*, **62**, 218–222.

23 Bernier, J., Bonner, J., Vermorken, J.B., Bensadoun, R.J., Dummer, R., Giralt, J. *et al.* (2008) Consensus guidelines for the management of radiation dermatitis and coexisting acne-like rash in patients receiving radiotherapy plus EGFR inhibitors for the treatment of squamous cell carcinoma of the head and neck. *Annals of Oncology*, **19**, 142–149.

24 Bennett, M.L. & Petraxxuoli, M. (2001) What patients should know about sunscreens. *Skin and Aging*, **9**, 50–57.

25 Schneider, J. (2002) The teaspoon rule of applying sunscreen. *Archives of Dermatology*, **138**, 838–839.

26 Wolf, R., Matz, H., Orion, E. & Lipozenćić, J. (2003) Sunscreens: the ultimate cosmetic. *Acta Dermatovenerologica Croatica*, **11**, 158–162.

27 Wolverton, S. (2007) *Comprehensive Dermatologic Drug Therapy*, W.B. Saunders, Philadelphia.

28 Rietschel, R.L. & Fowler, J. (2007) *Fisher's Contact Dermatitis*, 6th ed. Lippincott Williams & Wilkins, Philadelphia.

29 Kewka, E.J., Munga, S., Mahande, A.M., Msangi, S., Mazigo, H.D., Adrias, A.Q., Matias, J.R. (2012) Protective efficacy of menthol propylene glycol carbonate compared to N, N-deithyl-methylbenzamide against mosquito bites in Northern Tanzania. *Parasites & Vectors*, **5**, 189.

30 Maibach, H.I., Khan, A.A. & Akers, W. (1974) Use of insect repellents for maximum efficacy. *Archives of Dermatology*, **109**, 32–35.

31 Maibach, H.I., Akers, W.A., Johnson, H.L., Khan, A.A. & Skinner, W.A. (1974) Insects. Topical insect repellents. *Clinical Pharmacology and Therapeutics*, **16**, 970–973.

32 Katz, T.M., Miller, J.H. & Hebert, A.A. (2008) Insect repellents: historical perspectives and new developments. *Journal of the American Academy of Dermatology*, **58**, 865–871.

33 Brown, M. & Hebert, A.A. (1997) Insect repellents: an overview. *Journal of the American Academy of Dermatology*, **36**, 243–249.

34 Fradin, M.S. & Day, J.F. (2002) Comparative efficacy of insect repellents against mosquito bites. *New England Journal of Medicine*, **347**, 13–18.

35 Barnard, D.R., Bernier, U.R., Posey, K.H. & Xue, R.D. (2002) Repellency of IR3535, KBR3023, para-menthane-3,8-diol, and deet to black salt marsh mosquitoes (Diptera: Culicidae) in the Everglades National Park. *Journal of Medical Entomology*, **39**, 895–899.

36 Schmidt, C.W. (2005) Outsmarting olfaction: the next generation of mosquito repellents. *Environmental Health Perspectives*, **113**, A468–A471.

37 Kennedy, R.M. & Luhmann, J.D. (1999) The "ouchless emergency department". Getting closer: advances in decreasing distress during painful procedures in the emergency department. *Pediatric Clinics of North America*, **46**, 1215–1247, vii–viii.

38 Eichenfield, L.F., Funk, A., Fallon-Friedlander, S. & Cunningham, B.B. (2002) A clinical study to evaluate the efficacy of ELA-Max (4% liposomal lidocaine) as compared with eutectic mixture of local anesthetics cream for pain reduction of venipuncture in children. *Pediatrics*, **109**, 1093–1099.

39 Papoiu, A.D. & Yosipovitch, G. (2010) Topical capsaicin. The fire of a 'hot' medicine is reignited. *Expert Opinion on Pharmacotherapy*, **11**, 1359–1371.

40 Jatoi, A., Rowland, K., Sloan, J.A., Gross, H.M., Fishkin, P.A., Kahanic, S.P. *et al.* (2008) Tetracycline to prevent epidermal growth factor receptor inhibitor-induced skin rashes: results of a placebo-controlled trial from the North Central Cancer Treatment Group (N03CB). *Cancer*, **113**, 847–853.

41 Scope, A., Agero, A.L., Dusza, S.W., Myskowski, P.L., Lieb, J.A., Saltz, L. *et al.* (2007) Randomized double-blind trial of prophylactic oral minocycline and topical tazarotene for cetuximab-associated acne-like eruption. *Journal of Clinical Oncology*, **25**, 5390–5396.

42 Tan, H.H. (2004) Topical antibacterial treatments for acne vulgaris : comparative review and guide to selection. *American Journal of Clinical Dermatology*, **5**, 79–84.

43 Potthoff, K., Hofheinz, R., Hassel, J.C., Volkenandt, M., Lordick, F., Hartmann, J.T. *et al.* (2010) Interdisciplinary management of EGFR-inhibitor-induced skin reactions: a German expert opinion. *Annals of Oncology*, **22**, 524–535.

44 McGehee, R.F., Jr., Smith, C.B., Wilcox, C., & Finland, M. (1968) Comparative studies of antibacterial activity in vitro and absorption and excretion of lincomycin and clinimycin. *American Journal of the Medical Sciences*, **256**, 279–292.

45 Lacouture, M.E. (2007) Insights into the pathophysiology and management of dermatologic toxicities to EGFR-targeted therapies in colorectal cancer. *Cancer Nursing*, **30**, S17–S26.

46 Clindamycin topical [package insert]. Peapack, NJ, Greenstone LLC.

47 Parry, M.F. & Rha, C.K. (1986) Pseudomembranous colitis caused by topical clindamycin phosphate. *Archives of Dermatology*, **122**, 583–584.

48 Erythromycin [package insert]. Melville, New York, E. Fougera & CO., A division of Nycomed US Inc.

49 Metronidazole cream [package insert]. South Plainfield, NJ, GW Laboratories Inc.

50 Adderley, U., Smith, R. (2007) Topical agents and dressings for fungating wounds. *Cochrane Database of Systematic Reviews*. **18** CD003948. Review.

51 Pace, W.E. (1965) A benzoyl peroxide-sulfur cream for acne vulgaris. *Canadian Medical Association Journal*, **93**, 252–254.

52 Benzoyl peroxide topical solution [package insert]. Fairfield, NJ.

53 Spann, C.T., Taylor, S.C. & Weinberg, J.M. (2004) Topical antimicrobial agents in dermatology. *Disease-A-Month*, **50**, 407–421.

54 Kaye, E.T. (2000) Topical antibacterial agents. *Infectious Disease Clinics of North America*, **14**, 321–339.

55 Gunjan, K., Shobha, C., Sheetal, C., Nanda, H., Vikrant, C., Chitnis, D.S. (2012) A comparative study of the effect of different topical agents on burn wound infections. *Indian Journal of Plastic Surgery*. **45**, 374-8.

56 Saryan, J.A., Dammin, T.C. & Bouras, A.E. (1998) Anaphylaxis to topical bacitracin zinc ointment. *American Journal of Emergency Medicine*, **16**, 512–513.

57 Macdonald, R.H. & Beck, M. (1983) Neomycin: a review with particular reference to dermatological usage. *Clinical and Experimental Dermatology*, **8**, 249–258.

58 de Groot, A.C. & Maibach, H.I. (2010) Frequency of sensitization to common allergens: comparison between Europe and the USA. *Contact Dermatitis*, **62**, 325–329.

59 Parenti, M.A., Hatfield, S.M. & Leyden, J.J. (1987) Mupirocin: a topical antibiotic with a unique structure and mechanism of action. *Clinical Pharmacy*, **6**, 761–770.

60 Bactroban nasal ointment [package insert]. Research Triangle Park, NC.

61 Minocycline [package insert]. Sellersville, PA.

62 Tetracycline [package insert]. Sellersville, PA.

63 Cleach, L.L., Bocquet, H. & Roujeau, J.C. (1998) Reactions and interactions of some commonly used systemic drugs in dermatology. *Dermatologic Clinics*, **16**, 421–429.

64 Sapadin, A.N. & Fleischmajer, R. (2006) Tetracyclines: nonantibiotic properties and their clinical implications. *Journal of the American Academy of Dermatology*, **54**, 258–265.

65 Bartlett, J.G. (1981) Antimicrobial agents implicated in *Clostridium difficile* toxin-associated diarrhea of colitis. *Johns Hopkins Medical Journal*, **149**, 6–9.

66 Acyclovir cream [package insert]. Bridgewater, NJ.

67 Acyclovir ointment [package insert]. Bridgewater, NJ.

68 Penciclovir cream [package insert]. Parsippany, NJ.

69 Gibbs, S. & Harvey, I. (2006) Topical treatments for cutaneous warts. *Cochrane Database of Systematic Reviews*, 3, CD001781.

70 Rivera, A. & Tyring, S.K. (2004) Therapy of cutaneous human papillomavirus infections. *Dermatologic Therapy*, **17**, 441–448.

71 Gladsjo, J.A., Alio Saenz, A.B., Bergman, J., Kricorian, G. & Cunningham, B.B. (2009) 5% 5-Fluorouracil cream for treatment of verruca vulgaris in children. *Pediatric Dermatology*, **26**, 279–285.

72 Arany, I., Tyring, S.K., Stanley, M.A., Tomai, M.A., Miller, R.L., Smith, M.H. *et al.* (1999) Enhancement of the innate and cellular immune response in patients with genital warts treated with topical imiquimod cream 5. *Antiviral Research*, **43**, 55–63.

73 Ganjian, S., Ourian, A.J., Shamtoub, G., Wu, J.J. & Murase, J.E. (2009) Off-label indications for imiquimod. *Dermatology Online Journal*, **15**, 4.

74 Ebrahimi, S., Dabiri, N., Jamshidnejad, E. & Sarkari, B. (2007) Efficacy of 10% silver nitrate solution in the treatment of common warts: a placebo-controlled, randomized, clinical trial. *International Journal of Dermatology*, **46**, 215–217.

75 Acyclovir capsules [package insert]. Rockford, IL.

76 Wald, A., Zeh, J., Barnum, G., Davis, L.G. & Corey, L. (1996) Suppression of subclinical shedding of herpes simplex virus type 2 with acyclovir. *Annals of Internal Medicine*, **124**, 8–15.

77 Huff, J.C., Drucker, J.L., Clemmer, A., Laskin, O.L., Connor, J.D., Bryson, Y.J. *et al.* (1993) Effect of oral acyclovir on pain resolution in herpes zoster: a reanalysis. *Journal of Medical Virology*, **Suppl. 1**, 93–96.

78 Famcyclovir tablets [package insert]. Sellersville, PA.

79 Tyring, S.K. (1998) Advances in the treatment of herpesvirus infection: the role of famciclovir. *Clinical Therapeutics*, **20**, 661–670.

80 Pue, M.A., Pratt, S.K., Fairless, A.J., Fowles, S., Laroche, J., Georgiou, P. *et al.* (1994) Linear pharmacokinetics of penciclovir following administration of single oral doses of famciclovir 125, 250, 500 and 750 mg to healthy volunteers. *Journal of Antimicrobial Chemotherapy*, **33**, 119–127.

81 Millikan, L.E. (2010) Current concepts in systemic and topical therapy for superficial mycoses. *Clinics in Dermatology*, **28**, 212–216.

82 Vyas, K.S., Bariola, J.R. & Bradsher, R.W. Jr. (2010) Treatment of endemic mycoses. *Expert Review of Respiratory Medicine*, **4**, 85–95.

83 Redmond, A., Dancer, C. & Woods, M.L. (2007) Fungal infections of the central nervous system: a review of fungal pathogens and treatment. *Neurology India*, **55**, 251–259.

84 Baginski, M. & Czub, J. (2009) Amphotericin B and its new derivatives: mode of action. *Current Drug Metabolism*, **19**, 459–469.

85 Lopez-Martinez, R. (2010) Candidosis, a new challenge. *Clinics in Dermatology*, **28**, 178–184.

86 Chen, S.C. & Sorrell, T.C. (2007) Antifungal agents. *Medical Journal of Australia*, **187**, 404–409.

87 Boucher, H.W., Groll, A.H., Chiou, C.C. & Walsh, T.J. (1997) Newer systemic antifungal agents: pharmacokinetics, safety and efficacy. *Drugs*, **64**, 2020–2004.

88 Gupta, A.K. & Nicol, K.A. (2006) Ciclopirox 1% shampoo for the treatment of seborrheic dermatitis. *International Journal of Dermatology*, **45**, 66–69.

89 Subissi, A., Monti, D., Togni, G. & Mailland, F. (2010) Ciclopirox: recent nonclinical and clinical data relevant to its use as a topical antimycotic agent. *Drugs*, **70**, 2133–2152.

90 Gupta, A.K., Einarson, T.R., Summerbell, R.C. & Shear, N.H. (1998) An overview of topical antifungal therapy in dermatomycoses: a North American perspective. *Drugs*, **55**, 645–674.

91 Tadicherla, S., Ross, K., Shenefelt, P.D. & Fenske, N.A. (2009) Topical corticosteroids in dermatology. *Journal of Drugs in Dermatology*, **8**, 1093–1105.

92 Giannotti, B. (1988) Current treatment guidelines for topical corticosteroids. *Drugs*, **36** (Suppl. 5), 9–14.

93 Maibach, H. (1976) In vivo percutaneous penetration of corticosteroids in man and unresolved problems in the efficacy. *Dermatologica*, **152**, 11–25.

94 Melby, J.C. (1977) Clinical pharmacology of systemic corticosteroids. *Annual Review of Pharmacology and Toxicology*, **17**, 511–527.

95 Moghadam-Kia, S. & Werth, V.P. (2010) Prevention and treatment of systemic glucocorticoid side effects. *International Journal of Dermatology*, **49**, 239–248.

96 Williams, L.C. & Nesbitt, L.T. Jr. (2001) Update on systemic glucocorticosteroids in dermatology. *Dermatologic Clinics*, **19**, 63–77.

97 Hercogova, J. (2005) Topical anti-itch therapy. *Dermatologic Therapy*, **18**, 341–343.

98 Bigby, M., Stern, R.S. & Arndt, K.A. (1989) Allergic cutaneous reactions to drugs. *Primary Care*, **16**, 713–727.

99 Patel, T. & Yosipovitch, G. (2010) Therapy of pruritus. *Expert Opinion on Pharmacotherapy*, **11**, 1673–1682.

100 Kang, S., Lucky, A.W., Pariser, D., Lawrence, I. & Hanifin, J.M. (2001) Long-term safety and efficacy of tacrolimus ointment for the treatment of atopic dermatitis in children. *Journal of the American Academy of Dermatology*, **44**, S58–S64.

101 Kapp, A., Papp, K., Bingham, A., Fölster-Holst, R., Ortonne, J.P., Potter, P.C. *et al.* (2002) Long-term management of atopic dermatitis in infants with topical pimecrolimus, a nonsteroid anti-inflammatory drug. *Journal of Allergy and Clinical Immunology*, **110**, 277–284.

102 Fleischer, A.B. Jr. & Boguniewicz, M. (2010) An approach to pruritus in atopic dermatitis: a critical systematic review of the tacrolimus ointment literature. *Journal of Drugs in Dermatology*, **9**, 488–498.

103 Leurs, R., Church, M.K. & Taglialatela, M. (2002) H1-antihistamines: inverse agonism, anti-inflammatory actions and cardiac effects. *Clinical and Experimental Allergy*, **32**, 489–498.

104 Dhanya, N.B., Rai, R. & Srinivas, C.R. (2008) Histamine 2 blocker potentiates the effects of histamine 1 blocker in suppressing histamine-induced wheal. *Indian Journal of Dermatology, Venereology and Leprology*, **74**, 475–477.

105 Greaves, M.W. (2010) Pathogenesis and treatment of pruritus. *Current Allergy and Asthma Reports*, **10**, 236–242.

106 Cowden, J.M., Zhang, M., Dunford, P.J. & Thurmond, R.L. (2010) The histamine H4 receptor mediates inflammation and pruritus in Th2-dependent dermal inflammation. *Journal of Investigative Dermatology*, **130**, 1023–1033.

107 Dunford, P.J., Williams, K.N., Desai, P.J., Karlsson, L., McQueen, D. & Thurmond, R.L. (2007) Histamine H4 receptor antagonists are superior to traditional antihistamines in the attenuation of experimental pruritus. *Journal of Allergy and Clinical Immunology*, **119**, 176–183.

108 Choi, Y.S., Hann, S.K. & Park, Y.K. (1993) The effect of cimetidine on verruca plana juvenilis: clinical trials in six patients. *Journal of Dermatology*, **20**, 497–500.

109 Gupta, M.A. & Gupta, A.K. (2001) The use of antidepressant drugs in dermatology. *Journal of the European Academy of Dermatology and Venereology*, **15**, 512–518.

110 Eschler, D.C. & Klein, P. (2010) An evidence-based review of the efficacy of topical antihistamines in the relief of pruritus. *Journal of Drugs in Dermatology*, **9**, 992–997.

111 DiGiovanna, J.J. (2001) Systemic retinoid therapy. *Dermatologic Clinics*, **19**, 161–167.

112 George, R., Weightman, W., Russ, G.R., Bannister, K.M. & Mathew, T.H. (2002) Acitretin for chemoprevention of non-melanoma skin cancers in renal transplant recipients. *Australasian Journal of Dermatology*, **43**, 269–273.

113 Kang, S. (2005) The mechanism of action of topical retinoids. *Cutis*, **75**, 10–13, discussion 13.

114 Bavinck, J.N., Tieben, L.M., Van der Woude, F.J., Tegzess, A.M., Hermans, J., ter Schegget, J. *et al.* (1933) Prevention of skin cancer and reduction of keratotic skin lesions during acitretin therapy in renal transplant recipients: a double-blind, placebo-controlled study. *Journal of Clinical Oncology*, **13**, 8–1995.

115 de Sevaux, R.G., Smit, J.V., de Jong, E.M., van de Kerkhof, P.C. & Hoitsma, A.J. (2003) Acitretin treatment of premalignant and malignant skin disorders in renal transplant recipients: clinical effects of a randomized trial comparing two doses of acitretin. *Journal of the American Academy of Dermatology*, **49**, 407–412.

116 Pomerantz, R.G., Chirinos, R.E., Falo, L.D. Jr., Geskin, L.J. (2008) Acitretin for treatment of EGFR inhibitor-induced cutaneous toxic effects. *Archives of Dermatology*, **144**, 949-50

117 Duvic, M., Martin, A.G., Kim, Y. *et al.* (2001) Phase 2 and 3 clinical trial of oral bexarotene (Targretin capsules) for the treatment of refractory or persistent early-stage cutaneous T-cell lymphoma. *Archives of Dermatology*, **137**, 581–593.

118 American Academy of Pediatrics Committee on Drugs (1992) Retinoid therapy for severe dermatological disorders. *Pediatrics*, **90**, 119–120.

35 Dermatologic Techniques and Procedures

Robert Eilers Jr.[1], Kishwer S. Nehal[2] and Erica H. Lee[2]

[1]University of Michigan, Ann Arbor, MI, USA
[2]Dermatology Service, Memorial Sloan-Kettering Cancer Center, New York, NY, USA

Introduction

Cutaneous manifestations of internal malignancy and anticancer treatments are frequent. In order to diagnose the cutaneous findings accurately and guide overall oncologic management, obtaining skin tissue samples are often necessary. To facilitate the timely diagnosis of skin findings, the oncologist may choose to integrate certain dermatologic procedures into practice to expedite management decisions.

Diagnostic techniques in dermatology are typically performed in the outpatient setting. The most commonly performed procedure is the skin biopsy to obtain tissue for pathologic examination. Skin cultures for bacterial, fungal, and other atypical organisms are also performed because of the predisposition of the oncologic population to dermatologic infections [1].

In this chapter, common dermatologic procedures are reviewed. An overview of common skin cancers is also discussed. In order to perform dermatologic procedures in critically ill patients efficiently and effectively, a thorough understanding of preoperative evaluation, instruments, local anesthetics, antisepsis, and hemostatic agents is recommended.

Preoperative evaluation

Preoperative considerations for invasive skin procedures include a review of the patient's medical history, laboratory results, medications, and allergies (Table 35.1). A standard set of questions will assist the clinician in performing the procedure with minimal risk. Informed consent should be discussed with the patient. Risks of skin procedures include bleeding, infection, mild pain, scarring, and potential for an inconclusive diagnosis. In addition, a "time out" protocol will help ensure proper patient identity and safety.

As a general rule, in a neutropenic patient, sterile technique is recommended. Prophylactic antibiotics are a consideration prior to procedures involving infected skin or in patients with artificial prostheses or heart valves [2]. The American Heart Association recommends a preoperative dose of 2 g cephalexin or dicloxacillin orally 30–60 minutes prior to the procedure. In patients with a penicillin allergy, 600 mg clindamycin orally is an alternative [3]. Most simple skin procedures can be performed while the patient remains on anticoagulation but careful attention to hemostasis is necessary.

Antiseptics

Antiseptics are used to prepare the skin prior to an invasive skin procedure. Isopropyl alcohol 70% has weak antimicrobial activity but is the most commonly used antiseptic. Because of its flammable property, skin prepped with alcohol must be dry prior to use of electrosurgery. However, povidone-iodine (Betadine®) and chlorhexidine 4% (Hibiclens®) provides broad antimicrobial coverage, including fungi. These antiseptics should be used in neutropenic or immunocompromised patients or when a procedure is performed in areas such as the groin or lower extremity. Chlorhexidine should not be used around the eyes or ears because of the risk of keratitis and otitis, respectively [4].

Local anesthetic and technique

Local anesthetics are divided into two categories, amides and esters, and differ in their metabolism. Ester anesthetics such as procaine and tetracaine are metabolized by plasma pseudocholinesterase, whereas amides such as lidocaine and bupivacaine are metabolized by the liver. The most commonly

Dermatologic Principles and Practice in Oncology: Conditions of the Skin, Hair, and Nails in Cancer Patients, First Edition. Edited by Mario E. Lacouture.
© 2014 John Wiley & Sons, Inc. Published 2014 by John Wiley & Sons, Inc.

Table 35.1 Preoperative evaluation for skin procedures.

Is the patient thrombocytopenic?	Check platelet levels, consider platelet transfusion if <10 000
Is the patient immunosuppressed?	Check CBC for WBC count
Review current medications	Monoamine oxidase inhibitors are a contraindication with epinephrine in the local anesthetic
	Determine if patient has increased risk for bleeding (i.e., NSAIDs, clopidogrel, warfarin or aspirin, dalteparin)
History of drug or topical allergy?	Allergy to local anesthesia
	Allergy to bacitracin or antiseptic
	Allergy to oral antibiotics
	Allergy to latex
	Sensitivity to adhesives
Is the patient pregnant?	Avoid use of epinephrine in local anesthetic
Artificial joints or heart valve?	Consider prophylactic antibiotic treatment
History of IE or a cardiac condition associated with high risk for an adverse effect from IE	
Pacemaker or ICD?	Use heat cautery with ICDs
	Use heat cautery or electrosurgery in small bursts with pacemakers

CBC, complete blood count; ICD, implantable cardiac defibrillator; IE, infective endocarditis; NSAID, nonsteroidal anti-inflammatory drug; WBC, white blood cell.

used anesthetic in dermatologic procedures is lidocaine in a 1% solution with or without epinephrine. Epinephrine (1 : 100 000) is often added to promote vasoconstriction and prolong the anesthetic effect. It is important to note the vasoconstrictive effect of epinephrine requires approximately 15 minutes after injection to become effective. There is also some controversy regarding use of epinephrine in the ear or digits because of potential vasoconstriction and necrosis. Numerous recent studies demonstrate epinephrine is safe in these areas [5]; however, care should be taken to minimize the volume of anesthetic used especially on a digit to prevent local compressive effects.

True allergic reactions to local anesthetics are rare and represent less than 1% of adverse reactions to local anesthesia. Allergic reactions documented in the literature are primarily associated with the ester (e.g., procaine and tetracaine) type of local anesthetic [6]. There is no cross-reactivity between the amide or esters forms; therefore in allergic patients, the other anesthetic category may be used. In the event a patient is allergic to both

types of local anesthetic or a true allergy cannot be confirmed, intradermal injections of normal saline with benzyl alcohol preservative or 1% diphenhydramine solution are alternatives. Ethyl chloride is an easy-to-use topical vapocoolant (skin refrigerant) anesthetic that may also be used for shave biopsies in the event an alternative anesthetic is needed. Vasovagal reactions during injection of local anesthesia are common and steps to keep the patient calm and in a comfortable recumbent position can help minimize this problem.

The area to be biopsied is infiltrated with local anesthesia, ranging 1–3 mL in volume. In general, a slow injection will minimize pain because of less immediate tissue distension. Injection in the subcutis is also less painful than a dermal injection but requires more time for the anesthetic to take effect. The anesthetic can be injected into the dermis for an instantaneous effect by directing a 30-gauge needle at a shallow angle, creating a wheal. This method is recommended for shave biopsies, as the wheal also creates an elevated platform for the blade that is advantageous for obtaining an adequate tissue sample.

Hemostasis

Chemical hemostatic agents, also called styptics, include aluminum chloride or ferric subsulfate (Monsel solution) and are typically used on shave biopsy wounds. Aluminum chloride is preferred, as Monsel solution is a dark brown solution and may lead to permanent dermal staining. The styptic is applied with a cotton tip applicator and rolled along the wound bed with pressure. If hemostasis cannot be achieved, electrosurgery or heat cautery may be used. Another option for hemostasis is a white porous hemostatic sponge (Gelfoam®); the Gelfoam® is cut to size and applied with a pressure dressing. For small wounds, direct manual pressure for several minutes is also effective. For punch biopsy wounds, the wound is usually closed with a suture which produces hemostasis by compression.

Electrosurgery utilizes high frequency electrical current to achieve hemostasis. In patients with pacemakers or implantable cardioverter-defibrillators (ICDs), there is a potential risk of interference with the device and caution should be used. In patients with an ICD, electrosurgery should not be used. In patients with a pacemaker, electrosurgery may be used if the power output is kept to a minimum and short bursts of less than 5 seconds are used [7]. Thermocautery or heat cautery is safe for individuals with a pacemaker or ICD [8].

Wound dressings

Randomized controlled trials comparing bacitracin with petrolatum demonstrate no significant difference in wound healing or the rate of wound infections [9]. In the general population, 8% of patients develop an allergic contact dermatitis to bacitracin in patch testing [10]; therefore many dermatologists

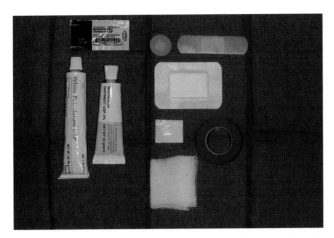

Figure 35.1 Wound dressing materials. Examples of topical ointments from the top left, clockwise: bacitracin ointment, mupirocin 2%, or petrolatum. Adhesive bandages come in varying sizes and are chosen based on anatomic location. For adhesive sensitive patients, nonstick Telfa with gauze and paper tape (lower right) may be used.

prefer petrolatum for clean wounds. An alternative antibiotic ointment with broad coverage is mupirocin (Bactroban®). A Band-aid® or a nonstick dressing such as Telfa® with gauze and adhesive tape is then applied to the wound (Figure 35.1). Applying a dressing with good pressure is important in patients at higher risk for bleeding.

Patients who undergo punch biopsy usually require sutures. The sutures may be removed in the office after 5–7 days from the face and neck and 10–14 days from the trunk and extremities. Steri-strips can be applied to sutured wounds if there is minimal bleeding.

Skin biopsy

There are four major types of skin biopsies:
1 Shave biopsy;
2 Punch biopsy;
3 Incisional biopsy; and
4 Excisional biopsy.
Characteristics of the skin lesion will determine the type of biopsy to be used. A shave biopsy is performed when the epidermis and superficial or mid dermis is sampled. A punch biopsy is performed to obtain a full-thickness specimen. Incisional and excisional biopsies are full-thickness elliptical-shaped biopsies often used to sample larger areas of involvement. General guidelines for performing a skin biopsy are outlined in Box 35.1. The procedure materials should be organized and placed on a sterile drape covering a Mayo stand (Box 35.2) [11].

Shave biopsy
A shave biopsy may be performed with a number 10 or 15 scalpel blade or curved blade specifically designed for shave biopsies, called a Dermablade® (Figure 35.2). Shave biopsies create

Box 35.1 Skin biopsy protocol

- Mark the lesion to be biopsied with a skin marker prior to injection of local anesthetic
- Perform "time out"
- Consider photography
- Select good lighting for visualization
- Position patient in a comfortable manner
- Use personal and patient safety precautions
- Apply antiseptic agent
- Inject local anesthesia
- Select best biopsy method/choose lesion
- Handle tissue carefully
- Place specimen directly into labeled specimen bottle
- Dispose of sharp instruments

Box 35.2 Equipment and materials for skin biopsies

Supplies:
- Sterile or nonsterile gloves
- Eye protection and face mask
- Marking pen
- Gauze
- Isopropyl alcohol, povidone-iodine solution or chlorhexidine 4%
- 1 or 3 mL syringe of 1% lidocaine with or without epinephrine and a 30-gauge needle
- Sterile fenestrated drape
- Specimen container labeled with patient identification/site (formalin or saline)
- Wound dressing materials

Materials required for punch biopsy (Figure 35.4):
- Punch biopsy instrument (2–6 mm)
- Needle holder and forceps
- Iris scissors or disposable blade
- Suture (4-0, 5-0, or 6-0 nonabsorbable nylon or polypropylene, or absorbable polyglactin 910)

Materials required for shave biopsy (Figure 35.2):
- No. 15 blade or Dermablade®
- Forceps
- Chemical hemostatic agent

superficial wounds that heal by second intention over several weeks through development of granulation tissue, wound contraction, and epidermal re-epithelialization.

To perform a shave biopsy, the curved or scalpel blade is passed at an angle almost parallel to the skin (Figure 35.3). Simple

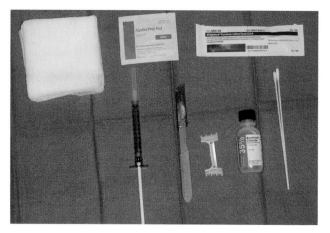

Figure 35.2 Shave biopsy tray setup. Biopsy tray with gauze and antiseptic agent (top row, left to right); local anesthetic, 15-blade or Dermablade® and aluminum chloride with cotton tip applicators for hemostasis (bottom row, left to right).

changes in angulation of the blade allow the clinician to obtain superficial dermis or deeper reticular dermis in the biopsy. Because of the subtle changes with angulation, the technique is skill dependent and may be initially challenging. However, as the physician performs more shave biopsies, the comfort level will also increase. The specimen is then placed in a vial of solution such as 10% formaldehyde for histopathologic assessment. Hemostasis is achieved with aluminum chloride or Monsel solution.

Punch biopsy

The punch instrument is a circular metal disposable blade with a diameter ranging 2–8 mm (Figure 35.4 standard size is 4 mm). The punch instrument is placed over the skin and advanced into the skin as the clinician twists the punch tool between their thumb and index finger, creating a twisting motion between the blade and the skin. The anatomic site will determine how deep the metal barrel is advanced. When there is a loss of resistance this signifies the subcutis has been reached. The cylindrically

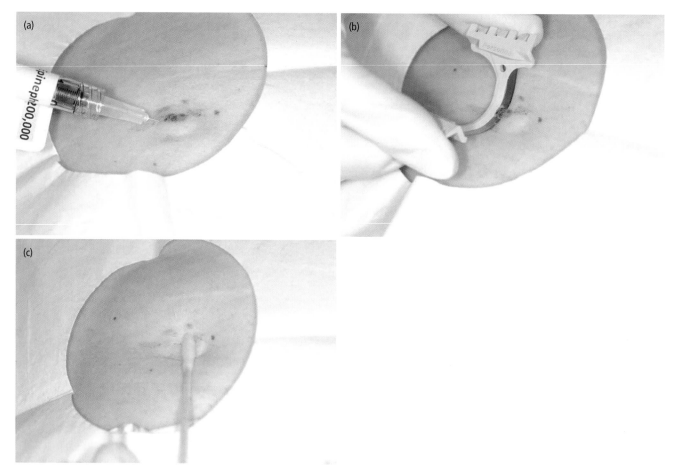

Figure 35.3 Shave biopsy procedure. (a) Local anesthetic is infiltrated, creating a wheal. (b) The blade is held parallel to the skin surface beneath the lesion. Smooth cutting of the tissue while advancing the blade in a swinging motion separates the lesion from the underlying reticular dermis. (c) Hemostasis is achieved with aluminum chloride.

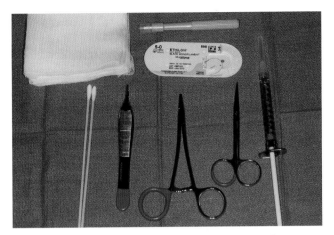

Figure 35.4 Punch biopsy tray setup. Biopsy tray with gauze, punch instrument, and nonabsorbable suture (top row, left to right); cotton tip applicator, forceps, suture needle holder, Iris scissors, and local anesthesia (bottom row, left to right).

shaped specimen is then gently lifted with tissue forceps, and cut with sterile scissors at the level of the subcutaneous fat (Figure 35.5). It is important to handle the tissue with care to avoid crush artifact. The specimen is placed in a vial of solution of 10% formaldehyde or in a sterile container with (antiseptic-free) saline-impregnated gauze for tissue culture. The wound is re-approximated with one or two interrupted sutures.

To perform an interrupted suture, the suture needle is loaded on to the needle holder and enters the skin 2–3 mm from the biopsy defect perpendicular to the line of closure. The needle enters the skin at a 90° angle and is guided through the base of the wound to emerge from the opposite wound edge. The suture is then tied with a series of square knots using the instrument tie [12].

Incisional biopsy and excisional biopsy

An incisional biopsy involves removal of a portion of a skin lesion or affected area. A clinician may elect to perform an incisional biopsy when a punch biopsy does not yield sufficient information of the deeper layers of skin or the area of involvement is large. The skin defect is re-approximated with sutures.

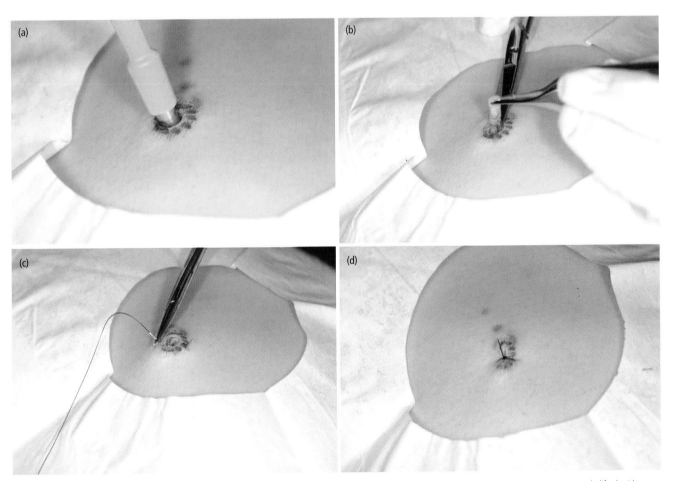

Figure 35.5 Punch biopsy procedure. (a) The punch biopsy instrument is advanced into the skin until there is a loss of resistance. (b) The tissue is gently lifted with forceps and cut at the level of the subcutaneous fat. (c,d) The resulting defect is sutured with a nonabsorbable suture to approximate the epidermal edge.

Excisional biopsies involve elliptical excision of an entire skin lesion down to the subcutaneous fat. This may be performed where histopathologic examination of the entire lesion is critical for appropriate diagnosis and staging, such as suspected melanoma.

Because of the invasive nature of these procedures, incisional and excisional biopsies may not be routinely performed by the oncologist. Consideration for referral to a dermatologist or plastic surgeon for suspicious lesions may be required.

Nail plate avulsion and chemical cauterization

Acute paronychia is usually caused by a bacterial infection, commonly *Staphylococcus aureus*, and presents as a painful swollen nail fold. It may also result from therapy with epidermal growth factor receptor (EGFR) inhibitors, mTOR inhibitors, and systemic retinoids. Treatment includes bacterial culture, antibiotics with Gram-positive coverage such as cephalexin or dicloxacillin, surgical incision and drainage, and in intolerable grade 2 or 3 paronychia (Common Terminology Criteria for Adverse Events version 4.0), or nail avulsion [13].

Nail plate avulsion may be partial or total. The avulsion will separate the nail plate from the underlying nail bed and adjacent nail folds. A digital block is performed utilizing 1% or 2% lidocaine without epinephrine. At the lateral base of the digit near the web space, the 30-g needle is advanced until the bone is touched and slightly withdrawn. The anesthetic is injected with a subtle angulation dorsally, then ventrally while aimed at the distal tip. A maximum of 1–1.5 mL is injected on each side to prevent mechanical compression. Alternatively, local anesthesia may be infiltrated at the site of the nail avulsion.

Following infiltration of local anesthesia, the Freer elevator is gently advanced underneath the nail plate in a distal to proximal direction. Multiple passes in a parallel direction are made to loosen the nail plate attachment. The elevator is then passed over the nail plate to loosen the attachments of the lateral and proximal nail fold. Once there is no resistance below the nail plate, the nail is removed in a rotating movement using a hemostat or platypus nail pulling forcep to release pressure and allow drainage of the underlying purulence (Figure 35.6).

Pyogenic granuloma is a benign vascular skin tumor composed of numerous well-differentiated blood vessels. These lesions appear as erythematous pedunculated painful papules at the

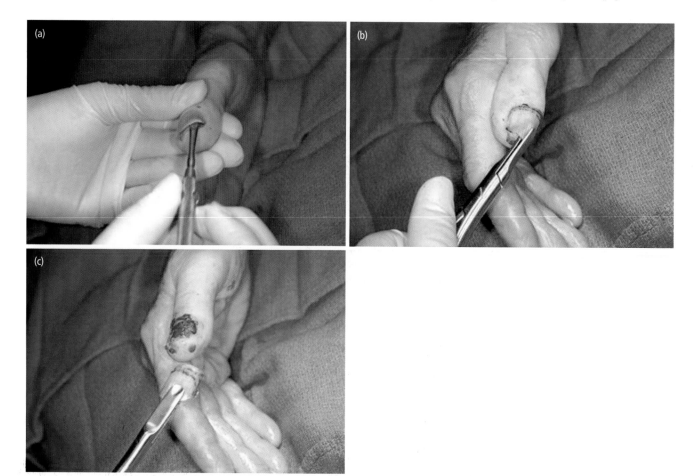

Figure 35.6 Nail plate avulsion. (a) The Freer elevator is gently advanced from a distal to proximal direction to separate the nail plate from the underlying nail bed. (b) The nail plate is then removed with a platypus nail pulling forcep to reveal the underlying nail bed (c).

lateral edges of the nail plate. Paronychia and pyogenic granuloma is a well-documented complication occurring in up to 56% of patients undergoing treatment with EGFRIs [14]. Treatment options for pyogenic granuloma include curettage and silver nitrate application, injection of 0.5% sodium tetradecyl sulfate, and nail avulsion [15]. Silver nitrate cauterization is a commonly performed procedure for these tumors. The applicator stick resembles a large matchstick and is composed of 75% silver nitrate and 25% potassium nitrate. When the silver nitrate contacts fluid (water or blood), the compound will activate and form nitric acid for hemostasis. The applicator is applied with pressure to the lesion for 20–30 seconds and will turn the treated area dark gray or black, a temporary discoloration.

Skin cultures

Bacterial culture

A bacterial culture kit consists of a sterile cotton swab and vial (Figure 35.7). For areas of frank purulence, the cotton swab is gently rolled across the pus. If pustules are present, they should be gently ruptured with a 30-gauge needle or a scalpel blade to expose the underlying exudate. Interpretation of the Gram stain, organism identification, and antibiotic sensitivities are used to guide antibiotic treatment. For recurrent skin infections, culture of the nares or unaffected areas of the skin may be performed to determine the presence of bacterial colonization.

Viral culture

The viral culture kit contains a sterile cotton swab and specialized transport medium (Figure 35.7). The ideal source for a culture is early vesicles. If there is a crust, removal for access to the underlying fluid is recommended. The sterile swab is gently rolled across the affected area of the skin. It is then placed in the transport medium and sent for microbiologic analysis. Viral cultures typically require

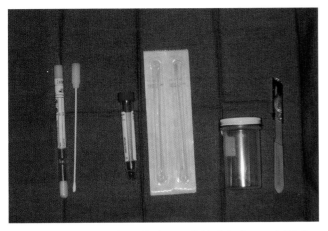

Figure 35.7 Culture sets. Bacterial culture set (left), viral culture set (middle), and 15-blade, microscope slides, and transport container for viral direct immunofluorescence (right).

2–5 days to identify the herpes simplex virus (HSV) and 7–10 days for varicella zoster virus (VZV).

Direct fluorescent antibody assay (DFA) is a diagnostic test frequently used for its rapid 24-hour turnaround time. DFA can identify VZV and HSV and differentiate HSV types 1 and 2 with 84.6% sensitivity and 95.7% specificity, respectively [16]. If a vesicle is present, the roof is removed from one side and the base gently scraped with a 15-blade or curette. The scrapings are smeared evenly on to a glass slide and sent for analysis. Fluorescent monoclonal viral antibodies are added to the sample and, if infected, will fluoresce under microscopy.

An alternative diagnostic test is the Tzanck smear. The Tzanck smear is performed within minutes and is positive in 50% of HSV infections and 80% of VZV infections [17]. To perform a Tzanck smear, the vesicle roof is removed and the base scraped. The material is smeared on to a microscope slide, allowed to dry, and stained with a Giemsa or Wright stain. The presence of the multinucleated giant cell, an epithelial cell with multiple nuclei and viral inclusions, confirms the diagnosis. Although the Tzanck smear can be performed within minutes, it does not differentiate between HSV and VZV. Furthermore, the accuracy of the test is dependent on the interpretation skills and comfort level of the individual carrying out the test. Therefore, in cases where a Tzanck smear is performed, a confirmatory DFA or viral culture is recommended.

Diagnosis of fungal infection

For a suspected fungal infection, skin scrapings are best obtained from the periphery of the rash. The area is gently scraped with a 15-blade or a glass slide to obtain scale. For microscopic examination, small fine scale is preferred over large thick scales. The scrapings are placed on to a glass slide and 1–2 drops of 10–20% potassium hydroxide with dimethylsulfoxide are added to destroy the epithelial cell wall. The presence of septated or pseudohyphae confirms the presence of a fungal infection. To specify the dermatophytic species, additional scrapings are sent for culture.

Treatment of limited superficial dermatophytic infections includes topical antifungal creams such as econazole, miconazole, terbinafine, or ciclopirox (which also has antibacterial activity). More extensive fungal infections or infections resistant to topical therapy require oral therapy with ketoconazole, itraconazole, fluconazole, or terbinafine. The newer oral antifungals require shorter treatment periods to achieve remission [18].

Atypical mycobacterial and deep fungal culture

Deep tissue infections are more common in the immunocompromised population and typically present as erythematous nodules. For diagnosis, tissue for histologic assessment and skin culture is required and two punch biopsies are recommended (see section on punch biopsy). A 3 or 4-mm punch biopsy is usually adequate. The skin specimen is placed in the appropriate transport medium and sent for both pathologic and microbiologic analysis.

Management of common cutaneous neoplasms

The incidence of cutaneous neoplasms is often higher in the immunocompromised population and may have a more aggressive clinical course. Particularly, patients with chronic lymphocytic leukemia (CLL), treated with RAF inhibitors (vemurafenib, dabrafenib, sorafenib), total body irradiation, or hematopoietic and solid organ transplantation are at increased risk of developing skin cancers [19]. The most common cutaneous neoplasms are basal cell carcinoma, squamous cell carcinoma (SCC), and malignant melanoma. Of these, the risk of developing an SCC or melanoma is higher after hematopoietic stem cell transplantation and in patients with chronic graft versus host disease [20]. In patients with CLL, cutaneous SCC act more aggressively and are associated with higher levels of metastasis and death [21]. Therefore, physicians should have a high index of suspicion when an immunocompromised patient presents with a nonhealing, enlarging, or tender growth.

Keratoacanthoma is a low-grade malignancy considered to be a variant of SCC. Keratoacanthomas, keratoacanthoma-like SCC, and invasive SCC have increasingly been associated with vemurafenib and other RAF inhibitors [22,23]. The lesions clinically present as rapidly growing papules and nodules with a central crust. Early detection and management is recommended to limit interruptions in antineoplastic treatment and minimize patient morbidity.

For a lesion suspicious for skin cancer, a shave or punch biopsy is performed. Following the diagnosis of a cutaneous malignancy, referral to a dermatologist, surgeon, or radiation oncologist is recommended for definitive management. There are various treatment modalities depending on the type and depth of the cancer. Excisional biopsy of the lesion is both diagnostic and curative if clear margins are obtained; if not, wide local excision is a treatment option. Destructive modalities such as cryosurgery and electrodessication and curettage are restricted to superficial nonmelanoma skin cancers. These techniques are commonly performed by a dermatologist and greater in-depth review is recommended prior to initiating these procedures [24]. Mohs micrographic surgery, a tissue-sparing surgical technique is indicated for recurrent or high risk [25] nonmelanoma skin cancers in cosmetically sensitive areas such as the face or the genitals [26].

Conclusions

The dermatologic procedures outlined in this chapter can be performed by an oncologist in the outpatient setting. These procedures and techniques enable the oncologist to sample and diagnose cutaneous manifestations for timely management and treatment.

Acknowledgments

Special thanks to Indira Singh and Desiree Kingston for assistance with photography.

References

1 Eilers, R.E. Jr., Gandhi, M., Patel, J.D. et al. (2010) Dermatologic infections in cancer patients treated with epidermal growth factor receptor inhibitor therapy. *Journal of the National Cancer Institute*, **102**, 47–53.

2 Wilson, W., Taubert, K.A., Gewitz, M. et al. (2007) Prevention of infective endocarditis. Guidelines from the Americal Heart Association. A Guideline From the American Heart Association Rheumatic Fever, Endocarditis, and Kawasaki Disease Committee, Council on Cardiovascular Disease in the Young, and the Council on Clinical Oncology, Council on Cardiovascular Surgery and Anesthesia, and the Quality of care and Outcomes Research Interdisciplinary Working Group. *Circulation*, **116** (15), 1736–1754.

3 Wright, T.I., Baddour, L.M., Berbari, E.F. et al. (2008) Antibiotic prophylaxis in dermatologic surgery: advisory statement 2008. *Journal of the American Academy of Dermatology*, **59** (3), 464–473.

4 Leffell, D.J. & Brown, M. (1997) *Manual of Skin Surgery*, p. 155. Wiley-Liss, New York.

5 Bruce, A.M. & Spencer, J.M. (2010) Surgical myths in dermatology. *Dermatologic Surgery*, **36** (4), 512–517.

6 Fuzier, R., Lapeyre-Mestre, M., Mertes, P.M. et al. (2009) Immediate- and delayed-type allergic reactions to amide local anesthetics: clnical features and skin testing. *Pharmacoepidemiology and Drug Safety*, **18**, 595–601.

7 Senthuran, S., Toff, W.D., Vuylsteke, A., Solesbury, P.M. & Menon, D.K. (2002) Implanted cardiac pacemakers and defibrillators in anaesthetic practice. *British Journal of Anaesthesia*, **8** (5), 627–631.

8 Lane, J.E., O'Brien, E.M. & Kent, D.E. (2006) Optimization of thermocautery in excisional dermatologic surgery. *Dermatologic Surgery*, **32** (5), 669–675.

9 Smack, D.P., Harrington, A.C., Dunn, C. et al. (1996) Infection and allergy incidence in ambulatory surgery patients using white petrolatum vs bacitracin ointment: a randomized controlled trial. *Journal of the American Medical Association*, **276** (12), 972–977.

10 Sheth, V.M. & Weitzul, S. (2008) Postoperative topical antimicrobial use. *Dermatitis: Contact, Atopic, Occupational, Drug*, **19** (4), 181–189.

11 Zuber, T.J. (2002) Punch biopsy of the skin. *American Family Physician*, **65** (6), 1155–1158.

12 Wiggan, J. & Ratner, D. (2012) Suturing techniques. Emedicine online. Available from: http://emedicine.medscape.com/article/1824895-overview (accessed 5 May 2013).

13 Lacouture, M.E. (2007) Clinical management of EGFRI dermatologic toxicities: US perspective. *Oncology*, **21** (11 Suppl. 5), 17–21.

14 Segaert, S. & Cutsem, E.V. (2005) Clinical signs, pathophysiology and management of skin toxicity during therapy with epidermal growth factor receptor inhibitors. *Annals of Oncology*, **16** (9), 1425–1433.

15 Moon, S.E. (2005) Subungual pyogenic granuloma treated by sodium tetradecyl sulfate sclerotherapy. *Dermatologic Surgery*, **34** (6), 846–847.

16 Pouletty, P., Chomel, J.J., Thouvenot, D., Catalan, F., Rabillon, V. & Kadouche, J. (1987) Detection of herpes simplex virus in direct specimens by immunofluorescence assay using a monoclonal antibody. *Journal of Clinical Microbiology*, **25** (5), 958–959.

17 Nahass, G.T., Goldstein, B.A., Zhu, W.Y., Serling, U., Penneys, N.S. & Leonardi, C.L. (1992) Comparison of tzanck smear, viral culture, and DNA diagnostic methods in detection of herpes simplex and varicella-zoster infection. *Journal of the American Medical Association*, **268** (18), 2541–2544.

18 Millikan, L.E. (2010) Current concepts in systemic and topical therapy for superficial mycoses. *Clinics in Dermatology*, **28**, 212–216.

19 Lichter, M.D., Karagas, M.R., Mott, L.A., Spencer, S.K., Stukel, T.A. & Greenberg, E.R. (2000) Therapeutic ionizing radiation and the incidence of basal cell carcinoma and squamous cell carcinoma. The New Hampshire Skin Cancer Study Group. *Archives of Dermatology*, **136**, 1007–1011.

20 Deeg, J.H. & Socie, G. (1998) Malignancies after hematopoietic stem cell transplantation: many questions, some answers. *Blood*, **91**, 1833–1844.

21 Mehrany, K., Weenig, R.H., Lee, K.K., Pittelkow, M.R. & Otley, C.C. (2005) Increased metastasis and mortality from cutaneous squamous cell carcinoma in patients with chronic lymphocytic leukemia. *Journal of the American Academy of Dermatology*, **53**, 1067–1071.

22 Smith, K.J., Haley, H., Hamza, S. & Skelton, H.G. (2009) Eruptive keratoacanthoma-type squamous cell carcinomas in patients taking sorafenib for the treatment of solid tumors. *Dermatologic Surgery*, **35** (11), 1766–1770.

23 Kwon, E.J., Kish, L.S. & Jaworsky, C. (2009) The histologic spectrum of epithelial neoplasms induced by sorafenib. *Journal of the American Academy of Dermatology*, **61**, 522–527.

24 Bolognia, J.L., Jorizzo, J.L. & Rapini, R.P. (eds) (2003) *Dermatology*, 1st edn, Mosby, St. Louis.

25 Brantsch, K.D., Meinsner, C., Schonfisch, B. *et al.* (2008) Analysis of risk factors determining prognosis of cutaneous squamous-cell carcinoma: a prospective study. *Lancet Oncology*, **9**, 713–720.

26 Shriner, D.L., McCoy, D.K., Goldberg, D.J. & Wagner, R.F. Jr. (1998) Mohs micrographic surgery. *Journal of the American Academy of Dermatology*, **39**, 79–97.

36 Appearance-Related Concerns in the Cancer Patient

Amy J. Derick

Northwestern University, Feinberg School of Medicine, Chicago; Derick Dermatology LLC, Barrington, IL, USA

Introduction

Cancer treatments can cause dermatologic adverse events (AEs) that are cosmetically unappealing and a daily visual reminder of a patient's illness. Unfortunately, cosmetically unappealing AEs can erode a patient's self-esteem, but fortunately treatments are available.

This chapter discusses options for optimizing the appearance of the following concerns:
- Scarring from cancer-related surgery;
- Radiation tattoos;
- Areola tattoos;
- Hypertrichosis resulting from epidermal growth factor receptor (EGFR) inhibitors;
- Sensitive skin from chemotherapy;
- Bruising (purpura);
- Radiation-induced telangiectasias; and
- Hyperpigmentation from therapy.

Limitations to this chapter arise from a scarcity of incidence data related to these conditions. Also, there are few randomized trials dedicated to the treatments discussed in the oncology setting. In light of these limitations, this chapter focuses on problems and treatments for which the data are more robust. Some recommendations are based on the author's professional experience.

Scarring from cancer-related surgery

Cancer patients may undergo surgeries connected to their treatment. Examples include mastectomy, port placement, and device implantation. Post-procedural scars can be both cosmetically unappealing and symptomatic. Scars may be tender, painful, pruritic, or cause a burning sensation [1], and impede functionality if they limit range of motion.

Scars can become hypertrophic. If a scar spreads beyond the original wound surface, it is called a keloid scar. Warning signs for impending hypertrophic or keloid scarring can appear within the first several weeks post-incision. Warning signs include excessive redness, itching, or tenderness of the wound. Early treatment may prevent wound over-healing [2].

The incidence of keloid and hypertrophic scarring in cancer patients is unknown. Radiation therapy is known to reduce the risk of keloids and hypertrophic scars. For this reason, it is thought the incidence of keloid formation and hypertophic scarring may be lower for those patients receiving radiation therapy concomitant to surgery than for those patients who receive surgery alone (Figure 36.1) [3].

Treatment options

In the context of an impending hypertrophic or keloid scar, mid to high potency topical steroids can be applied three times per week starting 2 weeks post-procedure. Vascular laser treatments may also begin at this time and continue twice per week until erythema resolves [2]. Depending on the patient's skin color, either a pulsed-dye or neodymium:yttrium-aluminum-garnet (Nd:YAG) laser would be appropriate (Figure 36.1b) [4,5]. Treatment with these lasers is thought to decrease the vascularity that plays a part in causing scars to thicken.

In nonfacial hypertrophic or keloid scars that are already thickened, it is appropriate to start with interlesional corticosteroids. Adding 5-fluorouracil (5-FU) to triamcinolone may decrease the local AEs of interlesional steroid injections, including skin and subcutaneous tissue atrophy. In one study, 1 mL of 20 mg/mL triamcinolone acetonide is combined with 1 mL of

Dermatologic Principles and Practice in Oncology: Conditions of the Skin, Hair, and Nails in Cancer Patients, First Edition. Edited by Mario E. Lacouture.
© 2014 John Wiley & Sons, Inc. Published 2014 by John Wiley & Sons, Inc.

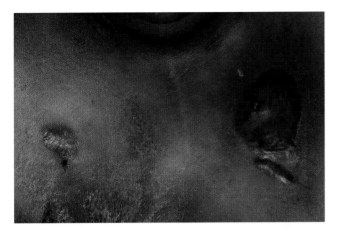

Figure 36.1 Hypertrophic scarring after port placement. Photo courtesy of Dr. Mario E. Lacouture.

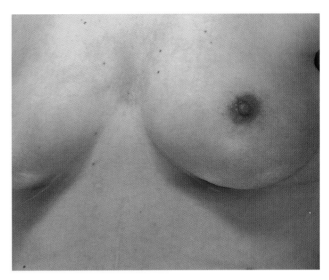

Figure 36.2 Radiation tattoos on the torso post-radiation therapy.

50 mg/mL 5-FU. The resulting combination yields a dilution of 10 mg/mL triamcinolone acetonide and 25 mg/mL of 5-FU. Injections may be performed every 2–4 weeks [6]. Another study calls for an alternative dilution of 0.1 mL of 40 mg/mL triamcinolone acetonide combined with 0.9 mL of 50 mg/mL 5-FU. This dilution would yield a final dilution of 4 mg/mL triamcinolone acetonide and 45 mg/mL 5-FU [7]. It should be noted that the use of 5-FU in conjunction with triamcinolone acetonide is not universally considered superior than treatment with triamcinolone acetonide alone. The addition of 5-FU increases the risk of hyperpigmentation and makes the treatments more painful for the patient.

Once the scar is flat, vascular lasering and topical steroids can be used to reduce erythema. Laser treatments are typically performed every 2–4 weeks. Laser resurfacing, using ablative and nonablative wavelengths, may improve textural abnormalities [8].

Radiation tattoos

Radiation tattoos are permanent markers designed to assist radiation oncologists and their technicians in planning radiation treatments for cancer patients. These blue or black tattoos are created by the implantation of india ink into the skin. These tattoos can be placed in cosmetically sensitive areas. Patients with radiation tattoos may seek tattoo removal once their treatment is concluded. Although the precise incidence of radiation tattoos is not known, it may be high due to the number of cancer patients undergoing radiation therapy.

Whether or not it is appropriate to remove a patient's tattoo is best decided by the patient and radiation oncologist. There has been some concern about removing these tattoos. Radiation tattoos are functional and once they are removed that function is lost. If the patient requires additional rounds of radiation after the removal of radiation tattoos, some areas could be inadvertently irradiated again (Figure 36.2).

Treatment options

If the patient and radiation oncologist agree that removal of a tattoo is indicated, the patient has options for removal. In a study of patients undergoing radiation tattoo removal, laser therapy removal was preferred to punch biopsy removal. Each study participant had two tattoos treated. One tattoo was treated by laser and the other by punch biopsy. Although both treatments had excellent cosmetic outcomes, patients preferred three Q-switched laser treatments to one punch biopsy removal with stitches. Blinded photographic evaluations showed overall excellent clearance (75–100%) and similar patient satisfaction in both laser and surgical treatments. The majority of the patients preferred laser tattoo removal because AEs such as hypopigmentation and scarring were less than for excision at the 12-week mark [9].

When advising patients regarding tattoo removal, it is important to guide patients to qualified medical physicians, such as board-certified dermatologists or plastic surgeons. The standard laser for tattoo removal has been the Q-switched laser. However, in 2013, the FDA approved a novel tattoo removal device with a picosecond pulse duration. Either laser should be viewed as standard for tattoo removal; although the picosecond laser may remove the tattoo more quickly. The use of other lasers not designed for tattoo removal may have unwanted AEs [10]. Also, the use of a wavelength suitable for the patient's skin type is important. Tan skin should not be treated.

Areola tattoos

After breast reconstruction, the breast mounds that are created do not have areolas or nipples. Patients may opt for cosmetic tattooing of the breast to make the nipple–areola complex look more realistic. The technician who places these tattoos can be a

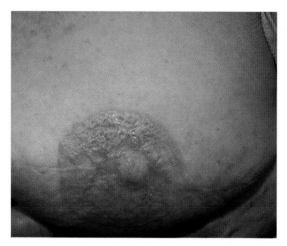

Figure 36.3 Patient unhappy with appearance of areola tattoo. Picture courtesy of Dr. Anne Laumann.

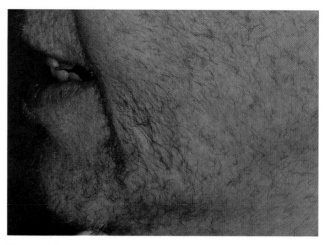

Figure 36.4 Hypertrichosis resulting from epidermal growth factor receptor inhibitor therapy. Photo courtesy of Dr. Mario E. Lacouture.

plastic surgeon or a micropigmentation specialist. These practices are regulated at the state level and therefore specific requirements for training and regulation vary. The process is similar to decorative tattooing, but flesh-colored pigments are used. These pigments may contain ferric oxide and titanium dioxide in order to simulate realistic areolas.

Treatment options

Nipple–areola tattooing is a well-accepted step in breast reconstruction, and patient satisfaction is typically high [11–14]. However, patients may choose to remove these tattoos for various reasons. Once the decision has been made, Q-switched or picosecond laser therapy is the treatment of choice. A laser test spot should be performed on the tattoo prior to the initiation of a complete treatment. Certain tattoo pigments, especially iron oxide and titanium dioxide, found in cosmetic tattoos, can oxidize when lasered. Oxidization causes the tattoo to change color from flesh-colored to black [15,16]. This has been reported in context of areola cosmetic tattoo removal [17]. The treating physician may review the material safety data sheets of the pigment (if known) to screen for these types of ingredients.

If darkening should occur, subsequent treatments can be performed with the Q-switched or picosecond laser. It may require many treatments to achieve clearance. One study showed that 26 monthly treatments with a Q-switched alexandrite and Nd:YAG laser completely cleared a cosmetic tattoo of the upper lip that had darkened after laser treatment (Figure 36.3 [18].

Hypertrichosis resulting from epidermal growth factor receptor inhibitors

EGFR inhibitors are a class of medications used to treat various solid tumors. The incidence of cutaneous AEs in patients receiving long-term (more than 2 months) therapy is high. Fifty-six

percent of patients report facial hypertrichosis (excess hair) while undergoing EGFR inhibitor therapy (Figure 36.4). This AEs is reported to have a moderate to strong effect on the quality of life of afflicted patients [19]. This AE can be seen after several weeks to months of EGFR inhibitor treatment. One case report noted excess hair growth in patients after 5–6 weeks of therapy [20].

Treatment options

There are no studies available for the best method to remove excess hair resulting from EGFR inhibitor therapy. Chemical depilatories, shaving, or waxing may be suboptimal because of skin sensitivities commonly associated with these treatments. Some success has been reported with laser hair removal [20]. This may be a viable option for patients and needs further safety testing.

If laser hair removal is the methodology selected, the patient should be referred to an experienced care provider, such as a board-certified dermatologist or plastic surgeon. The standard lasers for removing unwanted hair are the long-pulsed alexandrite, long-pulsed Nd:YAG, and diode lasers. The patient's skin type and level of tan determine which laser should be used. Patients with light untanned skin are ideal candidates for treatment using the long-pulsed alexandrite laser. Patients with dark untanned skin are better suited to treatment with the long-pulsed Nd:YAG or diode lasers. Patients with tanned skin should not undergo laser hair removal until the tan has resolved.

Sensitive skin from chemotherapy

When patients undergo chemotherapy their skin may become more sensitive to external irritants. For example, acne is one common AE of some chemotherapy agents. Patients undergoing chemotherapy must be cautious using over-the-counter products to treat their acne. One case report noted an instance of mild acne turning into a toxic rash after exposure to common over-the-counter treatments [21]. In consideration of this sensitivity, patients should consider the following suggestions.

Facial cleansing:
- Use synthetic detergent cleanser instead of soap.
- Avoid scrubs or other sources of mechanical irritation.
- Use lukewarm water to rinse off cleanser completely.
- Use a gentle fragrance-free moisturizer at bed time to prevent trans-epidermal water loss (dehydration) at night.

Sunscreen:
- Apply daily sunscreen to all exposed areas. Not only does sunscreen protect from skin cancer, but it may also help protect from drug-induced staining of photo-exposed skin.
- Choose chemical-free sunscreen formulations such a zinc or titanium dioxide [22].
- Use a sunscreen with an SPF 30 or higher and reapply every 1–2 hours.
- Wear a hat or seek shade, when possible.

Bruising (purpura)

Bruising is a common complaint of cancer patients. They may be taking prescription anticoagulants for deep vein thrombosis prophylaxis or treatment and oral corticosteroids for various numerous indications. In addition, they experience frequent iatrogenic trauma (blood draws and infusions). This combination leads to a high incidence of bruising – potentially more pronounced on sun-damaged skin (actinic purpura) on the forearms and hands.

Treatment options
The pulsed-dye laser is a way to speed resolution of bruising. The exact mechanism by which the laser accelerates resolution is unknown but it is thought to target the hemoglobin that is present in bruised skin. The wavelength of the 595 nm pulsed-dye laser matches the absorption peak for oxyhemoglobin (Figure 36.5).

Two studies documenting this phenomenon have been published. The first was a study carried out 6 days post facial plastic surgery. The treated patients found a 63% mean improvement within 48–72 hours. Bruising from facial plastic procedures decreased from 2 weeks to 7–8 days with this treatment [23]. The second study focused on more superficial bruising from nonsurgical cosmetic procedures or trauma. In this study, bruises were lasered 48 hours after onset. Compared with untreated ecchymosis, the treated area resolved more quickly. Twenty four hours after treatment, lasered bruises had 62% improvement compared with 13% of untreated bruises. Forty eight hours later, average improvement was 76% and 37%, respectively [24].

Radiation-induced telangiectasias

Long after the completion of radiation treatments to the body, the skin may remain damaged. Damage from radiation causes atrophy and prominent telangiectasias. These changes may not develop for months to years after radiation exposure (Figure 36.6) [25].

Treatment options
There are several ways to treat the prominent telangiectasias associated with radiation dermatitis. One cost-effective option is to destroy the blood vessels using a hyfrecator. In a study treating patients with breast and chest wall telangiectasias with the hyfrecator, the majority (88%) had complete resolution after a median of six sessions. All but one (93%) considered the treatment to be worthwhile. These treatments were viewed as painless or mildly painful (69%). A majority of patients (73%) also reported an increase in self-confidence [26].

Pulsed-dye laser treatment has also been beneficial in clearing radiation-induced telangiectasia. In one study, all telangiectasias showed complete clearance with high satisfaction [27]. Compared with another source of energy, the intense pulsed light device, the

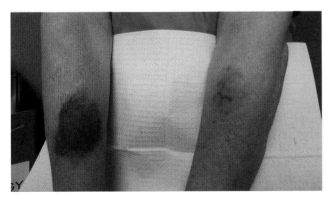

Figure 36.5 Originally identical purpura shown here 2 days after the left arm was treated with a pulsed-dye laser.

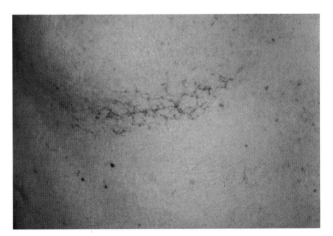

Figure 36.6 Telangiectasias post-radiation treatment. Photo courtesy of Dr. Mario E. Lacouture.

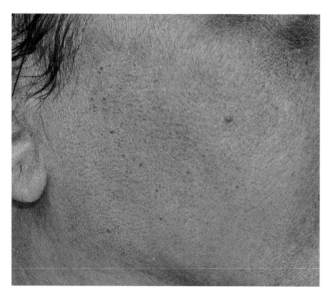

Figure 36.7 Hyperpigmentation resulting from epidermal growth factor receptor inhibitor therapy. Photo courtesy of Dr. Mario E. Lacouture.

pulsed-dye laser was seen as superior in terms of vessel clearance and patient satisfaction. In this study, three treatments of pulsed-dye laser were performed at 6-week intervals [28].

Hyperpigmentation from therapy

While undergoing anticancer therapy, patients may experience photosensitivity and diffuse or localized hyperpigmentation of the skin, nails, and mucous membranes. The pathogenesis underlying therapy-related dyspigmentation is not completely known. Many agents are known to cause skin dyspigmentation, both from direct pigment deposition and phototoxic drug reaction (Figure 36.7) [21].

Treatment options
There are few published data related specifically to the treatment of therapy-induced hyperpigmentation. However, there are data related to the treatment of other drug-induced hyperpigmentation as well as treatment of hyperpigmentation in general [29–34]. Most discoloration is reversible and resolves if the chemotherapeutic medication is discontinued [35]. UV radiation can increase pigmentation, especially with photosensitizing medication. To protect the skin, patients should apply a broad-spectrum daily sunscreen for exposed areas of at least SPF 30. Physical block sunscreens, such as zinc oxide and titanium dioxide, are preferred to chemical sunscreens because they are less irritating [21].

Topical depigmenting agents, such as hydroquinone, or laser treatments may also be an option for treating chemotherapy-induced hyperpigmentation. Treatments with the Q-switched alexandrite and ruby lasers have been studied for other kinds of drug-induced hyperpigmentation [29–34]. However, inconsistent results have been reported.

Conclusions

In an effort to manage the human element of cancer treatment, it is important to consider the impact appearance-related AEs may have on patients' self-esteem and psychosocial well-being. Evidence shows patients who have received treatments to improve the appearance of cosmetic AE are happier [19,26]. Viable options exist to manage cosmetic concerns. Patients and providers should be aware of these options, so an optimal course of treatment can be designed. Additional research needs to be done on how to treat these appearance-related AEs safely and effectively.

References

1 English, R.S. & Shenefelt, P.D. (1999) Keloids and hypertrophic scars. *Dermatologic Surgery*, **25**, 631–638.
2 Kranendonk, S. & Obagi, S. (2011) An algorithmic approach to hypertrophic scars and keloids: maximizing nonsurgical options. *Cosmetic Dermatology*, **24**, 28–39.
3 Bölke, E., Peiper, M., Budach, W. et al. (2007) Unilateral keloid formation after bilateral breast surgery and unilateral radiation. *European Journal of Medical Research*, **12** (7), 320–322.
4 Alster, T. (2003) Laser scar revision: comparison study of 585-nm pulsed-dye laser with and without intralesional corticosteroids. *Dermatologic Surgery*, **29** (1), 25–29.
5 Badawi, A., Tome, M.A., Atteya, A., Sami, N. & Morsy, I.A. (2011) Retrospective analysis of non-ablative scar treatment in dark skin types using the sub-millisecond Nd:YAG 1,064 nm laser. *Lasers in Surgery and Medicine*, **43** (2), 130–136.
6 Mansukiatti, W. & Fitzpatrick, R.E. (2002) Treatment response of keloidal and hypertrophic sternotomy scars: comparison among intralesional corticosteroid, 5-fluorouracil, and 585-nm flashlamp-pumped pulsed-dye laser treatments. *Archives of Dermatology*, **138**, 1149–1154.
7 Asilian, A., Darougheh, A. & Shariati, F. (2006) New combination of triamcinolone, 5-fluorouracil, and pulsed-dye laser for treatment of keloid and hypertophic scars. *Dermatologic Surgery*, **32**, 907–915.
8 Cervelli, V., Gentile, P., Spallone, D. et al. (2010) Ultrapulsed fractional CO2 laser for the treatment of post-traumatic and pathological scars. *Journal of Drugs in Dermatology*, **9** (11), 1328–1331.
9 Bregnhøj, A. & Haedersdal, M. (2010) Q-switched YAG laser vs. punch biopsy excision for iatrogenic radiation tattoo markers: a randomized controlled trial. *Journal of the European Academy of Dermatology and Venereology*, **24** (10), 1183–1186.
10 Wenzel, S., Landthaler, M. & Baumler, W. (2009) Recurring mistakes in tattoo removal: a case series. *Dermatology (Basel, Switzerland)*, **218** (2), 164–167.
11 El-Ali, K., Dalal, M. & Kat, C.C. (2006) Tattooing of the nipple-areola complex: review of outcome in 40 patients. *Journal of Plastic, Reconstructive and Aesthetic Surgery*, **59** (10), 1052–1057.
12 Bhatty, M.A. & Berry, R.B. (1997) Nipple-areola reconstruction by tattooing and nipple sharing. *British Journal of Plastic Surgery*, **50** (5), 331–334.

13 Clarkson, J.H., Tracey, A., Eltigani, E. & Park, A. (2006) The patient's experience of a nurse-led nipple tattoo service: a successful program in Warwickshire. *Journal of Plastic, Reconstructive and Aesthetic Surgery*, **59** (10), 1058–1062.

14 Spear, S.L. & Arias, J. (1995) Long-term experience with nipple-areola tattooing. *Annals of Plastic Surgery*, **35** (3), 232–236.

15 Kirby, W., Kaur, R.R. & Desai, A. (2010) Paradoxical darkening and removal of pink tattoo ink. *Journal of Cosmetic Dermatology*, **9** (2), 149–151.

16 Anderson, R.R., Geronemus, R., Kilmer, S.L., Farinelli, W. & Fitzpatrick, R.E. (1993) Cosmetic tattoo ink darkening: a complication of Q-switched and pulsed-laser treatment. *Archives of Dermatology*, **129** (8), 1010–1014.

17 Chang, S.E., Kim, K.J., Choi, J.H., Sung, K.J., Moon, K.C. & Koh, J.K. (2002) Areolar cosmetic tattoo ink darkening: a complication of Q-switched alexandrite laser treatment. *Dermatologic Surgery*, **28** (1), 95–96.

18 Fitzpatrick, R.E. & Lupton, J.R. (2000) Successful treatment of treatment-resistant laser-induced pigment darkening of a cosmetic tattoo. *Lasers in Surgery and Medicine*, **27**, 358–361.

19 Osio, A., Mateus, C. & Soria, J.C. (2009) Cutaneous side-effects in patients on long-term treatment with epidermal growth factor receptor inhibitors. *British Journal of Dermatology*, **161**, 515–521.

20 Vergou, T., Stratigos, A.J., Karapanagiotou, E.M. *et al.* (2010) Facial hypertrichosis and trichomegaly developing in patients treated with the epidermal growth factor receptor inhibitor erlotinib. *Journal of the American Academy of Dermatology*, **63**, e56–e58.

21 Waris, W., Naik, S., Idrees, I. *et al.* (2009) Severe cutaneous reaction to cetuximab with possible association with the use of over-the-counter skin care products in a patient with oropharyngeal cancer. *Cutaneous and Ocular Toxicology*, **28** (1), 41–44.

22 Susser, W.S., Whitaker-Worth, D.L. & Grant-Kels, J.M. (1999) Mucocutaneous reactions to chemotherapy. *Journal of the American Academy of Dermatology*, **40** (3), 367–398.

23 DeFatta, R.J., Krishna, S. & Williams, E.F., III. (2009) Pulsed-dye laser for treating ecchymoses after facial cosmetic procedures. *Archives of Facial Plastic Surgery*, **11** (2), 99–103.

24 Karen, J.K., Hale, E.K. & Geronemus, R.G. (2010) A simple solution to the common problem of ecchymosis. *Archives of Dermatology*, **146**, 94–95.

25 Hymes, S.R., Strom, E.A. & Fife, C. (2006) Radiation dermatitis: clinical presentation, pathophysiology, and treatment. *Journal of the American Academy of Dermatology*, **54**, 28–46.

26 Rowland Payne, C.M., Somaiah, N., Neal, A.J. & Glees, J.P. (2005) The hyfrecator: a treatment for radiation-induced telangiectasia in breast cancer patients. *British Journal of Radiology*, **78** (926), 143–146.

27 Lanigan, S.W. & Joannides, T. (2003) Pulsed dye laser treatment of telangiectasia after radiotherapy for carcinoma of the breast. *British Journal of Dermatology*, **148**, 77–79.

28 Nymann, P., Hedelund, L. & Haedersdal, M. (2009) Intense pulsed light vs. long-pulsed dye laser treatment of telangiectasia after radiotherapy for breast cancer: a randomized split-lesion trial of two different treatments. *British Journal of Dermatology*, **160** (6), 1237–1241.

29 Alster, T. & Gupta, S. (2004) Minocycline-induced hyperpigmentation treated with a 755-nm Q-switched alexandrite laser. *Dermatologic Surgery*, **30**, 1201–1204.

30 Green, D. & Friedman, K. (2001) Treatment of minocycline-induced cutaneous pigmentation with the Q-switched alexandrite laser and a review of the literature. *Journal of the American Academy of Dermatology*, **44**, 342–347.

31 Friedman, I., Shelton, R. & Phelps, R. (2002) Minocycline-induced hyperpigmentation of the tongue: successful treatment with the Q-switched ruby laser. *Dermatologic Surgery*, **28**, 205–209.

32 Wee, S. & Dover, J. (2008) Effective treatment of psychotropic drug-induced facial hyperpigmentation with a 755-nm Q-switched alexandrite laser. *Dermatologic Surgery*, **34**, 1609–1612.

33 Bellew, S. & Alster, T. (2004) Treatment of exogenous ochronosis with a Q-switched alexandrite (755 nm) laser. *Dermatologic Surgery*, **30**, 555–558.

34 Raulin, C., Werner, S. & Greve, B. (2001) Circumscripted pigmentations after iron injections-treatment with Q-switched laser systems. *Lasers in Surgery and Medicine*, **28** (5), 456–460.

35 Bronner, A. & Hood, A. (1983) Cutaneous complications of chemotherapeutic agents. *Journal of the American Academy of Dermatology*, **9**, 645–663.

Index

Page numbers in *italics* denote figures, those in **bold** denote tables.

Dermatologic Principles and Practice in Oncology: Conditions of the Skin, Hair, and Nails in Cancer Patients, First Edition. Edited by Mario E. Lacouture.
© 2014 John Wiley & Sons, Inc. Published 2014 by John Wiley & Sons, Inc.

Index

Index

Index